Brief Contents

Mental Health Nursing

DATE DUE

3-30-00			
MAR 2 2 2000			
12-05			
NOV 1 3 2002			
SEP 1 0 2012			
2-28-17			
FEB 0 2 2017			
GAYLORD			PRINTED IN U.S.A.

FOURTH EDITION

Mental Health Nursing

Karen Lee Fontaine, RN, MSN, AASECT

Professor
Purdue University–Calumet
Hammond, Indiana

J. Sue Fletcher, RN, EdD

Associate Professor
California State University, Stanislaus
Turlock, California

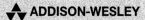
ADDISON-WESLEY

An imprint of Addison Wesley Longman, Inc.

Menlo Park, California • Reading, Massachusetts • New York • Harlow, England
Don Mills, Ontario • Sydney • Mexico City • Madrid • Amsterdam

Project Editor: Virginia Simione Jutson
Assistant Editor: Stephanie Kellogg
Managing Editor: Wendy Earl
Production Supervisor: David W. Rich
Text Designer: Carolyn Deacy
Cover Designer: Yvo Riezebos
Art Coordinator: David Novak
Artist: Shirley Bortoli
Copy Editor: Kristin Barendsen
Indexer: Sylvia Coates
Compositor: Fog Press

Care has been taken to confirm the accuracy of information presented in this book. The authors, editors, and the publisher, however, cannot accept any responsibility for errors or omissions or for the consequences from application of the information in this book and make no warranty, express or implied, with respect to its contents.

The authors and publishers have exerted every effort to ensure that drug selections and dosages set forth in this text are in accord with current recommendation and practice at time of publication. However, in view of ongoing research, changes in government regulations, and the constant flow of information relating to drug therapy and drug reactions, the reader is urged to check the package inserts of all drugs for any change in indications of dosage and for added warnings and precautions. This is particularly important when the recommended agent is a new and/or infrequently employed drug.

The quilt pictured on the cover is titled "Linen Closet." Acrylic on linen; silk; cotton batting; net backing. Hand appliquéd and quilted by Emily Richardson, Philadelphia, Pennsylvania. Photo courtesy of Lark Books, Asheville, North Carolina.

Library of Congress Cataloging-in-Publication Data

Fontaine, Karen Lee, 1943–
    Mental health nursing / Karen Lee Fontaine, J. Sue Fletcher. --
4th ed.
       p.   cm.
    Rev. ed. of: Essentials of mental health nursing. 3rd ed. c1995.
    Includes bibliographical references and index.
    ISBN 0-8053-1644-2 (alk. paper)
    1. Psychiatric nursing.   I. Fletcher, J. Sue. 1946–
II. Fontaine, Karen Lee, 1943–   Essentials of mental health
nursing.   III. Title.
    [DNLM: 1. Psychiatric Nursing.   WY 160 F678m 1999]
RC440.E82   1999
610.73'68--dc21
DNLM/DLC
for Library of Congress   98-23779

ISBN 0-8053-1644-2

2 3 4 5 6 7 8 9 10—RNV—02 01 00 99 98

Addison Wesley Longman, Inc.
2725 Sand Hill Road
Menlo Park, California 94025

This book is dedicated to Al Renslow for his unending cheerfulness and support. Everyone should have such a cheerleader!

Contributors

Suzanne C. Beyea, RN, CS, PhD
Co-Director Perioperative Nursing Research
Association of Operating Room Nurses
Denver, CO

Patriciann Furnari Brady, RN, EdD
Case Manager Youth Services
Sioux Valley Behavioral Health
Sioux Valley Hospital
Sioux Falls, SD

Carol Green, RN, PhD
Professor of Nursing
Johnson County Community College
Overland Park, KS

Kathryn Hopkins Kavanagh, RN, MSN, PhD
Associate Professor
University of Maryland, Baltimore
Baltimore, MD

Pamela Marcus, RN, MS, CS-P
Private Practice
Upper Marlboro, MD

Leslie Rittenmeyer, RN, MSN
Associate Professor
Department of Nursing
Purdue University–Calumet
Hammond, IN

Mary J. Roehring, RN, MSN, CS
Associate Professor
Ferris State University
Big Rapids, MI

Karen G. Vincent-Pounds, RN, MSN, CS
Coordinator of Geriatric Services
HRI Counseling Center
Franklin, MA

Preface

The fourth edition of *Mental Health Nursing* continues in the same spirit of the first three editions; that is, a spirit of helping students recognize that mental disorders are brain disorders and that there are many ways students can help individuals and families cope with these disorders. Mental health nursing is a wonderful practice specialty because it is so broad, diverse, and interesting. This text illustrates that breadth, the scientific basis of our knowledge, the diversity of clients we meet, and the exciting changes occurring in the practice of nursing. I have revised, reorganized, deleted, and added content based on my own use of the text, student input, peer and reviewer comments, clients in my private practice, and rapid proliferation in the knowledge of neurobiology.

Philosophical/Theoretical Frameworks

This text is based on the belief that the practice of mental health nursing means helping people manage difficulties, solve problems, decrease emotional pain, and promote growth, while respecting their rights to their own values, beliefs, and decisions. To that end, nursing students are encouraged to engage in self-analysis in order to increase their self-understanding and self-acceptance. This is important because nurses who are able to clarify their own beliefs and values are less likely to be judgmental or to impose their own values and beliefs on clients.

A variety of theories have been incorporated to help nursing students understand clients and their experiences. It is by applying neurobiological, psychological, sociological, and spiritual theories and concepts that nurses are able to respond as one human being to another and help clients engage in the healing process. A major focus of this text is the promotion of health and provision of opportunities for clients to maximize their ability to live, work, socialize, and learn in the communities of their choice. In addition, throughout the text I examine the impact of sexism, racism, ageism, and homophobia on the mental health of the members of our communities who suffer discrimination and prejudice.

Retained in This Edition

Mental Health Nursing retains, in the fourth edition, many of the strengths that have made it a "user-friendly" text for nursing students.

- There is a heavy emphasis throughout the text on the development of effective communication skills. Each chapter in Part III, *Mental Disorders*, features Clinical Interactions, illustrating a therapeutic interaction between a nurse and clients. Chapter 5, *Communicating and Teaching*, includes a new example of a student-client interaction and an analysis thereof in the form of a process recording. Appendix E provides five additional process recordings to bring to life the communication process with clients experiencing a variety of mental disorders.

- The nursing process is the organizing framework for the chapters in Part III, *Mental Disorders*, and Part IV, *Crisis*. This type of organizational consistency is extremely effective in helping students begin to assess, analyze, plan, implement, and evaluate in a systematic manner.

- The Focused Nursing Assessment tables are organized in the same pattern as the Knowledge Base sections of the text to help students correlate specific client responses with the general knowledge base. The Focused Nursing Assessment tables aid students in learning the type and range of assessment questions to ask particular clients.

New to This Edition

While retaining many of the strengths of the previous edition, this new fourth edition of *Mental Health Nursing* also includes much new and significantly updated material, new pedagogical features, and new emphases.

- New chapters include Chapter 2, *The Family and Community in Mental Health Nursing*, and Chapter 16, *Grief and Loss*.

- Chapters that have been extensively revised include Chapter 12, *Schizophrenic Disorders*; Chapter 20, *Disorders of Children and Adolescents*; and Chapter 21, *Disorders of Older Adults*.

- The emphasis throughout the text is community mental health nursing, to reflect today's changing health care environment, as opposed to the previous editions which were more focused on inpatient nursing care. Content includes community living, community settings, community-based services, advanced directives, and community-based nursing practice.

- The Nursing Interventions Classification (NIC) taxonomy is utilized in all chapters in Part III, *Mental Disorders*, and Part IV, *Crisis*. This is the first comprehensive standardized classification of nursing interventions that can easily be used with NANDA diagnoses and the DSM-IV.

- Critical thinking is introduced in Chapter 1, *Introduction to Mental Health Nursing*, and is continued throughout the text with critical thinking exercises in chapters 2, 5, 8, 12, 14, 16, 18, 20, and 23.

- Critical pathways have been added to chapters 9, 10, 11, 12, 13, and 15.

- Culture-specific content has been added to each of the disorders chapters.

- The Nursing Intervention sections have been expanded and organized according to NIC taxonomy.

- Internet addresses of major mental health organizations have been added to the Self-Help sections.

- Complementary/alternative medicine has been incorporated throughout the text.

Student Tutorial Disk

A new addition to the supplement package is a Student Tutorial Disk. This disk contains approximately 150 NCLEX-style multiple-choice questions which emphasize the application of nursing care. Students are able to test their knowledge and gain immediate feedback through rationales for right and wrong answers. This disk is packaged with every copy of the textbook and is free to students.

Instructor's Resource Manual

The Instructor's Resource Manual for *Mental Health Nursing*, which is free to adopters of the text, includes two distinct sections: a test bank and student exercises.

- The test bank portion consists of 400 multiple-choice questions and has been revised. Test items follow the NCLEX 2-column format and are classified by cognitive level, nursing process step, and client need. The test bank is also available on disk to decrease administrative time in formatting exams.

- The student exercises are designed to help students review and apply the text material and increase their critical-thinking and problem-solving skills. These exercises were developed by an outstanding and creative teacher in the field of mental health nursing to help professors promote active learning within the classroom setting or in small groups. The exercises use case studies and real-life situations to help students grasp abstract concepts discussed in the text.

Visit our website (www.awnursing.com) to download additional supplementary materials.

About the Unit and Chapter Opening Artwork

The artwork and commentary introducing each part were created by psychiatric clients at Stanford University Hospital in Palo Alto, California. The project grew naturally out of an existing expressive art program at Stanford, designed to help hospitalized people portray their private worlds—worlds often filled with despair, anxiety, confusion, anger, and apathy. Communication of these powerful feelings through writing and drawing helps decrease social isolation, as clients share common experiences with each other. Relief of inner tension is another frequent outcome; unmanageable emotions take form on paper, and containment of those emotions is achieved.

Participation in this project was voluntary. Written consent was required from both client and psychiatrist because of the highly revealing nature of the artwork. Clients who were overtly psychotic, dissociated, or paranoid were excluded, as a protective measure for them. Drawings and captions were contributed anonymously, to protect clients' rights to privacy.

Psychiatric clients often carry with them a very wounded self-image. Rehabilitation helps to alleviate despair and to restore hope through therapy, support, structure, medication, and the acquisition of improved coping strategies. In addition, expressive artwork is very effective; it helps channel overwhelming feelings into something constructive. In contributing to this textbook, clients experienced the opportunity to discover areas of personal strength, finding new avenues for individual expression along the way.

Goals

I have revised *Mental Health Nursing* to reflect the latest available information in neurobiology. My hope is that students begin to comprehend the inseparability of the mind and brain. "Mind" is our abstract term that refers to mental functions such as mood, memory, and thinking, while "brain" is the cells, chemicals, and circuits that produce those functions. The two are as inseparable as the song and the singer. To ask how much of a mental disorder is the brain and how much is the mind is as meaningless as to ask how much of the area of a rectangle is due to its width and how much to its height. The mind and brain are inseparable from one another and from the totality of every human being. Psychiatric nursing will always exist until mental disorders themselves cease to exist. My goal is that students respect and support clients' and families' struggles to cope with acute disorders or to live with psychiatric disabilities as they live, work, and study within a variety of community settings.

In closing, I have written this text with the understanding that students and clients encompass a wide range of ages and ethnic groups, both genders, and a variety of sexual identities. I have tried to reflect this diversity throughout.

Karen Lee Fontaine
Purdue University–Calumet

VISIT OUR WEBSITE!
www.awnursing.com

Acknowledgments

I would like to express thanks to many of those who have inspired, commented on, and in other ways assisted in the writing and publication of this book. On the production and publishing side at Addison-Wesley, I was most fortunate to have an exceptional team of editors and support staff. Sponsoring Editor, Ginnie Simione-Jutson, not only provided great assistance and support in the birthing of this text, but she concurrently birthed her new daughter, Hannah Faith. Stephanie Kellogg, Assistant Editor, was very organized in keeping track of everything in the final stages of manuscript preparation. A good deal of assistance goes into most scholarly writing projects, and my appreciation goes to Kristin Barendsen for her careful copy edit. A special thanks goes to Dave Rich, production editor, for his commitment to the project, attention to detail, and availability.

I am indebted to the contributors for sharing their special knowledge of the discipline: Suzanne Beyea, Patriciann Brady, Carol Green-Nigro, Kathryn H. Kavanagh, Pamela Marcus, Leslie Rittenmeyer, Mary J. Roehrig, and Karen G. Vincent-Pounds. I would also like to thank contributors for the first, second, and third editions: Ellen Marie Bratt, Brenda Lewis Cleary, Paula G. LeVeck, Valerie Mattheisen, Susan F. Miller, Mary D. Moller, Shirley Sennhauser, and Joseph E. Smith. A special thanks is due to the reviewers of all four editions, whose names appear on the facing page.

The opportunity to study at the Center for Human Caring at the University of Colorado School of Nursing was a godsend. I dedicate this book to those who touched my essence: Gena, Mary, Blu, Mary, Dorothy, and Sharon, as well as Janet Quinn and Jean Watson. I wish the best for the "fierce women," the Gtumo Healing Group, at the Mappleton Rehab Center in Boulder.

I appreciate the encouragement and support from many "old-time" friends, especially Beata, Bernie, and Ruth, and "new beach-friends," among them Jack, Paul, CD, Susie, Maryann, George, Liz, Jan, Jim, Brad, Betty, Karen, Matt, Geneie, and Anne. Unmeasurable thanks to the coffee house gang at Marquette Perk, who always help me keep my life (and sense of humor) in perspective!

Karen Lee Fontaine
Purdue University Calumet

Reviewers for the Fourth Edition

Robert Brautigan, RN, MSN
Assistant Professor
Nunn Dr. Department of Nursing
Northern Kentucky University
Highland Heights, KY

Bernice Wallace Carmon, RN, MPH, MS
Associate Professor
School of Nursing
University of Alaska-Anchorage
Anchorage, AK

Nancy Conrad, RN, EdD
Assistant Professor
Widener University
Chester, PA

Tobie Fleming Day, RN, BSN, MSN
Instructor
Bishop State Community College
Mobile, AL

Denise H. Elliott, BSN, MSN
Department Director
Wallace State College
Hanceville, AL

Bronwynne Evans, MSN
Department Head
Yakima Valley Community College
Yakima, WA

Carol Fountain, AS, BS, MN
Associate Professor
Department of Nursing
Boise State University
Boise, ID

Alison Pyke Harrigan, BSN, MSN
Junior Level Coordinator
College of Nursing
Mary Gladwin Hall
University of Akron
Akron, OH

E. Gloria Stewart Jones, RN, MAed, MSN
Assistant Professor
Coordinator of Mental Health Nursing
Gwynedd-Mercy College
Gwynedd Valley, PA

Patricia A. Parsons, MSN, MN
Instructor Riverland Community College
Austin, Minnesota

Kathleen Patterson, BSN, MSN
Assistant Professor
Department of Nursing
University of Pittsburgh
Bradford, PA

Marjorie Ryan, BSN, MSN
Associate Professor
Miami University
Hamilton, OH

Linda Servidio, RN, MSN
Associate Professor
Brookdale Community College
Lincroft, NJ

Norma A. Smith, BA, MS
School of Nursing
Mercer Medical Center
Trenton, NJ

Lois W. Witney, RN, EdD, CS
Associate Professor
College of Nursing
East Tennessee State University
Johanson City, TN

Contents

Preface vii

PART II

Skills for Clinical Practice

CHAPTER 8

Psychopharmacology 145

PART II1

Mental Disorders

CHAPTER 9

Anxiety Disorders 169

continued on page xviii

CHAPTER 14

Personality Disorders 353

CHAPTER 15

Cognitive Impairment Disorders 373

PART IV

Crisis

contents continued on page xxii

PART V

Special Populations and Topics

PART I

Foundations of Mental Health Nursing

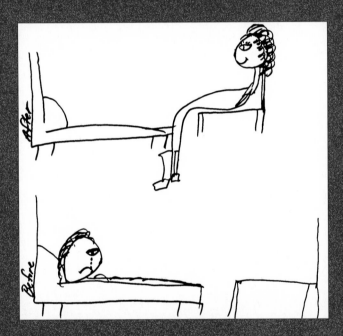

WHAT HELPS ME GET BETTER: *When I first came into the Hospital in order for asking for help! I had to first claim I had a illness or some thing like that. At first I didn't have any kind of feelings or thoughts of my own. All I thought or felt was darkness and sadness.*

This Hospital that I went to really helped me out. I really thank my doctor but most of all I thank the Nurses for being so understanding warm and kind to understand my sickness. I Thank you Medical people for learning and understanding Mental Illness.

CHAPTER 1

Introduction to Mental Health Nursing

Karen Lee Fontaine

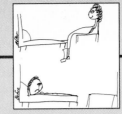

Objectives

After reading this chapter, you will be able to:

- Describe the continuum of mental illness–mental health.
- Describe the value of theories and models to mental health nursing practice.
- Explain the basic theoretical assumptions of the intrapersonal, social-interpersonal, behavioral, cognitive, and biogenic models.
- Relate the theories presented to the practice of mental health nursing.
- Discuss personal concerns about the clinical setting.
- Specify ways to care for yourself.
- Assess clients using psychosocial assessment and neuropsychiatric assessment.
- Differentiate between nursing diagnoses and *DSM-IV* diagnoses.
- Identify the most common priorities of care in mental health nursing.
- Identify a variety of nursing roles.
- Evaluate care on the basis of identified outcomes.

Key Terms

anxiety
biogenic theory
circadian rhythms
cognitive processes
conscious
countertransference
crisis
defense mechanisms
dynamism
ego
id
pleasure principle
personification
preconscious
psychosexual development
reality principle
superego
therapeutic alliance
therapeutic milieu
transference
unconscious

*O*ne of the first questions students ask at the beginning of their psychiatric nursing course is, "What is mental illness, or, for that matter, what is mental health?" It is not an easy question to answer. Cultural, family, and individual beliefs strongly influence what is defined as mental illness or mental health. For example, in one culture, seeing things others do not see (hallucinations) is a valued part of religious experience and something to be desired. In another culture, hallucinating is considered evidence of insanity and is something to be avoided. Cultures, families, and individuals often define mental illness as behaviors, feelings, or ways of thinking that are unusual to them or not easily understood by them.

This lack of understanding often leads to moral judgments about people who are labeled "mentally ill." American attitudes toward and stereotypes about mental illness include the belief that it is incurable or that people are capable of bringing on, or turning off, their illness at will—and that it is caused by bad parenting or sinful behavior. These social attitudes determine how people with mental illness are treated. For example, if we believe someone is evil, we will punish her or him. Other examples of attitudes and resulting treatment are:

Attitude	Treatment
Evil	Punish
Possessed	Exorcise
Inhuman	Abandon, disenfranchise
Bizarre	Avoid, degrade
Weak	Institutionalize
Sick	Medicate, hospitalize
Dangerous	Confine, control
Incompetent	Assume responsibility

Unfortunate stereotypes like these often keep people from seeking treatment or contribute to feeling ashamed of needing treatment.

As you begin the study of mental health nursing, you may believe many of society's myths and stereotypes about psychiatric consumers. As you progress through your course, you will begin to realize that there is neither a universally accepted definition of "normal" or "abnormal" nor clear parameters of mental health versus mental illness.

Mental health and mental illness can be viewed as end points on a continuum, with movement back and forth throughout life. You will be studying the continuum from several levels:

- Physical level, in the structure and function of the brain.
- Personal level, in caring for and about the self.
- Interpersonal level, in interactions with others.
- Societal level, in social conditions and the cultural context.

These levels interact in such a way that it is often difficult to separate the impact of each level. If a person's neurotransmitters are not functioning correctly, that person may have great difficulty organizing his or her thoughts. Disorganized thinking may interfere with the ability to perform activities of daily living (ADLs). Because of poor hygiene and the inability to communicate clearly, this individual may be shunned by others. As the person becomes more isolated, there may be a further loss of contact with reality. If adequate community resources are not available, the person may become homeless. In some cases, disruption to mental health may begin at the cultural level. An example is the impact of sexism on the mental health of women. Cultural sexism allows men to treat women as less worthy members of society. This treatment contributes to low self-esteem. Negative thoughts about oneself alter the amount and function of the neurotransmitters. Disruptions can occur at any level; however, each level is so intertwined with the others that it is often difficult to pinpoint the original source of the distress. Figure 1.1 illustrates how personal, interpersonal, and cultural factors interact in ways that produce movement toward mental health or mental illness. If there are more factors on the mental illness side of the continuum, the balance will shift toward that end of the continuum. Likewise, the presence of more factors associated with mental health will shift the balance toward mental health.

Movement toward the mental illness end of the continuum may begin with a sense of disharmony with aspects of living that may be distressing to the individual, family, friends, or community. Some aspects may be primarily distressing to the *individual,* such as feeling miserable, spending a great deal of time worrying, and suffering from multiple fears and anxieties. Other aspects may be distressing to *family and friends,* such as withdrawal from relationships,

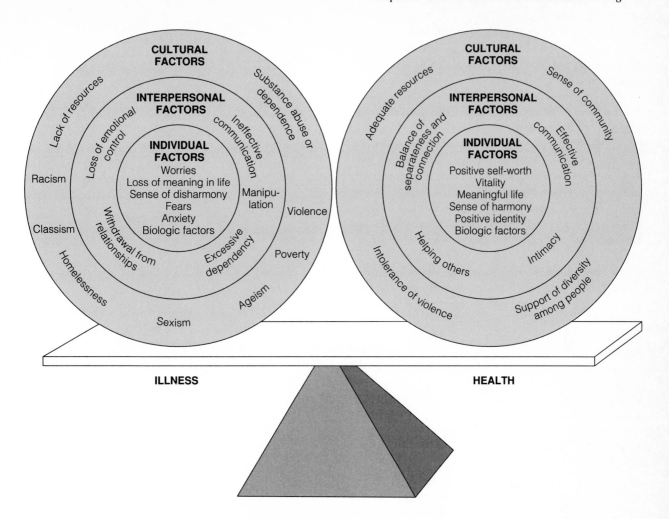

Figure 1.1 **Factors contributing to the mental health–mental illness continuum.**

an inability to communicate coherently, manipulation, and emotional outbursts. Other aspects are distressing to *society*, such as violence and substance abuse and dependence. Contributing cultural factors include racism, classism, sexism, inadequate access to health care, and disenfranchisement of many individuals and groups. All these aspects are interdependent and interactive. They influence the development of disorders, clinical pictures, the course and prognosis of the disorders, and responses to therapeutic interventions (Abraham, Fox, and Cohen, 1992).

Mental health is not a concrete goal to be achieved; rather, it is a lifelong process and includes a sense of harmony and balance for the individual, family, friends, and community. It differs from the mere absence of a mental disorder in that it is a growing toward potential, an inner feeling of aliveness. Movement toward the mental health end of the continuum brings with it a sense of harmony and balance, with a general feeling of vitality. *Individual* aspects may be a feeling of self-worth, a positive identity, and a sense of accomplishment. Aspects relating to *family and friends* may include a balance between separateness and connection, the ability to be intimate, and the desire or willingness to help others in need. *Societal* aspects may include tolerance for others who are different from oneself and the development of a sense of community. These aspects are also interdependent and interactive in the process of mental health.

To be healthy means to be whole and to be whole has a spiritual quality to it. Spirituality is that part of ourselves that deals with relationships and values and addresses questions of purpose and meaning in life. Spirituality unites people and is inclusive in nature, not exclusive. It is not loyal to one group, continent, or religion. Although spirituality is not a religion, being involved in a particular religion is a way some people enhance their spirituality. Yet people can be very spiritual and not religious (Seaward, 1997). Spirituality involves individuals, family, friends, and community. *Individual* aspects are the development of moral values and beliefs about the meaning and purpose of life and death. The development of our spirituality provides a grounding sense of identity and contributes to our self-esteem. Spiritual aspects relating to *family and friends* include the search for meaning through relationships, and the feeling of connectedness with others and with an external power often identified as God, a Supreme Being, or The Great Mystery. *Community* aspects of spirituality can be understood as a common humanity and a belief in the fundamental sacredness and unity of all life. It is that which motivates people toward truth and a sense of fairness and justice to all members of society. Our spiritual health is expressed through humor, compassion, faith, forgiveness, courage, and creativity. Spirituality enables us to develop healthy relationships based on acceptance, respect, and compassion (Seaward, 1997).

Spiritual activities may include meditating or praying, religious activities, mystical experiences, self-help groups, caring for others, or enjoying nature. Health care professionals often consider spiritual problems to be those that question spiritual values which may or may not be related to organized religion, the loss or questioning of faith, or problems associated with converting to a new faith (*DSM-IV*, 1994; North American Nursing Diagnosis Association, 1994). In a broader sense, spiritual problems are related to fear, anger, greed, guilt, and worry. These barriers can be described as those daily problems that drain our energy and immobilize us. Left unresolved, they can prevent our development as healthy, spiritual beings (Seaward, 1997).

Significance of Mental Disorders

Mental, behavioral, and social health problems are increasing throughout the world. According to recent world studies, mental health problems are one of the largest causes of lost years of quality life. Hundreds of millions of women, men, and children suffer from mental illnesses; others experience distress from the consequences of violence, abuse, dislocation, poverty, and exploitation. The number of persons with major mental illnesses will continue to grow in the decades to come. One contributing factor is the increase in population, which brings a corresponding increase in the number of people with mental illness. Also, the rates of depression have increased worldwide in recent decades. Depression is now being seen at younger ages and in greater frequency in countries as different as Lebanon, Taiwan, the United States, and countries of western Europe (Desjarlais et al, 1995; News, 1996).

In the United States, approximately one in four Americans will suffer a serious mental disorder during their lifetime, one in five children or adolescents may have a diagnosable mental disorder, and nearly one-third of the homeless population suffers from a psychiatric disability. More than 51 million Americans have a mental disorder in a single year, and a majority of the 29,000 Americans who commit suicide each year have a mental disorder.

Theories of Mental Disorders

Many theories and models are relevant to the practice of mental health nursing. One theory is not more "correct" than another, and practitioners choose the theory or model that is most appropriate for the client. The use of theories and models enables us to practice within a scientific framework, thereby providing scientifically based care. Using them also ensures humanistic practice because the concepts are rooted in humanistic philosophies. The theoretical models presented in this chapter are used in mental health nursing as guides for understanding clinical problems, as prescriptions for practice, and as aids in predicting outcomes of that practice. They focus on many different aspects of the person as a biopsychosocial being. Some focus on personality, others on behavior, and still others on learning. Some are based on principles of psychological development, and some on biogenic theories. They all provide a way of interpreting clinical data. The theories are organized under these headings, with representative theorists for each category: intrapersonal, social-interpersonal, behavioral, cognitive, and biogenic.

Intrapersonal Theory

Intrapersonal theory focuses on the behaviors, feelings, thoughts, and experiences of each individual person. Mental disorders are viewed as arising from within the individual. The intrapersonal theory of Sigmund Freud was the first to be developed. One of his great contributions was to identify components of the mind. The concepts of consciousness, id, ego, superego, and defense mechanisms are still widely used today. Erik Erikson expanded on Freud's theory of psychosexual development to include the entire life cycle.

Sigmund Freud

Freud divided all aspects of consciousness into three categories: conscious, preconscious, and unconscious. The first category, **conscious,** includes thoughts, feelings, and experiences that are easily remembered, such as certain addresses, phone numbers, anniversaries and birthdays, and recent enjoyable events. The second category, **preconscious** (sometimes called subconscious), includes thoughts, feelings, and experiences that have been forgotten but that can easily be recalled to consciousness. Examples are old phone numbers or addresses, the feeling a woman had during the birth of her first child, the name of a first girlfriend, and the animosity one felt toward a former boss. The third category, **unconscious,** encompasses thoughts, feelings, experiences, and dreams that cannot be brought to conscious thought or remembered (Freud, 1935).

Freud theorized that there were three components to the personality: the id, the ego, and the superego. Each component has individualized functions, but the three are so closely interrelated that it is difficult to separate their individual effects on a person's behavior.

The biologic and psychologic drives with which a person is born constitute the **id.** The id holds in reserve all psychic energy, which in turn furnishes the power for the operations of the ego and superego. It has no knowledge of outside reality and functions totally within its own subjective reality. The id is self-centered, and its major concern is the instant gratification of needs. The **ego** is the component of the personality that mediates the drives of the id with objective reality in a way that promotes well-being and survival. The ego does not concern itself with moral values or societal taboos. The **superego** is the component of the personality that is concerned with moral behavior. It is the accumulation of societal rules and personal values as interpreted by individuals. The emphasis of the superego is not reality but the ideal, and its goals are perfection as opposed to the id's pleasure or the ego's reality (Freud, 1935).

The id operates according to what Freud called the **pleasure principle:** the tendency to seek pleasure and avoid pain. As this is not always possible, the demands of the id must be modified by the reality principle. The ego has learned to use the **reality principle** to delay the immediate achievement of pleasure. It also functions to keep tension at a manageable level until an appropriate object can be found to meet the person's needs.

Freud saw the interplay between the three components of the personality as having great significance in determining human behavior. He also saw conflict arising when the components tried to meet different goals. Freud believed that the way in which people resolved these conflicts determined the status of their mental health.

The concept of anxiety is a thread that runs consistently through Freud's intrapersonal theory. **Anxiety** is defined as a feeling of tension, distress, and discomfort produced by a perceived or threatened loss of inner control rather than from external danger. The feelings brought about by anxiety are so uncomfortable that they force a person to take some type of corrective action. Anxiety is a warning of impending danger and a clear message to the ego that unless some palliative steps are taken, it is in danger of being overcome. The ego copes with anxiety by consistently applying rational measures to reduce feelings of discomfort. This process is often successful in healthy people, but there are times in the lives of all of us when the ego is unable to cope and resorts to less rational ways of handling anxiety. These processes are called defense mechanisms. **Defense mechanisms** alleviate anxiety by denying, misinterpreting, or distorting reality. Defense mechanisms create an incongruity between reality and the person's perception of reality. For the most part, they operate at an unconscious level. Table 1.1 lists and describes the most common defense mechanisms.

Freud called the process by which personality develops from birth to adolescence **psychosexual development.** Each of five stages is differentiated by characteristic ways of achieving libidinal, or sexual, pleasure. The psychosexual stages correspond to the maturational stages of the body: the oral stage, anal stage, phallic stage, latency stage, and genital stage. Readiness to move through each depends on how well the needs of the previous stage were met. For a summary of the defining characteristics of psychosexual development according to Freud, see Table 1.2.

Erik Erikson

Erik Erikson saw personality as developing throughout the entire life span rather than stopping at adolescence. He differed with Freud in that he believed people could move backward to achieve developmental tasks they were unable, for whatever reason, to achieve earlier. Erikson's perspective, the *developmental theory* of personality, offered the hope of achieving a healthy development pattern sometime during a life span.

Although Erikson accepted Freud's intrapersonal perspective of the importance of basic needs and drives in children, he felt personality was shaped more by conflict between needs and culture than by conflict between the id, ego, and superego. He based this philosophy on the assumption that drives are much the same from one child to another, and cultures differ from one part of the world to another. He also felt that cultures, like humans, are capable of developing.

Erikson believed that the ego is much more important than the id or superego in determining personality. He saw the ego as the mediating factor between the individual and society and felt that this relationship is at least as important as the influence of the basic drives. He also believed in the importance of social relationships in the development of individuals. Erikson expanded the determinants of personality development from merely instinctual and biological to social and cultural.

Another area where Erikson expanded intrapersonal theory is in his view of the future. Whereas Freud saw the most significance in past events, Erikson felt there was more significance in the future. He felt people's abilities to anticipate future events made a difference in the way they acted in the present. Many feel Erikson's theory is more hopeful and positive than Freud's. By expanding on the intrapersonal perspective, Erikson acknowledged the chance to develop through the life span and to grow in a variety of ways.

According to Erikson, every person passes through eight developmental stages: sensory, muscular, locomotor, latency, adolescence, young adulthood, adulthood, and maturity. Each stage is characterized by conflicts and a set of tasks that a person must accomplish before moving on to the next developmental stage. Erikson believed people had difficulty developing normally if they were unable to accomplish the tasks of the previous stage (Erikson, 1963). For a description of the eight stages of development according to Erikson, see Table 1.3.

Importance of the Intrapersonal Model

Freud's intrapersonal theory provides a systematic way of looking at how people develop in the early years of their lives and how they learn to cope with uncomfortable feelings of anxiety. Understanding this theory is beneficial for you because it provides a framework for assessing behavior. For example, using this theory makes it possible for you to distinguish clients' use of defense mechanisms. Anger, directed at you, is much easier to understand when you can identify the use of displacement or projection.

Using Erikson's developmental stages, you will discover that many of your clients are still trying to achieve developmental tasks in any number of stages. With this recognition and understanding, you can help them achieve tasks so they can move on to a higher level of development.

Social-Interpersonal Theory

The theories of Freud started a revolution in the field of psychology. During the late nineteenth century, other disciplines began to emerge and develop their own scientific bodies of knowledge. Sociologists and

Table 1.1 Defense Mechanisms

Defense Mechanism	Example(s)	Use/Purpose
Compensation Covering up weaknesses by emphasizing a more desirable trait or by overachievement in a more comfortable area.	A high school student too small to play football becomes the star long-distance runner for the track team.	Allows a person to overcome weakness and achieve success.
Denial An attempt to screen or ignore unacceptable realities by refusing to acknowledge them.	A woman, though told her father has metastatic cancer, continues to plan a family reunion 18 months in advance.	Temporarily isolates a person from the full impact of a traumatic situation.
Displacement The transferring or discharging of emotional reactions from one object or person to another object or person.	A husband and wife are fighting, and the husband becomes so angry he hits a door instead of his wife. A student gets a C on a paper she worked hard on and goes home and yells at her family.	Allows for feelings to be expressed through or to less dangerous objects or people.
Identification An attempt to manage anxiety by imitating the behavior of someone feared or respected.	A student nurse imitates the nurturing behavior she observes one of her instructors using with clients.	Helps a person avoid self-devaluation.
Intellectualization A mechanism by which an emotional response that normally would accompany an uncomfortable or painful incident is evaded by the use of rational explanations that remove from the incident any personal significance and feelings.	The pain over a parent's sudden death is reduced by saying, "He wouldn't have wanted to live disabled."	Protects a person from pain and traumatic events.
Introjection A form of identification that allows for the acceptance of others' norms and values into oneself, even when contrary to one's previous assumptions.	A 7-year-old tells his little sister, "Don't talk to strangers." He has introjected this value from the instructions of parents and teachers.	Helps a person avoid social retaliation and punishment; particularly important for the child's development of superego.
Minimization Not acknowledging the significance of one's behavior.	A person says, "Don't believe everything my wife tells you. I wasn't so drunk I couldn't drive."	Allows a person to decrease responsibility for own behavior.
Projection A process in which blame is attached to others or the environment for unacceptable desires, thoughts, shortcomings, and mistakes.	A mother is told her child must repeat a grade in school, and she blames this on the teacher's poor instruction. A husband forgets to pay a bill and blames his wife for not giving it to him earlier.	Allows a person to deny the existence of shortcomings and mistakes; protects self-image.
Rationalization Justification of certain behaviors by faulty logic and ascription of motives that are socially acceptable but did not in fact inspire the behavior.	A mother spanks her toddler too hard and says it was all right because he couldn't feel it through the diapers anyway.	Helps a person cope with the inability to meet goals or certain standards.

continued ➤

Table 1.1 Defense Mechanisms *continued*

Defense Mechanism	Example(s)	Use/Purpose
Reaction Formation A mechanism that causes people to act exactly opposite to the way they feel.	An executive resents his bosses for calling in a consulting firm to make recommendations for change in his department but verbalizes complete support of the idea and is exceedingly polite and cooperative.	Aids in reinforcing repression by allowing feelings to be acted out in a more acceptable way.
Regression Resorting to an earlier, more comfortable level of functioning that is characteristically less demanding and responsible.	An adult throws a temper tantrum when he does not get his own way. A critically ill client allows the nurse to bathe and feed him.	Allows a person to return to a point in development when nurturing and dependency were needed and accepted with comfort.
Repression An unconscious mechanism by which threatening thoughts, feelings, and desires are kept from becoming conscious; the repressed material is denied entry into consciousness.	A teenager, seeing his best friend killed in a car accident, becomes amnesic about the circumstances surrounding the accident.	Protects a person from a traumatic experience until he or she has the resources to cope.
Sublimation Displacement of energy associated with more primitive sexual or aggressive drives into socially acceptable activities.	A person with excessive, primitive sexual drives invests psychic energy into a well-defined religious value system.	Protects a person from behaving in irrational, impulsive ways.
Substitution The replacement of a highly valued, unacceptable, or unavailable object by a less valuable, acceptable, or available object.	A woman wants to marry a man exactly like her dead father and settles for someone who looks a little bit like him.	Helps a person achieve goals and minimizes frustration and disappointment.
Undoing An action or words designed to cancel some disapproved thoughts, impulses, or acts in which the person relieves guilt by making reparation.	A father spanks his child and the next evening brings home a present for him. A teacher writes an exam that is far too easy, then constructs a grading curve that makes it difficult to earn a high grade.	Allows a person to appease guilty feelings and atone for mistakes.

anthropologists started to believe that human development was more complex than previously thought. It was not long before these beliefs started filtering into the knowledge that had come primarily from the advances in psychology. A number of theorists began to recognize the importance of the social context of personality development. The focus shifted away from forces within the individual to interpersonal relationships and events in the social context. *Social-interpersonal theory* was the result of this broader perspective.

Harry Stack Sullivan

The work of Harry Stack Sullivan had its beginnings under the umbrella of the intrapersonal perspective. But Sullivan created a developmental system markedly different from that of Freud. Sullivan believed personality was an abstraction that could not be observed apart from interpersonal relationships. Therefore, the unit of study for Sullivan was not the person alone but the person in the context of relationships. According to *interpersonal theory,* personality is manifested only in a person's interactions with another person or

Table 1.2 Stages of Psychosexual Development According to Freud

Stage of Development	Period	Defining Characteristics
Oral	Birth–18 months	Principal source of pleasure from mouth, lips, and tongue. Dependent on mother for care, so feelings of dependency are developed.
Anal	18 months–3 years	Focus on muscle control necessary to control urination and defecation. Expulsion of feces gives a sense of relief. Learns to postpone gratification by postponing the pleasure that comes from anal relief.
Phallic	3–6 years	Develops an awareness of the genital area. Sexual and aggressive feelings associated with functioning of the sexual organs are emphasized. Learns sexual identity during this stage. Masturbation and sexual fantasy are common.
Latency	6–12 years	Sexual development dormant. Focus of energy on cognitive development and intellectual pursuits.
Genital	12 years–early adulthood	Abundance of sexual drive. Primary goal is to develop satisfying relationships with members of the opposite sex.

Table 1.3 Stages of Social Growth and Development According to Erikson

Stage of Development	Period	Developmental Task	Defining Characteristics
Sensory	Birth–18 months	Trust versus mistrust	Child learns to develop trusting relationships.
Muscular	1–3 years	Autonomy versus shame and doubt	Child starts the process of separation; starts learning to live autonomously.
Locomotor	3–6 years	Initiative versus guilt	Learns about environmental influences; becomes more aware of own identity.
Latency	6–12 years	Industry versus inferiority	Energy is directed at accomplishments, creative activities, and learning.
Adolescent	12–20 years	Identity versus role confusion	Transitional period; movement toward adulthood. Starts incorporating beliefs and value systems that have been acquired previously.
Young adulthood	18–25 years	Intimacy versus isolation	Learns the ability to have intimate relationships.
Adulthood	24–45 years	Generativity versus stagnation	Emphasis on maintaining intimate relationships. Movement toward developing a family.
Maturity	45 years–death	Integrity versus despair	Acceptance of life as it has been; acceptance of both good and bad aspects of past life. Maintaining a positive self-concept.

Table 1.4 Stages of Interpersonal Development According to Sullivan

Stage of Development	Period	Defining Characteristics
Infancy	Birth–18 months	Oral zone is the main means by which baby interacts with environment. Breastfeeding provides the first interpersonal experiences. Having needs met helps develop trust.
Childhood	18 months–6 years	Transition to this stage is achieved by child's learning to talk. Starts to see integration of self-concept. Gender development during this time. Child is learning delayed gratification.
Juvenile	6–9 years	This is a time for becoming social. Child learns social subordination to authority figures. Social relationships give a sense of belonging.
Preadolescence	9–12 years	Need for close relationships with peers of same sex. Learns to collaborate. This stage marks the beginning of the first genuine human relationships.
Early adolescence	12–14 years	Development of a pattern of heterosexual relationships. Searching for own identity. Ambiguity about dependence-independence issues.
Late adolescence	14–21 years	Prolonged introduction to society. Self-esteem becomes more stabilized. Will learn to achieve love relationships while maintaining self-identity.

with a group. Sullivan acknowledged heredity and maturation as parts of development but placed far more emphasis on the organism as a social rather than a biological entity (Sullivan, 1953). Although Sullivan saw personality more abstractly than Freud, he still viewed it as the axis of human dynamics in the interpersonal sphere. He identified three principal components of this sphere: dynamisms, personifications, and cognitive processes.

A **dynamism** is a long-standing pattern of behavior. You may think of a dynamism as a habit. In Sullivan's theory, dynamisms highlight personality traits. For instance, a child who is mean can be said to have a dynamism of hostility. The important idea is that any habitual reaction of one person to another or to a situation constitutes a dynamism. Sullivan viewed most dynamisms as meeting the basic human needs of an individual by reducing anxiety.

Sullivan believed that an infant first feels anxiety as the anxiety is transferred from the mother. As the person grows older, anxiety is felt as a response to a threat to his or her own security. Sullivan called the dynamism that develops to reduce anxiety the dynamism of the self, or the *self system*. The self system is the protector of one's security.

A **personification** is an image people have of themselves and others. Every person has many such images, which are made up of attitudes, feelings, and perceptions formed from experiences. For example, a child develops a personification of a good teacher by having the experience of being taught by one. Any relationship that leads to a "good" experience results in a favorable personification of the person involved in that relationship. Unfavorable personifications develop in response to bad experiences. Sullivan believed that personifications are formed early in life to help people cope with interpersonal relationships. As a person gets older, however, very rigid personifications can interfere with interpersonal relationships.

The third component of the interpersonal sphere, **cognitive processes** are the development of the thinking process from unconnected to causal to symbolic. Sullivan believed that cognitive processes, like personifications, are functions of experiences. He believed experiences could be classified into three types. A *protaxic experience* is an unconnected experience that flows through consciousness. Examples are images, sensations, and feelings. Infants experience these most often, and protaxic experiences must occur before the other types. A *parataxic experience* is when a person sees a causal relationship between events that occur at about the same time but are not logically related. Suppose, for example, a child tells his mother he hates her and later she becomes ill.

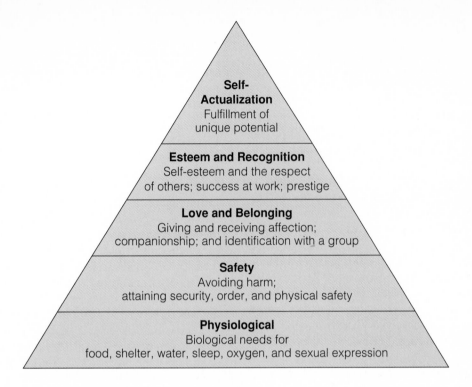

Figure 1.2 **Maslow's hierarchy of needs.**

Source: Adapted from Maslow, A. *Toward a Psychology of Being*, 2nd ed. Copyright 1968 by Van Nostrand Reinhold. Reprinted by permission.

Parataxic thinking leads him to conclude that every time he tells his mother he hates her, she will become ill. *Syntaxic experience*, the highest cognitive level, involves the validation of symbols, particularly verbal symbols. These symbols become validated when a group of people understands them and agrees on their meaning. This level of cognition gives a logical order to experiences and enables people to communicate.

Table 1.4 presents the six stages of development from childhood through adolescence according to Sullivan.

Abraham Maslow

Abraham Maslow viewed personality as self-actualizing; that is, the ideal individual is one who is at peak capacity for fulfilling his or her potential. However, before fulfillment can occur, more needs must be met. Maslow devised a hierarchy of needs (Figure 1.2). *Basic needs* are physiological such as the need for food, water, and sleep. *Metaneeds* are growth-related and include such things as love and belonging, esteem, and self-actualization. Under most circumstances, basic needs take precedence over metaneeds. A person who is hungry is going to be less concerned with truth and justice than a person whose basic needs have been met. Maslow felt that fulfilling metaneeds enables people to rise above an animal level of existence. People unable to meet their growth needs, Maslow postulated, have the potential of becoming psychologically disturbed (Maslow, 1968).

Maslow looked primarily at the healthy, strong side of human nature. His is a *humanistic theory,* in which people are defined holistically as dynamic combinations of physical, emotional, cognitive, and spiritual processes. Maslow emphasized health rather than illness, success rather than failure. He even viewed basic drives, such as sex drive, as natural rather than as unhealthy urges that should be controlled. Maslow felt people have an inborn nature that is essentially good or, at worst, neutral.

Hildegard Peplau

An early attempt to analyze nursing action using an interpersonal theoretical model was made by Hildegard Peplau in her 1952 book, *Interpersonal Relations in Nursing.* She defined nursing as a "significant therapeutic interpersonal process that makes health possible for individuals and groups" (p. xx). The major concepts of her theory include growth, development, communication, and roles.

Communication, described in detail in Chapter 5, is a problem-solving process that takes place within the nurse-client relationship. Problem solving is a collaborative process in which the nurse may assume many roles in helping clients meet their needs and continue their growth and development. As client conflicts and anxieties are resolved, their personalities are strengthened. Peplau noted that both nurses' and clients' culture, religion, ethnicity, education, past experiences, and preconceived ideas influence their interpersonal relationships. She believed that psychodynamic nursing liberated nurses from a tradition of being task-oriented and gave them permission to focus on their excellent interpersonal skills.

Feminist Theory

Feminist theory has evolved out of a new focus on the events and themes that are important in women's lives. Women have been labeled pathological when in fact many of their thoughts, feelings, and behaviors are the result of social, political, economic, psychological, and physical oppression. The consequences of this oppression are low self-esteem, powerlessness, and general unhappiness.

Feminist theory is a model of mental health for both women and men. The differences between nonfeminist and feminist approaches is in the definition of what it is to be a mentally healthy woman or man. For many years, there has been a double standard of mental health. Men and traditional male stereotypes were the model for a mentally healthy adult. Women and traditional female stereotypes were viewed as inadequate and mentally inferior. Feminist theory examines how gender roles limit the psychologic development of all people and inhibit the development of mutually satisfying and noncoercive intimacy. Feminist therapy is gender-sensitive family or relationship therapy and is not restricted to female therapists. Since women value and focus on relationships, feminist therapists are caring, empathetic, and nonauthoritarian. This sense of being cared about and well regarded helps women to achieve greater feelings of self-worth. The concept of self-help encourages women to be assertive and take control of their own lives (Cowan, 1996; Rosenblatt, 1995).

Crisis Theory

Crisis theory provides another perspective for understanding people's responses to life events. A **crisis** is a turning point in a person's life, a point at which usual resources and coping skills are no longer effective and the person enters a state of disequilibrium. All people experience psychological trauma at some point in their lives. Neither stress nor an emergency situation necessarily constitutes a crisis. It is only when an event is perceived subjectively as a threat to need fulfillment, safety, or a meaningful existence that the person enters a crisis state. A number of variables determine a person's potential for entering a crisis state (Aguiliera and Messick, 1990). These variables, known as *balancing factors,* include the following:

- How the person perceives the event.
- What experiences the person has had in coping with stress.
- The person's usual coping abilities.
- The support systems available to the person.

To understand the development of a crisis state, you must be aware of the process of a crisis. Initially, people experience increased anxiety about the traumatic event and are unable to adapt to the situation. As their anxiety increases to high levels, they recognize the need to reach out for help. When both inner resources and external support systems are inadequate, they enter an active crisis state. During this time, they have a short attention span and are unproductive and impulsive. They look to others to solve their problems because they are consumed with feelings of "going crazy" or "losing their mind." Often their interpersonal relationships deteriorate.

Because a state of disequilibrium is so uncomfortable, a crisis is self-limiting and usually lasts about 4–6 weeks. It is during this time that people are most receptive to professional intervention. Because people experiencing crisis are viewed as essentially healthy and capable of growth, changes may be made in a short period of time by focusing on the stressor and using the problem-solving process. The minimum goal of intervention is to help clients adapt and return to the precrisis level of functioning. The maximum goal is to help clients develop more constructive coping skills and move on to a higher level of functioning.

Importance of the Social-Interpersonal Model

Social-interpersonal theory provides another perspective from which you can view human behavior. This theory conceptualizes development within a social context and enables you to assess the influences of culture, social interaction, gender stereotypes, and support systems on the behavior of clients. The emphasis is on what is observable.

Behavioral Theory

The focus of behavioral theory is on a person's actions, not on thoughts and feelings. Behavioral theorists believe that all behavior is learned and can therefore be modified by a system of rewards and punishments. They think that undesirable behavior occurs because it has been learned and reinforced, and that it is possible for people to learn to replace undesirable behaviors with desirable ones.

B. F. Skinner

Behavioral theory, particularly that of B. F. Skinner, had a major impact on the way scientists looked at personality development. Like the social interpersonal theorists, Skinner rejected many of the conceptualizations of Freud and his followers. In addition, he questioned the validity of ideas such as instinctual drives and personality structure; he felt these could not be observed and therefore could not be studied scientifically.

The major emphasis of Skinner's theory is functional analysis of behavior, which suggests looking at behavior pragmatically. What is causing a person to act in a particular way? What factors in the environment reinforce that behavior? Behavioral theory is less concerned with understanding behavior in relation to past events than with the immediate need to predict a trend in behavior and control it. Skinner did not attribute much importance to unconscious motivations, instincts, and feelings; he did attribute importance to a person's immediate actions.

Skinner thought a person's behavior could be controlled by rewards and punishments, that all behavior has specific consequences. Consequences that lead to an increase in the behavior he called *reinforcements,* or *rewards,* and consequences that lead to a decrease in the behavior he called *punishments.*

One of the assumptions of the behavioral perspective is that behavior is orderly and can be controlled. Skinner believed people become who they are through a learning process and by interacting with the environment. Personality problems are the result of faulty learning and can be corrected by new learning experiences that reinforce different behavior.

One of the major concepts within Skinner's system is the *principle of reinforcement* (sometimes referred to as operant reinforcement theory). The ability to reinforce behavior is the ability to change the number of times a particular behavior occurs in the future. Skinner believed certain operations would decrease certain behaviors and increase other behaviors. According to the principle of reinforcement, a response is strengthened when reinforcement is given. Skinner referred to this as an *operant response,* that is, a response that works on the environment and changes it. An example of *operant conditioning* results when a nursing instructor teaches students it is all right to hand in papers late by always accepting late papers. However, handing in papers late can be minimized if the instructor prohibits this behavior. Another way for the instructor to diminish the behavior is by handing out punishments for it; this is called a *punishing response* (Skinner, 1953).

Skinner's theories have been criticized by some and embraced by others. To some, the idea of controlling people's behavior by a systematically applied reward-punishment system is abhorrent. One argument in defense of the theory is that using punishment is not necessary to reinforce desirable behaviors. In other words, a systematic application of rewards can reinforce desirable behaviors, and punishment does not necessarily have to be part of the process.

Importance of the Behavioral Model

Skinner's theories can be beneficial to you in two major areas. The first area is client education. One of the ways people learn is through positive reinforcement of correct responses. One of Skinner's philosophies is that people do not usually fail to learn, but that teachers fail to teach. If the client receives praise and nurturing feedback from you, success will be more likely. For this principle to work, goals must be clearly established so that success can be measured.

The second area in which behavioral principles might be applied is in the practice of mental health nursing. Behavioral therapies are frequently used with adolescents, with those who abuse alcohol or drugs, and with those who wish to control eating or smoking behavior. Behavioral theory can help both you and your clients understand more clearly what is being gained by acting a certain way.

Cognitive Theory

Cognitive theory gives us a blueprint for the process of learning. The ability to think and learn makes us uniquely human. It enables us to be rational, make good judgments, interpret the world around us, and learn new skills. Without cognitive functions, we could not interpret our daily lives, adapt and make changes, and develop the insights to make those changes.

Jean Piaget

Jean Piaget believed that intelligence grows by exposing children to the world around them. He hypothesized that children's experiences and perceptions are challenged by constantly changing stimuli, whereby they recognize discrepancies between their own reality and the environment. Resolving these discrepancies helps children learn new relationships between objects and therefore develop a more mature understanding (Piaget, 1972).

Piaget identified four major stages of cognitive development: the sensorimotor stage, preoperational stage, concrete operational stage, and formal operational stage. Piaget emphasized the range of personal differences in rates of development. The speed by which a child moves through each period depends on biological, intrapersonal, and interpersonal factors.

Aaron Beck

Cognitive theory according to Aaron Beck focuses not on what people do but rather on how they view themselves and their world. He believed that much emotional upset and dysfunctional behavior is related to misperceptions and misinterpretations of experiences. Cognitive theory does not speak to ultimate "causes" of mental disorders but describes how negative thinking (cognitions) can be the first link in the chain of symptoms of mental disorders.

Two important constructs of Beck's cognitive theory are schemas and the cognitive triad. *Cognitive schemas* are personal controlling beliefs that influence the way people process data about themselves and others. For example, you may believe that you are unlovable. When your partner left for work this morning, he slammed the door. The way you processed this event was: "If John slams the door, it means he is angry with me. If he is angry with me, he will reject me. If he rejects me, I will be all alone. If I am all alone, I will not survive." In this example, your core belief led you to misinterpret the significance of the slamming door, which, in fact, was caused by a sudden gust of wind. It is thought that cognitive schemas become activated during depression, anxiety, panic attacks, and personality disorders. These distorted views of the self and the world appear to be reality to a person who is ill.

Cognitive schemas contribute to the development of Beck's *cognitive triad*. Included in this process is (1) a view of the self as inadequate, (2) a negative misinterpretation of current experiences, and (3) a negative view of the future. When clients become caught up in this process, a number of cognitive distortions may occur (Beck and Freeman, 1990). One type of distortion is selective abstraction, or focusing on certain information while ignoring contradictory information. Another distortion is overgeneralization, in which the person takes information or an impression from one event and attaches it to a wide variety of situations. Using such words as "always," "never," "everybody," and "nobody" indicates that the client is overgeneralizing. People who use magnification attribute a high level of importance to insignificant events. Through the distortion of personalization, or ideas of reference, clients believe that what occurs in the environment is related to them, even when no obvious relationship exists. There is also a tendency for superstitious thinking, in which the person believes that some unrelated action will magically influence a course of events. A further distortion is dichotomous thinking, an all-or-none type of reasoning that interferes with people's realistic perception of themselves. Dichotomous thinking involves opposite and mutually exclusive categories such as all good or all bad, celibacy or promiscuity, or depressed or euphoric. Table 1.5 gives examples of cognitive distortions.

Importance of the Cognitive Model

Cognitive theory provides a framework for assessment and intervention. It focuses on the educative nature of nursing practice. Because client/family education is extremely important, it is vital for you to be proficient in the assessment of the learning capabilities of consumers. Cognitive theory provides criteria on which to base these judgments. Cognitive distortions are symptoms of a number of mental disorders. Analyzing clients' cognitive schemas and triads will help you design individualized plans of care.

For assessment questions based on the theories of Freud, Erikson, Sullivan, Maslow, Skinner, and Beck, see Box 1.1.

Biogenic Theory

Biogenic theory focuses on genetic factors, neuroanatomy, neurophysiology, and biological rhythms as they relate to the cause, course, and prognosis of mental disorders. (See Chapter 4 for a review of neurobiology.) In the past, nurses have talked about psychological problems as separate from biological processes in the brain. It was as if the mental and the physical were separate entities, and the symptoms of mental illness existed in the mind but not in the brain. The more current view is that every thought or feeling creates a change in every cell of the body, including the brain. Although we speak of the mind-body-spirit interaction, they are in fact inseparable.

Genetic Factors

We must be careful not to equate "running in families" with hereditary causation. For example, if one of your parents is a nurse, there is a higher chance you will end up being a nurse. The simplistic and erroneous conclusion is that being a nurse is genetically determined. In studying the genetic factors in mental disorders, researchers must first establish that there is a higher-than-expected rate of incidence within families. The next step is identifying what parts are due to genetic factors and what parts are due to environmental factors. Studying monozygotic (identical) and dizygotic (fraternal) twins helps deter-

Table 1.5 Examples of Cognitive Distortions

Distortion	Example
Selective abstraction	"Even though my husband says he loves me, I don't believe him. Look at how he never picks up his laundry."
Overgeneralization	"Women always turn mean after you marry them."
Magnification	"I know he saw the spot of coffee on my tie. Now I'll never get the job because he thinks I'm a slob."
Personalization	"I walked into the classroom and everyone stopped talking. I know they were talking about me."
Superstitious thinking	"If I never take off my wedding ring, my husband will never leave me."
Dichotomous thinking	"Either my life has to be absolutely perfect or I will commit suicide."

mine possible genetic influences. If the incidence of a mental disorder is greater among monozygotic twins than dizygotic twins, there is at least some degree of genetic influence. However, environmental variables are also a factor, even with monozygotic twins. The best twin studies available at this time are those in which monozygotic twins have been separated at birth and reared separately. When these twins demonstrate a higher-than-expected incidence of a mental disorder, a strong degree of genetic influence is likely. It is important to understand the genetic mapping, since hereditary factors appear to play a role in the development of many mental disorders. However, there is something else involved in the etiology of these disorders. Most likely, it is a combination of genes and environment. It is as if there needs to be a "second hit" to convert genetic vulnerability into these brain disorders. This "second hit" could be a perinatal injury, a toxin, and/or life experiences. It is noteworthy that genetic influence is not static but rather reacts to and interacts with environmental experiences.

Box 1.1

Assessment Questions Using Specific Models

Freud's Intrapersonal Theory

What is the developmental stage of the client?

What tasks should the client be accomplishing?

Is there anything that is preventing the accomplishment of tasks?

What are the biological and psychological threats to the client?

What needs of the client are not being met?

What are the client's perceptions of his or her personal situation?

Is there an obvious use of defense mechanisms?

What purpose are those defense mechanisms serving for the client?

What signs of anxiety can be observed in the client?

Can the client's anxiety be validated?

Erikson's Developmental Theory

What is the developmental stage of the client?

What tasks should the client be accomplishing?

Was the client successful in accomplishing the tasks of previous developmental stages?

During what stages did the client fail to accomplish the developmental tasks?

What effect does this have on the client's psychosocial development?

How is this affecting the immediate problems confronting the client?

What are the environmental factors affecting the client and the client's present problems?

Sullivan's Interpersonal Theory of Development

At what stage of development is the client?

What development tasks should the client be accomplishing?

Did accomplishing previous developmental tasks meet the interpersonal needs of the client?

If interpersonal needs were not met, what effect did this have on the client?

What is the client's personification of self? How does the client describe self?

In what way does the client exhibit anxiety?

What are the client's coping mechanisms?

How does the client relate to other people?

What social networks are available to the client?

How can these social networks affect outcomes of the present situation?

Maslow's Humanistic Theory

Is the client meeting his or her basic needs?

How does the client describe these basic needs?

What obvious needs are being frustrated at this time?

Other than basic needs, what needs does the client consider important?

What is your description of the metaneeds being met by the client?

How does the client express self creatively?

What types of behaviors can be described that indicate the client is moving toward self-actualization?

How does the client describe his or her capabilities and resources?

Skinner's Behavioral Theory

What specific behaviors of the client need to be changed?

What new behaviors are desired to replace the old ones?

Does the client agree that certain behaviors need to be changed?

How is the behavior that needs to be changed reinforced?

Who or what is doing the reinforcing?

What types of things are important to the client?

What types of rewards would reinforce the new, desired behaviors?

Is the client willing to do mutual goal setting?

Does the client clearly understand the goals?

Box 1.1 continued

Beck's Cognitive Theory

What are the cognitive schemas or controlling beliefs that the client holds about self and others?

In what ways does the client have inadequate views of self?

What evidence is there that the client misinterprets current experiences?

How positively or negatively does the client view the future?

Is there evidence of cognitive distortions?

Neurotransmission

Theories of neurotransmission in mental disorders are concerned with the levels of norepinephrine (NE), serotonin (5-HT), dopamine (DA), acetylcholine (ACH), and gamma aminobutyric acid (GABA) in the brain. As an electrical impulse travels to the nerve endings, neurotransmitters (chemical messengers) are released at the synaptic junction. These neurotransmitters react with the neuronal receptors, which allow the impulse to be conducted through the next nerve cell. Brain disorders, commonly referred to as mental disorders, are often related to either a deficiency or an excess of neurotransmitters, or to an imbalance among the various neurotransmitters. In other cases, there is a change in the sensitivity or the shape of the neuronal receptors, resulting in altered transmission of impulses. Neurotransmission is described in greater detail in Chapter 4.

Biological Rhythms

Circadian rhythms are regular fluctuations of a variety of physiological factors over a period of 24 hours. Temperature, energy, sleep, arousal, motor activity, appetite, hormones, and mood all demonstrate circadian rhythms. The "biological clock" is located in the hypothalamus and may be desynchronized by external or internal factors. An example of external desynchronization is jet lag: decreased energy level, reduced ability to concentrate, and mood variations resulting from rapid time zone changes. Some mental disorders demonstrate alterations in adrenal rhythm, temperature patterns, and sleep patterns.

Importance of the Biogenic Model

Our understanding of mental disorders has been revolutionized by contemporary knowledge of the biological components of behavior, affect, cognition, and interpersonal relationships. Recognizing genetic factors in mental disorders minimizes the tendency to blame the victim or family for the disorder. Understanding neurotransmission helps you comprehend how psychotropic drugs affect the brain to reduce or eliminate the symptoms of many mental disorders. It is impossible to practice mental health nursing without knowing and applying biological principles.

The Therapeutic Relationship

Therapeutic relationships are established to help the client. The way you establish the relationship depends on your reactions to the clinical setting and how you are able to care for clients. In mental health nursing, you examine the relationship to ensure that it is goal-directed and therapeutic.

Student Concerns

At the onset of your course in mental health nursing, you may be quite comfortable in the clinical setting, or you may experience uncertainties and concern relating to both yourself and your clients. Your personal concerns may stem from being in an unfamiliar environment, not knowing what to talk about, believing you have nothing to offer, and/or thinking you might say the wrong thing. Your concerns about clients may be rooted in your stereotypes of people with mental illness, your fear of rejection, your discomfort with anger, or your fear of being physically harmed by a client. Box 1.2 lists common student concerns and strategies for dealing with them.

Caring: The Art and Essence of Nursing

Caring is the essence of nursing and the foundation upon which the nursing process is based. It is more than merely liking or comforting other people. It involves commitment and a binding together of individuals in interpersonal connections. Before nurses can care for clients, they must first learn to value and care for themselves. As Keen (1991) states: "If we are unable to care first for ourselves as individuals, and then for our nursing colleagues, the caring we give to our patients is not as good as it could be" (p. 173). One of your educational goals in mental health nursing might be discovering how to care for yourself more effectively. Caring for yourself means reducing unnecessary stress, managing conflict more effectively, communicating with family and friends more clearly, and taking time out for yourself. Caring for your colleagues means respecting cultural differences, asking for collaboration, and responding to constructive criticism.

The art of nursing is in being there, with another person or persons, in a context of caring. It is the capacity "to receive another human being's expression of feelings and to experience those feelings for oneself" (Chinn and Watson, 1994, p. xvi). Caring involves compassion and sensitivity to each person within the context of her or his entire life. In the past, nurses have been urged not to care too much or get too involved. However, caring, successful nurses do get involved with clients because they practice nursing as an art instead of nursing as just a day-to-day job. Clients have a right to competent nursing care, but they also desire a nurse who is committed to clients. In many schools of nursing over the past 50 years, the art of nursing has been devalued and separated from the science of nursing. Consequently, caring has often been a minimal part of the curriculum. With consumer expectations and demand, nursing is beginning to restore its caring-healing art as the basis of nursing practice (Appleton, 1994; Montgomery, 1996).

The Nurse-Client Relationship

Throughout the text, the terms *client* and *consumer* refer to individuals experiencing mental disorders as well as their families and significant others. The nurse-client relationship is the key factor throughout the nursing process. It is the means by which nurses are able to assess clients accurately, formulate diagnoses, help them establish outcomes, plan and implement interventions, and evaluate the effectiveness of the nursing process. The nurse-client relationship is therapeutic, not social. Social relationships are reciprocal in that both people expect their individual needs to be met as fully as possible. The therapeutic relationship, on the other hand, exists for clients, and the focus is on their needs. To minimize the possibility of client dependency, do not try to meet all the needs of every client; support them in meeting their own needs whenever possible. In the professional role, you collaborate with your client as a team, forming a therapeutic alliance with the goal of the client's growth and adaptation. The therapeutic relationship is client-centered, goal-specific, theory-based, and open to supervision by your peers, instructors, and supervising nurses.

The therapeutic relationship has three phases: introductory, working, and termination. These phases are more easily identified in nurse-client relationships that last more than a few days. The phases often overlap and are thought of as interlocking. There are goals to be achieved in each phase of the relationship.

Introductory Phase

The introductory phase usually begins when you initiate the therapeutic relationship with your client. Start by introducing yourself by name and position. Suggest helping the client identify problems, and work toward resolving them. Establish a mutually acceptable agreement or contract to guide the relationship. This contract, which is typically verbal, should include the purpose of the relationship; the duration of the relationship; and where, when, and for how long you will meet. It is critical that the issue of confidentiality be discussed. (See Chapter 23 for guidelines on confidentiality.)

Although client assessment continues throughout the therapeutic relationship, it is extremely important during the introductory phase. The introductory phase ends with the development of preliminary diagnoses and outcome identification.

Working Phase

The second phase of the therapeutic relationship is the working phase. The nursing process is dynamic; assessment, diagnosis, outcome identification, planning,

Box 1.2

Student Concerns and Strategies for Dealing with Them

Stereotypical ideas about people with mental health problems.

Identify cultural stereotypes and discuss your expectations in the first clinical preconference.

Identify specific concerns about clients and/or their families of origin or their current families.

Approach the client as a person rather than as a diagnosis.

Identify healthy aspects and resources of clients; they *are* able to cope effectively in many areas of life.

Fear of not knowing what to talk about.

When first meeting a client, introduce yourself by name and position.

Follow the client's lead in topics to be discussed in the initial interaction; pay attention to the client's nonverbal communication signals indicating comfort or discomfort.

Give up the unrealistic expectation that you have to be absolutely right before you offer any observations to clients.

Share your perceptions with clients and seek validation, by asking, for example, "Am I hearing you correctly, that you are very frustrated over this situation?" or "It sounds as if you are becoming more comfortable with being in the hospital."

Using your nursing care plan, decide on specific topics and goals for your one-to-one interaction; be flexible if the client has different priorities.

Concern about having nothing to offer.

Identify your own fears of inadequacy by listening to your self-statements: "How can I help this person when I don't know what's wrong with him?" "These clients are too sick/well, so how can I help them?"

If clients question your qualifications, simply state why you are here and what your role is on the unit.

Recognize that your knowledge and theory base will be increasing throughout the course.

Identify the energy and enthusiasm you bring as a positive quality to be used therapeutically.

Recognize that a positive interpersonal relationship is therapeutic because it increases self-esteem, develops interactional skills for clients, and promotes your own professional growth.

Involve clients in the nursing process and work together as a team toward specific goals; solutions come from working *with* clients, not from doing something *to* clients.

Concern about hurting clients by saying the wrong thing.

The quality of a caring relationship overcomes verbal mistakes; you will not destroy a client with a few ill-chosen words.

Recognize that clinical experience is an opportunity to learn and that verbal mistakes will be made; opportunities for more appropriate interventions are seldom lost—they're just postponed.

If you have made a mistake, apologize to the client and identify what would have been a more therapeutic response.

Use process recordings or audiotapes to evaluate, improve, and increase your communication skills.

Concern about rejection by the client.

Identify your own characteristic response to rejection. Do you become angry? Feel hurt? Feel resigned to it? Withdraw from the person? In what other ways might you respond?

Identify what is the worst thing that will happen to you if a client refuses to work with you.

If a client is exhibiting behavior that indicates unwillingness to work with you, validate this behavior with her or him.

Remember that you will have opportunities to work with other clients.

Concern about client anger.

Know and understand your own response to the feeling and expression of anger: "Nice people don't get angry," "It's okay to feel angry but it should be talked about calmly," "I'm uncomfortable if people shout when they are angry."

Accept the client's right to be angry; feelings are real and cannot be discounted or ignored.

Try to understand the meaning of the client's anger.

Ask the client in what way you have contributed to the anger; help the client "own" the anger—do not assume responsibility for her or his feelings.

continued ➤

■ *Box 1.2 continued*

Student Concerns and Strategies for Dealing with Them

Let clients talk about their anger.

Listen to the client, and react as calmly as possible.

After the interaction is completed, take time to process your feelings and your responses to the client with your peers and instructor.

Concern about physical harm from clients.

Ask your instructor about the reality of this concern.

Avoid being in a "trapped" position, e.g., isolated in a client's room.

Recognize the early signs of an impending violent outburst.

Seek help immediately from a staff member or instructor before a client gets out of control.

If a client begins to act out physically, stay out of the staff members' way as they implement their plan of action.

---

implementation, and evaluation are continuous throughout this phase. Parts of the care plan are revised, expanded, or eliminated according to the individual client's needs. The conscious process of working together toward mutually established goals is referred to as the **therapeutic alliance.** Ineffective behaviors and thoughts are identified as problems, and you and your clients work together to establish more effective ways of coping. It is during the working phase that the bulk of client education and problem solving is accomplished.

Two phenomena that may occur during any phase of the relationship (but that are more likely to be noticed during the working phase) are transference and countertransference. **Transference** is a client's unconscious displacement of feelings for significant people in the past onto the nurse in the current relationship. These displaced feelings can be positive or negative and may be highly emotional. Transference that is not identified and managed may decrease the effectiveness of the working phase because the meaning of the nurse-client relationship becomes misinterpreted. When transference occurs, the nurse and client must explore it and separate past relationships from the present one.

> Sue, 20 years old, is being seen in the clinic for depression. She was sexually abused by her father from age 7 to 12. Miguel is Sue's nurse-therapist. Sue states that she trusts Miguel, but her nonverbal communication indicates a great deal of fear and suspicion. Sue's feelings about

her father have been unconsciously displaced onto Miguel.

Countertransference is the nurse's emotional reaction to the client based on significant relationships in the nurse's past. Countertransference may be conscious or unconscious, and the feelings may be positive or negative. Awareness of countertransference is critical because it could interfere with understanding the client and providing effective care. Discussing your feelings about your client with your instructor will help bring countertransference into conscious awareness.

> Collen's son was killed in an accident several years ago when he was 15 years old. Collen is taking a course in psychiatric nursing and has been assigned to work with Brendan, who is 15 years old. Brendan is very manipulative, but Collen has difficulty setting limits on his behavior. Through the process of supervision with her instructor, Collen begins to realize that her inability to recognize Brendan's manipulation is because he reminds her of her dead son. She has displaced her feelings about her son onto Brendan and has attributed to him positive qualities he really doesn't have at this time.

Termination Phase

The third phase of the therapeutic relationship is the termination phase. Information about when and how this will occur is included in the introductory phase and discussed at times during the working phase. The primary goal of the termination phase is to reminisce about the relationship experiences in order to review the client's progress. With the client, review plans for the immediate future. Termination can be a traumatic experience for clients. Those who have had difficulty ending other relationships will likely have problems ending your shared therapeutic relationship. You must understand their sense of loss and help them express and cope with their feelings. In an effort to continue the relationship, clients may introduce new problems or try to extend the relationship beyond the clinical setting. Here is an example of part of the termination process between Collen (the nurse) and Brendan (the client):

> Brendan: Collen, I know this is your last day on the unit, and I'm going to be out of here next week. How about if you give me your phone number so I can call you up sometime?
>
> Collen: Our relationship was a professional one and is restricted to the time we worked together here at the hospital.
>
> Brendan: But Collen, you really understand me. My own mother doesn't understand me. I just want to be able to call you if things get a little tough. Is that too much to ask?
>
> Collen: Yes, Brendan, it is. I cannot continue to be your nurse outside of the hospital. Let's talk about choices you do have if things get tough when you go home. I would also like to talk about feelings you're having right now as we are about to end our time together.

The physical component of the nurse-client relationship includes all the procedures and technical skills that you do with or for clients. This technological component of nursing education is easily defined and described for you. As a student, you are praised and evaluated for tasks that can be observed, which reinforces the task orientation prevalent in the medical model of health care.

The psychosocial component of the nurse-client relationship, which is as important as the physical component, involves your response to the client as one human being to another. You bring many qualities to these relationships: positive regard, a nonjudgmental attitude, acceptance, warmth, empathy, authenticity, and congruity of communication. You encourage clients to share their thoughts on how they perceive the world, their past experiences and expectations, and their hopes and dreams for the future.

Together with the psychosocial component, the spiritual component of the nurse-client relationship comprises the caring relationship. The spiritual component is the feeling of connectedness between you and the client. It is that inner sense of being a part of something more than yourself. It is respect for the client's cultural values and religious views. Spirituality is what allows us to connect with clients who may be very different from ourselves. We may not be able to see clearly the person who lives behind the mask of substance abuse or who is experiencing delusions or who has been forced into living on the streets, but responding to that person's spirit is what allows us to connect to them. Your role in providing spiritual care includes allowing clients to express important spiritual needs, such as the need for meaning in life, belief in God, or relief from fear, doubt, or loneliness. The important point is to recognize that spiritual needs are as diverse as our clients, their cultures, and their illnesses.

The power component of the nurse-client relationship is related to your and your clients' beliefs in locus of control. If you reflect an *external locus of control* you expect clients to give up control to the staff, who then do "to" and "for" clients, stripping from them the right to choose their own healing journey and the quality of their life experiences. The focus of the nurse-client relationship has traditionally been one of curing, with health care professionals as the heroes. When clients have an external locus of control, they view their disease or disability as a "thing" that has been imposed upon them and believe they are not responsible for either the cause or the cure.

If you believe in an *internal locus of control* you welcome your clients' feelings, respect their wishes, and honor their needs for self-expression. Your role is to empower consumers through providing skills, information, and support as they choose options that are in their best interests. The relationship is built around clients' needs to shape and control their own lives as much as possible. Clients who have an internal locus of control feel powerful rather than victimized and are participants in their own healing process. They recognize behaviors, thoughts, and feelings that influence their own movement towards health or illness.

Nursing Process in Mental Health Nursing

Critical Thinking

As nurses, we must be critical thinkers because of the nature of the discipline and the nature of our work. We are expected to solve client problems by performing critical analyses of the factors associated with the problems. This analytical process, or *critical thinking*, enables us to make better decisions. Thus, critical thinking, problem solving, and decision making are interrelated processes, with creativity enhancing the result.

Because nursing decisions may profoundly affect the lives of our clients and their families, we must think critically. But critical thinking is not limited to problem solving or decision making; we use critical thinking to make reliable observations, draw sound conclusions, create new ideas, evaluate lines of reasoning, and improve our self-knowledge.

To think critically, you must have cognitive skills and be willing to use them. Critical thinking attitudes provide the motivation to use cognitive skills. These attitudes are interrelated and integrated, rather than used in isolation. For instance, it takes courage to acknowledge that you do not know something and to develop an inquiring attitude.

Characteristics of Critical Thinking

Thinking Independently   Critical thinking requires that we think for ourselves. As we mature and acquire knowledge, we must examine beliefs we acquired as children, holding those we can rationally support and rejecting those we cannot.

Humility   Intellectual humility means having an awareness of the limits of our own knowledge. As critical thinkers we are willing to admit what we don't know; we are willing to seek new information and to rethink our conclusions in the light of new knowledge.

Courage   With an attitude of courage, we are willing to consider and fairly examine ideas or views, especially those to which we may have a strongly negative reaction. This type of courage comes from recognizing that our own beliefs are sometimes false, misleading, and prejudicial.

Integrity   Intellectual integrity requires that we question our own knowledge and beliefs as quickly and as thoroughly as we will challenge those of another.

Perseverance   As critical thinkers, we strive to find effective solutions to client and nursing problems. We resist the temptation to find a quick and easy answer. Important questions tend to be complex and therefore often require a great deal of thought and research.

Empathy   It is easy to misinterpret the words or actions of a person who is from a different cultural, religious, or socioeconomic background. It is also difficult to understand the beliefs or actions of a person experiencing a situation that you have never experienced. Empathy is the ability to see the world from another's perspective and to communicate this understanding for validation or correction.

Fair-Mindedness   As critical thinkers, we are fair-minded, assessing all viewpoints with the same objectivity. Fair-mindedness helps us consider opposing points of view and work to understand new ideas before rejecting or accepting them.

See Table 1.6 for characteristics that are important for critical thinking.

After gaining an idea of what it means to think critically, solve problems, and make decisions, you need to become aware of your own thinking style and abilities. Acquiring critical-thinking skills and an attitude of inquiry then becomes a matter of practice. Critical thinking is not an "either-or" phenomenon; it exists on a continuum, along which people develop and employ the process of inquiry. Solving problems and making decisions are risky. Sometimes the outcome is not what was desired. With effort, however, everyone can achieve some level of critical thinking in order to become effective problem solvers and decision makers (Kozier et al, 1998).

The nursing process is the same in all clinical areas of professional practice. In the 1994 *Standards of Psychiatric and Mental Health Nursing Practice*, the American Nurses' Association (ANA) delineates the standards to which nurses are held, both legally and ethically. These standards, based on the steps of the nursing process, are covered in Box 1.3.

Table 1.6 Characteristics of Critical Thinking

Characteristic	Description
Rational	Based on logic rather than prejudice or fear
Reflective	Collect data; think through in disciplined manner
Inquiring	Examine claims; determine truth and validity
Analytical	Analyze issues for understanding; decide which authorities are credible
Objective	Attempt to remove bias from own and others' thinking; aware of own values and feelings
Evaluative	Evaluate arguments; decide on course of action; solve problems; use accepted standards

Box 1.3

1994 ANA Standards of Psychiatric–Mental Health Clinical Nursing Practice

Standard I Assessment: The nurse collects client health data.

Standard II Diagnosis: The nurse analyzes the assessment data in determining diagnoses.

Standard III Outcome Identification: The nurse identifies expected outcomes individualized to the client.

Standard IV Planning: The nurse develops a plan of care that prescribes interventions to attain expected outcomes.

Standard V Implementation: The nurse implements the interventions identified in the plan of care.

Standard VI Evaluation: The nurse evaluates the client's progress in attaining expected outcomes.

The Nursing Process

Standard I: Assessment

Assessment in mental health nursing is based on the collection of data from multiple sources, such as the client, family and friends, other health care providers, past and current medical records, and community agencies. The client's immediate condition or needs determine the order in which assessment data is collected. Assessment tools you will use are psychosocial assessments and neuropsychiatric assessments.

Observation   Careful, accurate observation is vital during the psychosocial and neurophsyciatric assessment. You begin to observe the moment you meet the person and their family. Observation involves all the senses, but seeing and hearing are the most critical. In the chapters on disorders (Part III) and crisis (Part IV), you will learn how to assess clients for the behavioral, affective, cognitive, sociocultural, and physiological characteristics of each disorder or crisis situation. In general, here is how observations are used in each of those categories.

When observing clients behaviorally, answer the following questions:

- Where is the client, and what is she or he doing?
- Is the behavior appropriate to the setting (own home, public place)?
- Is the client dangerous to self or others?
- Is any bizarre or unusual behavior occurring?

When observing for affective characteristics, answer the following questions:

- Is there any evidence of intense emotions, such as loud laughter, crying, yelling, or screaming?
- Is the affect appropriate to the situation?

When observing for cognitive characteristics, answer the following questions:

- Is the client going over and over the same topic (ruminating)?
- Can you follow what the client is saying?
- Are there themes recurring during the interaction?

When observing for sociocultural characteristics, answer the following questions:

- Does the client interact with others? Who? Staff? Peers? Family?

Box 1.4

Neuropsychiatric Assessment

General
- Age
- Relationship status
- Family composition
- Employment
- Living situation

Appearance
- Apparent age
- General state of health
- Grooming and hygiene

Activity
- Motor activity (appropriate, increased, decreased)
- Tremors, dystonias
- Hyperactivity (activity is purposeful)
- Agitation (activity is purposeless)

Speech and Language
- Fluency
- Comprehension
- Pace (fast, slow)
- Volume
- Tone (calm, hostile)

Emotional State
- Mood (sustained emotional state; what client describes; depression, anxiety, sadness, calmness, anger)
- Affect (immediate emotional expression; what others observe; appropriateness, intensity, lability, range of expression)

Form of Thought
Signs of pathology
- Blocking (sudden stop in speech or train of thought)

- Circumstantiality (overly detailed, tedious; eventually reaches goal)
- Confabulation (unconsciously filling in memory gaps with imagined material)
- Derailment (speech is blocked and then begins again on unrelated topic)
- Flight of ideas (rapid, fragmented thoughts manifested in pressured speech)
- Loose association (disconnected thoughts)
- Neologism (making up new words; not understood by others)
- Tangential (thoughts veer from main idea and never get back to it)

Content of Thought
Disorders range from transient preoccupations to intractable delusions
- Ruminations (recurring mood-congruent concerns usually related to anxiety or depression)
- Obsessions (unwanted, repetitive thoughts that lead to feelings of fear or guilt)
- Compulsions (thoughts or behaviors used to decrease the fear or guilt associated with obsessions)
- Delusions (grandiosity, persecution, control, sin and guilt; religious, erotomanic, somatic)
- Experiences of influence (ideas of reference, thought broadcasting, thought withdrawal, thought insertion)

Perception
Signs of pathology
- Illusions (the misintrepretation of an environmental stimulus of sight, sound, touch, smell, or taste)
- Hallucination (occurence of a sight, sound, touch, smell, or taste without any external stimulus)
- Depersonalization (feel sense of identity has been altered and therefore feel strange and unreal)
- Derealization (feel the environment has changed and is unreal)

- Is the client assertive or passive with others?
- Is the client having any problems in living at home, in a residential setting, or on the inpatient unit?
- How does the client manage conflict with others?

When observing for physiological characteristics, answer the following questions:

- What is the client's motor behavior—for example, pacing, sitting in one position for a long period of time, foot swinging, teeth grinding?
- What does the client's nutritional status appear to be?
- Is the client sleeping at night? Taking naps during the day?
- Are there any physical complaints?

The above question sets are general guidelines. As you learn about the mental disorders and crisis situations, you will gather more specific information to guide your observations.

Psychosocial Assessment The interview is often the initial step in the assessment process. The setting for the interview and the length of time are determined by the client's mental and physical status. Agencies often have specific forms to be completed as part of the psychosocial assessment. In general, the following information is gathered from the client and significant others:

- client and family's definition of present problem
- history of present problem, including health beliefs and practices
- family history, including support systems and ethnic and cultural factors
- social history, including communication skills, social networks, work/school roles, economic stressors, and legal stressors
- spiritual considerations, including beliefs, values, and religious concerns
- physical and neurological assessment
- strengths and competencies

In each chapter in Parts III and IV, you will find a Focused Nursing Assessment table to help you learn the types of questions to ask and the particular characteristics for which to assess. Observing experienced nurses is a great way to learn basic interviewing skills, as well as seeing more advanced techniques implemented. Be sure to discuss with the nurse what you observed, and clarify anything you did not understand.

Neuropsychiatric Assessment The neuropsychiatric assessment provides information about the client's appearance, speech, emotional state, and cognitive functioning. See Box 1.4 for the neuropsychiatric assessment.

Following the collection of data from observations and assessments, you will review the data and formulate an initial nursing care plan or critical pathway.

Standard II: Diagnosis

Analysis of the significance of the assessment data results in the formulation of nursing diagnoses.

Psychiatric Nursing Diagnosis Standardized labels are applied to clients' problems and responses to mental disorders. These standardized labels come from the list of approved nursing diagnoses accepted by the North American Nursing Diagnosis Association (NANDA). Appendix B contains the current list of approved NANDA diagnoses. When we use standardized language to document the diagnoses of our clients, we can begin to build large databases that will expand nursing knowledge.

In developing the nursing diagnoses further, it is necessary to describe the related or contributing factors. These include behavioral symptoms, affective changes, and disrupted cognitive patterns that accompany the mental disorders. Spiritually, people with psychiatric disabilities often have difficulty with interpersonal relationships and may feel a lack of connectedness with others. Some people suffer from a lack of meaning in life, while others attempt to find meaning in their response to their mental disorder. Cultural pressures and expectations may be contributing factors in the development and prognosis of mental disorders. Signs and symptoms, referred to as *defining characteristics*, are subjective and objective data that support the nursing diagnosis. Defining characteristics are identified during the assessment process but are not usually written as part of the diagnostic statement. The following are examples of nursing diagnoses you may use during your clinical experience:

- *Hopelessness* related to chronic effects of poverty and racism; dire expectations of the future.
- *Self-care deficit: bathing/hygiene* related to low energy and decreased desire to care for self; distractibility in *completing ADLs.*
- *Impaired verbal communication* related to retardation in flow of thought; flight of ideas; altered thought processes; obsessive thoughts; panic level of anxiety.
- *Altered family processes* related to rigidity in functions and roles; enmeshed family system; demands of caring for a family member with dementia; use of violence to maintain family relationships.

Nursing Diagnoses Versus DSM-IV Diagnoses   Mental disorders are classified in the *Diagnostic and Statistical Manual of Mental Disorders, Fourth Edition (DSM-IV)*, published by the American Psychiatric Association. The *DSM-IV* is used by all members of the health care team. It groups client information into five categories, called axes. (See Box 1.5 for a listing of the axes.) Axis I includes the majority of the mental disorders. Axis II lists long-lasting problems, including personality disorders and developmental disorders. Both Axis I and Axis II describe the intrapersonal area of functioning. Axis III describes the physical problems of disorders that must be considered when planning the client's treatment program. If there are no physical problems, the diagnosis on Axis III will be stated as "none." Axis IV describes the psychosocial stressors (acute and long-lasting) occurring in the past year that have contributed to the current mental disorder. Nurses should be aware of how many stressors have occurred and how much change each stressor caused in the life of the client. Axis V rates the highest level of psychological, social, and occupational functioning the client has achieved in the past year, as well as the current level of functioning. It is especially important to be sensitive to cultural differences and expectations when rating clients on Axis V. Appendix A lists and describes the diagnostic categories of the *DSM-IV*.

The basis of nursing diagnoses and *DSM-IV* diagnoses evolves from problem solving, which begins with data collection. Data collection includes reviewing signs and symptoms exhibited by clients. With nursing diagnoses, those signs and symptoms are translated into related to and contributing factors.

Box 1.5

DSM-IV Axes

Axis I:	Adult and child clinical disorders
	Conditions not attributable to a mental disorder that are a focus of clinical attention
Axis II:	Personality disorders
	Mental retardation
Axis III:	General medical conditions
Axis IV:	Psychosocial and environmental problems
Axis V:	Global assessment of functioning

With the *DSM-IV*, the signs and symptoms are translated into diagnostic criteria, including the essential and associated features of specific mental disorders, and a differential diagnosis ultimately results.

There are some similarities between psychiatric nursing diagnoses and the *DSM-IV* diagnoses. They both serve to guide practice by synthesizing data leading to appropriate interventions. They are both communication tools basic to client care and research activities, and they are both international in scope. There are also significant differences between the two. *DSM-IV* diagnoses are applicable only to individuals, while nursing diagnoses are applicable to individuals, families, groups, and communities. Nursing diagnoses are generally directed toward problems in daily living, while *DSM-IV* diagnoses are oriented toward the "disease and cure" model (Malone, 1991).

Standard III: Outcome Identification

Once you have established diagnoses, you and the client mutually identify goals for change. Mutual goal-setting is the process of collaborating with clients to identify and prioritize care goals and develop a plan for achieving those goals. Underlying this process is respect for clients' cultural values. You begin by assessing the clients' degree of insight into their problems. If clients are too acutely ill to be actively involved in the initial goal formulation, or if they are in denial of mental health problems, they must at least be informed of the goals and given an opportunity to express their opinions (McCloskey and Bulechek, 1996).

Clients are encouraged to identify strengths and abilities that they bring to this problem-solving process. You help them identify realistic, attainable goals and break down complex goals into small, manageable steps. After goals become manageable, work with clients on prioritizations so they try to modify only one behavior at a time. Finally, help clients develop a plan to meet their goals which includes identifying available resources, setting realistic time limits, and clarifying the roles of the nurse and client (McCloskey and Bulechek, 1996).

Client outcomes are specific behavioral measures by which you, clients, and significant others determine progress toward goals. Outcomes are selected in relationship to a particular nursing diagnosis and are written in terms of client behavior or client status. Outcomes are specified before interventions are chosen and should be directed at improving mental health as well as minimizing problems. Consideration must be given to how realistic, attainable, and cost-effective the outcomes are. Regular review dates are established with clients and families to review progress toward outcomes and goals.

> Moune, a middle-aged woman who is depressed, has the following nursing diagnosis:
> *Bathing/hygiene self-care deficit* related to lack of interest in shampooing hair or washing clothes for one month.
> Goal: Will become independent in bathing and hygiene.
> Outcome criteria: Will verbalize need and desire for cleanliness, take a daily shower, wash hair, do laundry on Monday and Thursday.

Standard IV: Planning

Once the nursing diagnoses, goals, and outcome criteria have been identified, the plan of care is developed to assist the client toward a higher level of functioning and improved mental health. Planning consists of establishing nursing care priorities, identifying interventions, and selecting appropriate nursing activities.

Priorities of Care   In mental health nursing, safety needs are often more of a priority than physiological needs. There are many safety issues you need to be aware of at all times. Frequently ask yourself if the client is in danger of the following:

- Exhaustion related to excessive exercise; lack of sleep; panic level of anxiety
- Inability to exercise good judgment related to problems in thinking or perceiving
- Self-mutilation based on past or current behavior
- Violence directed toward others based on past or current behavior
- Suicide related to hopelessness; command hallucinations

Interventions   The widespread use of NANDA's nursing diagnoses has increased awareness of the need for standardized classifications of nursing interventions or treatments. Until very recently there has been no uniform way to define and document nursing care. The Nursing Interventions Classification (NIC) is the first comprehensive standardized classification of nursing interventions and is useful to nurses in all specialties and in all settings. Most of the interventions are for use with individuals, but many are for use with families, and a few are for use with entire communities (McCloskey and Bulechek, 1996). Appendix C is a partial list of the NIC taxonomy with the most common interventions used in mental health nursing. Definitions for each intervention are also supplied. NIC is a three-level taxonomy. The highest level contains six domains (or supercategories):

- Physiological: Basic
- Physiological: Complex
- Behavioral
- Safety
- Family
- Health System

Each domain includes *classes* (or subcategories), which are groups of related interventions. The third level in the taxonomy are the *interventions*. Supplementing the interventions are a list of nursing activities for each intervention. This is not a list of specific procedures as not all activities apply to every client. In addition, nurses may modify or add to the list of activities. The following is an example of the NIC taxonomy:

> Domain: Behavioral
> Class: Behavioral Therapy
> Intervention: Limit Setting

Definition: Establishing the parameters of desirable and acceptable patient behavior.

Activities: (sample from a list of 13 activities)

- Discuss concerns with patient about behavior.
- Identify undesirable patient behavior.
- Discuss what is desirable behavior in a given situation.
- Establish reasonable expectations.
- Establish consequences.

The taxonomy is not linked to any specific nursing theory and can easily be used with NANDA and *DSM-IV* diagnoses. You are encouraged to look over this classification system in Appendix C before reading any further.

This text uses the NIC format in organizing the planning and implementation of nursing care. You will find the domains, classes, and interventions in bold type. Each intervention is accompanied by text which describes the nursing activities you consider when planning and implementing your care.

Standard V: Implementation

Caring is a way of relating to people that enables them to grow toward their full potential. Your nursing interventions should be implemented in a manner that recognizes the worth and dignity of people and considers the physical, emotional, social, cultural, and spiritual needs of your clients and their families. No matter what mental disorder the client is experiencing, you will assume several roles in helping your clients grow and adapt. The appropriate role at any given time is determined by the planned interventions. The various roles of a nurse are described below.

Socializing Agent   The nurse functions as a socializing agent with clients. Working one-to-one with your client, you will focus on difficulties she or he may have in communicating thoughts and feelings to others. Socializing helps to model appropriate interpersonal behavior. Informal conversations such as these give clients the opportunity to discuss nonstressful topics and provide some relief from anxiety.

Teacher   Another nursing role is that of teacher. A great deal of teaching occurs in connection with the treatment plan (see Chapter 5 for information on client and family education). Depending on client diagnoses, you may be involved in teaching ADLs.

Some clients may need to learn basic cooking, laundry, or shopping skills in order to be able to live independently. Those who have no diversions or hobbies may need help selecting appropriate activities and learning the skills associated with them. Some clients will need to learn and practice assertiveness skills, anger management skills, and/or conflict resolution strategies. The problem-solving process is discussed in detail in Chapter 5.

You will also teach clients and families about the purpose of medication: expected therapeutic effects, the length of time after taking the medication before a change, and the usual side effects. Clients must be informed about any dietary or activity restrictions related to their medications, as well as what to do if they forget to take a dose. In addition, you must instruct clients about any related blood testing or situations in which the client should notify the physician immediately. In addition to oral instruction, written material (in the appropriate language) or pictures should be provided as a reference.

Model   People learn by imitating models. Modeling enables clients to observe and experience alternative patterns of behavior. It helps clients clarify values and communicate openly and congruently. As a student nurse, you are a model for your clients, and you must not impose your own value system on impressionable individuals.

Advocate   Nurses also act as advocates for clients. As an advocate, you will use a variety of communication techniques to reach clients in ways they can understand and to which they can respond. Nurse advocates serve as links between clients and other professionals or people in the community. As community members, nurses serve as advocates for all recipients of mental health care by striving to remove the stigma of mental illness.

Advocacy in nursing is based on a client's right to make decisions and a client's responsibility for the consequences of those decisions. You must respect the decisions even when you disagree with them. However, if the decisions involve danger to self or others, you must try to prevent the client from acting on the decision. As an advocate, you allow clients to express their feelings appropriately without censure or criticism. You teach responsible behavior of one person toward another, and you protect those clients temporarily unable to protect themselves.

Counselor   Another nursing role is that of counselor. The counseling role is most typically assumed during regularly scheduled one-to-one sessions. The counseling interaction is directed toward specific goals and is based on the nursing care plan. As a counselor, you will create opportunities for clients to talk about thoughts, feelings, and behaviors that affect themselves and others. Effective verbal and nonverbal communication is both modeled and practiced during the interactions. The effectiveness of counseling is seen when clients exhibit improved coping skills, increased self-esteem, and greater insight into and understanding of themselves.

Role Player   As role players, nurses help clients recreate and enact specific past or future situations as if they were occurring in the present. You will create an environment in which new behaviors can be practiced in a nonthreatening way. Role playing can strengthen a client's self-confidence in coping with problematic interactions, which in turn will increase the desire to implement what was learned in real-life situations. Through role playing, you will help clients express themselves directly, clarify feelings, act out fears, and become more assertive. Clients who think at a concrete level, however, may not be able to transfer the role-playing experience to real-life situations. Role playing is contraindicated with psychotic clients who are unable to comprehend "pretend" situations.

Milieu Manager   Because of the round-the-clock contact with clients in some residential or hospital clinical settings, nurses have a unique opportunity to become milieu managers. The **therapeutic milieu** refers to the client's physical environment as well as all the interactions with staff members and other clients. The unit or facility is not just a place but is an active part of the treatment plan for each client, where there is a balance between the needs of each individual and the needs of the group. The environment influences client and staff behavior, and client and staff behavior changes the environment. You must be aware of this interactive process at all times. Think about what you are doing and saying, and evaluate the impact on the therapeutic milieu.

The therapeutic milieu has many group activities and is as democratic as possible. In some settings, clients will elect officers from the client population. Community meetings provide opportunities for clients to solve problems related to living with a large group of people, to experience leadership, to help develop policies and rules, and to make decisions for themselves. As milieu manager, you will be providing clients with a safe environment in terms of self-mutilation, suicide, or violence to others. For some clients, you will have to set limits on behaviors that are not appropriate to the setting. Some clients require periods of privacy, while others need to be encouraged to socialize. You manage the milieu by your presence and your contact with clients. To help them learn new behaviors, you give support and direction, along with modeling appropriate behaviors. The goal of a therapeutic milieu is to increase clients' sense of belonging, improve their interpersonal skills such as socialization or conflict management, help them recognize the impact of their own behavior on others, and grow toward autonomy as much as possible. (Characteristics of the therapeutic milieu are covered further in Chapter 7.)

Standard VI: Evaluation

The final step in the nursing process is evaluation. In this step, nurses evaluate and document client progress toward the outcome criteria, as well as evaluate their own clinical practice.

Evaluation of Client Progress   As you compare client behavior to previously established goals and outcome criteria, you should be able to answer the following questions:

1. Was the assessment adequate?
2. Were the nursing diagnoses accurate?
3. Was the client involved in setting goals? Were the goals appropriate? Were the goals attained?
4. Were the planned interventions effective?
5. Were the outcome criteria demonstrated?
6. What changes took place in the client's behavior?
7. Which nursing interventions were effective?
8. Which nursing interventions need revision?
9. Was the client satisfied with the nursing care?
10. What plans need to be modified?
11. Are new care plans necessary?
12. Has adequate documentation of the client's progress been completed?

There are two types of evaluation: formative and summative. *Formative evaluation* is an ongoing process based on the client's responses to care. From the formative evaluation, you maintain, modify, or expand the nursing care plan. *Summative evaluation* is a terminal process and is used to determine whether the client has achieved the mutually set goals. Summative evaluations are done in the form of discharge summaries.

Documentation   Documentation is a critical component of nursing practice. The general rule is: If it is not documented, it has not occurred. All steps of the nursing process pertinent to the client must be documented in the client's record. *Documenting assessment* includes the recording of psychosocial histories, focused nursing assessments, neuropsychiatric assessments, and client/family education needs. *Documenting diagnosis and planning* is typically accomplished in one or more of the following formats: critical pathways, individual nursing care plans, standard nursing care plans, and multidisciplinary care plans. Further documentation includes specific plans for client/family education. *Documenting implementation* includes writing progress notes in the form of narrative and flow sheets. Inpatient agencies require that nursing progress notes be entered at specific times, such as once every shift or once every 24 hours. Any significant events must also be documented, as well as the client's participation in and influence on the therapeutic milieu. Some of the most critical documentation issues in inpatient nursing involve falls, seclusion, restraints, and suicidal or violent behavior. Each clinical setting has specific routines and forms for close observation of these episodes. *Documenting evaluation* is done when progress toward the outcome criteria and goals is charted in the record. The client's level of knowledge achieved through the teaching plan must be included in the documentation. Discharge summaries are written when contact with the client has ended.

Self-Evaluation   It is important not only to evaluate client progress but also to evaluate yourself. Self-evaluation will increase your self-understanding and improve your clinical practice. You may use a variety of methods in this process such as process recordings, one-to-one interactions with your instructor, and group supervision during preconferences and postconferences.

Dealing with client desires, needs, and emotions can lead to feelings of discomfort or burnout for mental health nurses. Therefore, both beginning and experienced nurses need support and supervision to maintain their effectiveness. Supervision is the process of having a peer, teacher, head nurse, clinical specialist, or mentor evaluate your clinical practice to increase your knowledge and competence. It is an opportunity to share your feelings about yourself and your clients and to receive emotional support and guidance. From peers, you can determine the image you project and how you are viewed by others. Supervisors can assist in your process of self-evaluation by sharing their perceptions and offering suggestions for change.

Key Concepts

Introduction

- Cultures, families, and individuals often define mental illness as behaviors, feelings, or ways of thinking that are unusual to them or not easily understood by them.
- Mental health and mental illness are end points on a continuum, with movement back and forth throughout life.
- Mental illness is a sense of disharmony with aspects of living that may be distressing to the individual, family, friends, and community.
- Mental health is a lifelong process and includes a sense of harmony and balance for the individual, family, friends, and community.
- Spirituality is a belief system that addresses questions of purpose and meaning in life, moral values, feelings of connectedness with others and an external power, and a belief in a common humanity.

Intrapersonal Theory

- Intrapersonal theory focuses on the behaviors, feelings, thoughts, and experiences of each individual.

- Freud divided all aspects of consciousness into three categories: conscious, preconscious, and unconscious. He theorized that there were three components to the personality: the id, ego, and superego.

- Freud defined anxiety as a feeling of tension, distress, and discomfort produced by a perceived or threatened loss of inner control. He identified processes called defense mechanisms, which alleviate anxiety by denying, misinterpreting, or distorting reality. For the most part, defense mechanisms operate at an unconscious level.

- Erikson saw personality as developing throughout the entire life span rather than stopping at adolescence. He felt personality was shaped by conflict between needs and culture. Erikson identified eight developmental stages: sensory, muscular, locomotor, latency, adolescence, young adulthood, adulthood, and maturity.

- Intrapersonal models provide a way of looking at how individuals develop, how they are still trying to achieve developmental tasks, and how they have learned to cope with anxiety.

Social-Interpersonal Theory

- The focus of social-interpersonal theory is on relationships and events in the social context.

- Sullivan believed that personality could not be observed apart from interpersonal relationships. He identified three principal components of the interpersonal sphere: dynamisms, personifications, and cognitive processes.

- Maslow identified basic physiological needs and growth-related metaneeds. His humanistic theory emphasizes health rather than illness.

- Peplau saw nursing as an interpersonal process, with the therapeutic nurse-client relationship at its core. The major components of her theory are growth, development, communication, and roles.

- Feminist theory is an androgynous model of mental health. Theorists examine how gender roles limit the psychological development of all people and inhibit the development of mutually satisfying and noncoercive intimacy.

- A crisis is a turning point in a person's life at which usual resources and coping skills are no longer effective and the person enters a state of disequilibrium. Variables, or balancing factors, determine a person's potential for entering a crisis state.

- Crises are self-limiting and usually last about 4–6 weeks. It is during this time that people are most receptive to professional intervention.

- Social-interpersonal models enable the nurse to assess the influences of culture, social interaction, gender stereotypes, and support systems on the behavior of clients.

Behavioral Theory

- The focus of behavioral theory is on a person's actions, not on thoughts and feelings.

- The major emphasis of Skinner's theory is the functional analysis of behavior. Reinforcements are consequences that lead to an increase in a behavior, and punishments are consequences that lead to a decrease in the behavior. The principle of reinforcement states that a response is strengthened when reinforcement is given.

- Behavioral models are helpful in planning client education and designing programs for a variety of mental health clients and families.

Cognitive Theory

- Cognitive theory explains how we interpret our daily lives, adapt and make changes, and develop the insights to make those changes.

- Piaget thought that children learn by the changing stimuli that challenge their experiences and perceptions. He identified four major stages of cognitive development: sensorimotor, preoperational, concrete operational, and formal operational.

- Beck's cognitive theory focuses on how people view themselves and their world. He identified cognitive schemas as personal controlling beliefs that influence the way people process data about themselves and others. Cognitive distortions result from the cognitive triad of an inadequate view of self, a negative misinterpretation of the present, and a negative view of the future.

- Cognitive models help you assess clients' learning capabilities. They also help you analyze cognitive distortions that are symptoms of a number of mental disorders.

Biogenic Theory

- Biogenic theory looks at how genetic factors, neuroanatomy, neurophysiology, and biological rhythms relate to the cause, course, and prognosis of mental disorders.

- Mental disorders are often related to dysfunctional neuronal receptors or a deficiency, excess, or imbalance of neurotransmitters.

The Therapeutic Relationship

- The art of nursing is the ability to be compassionate and sensitive to each client within the context of that person's life.

- A therapeutic relationship focuses on client needs and is goal-specific, theory-based, and open to supervision.

- The introductory phase of the therapeutic relationship includes establishing a contract, discussing confidentiality, assessing thoroughly, and developing the preliminary nursing care plan.

- During the working phase, the care plan is implemented through the process of therapeutic alliance.

- Client transference is the unconscious process of displacing feelings for significant people in the past onto the nurse in the present relationship.

- Countertransference is the nurse's emotional reaction to clients based on feelings for significant people in the past.

- The primary goal of the termination phase of the therapeutic relationship is to review the client's progress and plans for the immediate future.

- The physical component of the relationship includes all procedures and technical skills that you do for clients.

- The psychosocial component involves qualities such as positive regard, nonjudgmental attitude, acceptance, warmth, empathy, and authenticity.

- The spiritual component is the feeling of connectedness with your clients and the respect for the diversity of spiritual needs among clients.

- The power component includes beliefs about external and internal locus of control.

Nursing Process: Assessment

- Critical thinking helps us make reliable observations, draw sound conclusions, solve problems, create new ideas, evaluate lines of reasoning, and improve our self-knowledge.

- Observation is extremely important in assessing clients with mental illness. Clients are observed in terms of their behavior, affect, cognition, interpersonal relationships, and physiology.

- The psychosocial assessment includes the client's and family's definition of the problem, history of the present problem, family and social history, spiritual con-

siderations, physical assessment, and strengths and competencies.

- The neuropsychiatric assessment provides more specific information about the client's appearance, activity, speech, emotional state, cognitive functioning, and perception.

Nursing Process: Diagnosis

- The *DSM-IV* is used by all members of the health care team. It categorizes client information into five axes: mental disorders, personality or developmental disorders, complicating physical problems, psychosocial stressors, and the client's past and current level of functioning.

- Psychiatric nursing diagnoses are applicable to individuals, families, groups, and communities. They include the etiologies and standard nursing interventions.

Nursing Process: Outcome Identification

- Client outcomes are specific behavioral measures by which you, clients, and significant others determine progress toward a goal.

Nursing Process: Planning

- In mental health nursing, safety needs often are more of a priority than physiological needs. Clients must be assessed for exhaustion, poor judgment, self-mutilation, violence, and suicide potential.

- Ideally, goals are planned with client input, but some clients may be too ill to participate in this process.

Nursing Process: Implementation

- Nurses assume several roles in helping clients grow and adapt: socializing agent, teacher, model, advocate, counselor, role player, and milieu manager.

Nursing Process: Evaluation

- Formative evaluation is an ongoing process for maintaining, modifying, or expanding the nursing care plan.

- Summative evaluation is a terminal process; summative evaluations are written in the form of discharge summaries.

- All steps of the nursing process pertinent to the client must be documented in the client's record. Some of the most critical documentation involves falls, seclusion, restraints, and suicidal or violent behavior.

- Supervision by peers, teachers, or other nurses helps you evaluate your own professional practice.

Review Questions

1. You have assessed your client, Sue, as being on the mental health end of the continuum. Which of the following statements best supports your assessment?

    a. Sue says she continues to grow daily and is satisfied with life.

    b. Sue has no evidence of any organic disease.

    c. Sue is dissatisfied with her marriage.

    d. Sue says her life is boring but has little stress.

2. Which of the following illustrates the defense mechanism of rationalization?

    a. A man cheats on his income tax return and tells himself it's all right because everyone does it.

    b. A manager tells an employee he may have to fire him. On the way home, the employee shops for a new car.

    c. A man is jealous of a good friend's success but is unaware of his feelings.

    d. A woman who dislikes her aunt is always nice to her.

3. Feminist therapy is best described as

    a. male-bashing.

    b. done with women clients.

    c. gender-sensitive therapy.

    d. helping battered women.

4. Spiritual nursing care includes

    a. doing things for clients.

    b. allowing clients to search for meaning in life.

    c. having a nonjudgmental approach to clients.

    d. ensuring congruity of communication.

5. Charley tells you about his trip to the grocery store. He spends 10 minutes talking about the produce department in great detail. Ten minutes later he finally gets to the main point of the story, which was meeting an old friend. You describe Charley's form of thought as

    a. confabulation.

    b. blocking.

    c. circumstantiality.

    d. loose association.

References

Abraham, I. L., Fox, J. C., & Cohen, B. T. (1992). Integrating the bio into the biopsychosocial. *Arch Psychiatr Nurs, 6*(5), 296–305.

Aguiliera, D. C., & Messick, J. M. (1990). *Crisis Intervention: Theory and Methodology* (6th ed.). St. Louis, MO: Mosby.

American Psychiatric Association. (1994). *Diagnostic and Statistical Manual of Mental Disorders* (4th ed.). Washington, DC: APA.

Appleton, C. (1994). The gift of self: A paradigm for originating nursing as art. In P. L. Chinn & J. Watson (Eds.), *Art and Aesthetics in Nursing* (pp. 91–114). New York: NLN Press.

Beck, A., & Freeman, A. (1990). *Cognitive Therapy of Personality Disorders*. New York: Guilford Press.

Chinn, P. L., Watson, J. (Eds.). (1994). *Art and Aesthetics in Nursing*. New York: NLN Press.

Cowan, P. J. (1996). Women's mental health issues. *J Psychosoc Nurs, 34*(4), 20–24.

Desjarlais, R., Eisenberg, L., Good, B., & Kleinman, A. (1995). *World Mental Health*. Oxford, England: Oxford Univ Press.

Erickson, E. H. (1963). *Childhood and Society* (2nd ed.). New York: Norton.

Freud, S. (1935). *A General Introduction to Psychoanalysis*. New York: Simon & Schuster.

Keen, P. (1991). Caring for ourselves. In R. M. Neil & R. Watts (Eds.). *Caring and Nursing: Explorations in Feminist Perspective* (pp.173–188), Pub. No. 14-2369. New York: NLN Press.

Kozier, B., Erb, G., Blais, K., Wilkinson, J., & Van Leuven, K. (1998). *Fundamentals of Nursing* (5th ed. update). Menlo Park, CA: Addison-Wesley.

Malone, J. A. (1991). The DSM-III-R versus nursing diagnosis. *Issues Ment Health.* 13(12): 219–228.

Maslow, A. (1968). *Toward a Psychology of Being* (2nd ed.). New York: Van Nostrand Reinhold.

McCloskey, J., Bulechek, G. M. (Eds.). (1996). *Nursing Interventions Classification (NIC)* (2nd ed.). St. Louis: Mosby.

Montgomery, C. L. (1996). The care-giving relationship. *Altern Ther.* 2(2), 52–57.

North American Nursing Diagnosis Association. (1994). *Nursing Diagnoses, Definitions and Classification 1995–1996.* NANDA.

Peplau, H. E. (1952). *Interpersonal Relations in Nursing.* New York: Putnam.

Piaget, J. (1972). *The Psychology of the Child.* New York: Basic Books.

Rosenblatt, E. A. (1995). Emerging concepts of women's development. *Psychiatr Clin North Am, 18*(2), 95–106.

Seaward, B. L. (1997). *Stand Like Mountain, Flow Like Water.* Deerfield Beach, FL: Health Communications.

Skinner, B. F. (1953). *Science and Human Behavior.* Riverside, NJ: Macmillan.

Sullivan, H. S. (1953). *The Interpersonal Theory of Psychiatry.* New York: Norton.

CHAPTER 2

The Family and Community in Mental Health Nursing

Pamela Marcus
Karen Lee Fontaine

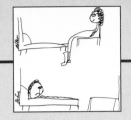

Objectives

After reading this chapter, you will be able to:

- Distinguish between functional and dysfunctional families.
- Assess the impact of culture on style of family functioning.
- Assist families through the process of family transformation.
- Design family nursing interventions.
- Identify the characteristics of community mental health nursing practice and discuss the advantages for the consumer and the community.

Key Terms

boundaries
egocentric self
family cohesion
family communication
family flexibility
family functioning
sociocentric self

The primary context of people is family and community. That understanding necessitates inclusion of consumers, family members, friends, and community resources in the planning and provision of mental health services. Community refers to the geographic area in which people live as well as relationships with others and the sense of affiliation among family, friends, and even strangers who participate in shared goals and activities. Families are considered to be all members of a social group who are living under the same roof. This definition includes couples, traditional families, lesbian and gay families, communal families, families with cohabiting parents, extended families, and even friends living together. Each of us is simultaneously independent of and part of our families. We are *both* individuals and family members. We are part of our family and the family is part of us.

Family and relationship distress is the most common problem of people seeking mental health care. Mental disorders and psychiatric disability are stressful, not only to individuals but for their families. Only 15% of consumers participate in mental health programs. Therefore, families are often forced to compensate for the deficiencies of the mental health system as they become the major source of support and rehabilitation. Of clients discharged from acute care, 65% return to their families. At any given time, 40–50% of the 48 million Americans who are psychiatrically disabled live with their families on a regular basis. Even when consumers do not live at home, their families are often the only source of support. This situation can result in overwhelming emotional and economic stress (Denton, 1996; Robinson, 1995; Saunders, 1997).

Family Assessment

As nurses we must focus our attention on the family both as the context for the individual as well as the unit of care. It is important to assess and involve families since they are in a position to be impacted by and to influence the course of individuals' problems. Assessment includes gathering information on how partners, parents, and children in the family experience or react to the client's symptoms. Together, clients, families, and nurses identify the family's strengths,

resources, and social support, and try to identify problems that might cause stress for any of the family members. Factors in assessing clients and their families include family communication, cohesion, boundaries, flexibility, and overall family functionality.

Family communication is measured by focusing on the family as a group with regard to their listening skills, speaking skills, self-disclosure, and tracking. The focus of listening skills is on empathy and attentive listening. Speaking skills include speaking for oneself and not speaking for others. Self-disclosure is the ability to share feelings about oneself and the relationship. Tracking is the capability to stay on topic. Family communication difficulties result in lower levels of expressiveness, more vague requests, inability to comprehend others' messages, frequent interruption of others, speaking for others, and high levels of verbalized hostility.

Another aspect of family communication is the family's strategies to resolve conflict. The ability to resolve differences is based on the family's capacity to talk about areas of disagreement and their mutual willingness to reach acceptable solutions. Problem-solving skills are critical to smooth family functioning. Without these skills, families seem to use strategies such as confrontation or avoidance, which are ineffective in reducing stress and do not resolve conflict satisfactorily.

Family cohesion is defined as the emotional bonding that family members have toward one another. There are four levels of cohesion, ranging from disengaged (very low) to separated (low to moderate), to connected (moderate to high), to enmeshed (very high). It is believed that the central ranges of cohesion (separated and connected) contribute to optimal family functioning. The extremes (disengaged or enmeshed) are generally seen as problematic (Olson, 1996). See Box 2.1 for characteristics of family cohesion.

Boundaries are the invisible lines that define the amount and kind of contact allowable between members of the family and between the family and outside systems. Boundaries determine the patterns of how, when, and to whom family members relate. Clear boundaries are firm yet flexible, and members are supported and nurtured but also allowed a certain degree of autonomy. Rigid boundaries isolate family members from one another; parents are parents and children are children, and there is little room for

Box 2.1

Characteristics of Family Cohesion

Disengaged
- Little closeness
- Little loyalty
- High independence

Separated
- Low-moderate closeness
- Some loyalty
- Interdependent with more independence than dependence

Connected
- Moderate-high closeness
- High loyalty
- Interdependent with more dependence than independence

Enmeshed
- Very high closeness
- Very high loyalty
- High dependency

Sources: Olson, 1996; Olson, Russell, and Sprenkle, 1989

Box 2.2

Characteristics of Family Flexibility

Chaotic
- Lack of leadership
- Dramatic role shifts
- Erratic discipline
- Too much change

Flexible
- Shared leadership
- Democratic discipline
- Role sharing change
- Change when necessary

Structured
- Leadership sometimes shared
- Somewhat democratic discipline
- Roles stable
- Change when demanded

Rigid
- Authoritarian leadership
- Strict discipline
- Roles seldom change
- Too little change

Sources: Olson, 1996; Olson, Russell, and Sprenkle, 1989

negotiation. Diffuse boundaries are the opposite, where everybody is into everybody else's business. There is little distinction between members and too much negotiation, resulting in a loss of autonomy.

Family flexibility is the amount of change in a family's leadership, role relationships, and relationship rules. There are four levels of flexibility, ranging from rigid (very low) to structured (low to moderate), to flexible (moderate to high), to chaotic (very high). As with cohesion, it is believed that the central ranges (structured and flexible) are more conducive to good family functioning, with the extremes (rigid and chaotic) being the most problematic (Olson, 1996). See Box 2.2 for characteristics of family flexibility.

Rules determine appropriate roles and relationship patterns within the family. Rules express the val-

ues of the family and form a boundary around each family which then screens outside information for compatibility with the family's value system. If the message is not congruent with the family's values, you will hear such statements as: "That is not the way we do things in this family" or "I don't care what Marc is allowed to do; in this family we . . . ." To understand rules more clearly, reflect for a moment on the family in which you grew up. There were certain things that you just did, that you knew were expected. There were other things that were not permitted. For purposes of assessing a few of the rules in your family of origin, complete the statements in Box 2.3.

Box 2.3

Assessing Rules in Your Family of Origin

In my family, we were never allowed to . . .

In my family, we were always expected to . . .

In my family, girls were required to . . .

In my family, girls were allowed to . . .

In my family, girls were forbidden to . . .

In my family, boys were required to . . .

In my family, boys were allowed to . . .

In my family, boys were forbidden to . . .

In my family, household responsibilities were determined by . . .

In my family, we handled conflict by . . .

In my family, the most important thing in life for women is . . .

In my family, the most important thing in life for men is . . .

The level of **family functioning** can be determined by assessing such areas as the family's ability to negotiate and change when appropriate, respect for individual's choices, and the absence of intimidation. High-functioning families have open and clear communication and members are able to be both independent from and connected to their families. It is important for you to recognize that the labels we use, such as "functional" and "dysfunctional," are beliefs about families that are consistent with our personal values and the values of the culture in which we live. Therefore, the terms are arbitrary and descriptions of a "functional family" vary a great deal from culture to culture.

Box 2.4 lists criteria for levels of family functioning ranging from Level 1, high-functioning families, to Level 5, severely dysfunctional families. Families at the higher levels of functioning are better able to manage the stress that comes when a family member is experiencing a mental disorder. Those at dysfunctional levels may be incapable of caring and providing support for their loved one.

Family Transformation and Family Coping

Badger (1996) describes the process of family transformation when living with a member who is experiencing a severe mental disorder. Three stages have been identified: acknowledging the strangers within, fighting the battle, and gaining a new perspective.

During the first stage, acknowledging the strangers within, individuals and their family members recognize that family functioning has changed. When people become psychiatrically disabled they often cannot carry out their family roles and responsibilities. Thus, other family members must assume those role functions and come to terms with an altered family lifestyle. As the family attempts to explain the altered lifestyle to others, they may attribute the changes to something more socially acceptable than mental illness. For example, they might tell others that the person is suffering from exhaustion or an endocrine problem or that stress at school or work is causing the difficulties. This avoidance of stigma and prejudice on the part of others can lead to family isolation and loss of extrafamily relationships. As it becomes more evident that there is a significant problem, the family begins to search for reasons and solutions by gathering available information. Families begin to develop their own image of the disease process and expectations of mental health professionals. Many families also hope for what was in the past and for what might be in the future. It is very sad to lose a close family member to the world of mental illness. Many people do not believe that mental illness is a brain disease. If the disorder begins in childhood, it is easier to think that it is a result of bad parenting because that means good parenting should fix it. That is like telling parents of a child with leukemia that if they were better parents they could stop the white cells from growing. When a person experiences a mental disorder, the loss of ideal family dreams occurs. The expectation of meaningful and productive individual and family life is shattered. All must be supported as they grieve the loss of their hopes and dreams (Badger, 1996). See Chapter 16 for further discussion of grief.

The second stage, fighting the battle, includes the day-to-day efforts to cope with all the changes that occurred during the first stage. Family members develop cognitive, emotional, and behavioral coping strategies to be able to live with their loved one who

Box 2.4

Levels of Family Functioning

Level 1: High-Functioning Family
- Good listening and speaking skills
- Appropriate self-disclosure
- Conflict is recognized and resolved through negotiation
- Clear hierarchical boundaries between generations
- Parents engage in joint decision making
- Roles are stable but some are shared
- Rules are enforced, age-appropriate, but can be changed
- Family members have time apart and time together

Level 2: Mild Impairment
- Parents are inconsistent in setting limits
- Members are manipulated to get needs met
- Household tasks are not consistently completed
- Opinions on important family matters are not shared
- Conflict emerges and is avoided

Level 3: Moderate Impairment
- Generational boundaries are fuzzy or inflexible
- Communication is confused
- Rules and roles are difficult to identify
- Increased blaming, manipulation, and resentment

- Lack of shared focus of attention
- Members begin to question each other's trust and caring
- Conflict is met with defensiveness, anger, and denial, which interferes with problem resolution

Level 4: Advanced Dysfunction
- Roles are increasingly blurred; children begin to play parental roles to their siblings
- Rules are very inconsistent; ignored at times and severely punished at other times
- Increased suspiciousness between members who question loyalty, love, and caring
- Frequent crises that are not attended to or resolved
- Household tasks become the focus of arguments and are frequently not completed

Level 5: Severely Dysfunctional
- Roles are completely blurred and often shift from person to person; or one individual is in charge and is highly controlling
- Decisions are impulsive or imposed by the leader
- Household is chaotic and basic needs of family neglected
- Members frequently attempt to obtain a power edge and to intimidate others
- High levels of verbalized hostility

is psychiatrically disabled. Coping strategies protect the affected family member and maintain the stability of family functioning. Some of these strategies include expressing affection, suggesting alternative choices, reducing conflict, and trying to make the best of their experiences by focusing on the positive parts of the relationship with the disabled family member.

Rose (1997) describes four family support sources: professional support, friend support, family support, and spiritual support. Professional support includes a nonblaming, respectful attitude toward families, information on how to respond to symptoms, and help in locating community resources such as housing or vocational training. Friend support

comes from non-family members such as close friends and coworkers. It is most valued when the concern is genuine and stigma is minimized. Family support often comes in the way of tangible assistance such as respite care for family members and physical presence in times of crisis. Many families find emotional strength from their religious faith. They find spiritual strength as they search for meaning through relationships and the feeling of connectedness with others.

Fighting the battle also involves working the mental health system to obtain treatment. Family members want to be seen as partners in treatment and do not want to be excluded from discussions and treatment recommendations. Ideally, professionals, clients, and families all work together in joint problem solving. At times the issue of client confidentiality is raised. Family members generally respect confidentiality but do need information about treatments, medications, and ways to cope with certain behaviors (Badger, 1996; Sveinbjarnardottir and de Casterle, 1997).

Assessment of Vulnerability to Relapse

Understandably, families are very concerned with their loved one's vulnerability to relapse. Although families are not to be blamed for mental disorders, their interactions may influence the course of the disorder. Relapse is less common in families who see the client as ill (rather than lazy or manipulative) and provide support to one another. Relapse is more common in families who are highly critical, highly anxious, and preoccupied with their problems. Researchers have studied two family patterns, family Expressed Emotion (EE) and family Affective Style (AS). Families rated as high EE tend to be hostile, critical, and emotionally overinvolved with the client. Families rated as high AS are intrusive and make guilt-inducing remarks during emotionally charged family discussions. Both high EE and SA families are predictors of relapse for people who are psychiatrically disabled. Families are more likely to be excessively critical or overinvolved when they lack information about the disorder and when they believe the symptoms are under the client's control. Family members who do not understand the nature of psychiatric disability may mistake the negative symptoms (see Chapter 12) as laziness (Denton, 1996).

Medication noncompliance and substance abuse are other changeable factors related to relapse. Medication noncompliance is linked to lack of insight into the disorder, medication side effects, cost of medication, missed outpatient appointments, and negative client/family attitudes toward medication. Mental health status is further compromised by the use of alcohol or drugs. Clients who abuse substances also tend to be noncompliant with medication (George and Howell, 1996).

Cultural Assessment

Our culture shapes our concept of self. One way to look at the cultural self is along a continuum between egocentric and sociocentric orientations. The **egocen-**

tric self, usually found in Western industrialized societies, exhibits characteristics such as individualism, separateness, autonomy, competition, and mastery of and control over one's environment. The **sociocentric self,** found in many non-Western societies, is interdependent and interconnected and values cooperation, cohesiveness, group identity, and harmony with one's environment. The person is defined by kinship and is seen in relationship terms.

African Americans, Asian Americans, Latinos, and Native Americans tend toward sociocentric orientations. There is a high value on interpersonal relationships, group membership, and cohesiveness. Relationships to others, family, and community, are central to one's sense of well-being. An extensive kin network provides both economic and emotional support to its members. Mental illness is often viewed as a family affair as it affects all family members. Cultural assessment of the family determines appropriate family-centered approaches to problem solving and treatment for mental disorders (Comas-Diaz, 1996).

Generalizations about ethnic group families increase our level of awareness and alert us to the possibility of differences. However, it is very important that you never assume that ethnic group generalizations accurately describe the family with whom you are working, as great variations exist. You must also recognize and understand that differences are not pathology or dysfunction but simply another way of life. As a nurse, you take your families where they are, help them achieve their goals, and facilitate health in the way that is most useful for them. See Chapter 3 for additional information on the role of cultural diversity.

Family Issues Across the Life Span

Pregnancy and Child Care

Pregnancy, childbirth, and parenting are major issues for all women. For the psychiatrically disabled woman, who already has problems in adjustment and coping, pregnancy and parenting can be sufficient strain to exacerbate symptoms of the mental illness. Women with a history of mental illness must be monitored closely throughout their pregnancy. Although 10–15% of pregnant women meet criteria for depression, they often remain undiagnosed because the symptoms of depression are similar to the somatic changes of pregnancy. For many women, the postpartum period is associated with mental health problems, including postpartum blues in as many as 80% of new mothers, postpartum depression in 10–15% of new mothers, and postpartum psychosis in about one in a thousand women (Blumenthal, 1996; Thurtle, 1995).

In the general U.S. population, 50% of pregnancies are unplanned; the rate is higher among women who are psychiatrically disabled. For women with bipolar disorder whose manic episodes increase their sexual activity and impair their judgment, the risk of unplanned pregnancy is high. It is not uncommon for women and their families to be unaware of a pregnancy until the pregnancy is far advanced, which places both the woman and fetus at risk. Other problems may include a diminished ability to comply with prenatal care, an inability to plan realistically for the baby, an increased risk of substance abuse during the pregnancy, and poor nutrition. The woman may also feel overwhelmed and ambivalent about motherhood and may fear losing custody of the baby (Finnerty, Levin, and Miller, 1996).

If the woman is pregnant and taking psychotropic medications, the primary health care provider must weigh the risk of fetal anomalies against the exacerbation of the illness, which may present a danger to herself and others, including the fetus. All effective mood-stabilizing agents pose risks during pregnancy. Carbamazepine and valproic acid are associated with increased risk of neural tube defects and an increased risk of neonatal hemorrhage due to low levels of vitamin K. The main risks of lithium are polyhydramnios, premature labor, neonatal toxicity, and neonatal hypothyroidism. Antipsychotic and antianxiety medications are often utilized, as they cause fewer fetal anomalies and problems with the pregnancy. Electroconvulsive therapy (ECT) is an effective and relatively safe treatment for some clients since uterine muscle does not contract as part of the generalized tonic-clonic seizure (Finnerty, Levin, and Miller, 1996).

Psychiatric disability among mothers of newborns and young children has far-reaching implications for the mother and the family. If the mother is acutely ill at childbirth, she is usually separated from her newborn, which may be deeply distressing for her and impede the bonding process. This separation may be temporary, but in some cases the loss of custody becomes permanent. Psychiatric hospitalization for acute illness leads to disruption of the family system as children suffer repeated separations and a chaotic and unpredictable environment.

Nursing interventions for young families include helping the family develop a social support system and use community resources. Programs such as Head Start, day care centers, and recreational programs can stimulate the children and provide a time of respite for the mother. Teaching includes providing information about normal growth and development, stress-management techniques, time-management skills, and problem-solving skills. Collaborating with the extended family may minimize the impact of psychiatric disability on the primary family (Mohit, 1996).

Youth

When a child or adolescent experiences a mental disorder, the entire family system is strained. Since caregiving usually falls to one person, the parental system is stressed, which may lead to increased conflict and a greater likelihood for parental separation. The siblings are often excluded, leading to confusion or misunderstanding of the problem. Siblings' feelings may range from shame to protectiveness. At times they may feel superior for not having "problems" while at other times they may feel neglected if the child with the disorder receives more parental attention.

Family turmoil can trigger the onset of a disorder in a biologically and genetically predisposed child. As discussed earlier, families' emotional and affective styles may be a factor in relapse. The parent-child relationship is often severely strained due to stressors related to the child's mental disorder. Some parents respond in ways that foster dependence, which contributes to separation/individuation problems or boundary issues. Some parents may be rejecting and critical of the child with the disorder. Other parents alternate between overprotection/overcontrol and rejection. Other families learn to adapt in ways that foster the growth and development of all the children. It must be remembered that family patterns are not the primary cause of childhood mental disorders; these have multiple etiologies, including the interaction of biological, genetic, psychological, and social factors (Kaslow, Deering, and Ash, 1996). See Chapter 20 for additional information on child and adolescent disorders.

Couples

Studies indicate that as many as half of individuals suffering from depression report serious couple difficulties and hope to resolve these relationship problems in therapy. In addition, couples who are experiencing relationship distress are at higher risk for developing depression. As discussed earlier in this chapter, one of the hallmarks of relationship distress is poor communication. Partners who are depressed behave in ways that discourage social interaction and increase relationship conflict. They are less skillful socially and more withdrawn; they seem to express more hostility and criticism of themselves and others; they may engage in long and hateful arguments; and they often express dissatisfaction with sexual activity. Living with a depressed person can also increase the nondepressed partner's susceptibility to depression. The goal of relationship therapy is to decrease conflict, increase the degree of intimacy and relationship satisfaction, and enhance effective coping and social competence (Gollan, Gortner, and Jacobson, 1996).

Adult Children

The current focus of mental health care is returning clients to their communities to live in the least restrictive environment that is realistic. As a result, at least half of the psychiatrically disabled adult population are living with their families on a regular basis. Professionals are beginning to look at and respond to the burden of family caregivers. Some of the problems that families of these adult children face are the need for daily caretaking, lack of freedom, emotional drain, stress of the unexpected, and financial strain. Client symptoms of illness such as inappropriate behavior, labile emotions, hallucinations, delusions, and outbursts of rage are often difficult for families to manage. Other symptoms that strain the family are dependency, poor social skills and outlets, and difficulties in finding employment. Financial considerations may force the parents to delay their expected retirement. They are often concerned about the welfare of their child after their death. Family caregivers need support and practical knowledge to enhance their ability to cope and their ability to support their loved one (Doornbos, 1997).

Family Nursing Practice

Until recently, family members were sometimes utilized as a source of information about their ill members but were rarely involved in treatment, psychoeducation, or family therapy and the idea of the family as a unit of care was controversial. With less restrictive environments, shorter hospital stays, and fewer community programs, nurses must now develop a collaborative partnership with clients and their families. This collaborative relationship means that the family is viewed as the unit of care and as partners in treatment and rehabilitation. Thus, programs must be in place to provide support, education, coping skills training, social network development, and family therapy. As family nurses, it is critically important that we take the time to be with families in deeply caring ways. As we share our ideas and our strengths, our shared goal is to help families develop as more balanced and caring systems.

The Nurse as Teacher

Psychoeducation has proven to be an important aspect of family nursing. (See Chapter 5 for more detailed information on psychoeducation.) We must be able to answer questions, help families identify feelings and reactions, and encourage them in their coping efforts. Illness education occurs in the context of the basic family unit and with multi-family groups. Information is provided on the disorder, symptoms, etiology, treatment, and relapse prevention and recognition. Families are helped to identify problems and work out solutions that fit the family's current patterns of living. Family education programs also include conflict-management skills and problem solving to help them resolve day-to-day living discord. Families can also benefit from stress-management programs, which include relaxation exercises, visualization, affirmations, meditation, and physical exercise. (See Chapter 7 for information on Alternative Therapies.) Families may find the following book by V. Secunda very helpful in their daily lives: *When Madness Comes Home: Help and Hope for the Children, Siblings, and Partners of the Mentally Ill* (Hyperion Books, 1997).

The Nurse as Referral Agent

Mental health nurses are expected to systematically assess families; identify their structure, development, communication, and decision-making patterns; and recognize and refer dysfunctional families for family therapy. In general, family therapists believe that the emotional symptoms or problems of an individual affect the family's ability to function while at other times the symptoms may be an expression of family problems. Family therapists should be specially educated in the practice of family therapy. Increasing numbers of psychiatric nurse practitioners and clinical specialists are being prepared in graduate programs that provide both theory and supervised clinical practice in this specialized area. Although undergraduate nursing programs focus on the importance of family nursing, they do not prepare nurses as family therapists.

Family nurses act as referral agents in making an effort to facilitate the transaction between family and community. As family advocates we must be familiar with our local community resources such as crisis centers, community mental health centers, telephone hotlines, support groups, religious institutions, acute care facilities, and specific names of mental health professionals. The goal is to provide opportunities for people who are psychiatrically disabled to maximize their ability to live, work, socialize, and learn in communities of their choice. Working together, consumers, families, and health care providers can develop strategies to help clients achieve lives of value, meaning, and better health, and become contributing members of their communities.

The National Alliance for the Mentally Ill (NAMI) is a grassroots, self-help, support and advocacy organization of people with mental illness and their families and friends. NAMI's mission is to eradicate mental illness and to improve the quality of life for those who suffer from these brain diseases. Local self-help support groups enable members to share concerns, learn about mental disorders, and receive practical advice on treatment and community resources. NAMI provides up-to-date scientific information through publications, the Helpline, and an annual Mental Illness Awareness Week campaign. At federal, state, and local levels, NAMI demands improved services for people who are psychiatrically disabled, such as greater access to treatment, housing, and employment, and better health insurance. NAMI actively supports increased federal and private funding for research into causes and treatments of severe mental illnesses. See the Self-Help Groups section at the end of this chapter for family resources.

The Nurse as Spiritual Caregiver

Any serious illness, but perhaps especially a mental illness, is really a dis-ease process. Both the illness and the associated stigma eat away at people's spirits, and they often feel beaten and broken. They begin to believe that their worth and value as a human being is diminished. As nurses, we must respond to the whole person, who is at once spirit, mind, and body. People who are psychiatrically disabled are entitled to dignified and meaningful lives.

Spiritual care includes developing caring and thoughtful relationships. We must foster family attitudes that arise out of people's spiritual dimension, such as love, forgiveness, hopefulness, and acceptance. Spiritual caregiving includes helping "patients" stop being patients and instead become active consumers and collaborators. Supporting individuals and families who seek ways to heal and achieve balance in their lives is an important aspect of spiritual nursing care.

Community Mental Health Focus

With the passage of the Americans with Disabilities Act in 1990, our society has made it a priority to promote full participation of people with psychiatric disabilities into the economic and social mainstream. To accomplish this goal, mental health services changed the focus from inpatient care to family and community care. In the past, professionals greatly underestimated the abilities of clients to make choices for themselves and determine the course of their lives. Through stressing the importance of consumer choice, the self-help and mental health consumer movements have demonstrated that psychiatrically disabled individuals can live successfully in local communities when given appropriate supports.

There are several principles that help guide how community mental health care is provided to consumers. The principle of *normalization* affirms that people with disabilities should be able to lead as normal a life as possible. This involves making modifications to both the physical environment, such as housing options, and the social environment, such as family respite care, community education, and employment opportunities. One goal of normalization is integration into the mainstream community. Integration is not simply physically housing disabled individuals within the community; it includes teaching necessary social skills to consumers as well as educating members of the community-at-large. With real integration comes destigmatization of those who are psychiatrically disabled. Another goal of normaliza-

tion is one of independence. This means creating opportunities for clients to develop their own senses of autonomy and self-help. Professionals and family members don't "do for" clients but rather help them with doing (Heaney and Burke, 1995).

Another principle of community mental health care is that of *contextualization*, or maintaining clients in their context. This means that clients are kept in as close contact as possible with their usual surroundings, both geographic and interpersonal. There may be temporary displacements, such as utilizing a transitional residential facility, but the long-range goal is living in their desired community. Another principle is *choice*. Consumer choice is critical to community mental health care. Having choice helps people cope with stressful situations and increases feelings of competence. The principle of *self-advocacy* arises out of the belief that those who are most affected by decisions should have the greatest impact on those decisions. This means advocating to be listened to when setting treatment goals and determining their own care.

In the recent past there has been a shift in relationships between mental health nurses and those who use their services. This shift is reflected in commonly used terms: Once it was "patients," then it was "clients," and now it is "consumers." This change in language demonstrates an increasing awareness of persons with mental illnesses as autonomous individuals who have preferences and make choices (Sullivan and Spritzer, 1997).

Community-based nurses have distinct advantages in providing care, including a first-hand opportunity to observe clients and their families in a natural setting. These nurses are able to more accurately assess and intervene with clients when they understand the problems that are troublesome to people in their daily living encounters in the community. Understanding the social context of specific stressors, nurses can also identify possible pitfalls to effective interventions. In addition, community-based nurses focus on those problems identified by clients as most important in their daily lives.

Community Living

Most consumers with psychiatric disabilities prefer their own residence and want autonomy over their housing choices. The greatest number prefer an apartment or a house that allows them to live independently. Consumers who live in transitional housing often see these arrangements as stepping stones to greater independence.

Studies have demonstrated that perceived choice over one's living arrangements is important to physical and psychological well-being. Increasing choice over housing can reduce the stress of repeated moves. When basic housing needs are satisfactorily met, consumers can begin to focus on other goals, such as employment, making friends, and participating in community activities (Schofield et al, 1997; Seilheimer and Doyal, 1996).

Supportive housing is used for consumers who do not live on their own or with their families and who benefit from some degree of assistance in self-care and self-management. These programs can increase social and vocational functioning, improve quality of life, and decrease homelessness and rehospitalization. Alternative housing often enables people with disabilities to increase their independence and develop the capacity to live as independently as possible. See Box 2.5 for descriptions of the types of residential facilities.

The goal of consumer choice in supported housing has not yet been achieved. Many consumers believe that they have little or no choice and that their choices are highly or completely influenced by others. People who are psychiatrically disabled may be living on SSI (Supplemental Security Income) or SSDI (Social Security Disability Insurance), which are inadequate to rent even "affordable housing" in the United States. The vast majority receive less than $600 per month for total living expenses, which includes supplements provided by most programs to help pay rent (Srebnik et al, 1995). As nurses we must become advocates at community, state, and federal levels to secure decent and affordable housing of choice in communities that consumers can call home.

Individuals who are psychiatrically disabled may need social skills training to enable them to live successfully in the community. Social skills training includes such things as personal hygiene and grooming skills, self-care, communication, time management, handling money, leisure activities, meal preparation, use of resources, and problem-solving skills. Consumers learn to interact appropriately with strangers, family members, and friends, both at work or at school. Social skills training fosters their ability to live and work in their communities just like anyone else.

Box 2.5

Types of Residential Facilities

Transitional Halfway Houses

- Provide room and board until suitable housing is available

Long-Term Group Residences

- On-site staff
- Appropriate for psychiatrically disabled person
- Length of stay is indefinite

Cooperative Apartments

- No on-site staff
- Staff members make regular visits to assist residents

**Intensive-Care
or Crisis Community Residences**

- Used to help prevent hospitalization or shorten length of hospitalization
- On-site nursing staff and counseling staff

Foster or Familiy Care

- In private homes
- Close supervsion of foster family to assure a therapeutic environment

Nursing Homes

- Appropriate for some geriatiric or medically disabled consumers
- Activity programs and psychiatric supervision

Community Settings

Prior to the 1950s, society believed that people with mental disorders could be treated only in hospitals. In the 1960s and 1970s, studies began to demonstrate that it was possible to treat even acutely ill people at home. Recent research provides evidence that community care is often as effective as hospital care and is significantly less costly. There are some situations in which inpatient care is the preferred setting: for consumers who are a danger to themselves or others, such as those who are acutely suicidal or homicidal;

for those who are acutely psychotic and thus a serious danger to themselves because of confusion and disorganization; and for treatment of acute intoxicated states and withdrawal from alcohol or drugs.

Home

Providing mental health services to consumers and their families in their homes is a fairly new initiative in the mental health field. Home treatment may be an alternative to inpatient treatment during the acute phase of a mental illness. Acute home care treatment involves the provision of intensive support through home visits by nurses, social workers, psychiatrists, and homemakers. Staff are available 24 hours per day and provide services such as medication management, interpersonal support for consumers and caregivers, behavioral management, maintenance of housing, assistance with ADLs, reality orientation, and social/recreational activities. Once clients stabilize, they return to their case manager team for continuing support (Wasylenki et al, 1997).

There are some distinct advantages of home care treatment. Consumers and families report more communication with staff, increased participation in treatment decisions, and being cared for with dignity and respect. Other advantages are that daily routines are less disrupted, relationships are less restricted, and levels of anxiety are minimized (Wasylenki et al, 1997).

Home health care nurses must always consider their own safety. If possible they should call ahead and let the client know their arrival time. Family members or friends may be called upon to escort the nurse from the car to the home if there are concerns about neighborhood safety. Portable phones should be turned on and programmed to speed-dial 911 in case of emergency. Once in the home, nurses must be alert to situations that might be risky, such as agitation, suspicious thinking, hostility, and threats. If calmness and nonthreatening support are ineffective in de-escalating the threatening behaviors, calling for emergency assistance may be necessary (Worley, 1997).

School

Nationwide, only one-third of the children who need mental health service receive it. The main barriers to care are availability, accessibility, and affordability. In some cases services may not be available, while in others, families may be unaware of the available services. There may also be cultural barriers such as language differences or a poor ethnic match between consumers and providers of care. Access is a major problem for children since they are unable to seek mental health services for themselves and are dependent on adults, such as parents or teachers, to recognize this need and to initiate contact. Other accessibility problems are transportation, day care, and parental schedules. Many children and families cannot afford services and are unaware that care may be available at adjusted rates or even no cost (Armbruster, Gerstein, and Fallon, 1997).

In a few locations, mental health services have teamed up with schools to provide services to behaviorally and emotionally disordered children. Services integrated into the school setting seem more natural for children and parents and improve access and limit barriers. Teachers often know the child and family well and are able to provide valuable information regarding strengths and weaknesses. The community mental health nurse is able to observe the child in the classroom, lunch room, and playground, which provides a broader and more useful picture of both problems and assets. As communities broaden their outreach into the school system, an increased number of children with a wide range of psychiatric and behavioral problems will have their mental health needs met regardless of their ability to afford or access mental health care.

Homeless Populations

The homeless include people of every race, ethnic background, and educational level. It is difficult to estimate the number of homeless people with mental illness, but it is believed that one-third have severe mental illness and up to one half of these have a concurrent substance use disorder (Worley, 1997). Chronic substance abusers may end up with no home if they are abandoned by families and friends. If the disease has interfered with the ability to maintain a job, the person may be forced to live on the streets. Many homeless families are headed by women who take their children and flee from an abusive husband or partner. Homeless families may lose their sense of identity as a family, parents lose their sense of competence, and children lose the idea of home. Many adolescents find themselves living on their own as a consequence of running away from home or being thrown out by their families. Some have been physically or sexually abused in their homes. In other situations, parents of acting-out adolescents may force the teenager out of the home as a way to gain control in their own lives. Adolescents also become homeless because of family conflict, chaotic family systems, and unsuccessful foster care situations.

Nurses help the homeless population through outreach, social support groups, case management, and provision of transitional housing. Outreach to homeless people includes advertising in missions and shelters, using former "street people" as liaison staff, and using mobile crisis services, as described in Chapter 7. The purpose of outreach is to explain the available services and help homeless consumers negotiate the system.

Social support groups are set up in shelters, soup kitchens, drop-in centers, transitional housing units, and single-room occupancy (SRO) houses. Through these groups, nurses can empower consumers, increase their problem-solving skills, help them develop self-confidence, and support their identity with a group of people.

Through case management, nurses can help consumers negotiate appointments and services from a variety of agencies. Nurse may also monitor medication compliance, assist with activities of daily living (ADLs), find appropriate shelter, and assist with the development of support systems.

Rural Settings

Increases in community-based services are needed in both rural and urban areas. However, rural communities face more severe challenges in meeting the mental health needs of their residents than do urban communities. Groups at greater risk for mental disorders, that is, those who are chronically ill, the poor, the dependent, and the elderly, are disproportionately represented in rural areas. Studies have consistently identified many rural services as fragmented, costly, and often ineffective. Poverty, inadequate transportation, and limited economic opportunities restrict treatment alternatives to the already insufficient numbers of mental health care providers (Kane and Ennis, 1996).

Although there are significant problems facing consumers who live in rural settings, there are also considerable community strengths in rural settings. Generally, rural communities have a strong loyalty to family, church, and community. This loyalty results in a higher degree of tolerance for perceived "abnormal behavior" among community members and a willingness to help those who are less fortunate. Depending on the rural community, there are indigenous care providers ranging from companion/aid to confidant/therapist to healer/shaman. These natural helpers within the community may complement professional mental health providers and may also serve as a "bridge" between consumers and professionals (Kane and Ennis, 1996).

Community-Based Nursing Practice

The goal of community mental health nursing is to promote health and provide opportunities for consumers to maximize their ability to live, work, socialize, and learn in the communities of their choice. Expanding consumer "voice" and choice continues to be the major focus for nurses working in the community. Successful support means that consumers of mental health services will be able to achieve lives of value and become contributing members of their communities.

Screening Programs

Community screening programs help provide early identification of mental health problems. Indications for using a screening test are that it is not readily apparent to people that they are suffering from the disorder, that the disorder is prevalent in the population and is treatable, and that early intervention will make a difference in the outcome. There must also be an accurate and cost-effective screening tool (Greenfield et al, 1997). A number of physical conditions meet these requirements, such as hypertension, breast cancer, lead screening, and stroke risk assessment. Screening for mental disorders is relatively new. National Depression Screening Day, begun in 1991, was the first national, community-based, voluntary screening program for mental illness. Research suggests that the program has been effective in bringing individuals with depression into treatment. Those who do not comply with screening recommendations to seek treatment often have misinformation about the disorder or lack financial means or insurance to seek additional evaluation and intervention. Other at-risk groups that would benefit from screening programs include single parents with young children, teen parents, victims of family and community violence, and older adults living alone. Community outreach must be increased to ensure that those who are at risk for or suffer from mental disorders receive appropriate and adequate assistance.

Community-Based Services

Community mental health services are often underused. In addition to the barriers previously mentioned, rigid bureaucratic guidelines and red tape are seen by consumers as derogatory or, at best, bothersome and unnecessary. Community-based services must be designed to minimize the problems of accessibility and promote entry into the care system. Staff must be educated about specific community issues. Treatment programs must actively involve consumers, such as developing outreach programs and home care programs, and offering comprehensive services, such as assistance with transportation and housing. Maintaining consumers in the community makes it possible for nurses to monitor the entire care process and remain involved until outcomes are achieved.

Psychosocial Rehabilitation

The field of psychosocial rehabilitation grew out of a need to create opportunities for people suffering from psychiatric disabilities. The rehabilitation approach emphasizes the development of skills and supports necessary for successful living, learning, and working in the community. This approach creates collaborative partnerships with all interested people—consumers, families, friends, and mental health care providers. It is assumed that the consumer will be "in charge" with regard to setting goals for where and how to live, work, learn, socialize, and recreate. Rehabilitation is a process, not a quick fix. This approach is also different from the traditional approach to long-term consumers, where the assumption was that people with psychiatric disabilities needed to have decisions made for them.

People with mental illness differ little from the general population. They want work that is meaningful and self-enhancing and the opportunity to socialize with others. Psychosocial rehabilitation is anchored in the values of hope and optimism that people can grow, learn, and make changes in their lives. One essential element is power. People who are psychiatrically disabled need power and control in their relationships with professionals, in their own lives, and in the way resources are allocated. This allows them to take personal responsibility for where they are in their lives and where they are going (Carling, 1995; Palmer-Erbs, 1996).

Social Network Interventions

Social support has an effect on physical and mental status. Research indicates that people with more social resources are better able to adapt to change and are in better health. Unfortunately, people who are psychiatrically disabled have fewer social networks and weaker support systems than people without mental illness. This restricted network may not be able to provide the amount and type of support necessary for consumers to live in the community. Thus case managers provide an important service: the enhancement of social support networks. Case managers accomplish this by reinforcing existing ties, improving family ties, and building new ties (Biegel, Tracy, and Song, 1995).

Social network interventions are designed to improve the relationships within the consumer's social network. These interventions include peer consumer support, connection with indigenous healers, volunteer matching, family education and support, social skills training groups, and linkage with community resources. As networks increase in size and strength, consumers will be more able to remain in their communities of choice.

Employment

The unemployment rate of people with psychiatric disabilities is 75–90% (Van Dongen, 1996; Worley, 1997). However, many of these same individuals would benefit from work, as it can provide needed daily structure and an opportunity for socialization and meaningful activity. Psychiatric disability and the accompanying unemployment, poverty, social stigma, hospitalizations, symptoms, and medication side effects contribute to lower quality of life. Being fired from a job or being persistently unemployed contribute to feelings of inadequacy and low self-esteem. Not all consumers want to be employed, but many desire work and may need support in locating positions, filling out applications, role-playing interviews, and learning job expectations and behaviors. Some community mental health centers provide job coaches if necessary; these coaches work alongside consumers on the job until they can gradually be self-sufficient in the job. The financial disincentives to employment have yet to be addressed. Individuals receiving SSI or SSDI funds risk losing this financial assistance when they become employed, even in entry-level, low-wage positions. A way must be found to encourage employment while at the same time providing enough support to maintain community living.

Self-Help Groups: Family Resources

National Alliance for the Mentally Ill (NAMI)
703-524-7600
e-mail NAMIofc@AOL.com
  Publications:
    Understanding Depression
    Surviving Schizophrenia: For Families, Consumers, and Providers (3rd Ed.)
    Neurobiological Disorders in Children and Adolescents
    The Family Face of Schizophrenia
    Mending Minds
    The Essential Guide to Psychiatric Drugs
    Anguished Voices: Personal Accounts of Siblings and Children of People with Mental Illness
    When Someone You Love Has a Mental Illness
National Empowerment Center
800-769-3728
  Videos:
    Self-Managed Care
    Recovery is for Everyone
    Recovery as a Journey of the Heart
  Printed Material:
    On Our Own
    Coping with Voices: Self-Help Strategies for People Who Hear Voices That Are Distressing

---

Key Concepts

Introduction

- Families include couples, traditional families, lesbian and gay families, communal families, families with cohabiting parents, extended families, and even friends living together.

- Family and relationship distress is the most common problem of people seeking mental health care.

Family Assessment

- Family communication is measured by focusing on the family as a group with regard to their listening skills, speaking skills, self-disclosure, tracking, and ability to resolve conflict.

- Family cohesion (emotional bonding) ranges from disengaged to separated, to connected, to enmeshed, with the central ranges being the most functional.

- Boundaries define the amount and kind of contact allowable between family members and between the family and outside systems. Boundaries are described as clear, rigid, or diffuse.

- Family flexibility in leadership, roles, and rules ranges from rigid to structured, to flexible, to chaotic, with the central ranges most functional.

- The terms "functional" and "dysfunctional" are based on personal values and the values of one's culture and are therefore arbitrary.

- Families at higher levels of family functioning are better able to manage the stress that comes with having a family member with a mental disorder. Those at dysfunctional levels may be incapable of caring and providing support for their loved one.

- Three stages of family transformation when living with a member experiencing a severe mental disorder have been identified: acknowledging the strangers within, fighting the battle, and gaining a new perspective.

- The four sources of support for families are professional support, friend support, family support, and spiritual support.

- Both high EE and SA families are predictors of relapse for people who are psychiatrically disabled.

- Medication noncompliance and substance abuse are other changeable factors related to relapse.

Cultural Assessment

- The egocentric self, usually found in Western industrialized societies, exhibits characteristics such as individualism, separateness, autonomy, competition, and mastery and control over one's environment.

- The sociocentric self, found in many non-Western societies, is interdependent and interconnected and values cooperation, cohesiveness, group identity, and harmony with one's environment.

Family Issues Across the Life Span

- Pregnancy may precipitate the onset of a mental illness or contribute to the exacerbation of a disorder.

- Problems to be addressed are medications and fetal defects, inadequate prenatal care, inability to care for a newborn, and disruption of the family system.

- When a child or adolescent experiences a mental disorder, the parental subsystem and the sibling subsystem may be severely strained.

- Depression can contribute to relationship problems and relationship problems can precipitate depression.

- The burden of family caregiving for adult children with mental disorders includes daily caretaking, emotional drain, and financial strain.

Family Nursing Practice

- Nurses must develop collaborative relationships with clients and families.

- Psychoeducation includes illness education, conflict management skills, problem solving, and stress management.

- Mental health nurses are expected to systematically assess families and make appropriate referrals to community resources and, if appropriate, for family therapy.

- Spiritual care giving includes developing caring and thoughtful relationships, fostering positive family attitudes, helping people become active consumers and collaborators, and supporting families who seek ways to heal and achieve balance in their lives.

Community Mental Health Focus

- The principle of normalization affirms that people with disabilities should be able to lead as normal a life as possible through integration into the mainstream community and support of independence.

- The principle of contextualization means that clients are kept in as close contact as possible with their usual surroundings.

- Advantages of community-based nursing is first-hand observation, more accurate assessment, and avoidance of pitfalls.

- Most consumers prefer their own residence and want autonomy over their housing choices.

- Social skills training may be necessary to enable consumers to live successfully in the community.

Community Settings

- Home treatment may be an alternative to inpatient treatment during the acute phase of a mental illness. This involves the provision of intensive support through home visits.

- Mental health services within school systems improves access and affordability to children and parents in need of service.

- A large number of homeless individuals are in need of community-based mental health services.

- Rural settings often have inadequate community-based services, but also provide more informal support to members of their communities.

Community-Based Nursing Practice

- Community screening programs help provide early identification of mental health problems.

- Psychosocial rehabilitation emphasizes the development of skills and supports necessary for successful living, learning, and working in the community.

- Case managers provide the enhancement of social support networks, an important service.

- Employment can provide needed structure and opportunity for socialization and meaningful activity.

Review Questions

1. In assessing the level of family cohesion, you have determined that the family is very close and has very high loyalty, and members are highly dependent on one another. You would document this as which level of cohesion?

   a. connected

   b. enmeshed

   c. disengaged

   d. separated

2. In assessing the level of family flexibility, you have determined that the family is rigid. Which of the following characteristics does the family exhibit?

   a. lack of leadership, erratic discipline

   b. shared leadership, role-sharing change

   c. leadership sometimes shared, somewhat democratic discipline

   d. authoritarian leadership, strict discipline

3. You have determined that the family you are caring for has a cultural value for the sociocentric self. The characteristics you observe in this family are

   a. interdependence, group identity.

   b. individualism, autonomy.

   c. separateness, mastery of environment.

   d. competition, self-reliance.

4. Relapse is more common in families who are

   a. emotionally disconnected, distant.

   b. able to have clear boundaries, good communication.

   c. able to have shared leadership, somewhat democratic discipline.

   d. critical, intrusive.

5. Carbamazepine and valproic acid taken during pregnancy are associated with

   a. premature labor.

   b. neonatal hypothyroidism.

   c. increased risk of neural tube defects.

   d. polyhydramnios.

References

Armbruster, P., Gerstein, S. H., & Fallon, T. (1997). Bridging the gap between service need and service utilization: A school-based mental health program. *Community Ment Health J, 33*(3), 199–210.

Badger, T. A. (1996). Living with depression. *J Psychosoc Nurs, 34*(1), 21–29.

Biegel, D. E., Tracy, E. M., & Song, L. (1995). Barriers to social network interventions with persons with severe and persistent mental illness. *Community Ment Health J, 31*(4), 335–349.

Blumenthal, S .J. (1996). Women and depression. *Decade of the Brain, 7*(3), 1–4.

Carling, P. J. (1995). *Return to Community.* New York: Guilford Press.

Comas-Diaz, L. (1996). Cultural considerations in diagnosis. In F. W. Kaslow (Ed.), *Handbook of Relational Diagnosis and Dysfunctional Family Patterns* (pp. 152–168). New York: Wiley & Sons.

Denton, W. H. (1996). Problems encountered in reconciling individual and relational diagnoses. In F. W. (Ed.), *Handbook of Relational Diagnosis and Dysfunctional Family Patterns* (pp. 35–45). New York: Wiley & Sons.

Doornbos, M. M. (1997). The problems and coping methods of caregivers of young adults with mental illness. *J Psychosoc Nurs, 35*(9), 22–26.

Finnerty, M., Levin, Z., & Miller, L. J. (1996). Acute manic episodes in pregnancy. *Am J Psychiatry, 153*(2), 261–263.

George, R. D., & Howell, C. C. (1996). Clients with schizophrenia and their caregivers' perceptions of frequent psychiatric rehospitalizations. *Issues Ment Health Nurs, 17*(6), 573–588.

Gollan, J. K., Gortner, E. T., & Jacobson, N. S. (1996). Partner relational problems and affective disorders. In F. W. Kaslow (Ed.), *Handbook of Relational Diagnosis and Dysfunctional Family Patterns* (pp. 322–337). New York: Wiley & Sons.

Greenfield, S. F., et al. (1997). Effectiveness of community-based screening for depression. *Am J Psychiatry, 154*(10), 1391–1397.

Heaney, C. A., & Burke, A. C. (1995). Ideologies of care in community residential services. *Community Ment Health J, 31*(5), 449–463.

Kane, C. F., & Ennis, J. M. (1996). Health care reform and rural mental health. *Community Ment Health J, 32*(5), 445–460.

Kaslow, N. J., Deering, C. G., & Ash, P. (1996). Relational diagnosis of child and adolescent depression. In F. W. Kaslow (Ed.), *Handbook of Relational Diagnosis and Dysfunctional Family Patterns* (pp. 171–185). New York: Wiley & Sons.

Mohit, D. L. (1996). Management and care of mentally ill mothers of young children: An innovative program. *Arch Psychiatr Nurs, 10*(1), 49–54.

Olson, D. H. (1996). Clinical assessment and treatment interventions using the family circumplex model. In F. W. Kaslow (Ed.), *Handbook of Relational Diagnosis and Dysfunctional Family Patterns* (pp. 59–77). New York: Wiley & Sons.

Olson, D. H., Russell, C. S., Sprenkle, D. H. (1989). *Circumplex Model: Systemic Assessment and Treatment of Families*. Haworth.

Palmer-Erbs, V. (1996). A breath of fresh air in a turbulent health-care environment. *J Psychosoc Nurs, 34*(9), 16–21.

Robinson, C. A. (1995). Beyond dichotomies in the nursing of persons and families. *Image, 27*(2), 116–120.

Rose, L. E. (1997). Caring for caregivers: Perceptions of social support. *J Psychosoc Nurs, 35*(2), 17–24.

Saunders, J. (1997). Walking a mile in their shoes . . . Symbolic interactionism for families living with severe mental illness. *J Psychosoc Nurs, 35*(6), 8–13.

Schofield, R., et al. (1997). Evaluation of bridging institution and housing: A joint consumer-care provider initiative. *J Psychosoc Nurs, 35*(10), 9–14.

Seilheimer, T. A. & Doyal, G. T. (1996). Self-efficacy and consumer satisfaction with housing. *Community Ment Health J, 32*(6), 549–559.

Srebnik, D., et al. (1995). Housing choice and community success for individuals with serious and persistent mental illness. *Community Ment Health J, 31*(2), 139–151.

Sullivan, G., & Spritzer, K. L. (1997). Consumer satisfaction with CMCH services. *Community Ment Health J, 33*(2), 123–131.

Sveinbjarnardottir, E., & de Casterle, B. D. (1997). Mental illness in the family: An emotional experience. *Issues Ment Health Nurs, 18*(1), 45–56.

Thurtle, V. (1995). Post-natal depression: The relevance of sociological approaches. *J Adv Nurs, 22*(3), 416–424.

Van Dongen, C. J. (1996). Quality of life and self-esteem in working and nonworking persons with mental illness. *Community Ment Health J, 32*(6), 535–548.

Wasylenki, D., et al. (1997). A home-based program for the treatment of acute psychosis. *Community Ment Health J, 33*(2), 151–162.

Worley, N. K. (1997). *Mental Health Nursing in the Community*. St. Louis: Mosby.

VISIT OUR WEBSITE!
www.awnursing.com

The Role of Cultural Diversity in Mental Health Nursing

Kathryn H. Kavanagh

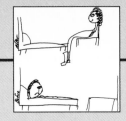

Objectives

After reading this chapter, you will be able to:

- Examine ways in which values, attitudes, beliefs, and behaviors are related to health and illness.
- Explain the importance of understanding cultural diversity in mental health nursing.
- Explore what happens when nurses and clients have different cultural values and social norms.

As a nation, the United States continues to change. By the year 2020, most U.S. residents will trace their ancestry to Africa, Asia, the Pacific Islands, or the Hispanic or Arab worlds, rather than to Europe. That is a radical change for a country in which European Americans have been the numerical majority and have held the bulk of the power, status, and wealth for several hundred years. Some people find the trend toward increased ethnic and racial diversity threatening. Others view it as an opportunity to make the United States the type of democracy that it has idealized, but that it has not, in fact, been. In any event, this transition, referred to as "the browning of America," is occurring. Nurses must be prepared to care for this diverse population, just as members of those diverse groups must be prepared to become nurses (Millet et al, 1996; Spector, 1996).

The United States has more than 100 ethnic groups, whose members have thousands of beliefs and practices related to health and illness. There are over 500 Native American and native Alaskan tribes and nations alone, plus dozens of different Asian and Pacific Island cultures. Various subgroups of African Americans live in the United States, as do different "black" cultures from Africa, the Caribbean, and other parts of the world. There are also numerous European American groups, each with its own ethnicity. The fastest-growing ethnic populations in the United States are Hispanic (also known as Latino), comprised of diverse nationalities, and Asian Pacific Americans, who include more than 50 distinct ethnic groups. Each of these major categories is so diverse that differences within groups may be as great as, or greater than, those between them. For instance, differences in the worldviews and experiences of Oglala Sioux and Lumbee Indians, or of Puerto Ricans and Bolivians, or African Americans who are poor and those who are middle class, are often greater than differences between such visibly different groups as blacks and whites. In addition, many Americans cross group lines and have blended the identities of more than one racial and/or ethnic group. It is easy to see the futility of trying to know everything about groups that number in the millions and have great internal variation.

Culture is a pattern of learned behavior based on values, beliefs, and perceptions of the world. More important than a specific behavior are the underlying values, beliefs, and perceptions that encourage or discourage that particular behavior. Culture is taught and shared by members of a group or society. It is always in process and constantly changing. A *subculture* is a smaller group within a large cultural group that shares values, beliefs, behaviors, and language. Although it is part of the larger group, a subculture is somewhat different. You may remember when you were a member of the teenage subculture. What you valued, what you believed in, and how you viewed the world may have been very different from your parents' subculture of adulthood. Your development and use of specific words, or informal language, may not have been understood by your parents. At the same time, both you and your family belonged to the larger cultural group with which you identified.

Ethnicity is ethnic affiliation, and a sense of belonging to a particular cultural group. Culture is so much a part of everyday life that it is taken for granted. We tend to assume that our own perspective is shared by others, including those for whom we care. When we believe that our own culture is more important than, and preferable to, any other culture, we are expressing ethnocentrism. It is impossible to provide sensitive nursing care from an ethnocentric position.

Nursing must change to meet the needs of an increasingly diverse population. *Diversity* refers to variation among people. Customs and lifestyles that may seem strange to those outside a client's cultural group may be very important to that client. Valuing diversity in practicing nursing means helping clients reach their full potential, preserving their ways of doing things, and helping them change only those patterns that are harmful (Spector, 1996).

As people throughout the world become more mobile, both in traveling and resettling, nurses are increasingly faced with the prospect of caring for people from a culture different than their own. More than ever, there is a need for nursing care designed around unique cultural beliefs and the values and practices of clients. Therefore, understanding and respecting cultural diversity is basic to the individualization of nursing care.

A main reason for being flexible in handling diversity is that culture is only one way in which people differ. There are also differences in ethnicity, age, health status, experience, gender, sexual orientation, and other aspects of social and economic position (Kavanagh and Kennedy, 1992). The same person might be Methodist, diabetic, Japanese American, a Democrat, a student, a sheet-metal worker, a bowler, and a parent. None of these characteristics describes the person's sex, family connections (being a son or daughter, sister or brother, cousin, and so on), educational level, socioeconomic status, or current health status. Yet just as each characteristic is part of who this person is, each is worthy of recognition, and each has a potential impact on his or her mental health situation.

Culture and Mental Health

Ideas about mental health, mental illness, psychiatric problems, and treatments are based on cultural values and understanding. These ideas, called explanatory models, make sense out of illness as it is understood by individual members of different groups. Models delineate what is considered "normal" and "abnormal" in a particular population, explain how things happen, shape clinical presentations of mental disorders, and determine culturally patterned ways that mental disorders are recognized, labeled, explained, and treated by other members of that group. By talking with clients, you can learn, for example, whether mental illness in their culture is considered psychological, emotional, spiritual, physical, or a combination of these categories. Many cultural groups do not view the body and mind as separate, but as one (Spector, 1996; Tseng and Straltzer, 1997).

What is considered normal or abnormal depends on the specific viewpoint. The same behavior may be seen as positive in one situation and pathological in another. Hallucinations, for instance, are typically viewed as abnormal by psychiatric standards but normal and even encouraged by certain Native American tribes as symbolic spiritual experiences called vision quests. Knowing about values and patterns of behavior helps us minimize the potential for imposing our expectations on people who come from different backgrounds and have different needs and goals.

Many beliefs about the cause of mental illness exist worldwide. Some people believe mental illness is a punishment for wrongdoing, the result of being "witched," or an illness that is "passed down" through the family. The belief that mental illness is a punishment for wrongdoing is quite common. Wrongdoings can range from minor infractions such as eating a taboo food to major violations such as killing a relative. Another type of wrongdoing is offending ancestors, gods, and goddesses. The belief that another person can "witch" a person to have a mental illness is also common. People who have been offended put a sign, or hex, on the person who is at fault, who then goes "crazy." "Down-the-line" or inherited mental illness is another cultural belief. This is thought to be passed through only the mother, since she is the one who gives birth to the child. While most people believe that mental illness is not contagious, they also believe that the mentally ill should be avoided (Hales, 1996).

Problems Related to Culture

Psychosocial problems can include problems related to culture. People can become alienated from their cultural group for any number of reasons, including geographical moves or marriage into a different group. They may also be expelled from their religious or ethnic associations for many reasons such as sexual orientation, interracial marriage, or other violations of cultural norms. These types of problems result in loss of social status and self-esteem. Accurate assessment of culture-related factors is important in providing holistic care to clients and their families.

Culture-Specific Syndromes

Certain forms of mental illness are restricted to specific areas or cultures. These well-defined syndromes occur in response to certain situations in a particular culture. They are a heterogeneous group that can be further subdivided into three groups. *True syndromes* are illnesses with specific symptoms. *Illnesses of attribution* have a presumed cause but no specific signs and symptoms. An example in Western medicine might be an illness classified only as "infectious disease." *Idioms of distress* occur in people who are especially vulnerable to stressful life events. This vulnerability makes them susceptible to a wide variety of physical and mental illnesses. See Box 3. 1 for information on culture-specific syndromes (Levine and Gaw, 1995).

Box 3.1

Culture-Specific Syndromes

True Syndromes—Dissociative Phenomena

Amok	Characterized by homicidal frenzy followed by amnesia; many different cultures.
Falling Out	Sudden collapse in which the eyes are open but the person cannot see or move; Southern USA and Caribbean.
Latah	Hypersensitivity to sudden fright with trance-like behavior; Malaysia.
Pibloktoq	Abrupt episodes of extreme excitement, followed by seizures, transient coma, and amnesia; Eskimo.
Grisi Siknis	Victim believes she is being attacked by devils and runs through the village; Nicaragua and Honduras.
Shin-Byung	Anxiety and somatic complaints followed by dissociation caused from possession by ancestral spirits; Korea.

True Syndromes—Anxiety States

Ataque de Nervios	Shaking, palpitations, flushing, and shouting or striking out; Latin America.
Dhat	Extreme anxiety associated with discharge of semen, which is thought to lead to depletion of physical and mental energy; Asia.
Koro	Man believes his penis is retracting into his body and that this will end in death; Asia.
Kayak Angst	Intense anxiety associated with fear of capsizing and drowning when going out to the open sea in a kayak; Eskimo.
Taijin Kyofusho	Intense anxiety about possibly offending, embarrassing, or displeasing others; Japan.

True Syndromes—Affective/Somatoform Disorders

Brain Fag	Pressure in the head, difficulty concentrating, anxiety, and visual complaints believed to result from too much thinking; West Africa.
Shenjing Shuairuo	Physical and mental exhaustion, difficulty concentrating, memory loss, sleeping and appetite problems, and irritability; China.
Anorexia Nervosa	Obsessive preoccupation with weight loss and delusional body image; Western cultures.

True Syndromes—Psychotic States

Boufee Delirante	Sudden outburst of aggressive behavior, confusion, agitation, paranoid ideation, and auditory and visual hallucinations; West Africa and Haiti.

Illnesses of Attribution—Induced by Anger

Bilis, Colera	Tension, somatic expressions, and fatigue; Latin America.
Hwa-Byung	Suppression of anger leads to indigestion, fatigue, fearfulness, and general dysphoria; Korea.

Illnesses of Attribution—Induced by Fright

Susto	Sudden fright believed to cause the soul to leave the body, leading to many physical and emotional symptoms; Latin America.

Illnesses of Attribution—Induced by Witchcraft

Ghost Sickness	An illness believed to be induced by witches, with symptoms such as delirium, nightmares, terror, anxiety, and confusion; Native American.

Box 3.1 continued

		Idioms of Distress	
Voodoo	Illness ascribed to hexing, witchcraft, or the evil influence of another person; believed to cause a variety of symptoms and even death; Caribbean, Southern USA, Latin America.	Nervios/Nevra	A term describing people who are vulnerable to stress and who display a wide variety of physical and emotional illnesses; Latin America, Greece.
Evil Eye	A fixed stare by an adult is believed capable of causing illness in a child or another adult; Mediterranean, Latin America.	Locura	The most severe form of chronic mental illness; victim is incoherent, agitated, unpredictable, and possibly violent; Latin America.

Sources: *DSM–IV*, 1994; Levine and Gaw, 1995.

Values

Values are a set of personal beliefs about what is meaningful and significant in life. Values provide general guidelines for behavior; they are standards of conduct that people or groups of people believe in. Values are the frame of reference through which we integrate, explain, and evaluate new ideas, situations, and relationships. Values may be intrinsic, internalized from a person's particular situation and experience, or extrinsic, derived from the culture's standards of right and wrong.

Value Orientations

It has long been recognized that in every society, basic values emphasize shared ideals about the following subjects (Kavanagh, 1991; Kluckholn et al, 1953):

- The relationship between humans and nature
- The relationship between humans and the universe
- A sense of time
- A sense of productivity and activity
- Interpersonal relationships

Values about the relationship between humans and nature fall along a continuum, as do values about each of the other subjects. The model relationship between humans and nature may be seen as predetermined, perhaps by God or fate or genetics, implying that some aspect of nature controls people. It may also be viewed as independent, with people controlling nature. Relationships with nature tend to reflect those between humans and the universe in being close and personal or distant and impersonal. Both orientations affect attitudes toward illness prevention and health care. For example, if we believe our fate is predetermined, we have little motivation for preventive strategies such as proper nutrition and immunization. In contrast, the more familiar value in the United States is mastery over nature, the attitude that nature can be conquered and controlled if and when we learn enough about it. This attitude has led to the development of extensive technology focused on health care, along with the assumption that it is appropriate to intervene in what were traditionally viewed as natural phenomena—disease and death.

People tend to be oriented toward the past, the present, or the future. The may emulate history and reclaim the past, such as through believing in ancestral spirits. Or they may live in the present moment, with little concern for the past or future. On the same continuum is an orientation toward the future that encourages people to save money, to get an education and qualify for a career, and to set other long-range goals such as preventing diseases.

Attitudes toward productivity are likewise varied. For some, it is enough to just exist; it is not necessary to accomplish great things in order to feel worthwhile.

For others, a desire to develop the self is its own reward and requires no outside recognition. For still others, however, there is a belief that hard work will pay off materially as well as psychologically. As a result of their attitude toward productivity in life, people are relatively passive or active.

Values about interpersonal relationships also exist on a continuum. Certain cultures, for example, think that some people are born followers and others are born leaders. This belief implies that the follower need not assume responsibility for the self and can and should rely on others, such as health care professionals. Other cultures believe that all people have equal rights and should control their own destinies, become assertive, and take the lead, at least over their own lives. Between those two extremes are people who take their problems to close friends or family members, sharing the problem but keeping responsibility for it within a close personal group. Values about interpersonal relationships are also reflected in the ideas people have about being individuals and members of groups, and who should interact with whom in what way. European Americans tend to value individualism highly, with members of families or communities a secondary priority.

Each of these sets of values exists along a continuum that illustrates wide human variation. No values are implicitly right or wrong; they simply shape ideas and responses. It is dangerously misleading if we assume that a given orientation is shared by all clients.

Predominant American Values

The most prominent values in the United States are reflected in our health care system, but those values tend to represent the dominant groups (European American, middle class, Judeo-Christian, and male) and not the numerous and diverse subgroups within the country. The dominant set of values is oriented toward individuals, who are viewed as accountable for decision making, self-care, and many other self-oriented tasks. Privacy rights and personal freedom are based on the value of individualism. However, in many American subcultures, being individualistic is not a primary value.

Parrillo (1990) has created a useful list of values that predominate in the United States, as shown in Box 3.2. Consider ways in which each of these values is promoted not only in society in general, but in nursing practice in particular.

Nursing Values

Nursing reflects the society in which it exists. Nursing would not be accepted and utilized if it did not reflect the cultural values and social norms that predominate. While American values generally reflect those of the dominant culture, in reality, many cultural subgroups have quite different values and norms (DeVita and Armstrong, 1993). Nursing as a discipline tends to have the same values as middle-class Americans of European American background. Yet, as nurses, we must be flexible enough to meet the needs expressed by a very diverse population with widely varying values. In other words, standard nursing practice exhibits less diversity than we or our clients possess. We must be aware of the "standard" values and avoid assuming that they apply to everyone.

Attitudes and Perceptions

Being knowledgeable about diversity includes understanding the attitudes and perceptions that perpetuate social equality and inequality. Attitudes and perceptions are formed from biases. Paul (1993) describes two different types of bias. The first type is natural bias, which refers simply to how our point of view causes us to notice some things and not others. The second type is negative bias: a refusal to recognize that there are other points of view. Natural and negative biases come into play when we organize or process information in such a way that we develop attitudes of open-mindedness and/or discrimination. As nurses, we must always be open-minded—learning what our natural and negative biases are, and changing those that prevent us from seeing and understanding the perspectives of other people.

Generalizations, Stereotypes, and Prejudice

We all work with huge amounts of information every day. To make it more manageable, we organize information into categories. One way we organize is through descriptive generalizations. *Generalizations,* which arise out of our natural biases, are changeable starting places for comparing typical behavioral patterns with what is actually observed, the facts of the situation. When we use generalizations to process

Box 3.2

Predominant American Values

Personal Achievement and Success

The emphasis is on competition, power, status, and wealth. What is good for the individual may be more important than what is good for the larger group, such as the community.

Activity and Work

People who do not work hard are considered lazy. It is assumed that hard work will be rewarded. Little consideration is given to people who have not had the same opportunities for success.

Moral Orientation

There is a tendency to moralize and to see the world in absolutes of right or wrong, good or bad. This pattern reinforces the inclination to stereotype.

Humanitarian Mores

Although quick to respond with charity and crisis aid, Americans often use these to limit deeper involvement with issues. Even professional "caring" relationships are typically kept impersonal.

Efficiency and Practicality

Solutions to problems are often based on short-term rather than long-term results.

Progress

Change is often seen as progress in which technology is highly valued and the focus is on the future rather than the present.

Material Comfort

The United States is a consumer-oriented society with a high standard of living.

Personal Freedom and Individualism

Individual rights are valued above the good of the group.

Equality

Personal freedom is a stronger value than equality, especially when there is competition for resources or opportunities.

External Conformity

Despite the value of personal freedom, there is pressure to conform to the European American, middle-class, Judeo-Christian, male values that predominate. Those differing are labeled deviant.

Science and Rationality

The medicalization of society has led to high expectations for "quick fixes," technology, and the efficiency of scientific medicine.

Source: Adapted from Parrillo, 1990.

information, we are more likely to remain open-minded: to develop open relationships with our clients, understand their point of view, and provide culturally sensitive nursing care.

Another way to organize information is by using *stereotypes*, which arise out of our negative biases. Stereotypes are images frozen in time that cause us to see what we expect to see, even when the facts differ from our expectations. Stereotypes often capture characteristics that are real and common to a group. However, stereotypes may also be out-of-date and dangerously limited. They are particularly dangerous when they involve negative beliefs about a person or group, leading to "prejudgment" (or prejudice) that ignores actual evidence. *Prejudice* is negative feeling about people who are different from us. Prejudicial attitudes are based on limited knowledge, limited contact, and emotional responses rather than on careful observation and thought. They are beliefs, opinions, or points of view that are formed before the facts are known, or in spite of them (Wells, 1995).

Stereotypes can be favorable as well as unfavorable, although even favorable ones disregard facts and rely on preconceived notions. For example, Asian American students are often expected to excel in mathematics because of the stereotype that associates

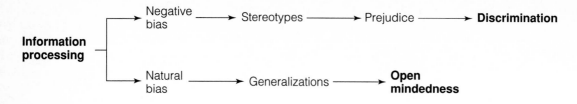

Figure 3.1 **Pathways to open-mindedness and discrimination.**

Asian Americans with technical accomplishments. Because every group has some individuals who do well in math and others who do not, Asian Americans who struggle with math must contend with a sense of failure. The same process occurs in many forms: A child is expected to do well because his or her older siblings did; people with glasses read a lot of books; all African Americans are good dancers or athletes. Although these are not negative stereotypes, they are potentially harmful because they impose expectations that are unrealistic.

The two pathways of information processing— one leading to open-mindedness and the other leading to discrimination—are shown in Figure 3. 1.

Discrimination

Several types of prejudice are commonly observed in health care settings and can lead to discriminatory behavior. Discrimination is prejudice that is expressed behaviorally. Racism is one example of discrimination. Differentiating people according to racial characteristics has always been a pervasive social process in the United States. Despite nurses' extensive knowledge of biology, we tend to leave incorrect ideas about race unchallenged.

We are all members of the human race. Nonetheless, we use racial terms to divide and separate people. We often refer to skin color to group people into different races. Imagine somehow lining up the more than 5 billion people on this planet, starting on one end with the darkest-skinned and ending with the lightest-skinned. The very dark individuals would seem quite different from the very light, yet the vast majority would be in between in every shade of brown. Based on skin color, no one would be able to tell where one "race" ends and the next begins.

The time when African Americans, Asian Americans, Hispanic Americans, and Native Americans were prevented from entering the social and economic mainstream is officially over. However, despite formal integration, stereotypes and prejudices associated with white versus nonwhite status remain. For instance, negative stereotypes that associate African Americans with poverty, drugs, and violence ignore the fact that most African Americans are not poor and have nothing to do with either drugs or violence. Assuming that a client is on welfare because he or she is African American, or that substance abuse exists or physical aggression is a likelihood, may result in treatment different from that given to clients who are not African American.

A number of other forms of discrimination may be observed in health care settings. These patterns of interaction have acquired the label "isms" because of their common word ending. Each ism involves a tendency to judge others according to similarity to or dissimilarity from a standard considered ideal or normal. Isms are shaped by personal or group judgment (Wells, 1995). For example, focusing on oneself is known as egocentrism. When an entire society promotes one way of behaving or thinking as the best way, it is called sociocentrism, as in Eurocentric or Afrocentric education. We frequently hear about ethnocentrism. Nearly every ethnic group sees itself as "best." However, in a society composed of multiple groups, we must counteract such biases, or isms, to prevent discrimination and social injustice.

For a description of the common forms of discrimination in health care settings, see Table 3.1. There is considerable evidence that even when the intent is to treat people fairly, they may be approached in ways that indicate subtle prejudice. In health care settings, one group tends to get treated well and

Table 3.1 Forms of Discrimination

Form	Description	Example
Ableism	The assumption that the able-bodied and sound of mind are superior to those who are disabled or mentally ill.	A person who is psychiatrically disabled is not offered treatment choices.
Adultism	The assumption that adults are superior to youths.	Children are ignored and not given opportunities to learn decision making.
Ageism	The assumption that members of one age group are superior to those of other age groups.	Older people are assumed to be senile and incompetent.
Classism	The assumption that certain people are superior because of their socioeconomic status or position in a group or organization.	A poorly dressed high school dropout is not offered the same treatment facility as a well-dressed college graduate.
Egocentrism	The assumption that one is superior to others.	A person who has never experienced a mental illness thinks he or she is better than those who are diagnosed with a mental disorder.
Ethnocentrism	The assumption that one's own cultural or ethnic group is superior to that of others.	Everyone is expected to speak English and to know the rules for living in America.
Heterosexism	The assumption that everyone is or should be heterosexual.	When gays or lesbians experience a mental disorder, the cause is assumed to be their sexual orientation.
Racism	The assumption that members of one race are superior to those of another.	The color of one's skin determines educational and career opportunities.
Sexism	The assumption that members of one gender are superior to those of the other.	Women are viewed as less rational and more emotional, and therefore more likely to have a mental illness, than men.
Sizism	The assumption that people of one body size are superior to those of other shapes and sizes.	Obese people have fewer job opportunities and advancements.
Sociocentrism	The assumption that one society's way of knowing or doing is superior to that of others.	Biomedicine is expected to be effective, while folk medicine is discounted.

another may get less attention, fewer choices, and generally less vigorous care. This unequal treatment is a reflection of the traits that society values (Kavanagh and Kennedy, 1992). The YAVIS are young, attractive, verbal, intelligent, and successful (or appear potentially successful). The QUOIDS, by contrast, are quiet, ugly, old, indigent (poor), dissimilar (in lifestyle, language, or culture), and thought to be stupid. Although someone carefully observing interactions in health care settings may readily discern preferential patterns involving YAVIS and QUOIDS, those who work there may be unaware of how their biases lead to behavior that is discriminatory.

Caring for a Diverse Population

To understand and care for diverse clients, you must learn to understand and appreciate multiple interpretations of events and behaviors. There are thousands of cultures and subcultures, and we cannot possibly know all there is to know about each one. Personal and group identities are very complex. Many people are exposed to or have been raised in more than one culture. Many others have altered their traditional cultural orientation to adapt to American society or specific life circumstances. We often hear about the importance of sensitivity to cultural differences. However, being *only* sensitive can leave you frustrated and powerless. You must also learn to become an advocate for diverse populations. Advocacy is supporting and defending people's rights to their beliefs, attitudes, and values. Effective advocacy depends on a balance of knowledge, sensitivity, and skills.

Knowledge

The first step in building knowledge is getting to know who *we* are. We cannot expect to understand others and help them achieve their full potential if we do not first develop an understanding of who we are as people and as nurses. This is not always simple, and it is an ongoing, never-ending process. Identifying our own attitudes, values, and prejudices helps us understand our feelings about people who are different. It helps us be nonjudgmental and may prevent us from exhibiting discriminating behavior when interacting with clients from a different cultural or subcultural group. Confronting our own ethnocentrism takes careful attention to our thoughts and behaviors. Self-understanding is enhanced when we ask for and listen carefully to feedback from clients, peers, faculty members, and supervisors. There is no easy way to acquire a depth of knowledge about cultural groups different from our own. Wherever we practice nursing, we must assume responsibility for learning about the culture of our clients. This can be done through reading, by talking to and listening to clients, and by attending workshops about diverse cultural groups.

Sensitivity

Knowing ourselves is critical to becoming sensitive nurses. Once we become aware of our own attitudes, values, and prejudices, we must examine how they affect our nursing practice. Ask yourself: Do I pay more attention to clients who have a background similar to mine? Do I approach clients from a different background with initial suspicion or distrust? Does my body language change when I interact with someone from a different background? What are the stereotypes I have of people from various cultures? When I don't understand a client's behavior, do I ask for clarification or do I make assumptions about that behavior? Am I open to learning about folk healing practices? Do I penalize clients whose values or behaviors are different from mine?

Skills in Implementing Nursing Interventions

Knowledge empowers us to understand cultural differences. Sensitivity enables us to respect and honor differences. Sensitivity and knowledge must be combined with skills for appropriate and effective nursing intervention to occur.

Communication is crucial to all nursing care, but it is especially important when caring for mental health clients from diverse backgrounds. To establish contact, present yourself in a confident way without seeming to be superior. Shake hands, if appropriate. Allow clients to choose their comfortable personal space. Respect their version of acceptable eye contact. Ask how they prefer to be addressed. Most people are pleased when others show sincere interest in them. Small things can often communicate acceptance. Making a setting comfortable by considering seating arrangements, background noises, and other environmental variables helps make clients feel welcome and recognized.

Talk with clients to determine their level of fluency in English, and arrange for an interpreter if needed. Speak directly to the client even if an interpreter is present. Choose a style of speech that promotes understanding and demonstrates respect for each client. Avoid the tendency to raise your voice, as if that will increase understanding or fluency. Avoid jargon, slang, complex sentences, and body language that may be offensive or misunderstood.

Before using any written materials, ask clients if they can read English. They may feel defensive about their reading ability. Softening the question can help. For example, asking "Are you comfortable reading this?" avoids the issue of ability and allows clients to say that they prefer to have printed materials read to them. The ability to read varies widely, and many people who speak English do not read it. Medications and the symptoms of mental disorders can also interfere with the ability and motivation to read.

To obtain information, use open-ended questions or questions phrased in several ways. Allow plenty of time for answers. Be aware that some people consider only open-ended questions to be acceptable, such as "How do you manage your job when you feel sick?" Others prefer closed-ended questions, such as "Do you sleep a lot when you feel sick?" Still others (members of certain Native American, Pacific Island, and African groups, for example) consider direct questions to be impolite. They may expect inquiries to be presented like a story, as in "One client told me that when he feels really bad, he wears a special shirt. I guess we all have things we do at certain times."

You may have to learn to use certain indirect styles of communication and wait to see if and how the client responds. Observe how the client communicates to others to learn what style is most appropriate. Ask family members or significant others if they can help with this information. It is important to avoid forcing clients to conform to communication patterns with which they are not comfortable.

Storytelling is a valuable approach to sharing views. Inviting clients to tell you stories about themselves and their problems is an excellent way to find out what is important to them and how they view their situations. "Can you tell me a story about when you were growing up?" "Would you tell me a story about coming to the hospital?" Communication is most productive when you acknowledge that clients know more about their personal situation than you do. Having clients tell the story of their life and of their illness often provides information that will help you understand their experiences and views. Although this approach requires good listening skills and adequate amounts of time, it forms the core of effective care and treatment in many societies (Leininger, 1991; Wells, 1995).

Client values, beliefs, and practices do not have to change simply because they are different from those of health care providers. You can help people recognize what to change and what not to change. To provide care that is both knowledgeable and sensitive, it is essential to identify the following (Leininger, 1991):

- Those aspects of the client's life that mean a lot, are valuable just as they are, and should be understood and preserved without change.

- Those that can be partially preserved but need some adjustment, to be negotiated with the client.

- Those that require change and repatterning.

Analysis of the situation to clarify what is happening, and the probable consequences of each type of intervention, helps you make informed decisions. If your relationship is mutual and communication open, it may quickly become clear that the client's value orientation can be maintained or will require only minor alteration. Lack of knowledge and insensitivity often leads to the conclusion that a client's approach is totally wrong and requires radical overhauling. In order to gain the client's cooperation, preserve the integrity of the client's view by being flexible, sensitive, knowledgeable, and skillful. On the other hand, at times you must take a stand for substantive change, as in cases of illegal or injurious behavior. It may be appropriate to consult the client's family or friends to help articulate a particular point of view. Many communities have rosters of organizations and individuals who will share information about the populations they represent. Getting help from these people is especially important when language or value differences create barriers between you and your clients.

Becoming competent and confident in managing diversity requires expertise and practice. Implementing knowledge, sensitivity, and skills in psychiatric nursing settings requires considerable time and energy. These efforts are rewarded, however, when difficult situations are handled as openly, mutually, and respectfully as possible, and by seeing clients respond favorably to such humanistic treatment.

Key Concepts

Introduction

- Each of the major ethnic groups is so diverse that differences within groups may be as great as, or greater than, those between them.

- Culture is a pattern of learned behavior based on values, beliefs, and perceptions of the world. It is taught and shared by members of a group or society.

- A subculture is a smaller group within a large cultural group that shares values, beliefs, behaviors, and language.

- Ethnicity is ethnic affiliation, and a sense of belonging to a particular cultural group.

- Ethnocentrism is the belief that one's own culture is more important than, and preferable to, any other culture.

Culture and Mental Health

- Ideas about mental health, mental illness, psychiatric problems, and treatments are based on cultural values and understanding.
- What is considered normal or abnormal depends on the specific cultural viewpoint.

Values

- Values are a set of personal beliefs about what is meaningful and significant in life. They provide general guidelines for behavior and are standards of conduct in which people or groups of people believe.
- Every society has basic values about the relationship between humans and nature, a sense of time, a sense of productivity, and interpersonal relationships.
- Values about the relationship between humans and nature vary from predetermined to independent. These reflect beliefs about humans and the universe.
- Predominant American values tend to represent European American, middle-class, Judeo-Christian, male values.
- Nursing as a discipline tends to have the same values as middle-class Americans of European American background.

Attitudes and Perceptions

- Natural bias refers to how our point of view causes us to notice some things and not others.
- Negative bias is a refusal to recognize that there are other points of view.
- Generalizations are a way of organizing information. Arising out of natural biases, they are changeable starting places for comparing typical behavioral patterns with what is actually observed.
- Stereotypes are a way of organizing information. Arising out of negative biases, they are images frozen in time that cause us to see what we expect to see, even when the facts differ from our expectations. Stereotypes can be favorable or unfavorable, and either kind is potentially harmful.
- Prejudice is negative feeling about people who are different from us.

- Discrimination is prejudice that is expressed behaviorally. Examples are racism, egocentrism, and sociocentrism.

Caring for a Diverse Population

- Effective advocacy depends on a balance of knowledge, sensitivity, and skills.
- The first step in building knowledge is understanding ourselves and confronting our own ethnocentrism.
- You must acquire knowledge about clients' cultural groups that are different from your own.
- When we know ourselves, we are able to be nonjudgmental and sensitive to other's beliefs, feelings, and behaviors.
- Sensitivity includes examining how our own attitudes, values, and prejudices affect our nursing practice.
- Communication is an important skill in caring for clients from diverse backgrounds. It includes learning their level of fluency in spoken and written English, and determining the most important style of communication.
- Many aspects of the client's life should be understood and preserved without change. Some can be partially preserved but need adjustment, which is negotiated with the client. Other aspects require change and repatterning.
- Becoming competent and confident in managing diversity requires practice and patience. The reward is seeing clients respond favorably to such humanistic treatment.

Review Questions

1. Valuing diversity in practicing nursing means
   a. being politically correct.
   b. helping people preserve their ways of doing things.
   c. suggesting to people that they become acculturated.
   d. acting ethnocentrically.

2. Discrimination is
   a. a way to organize information into categories.
   b. an image frozen in time that causes us to see what we expect to see.
   c. a negative feeling about people who are different from us.
   d. prejudice that is expressed behaviorally.

3. Which one of the following is a predominant value in the United States?

   a. personal achievement and success

   b. the good of the community

   c. long-term solutions to problems

   d. acceptance of nonconformity

4. As nurses, it is only when we know ourselves that we are able to be

   a. egocentric.

   b. ethnocentric.

   c. discriminating.

   d. nonjudgmental.

5. You believe that there is never a good reason for a person to commit suicide. Which predominant American value does this reflect?

   a. personal achievement

   b. external conformity

   c. humanitarian mores

   d. moral orientation

References

DeVita, P. R., Armstrong, J. D. (1993). *Distant Mirrors: America as a Foreign Culture.* Belmont, CA: Wadsworth.

Hales, A., (1996). West African Beliefs About Mental Illness. In *Perspectives in Psych Care, 32*(2), 23–29.

Kavanagh, K. H. (1991). Invisibility and selective avoidance: Gender and ethnicity in psychiatry and psychiatric nursing staff interaction. *Culture, Medicine and Psychiatry, 15,*245–274.

Kavanagh, K. H., Kennedy, P. H. (1992). *Promoting Cultural Diversity: Strategies for Health Care Professionals.* Thousand Oaks, CA: Sage.

Kluckholn, F. R., Kluckholn, C., & Murray, H. (Eds.) (1953). Dominant and variant value orientations. In *Personality in Nature, Society, and Culture.* (342–357). New York: Knopf.

Leininger, M. M. (Ed.) (1991). *Culture, Care, Diversity, and Universality: A Theory of Nursing.* New York: National League for Nursing Press.

Levine, R. E., & Gaw A. C. (1995). Culture-bound syndromes. *Psychiatric Clinics North America, 18*(3), 523–536.

Millet, P. E., et al. (1996). Black Americans' and white Americans' views of the etiology and treatment of mental health problems. *Community Ment Health J, 32*(3), 235–241.

Parrillo, V. N. (1990). *Strangers to These Shores: Race and Ethnic Relations in the United States.* Riverside, NJ: Macmillan.

Paul, R. W. (1993). *Critical Thinking: How to Prepare Students for a Rapidly Changing World.* Cotati, CA: Foundation for Critical Thinking.

Spector, R. E. (1996). *Cultural Diversity in Health & Illness* (4th ed.). Norwalk, CT: Appleton & Lange. 1996.

Tseng, W. S., & Straltzer, J. (Eds) (1997). *Culture and Psychopathology.* New York: Brunner/Mazel.

Wells, S. A. (1995). Creating a culturally competent workforce. *Caring, 14*(12), 50–53.

CHAPTER 4

Neurobiology and Behavior

Mary Moller
Karen Lee Fontaine

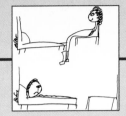

Objectives

After reading this chapter, you will be able to:

- Describe basic brain development.
- Discuss selected functions of the brain.
- Relate brain functions to major brain structures.
- Describe the clinical manifestations of brain dysfunction in mental disorders.
- Identify the role of neuroanatomy and neurophysiology in brain dysfunction.

Key Terms

abstract thinking
alexithymia
amino acids
biogenic amines
concrete thinking
circumstantial speech
illogical thinking
loose association
neuromodulators
peptides
pressured speech
proprioception
receptor agonists
receptor antagonists
tangential speech

The human brain is a highly complex and delicately balanced organ. It has become increasingly clear that this control center is not only a place but a process involving the interrelationship between the brain, our hormones, our biochemistry, and the environment. We still have a long way to go in understanding how mental disorders occur. But we do know that mental disorders, like strokes and brain tumors, are serious brain disorders.

Historically, lack of understanding of brain function led to separating mental disorders from other serious illnesses and to stigmatizing those who were suffering. Currently, biological psychiatry is focusing on the etiology and treatment of brain disorders frequently referred to as mental disorders. Biological psychiatry encompasses neuroanatomy, neurophysiology, neurochemistry, neurogenetics, neuroimmunology, neuropsychology, neuroendocrinology, neuroimaging, and neurocomputational sciences. Researchers hope to learn how the brains of those affected by mental disorders are different from the brains of those who are not.

What this means for you, as a nursing student, is that in addition to principles from the sociological and psychological sciences, nursing care of clients with mental disorders also includes principles from the biological sciences.

Development of the Brain

The brain develops through the constant interaction of genetic and environmental factors. Genes shape the structure of the infant brain, but the infant's environmental and social experiences fine-tune the brain's function. Studies indicate that the brain begins as random neural circuits that continue to be programmed throughout early life. There are three major developmental periods. *Organogenesis*, the first period, includes the development of the neural tube. This vital structure forms during the third week after conception. The closure of the neural tube is referred to as myerulation. Problems during this period are usually fatal to the fetus.

The second major developmental period, *rapid neuronal proliferation*, occurs during fetal weeks 12–20 during the second trimester. In this stage, the process of histogenesis occurs. Histogenesis refers to the laying down of nerve and glial cells, cell migration, and cell differentiation. After a cell is born, it migrates to where it is genetically programmed to go. When it gets to its predetermined location, it starts to differentiate and communicate with other cells. Histogenesis continues until the child is about 8 years old. Consequences of deficient cell differentiation can be devastating. Trauma or disruption during this process affects a cell's ability to communicate with other cells. Problems in cellular communication ultimately affect overall function of the structure. At present, we cannot predict deficits in a structure before the structure develops. For example, higher-level cognitive functions, such as planning and predicting, generally develop around the age of 16. If the frontal lobe structures of the brain are even slightly damaged, the deficit will not be apparent until that developmental stage (Hedaya, 1996).

The third major developmental period, the *brain growth spurt*, begins in the third trimester, reaches peak acceleration prior to full term, and continues at a gradually decreasing rate until around the age of 2. This is a critical period of brain development.

Brain functions continue to mature until well into the second decade of life. The brain begins shrinking around age 35, and adult function is determined by the brain's ability to repair itself (neuroplasticity), metabolism, and intact neuroanatomy and neurophysiology.

Scientists have found convincing evidence that brains of women and men work in dramatically different ways, at least in certain kinds of language functions and expression of emotion. The same emotion might trigger a man to fight and a woman to react with words, facial expressions, and gestures; this has a physical basis. There are gender differences in the size, form, and structure of the limbic system, cortical gray matter tissue, and cerebral blood flow. These disparities may help to explain gender-related differences in behavior (Gur et al, 1995).

Research suggests that regular physical exercise makes our bodies more adept at delivering oxygen and nutrients to the brain. Your brain is a hungry machine that makes up just 2 percent of your body weight but consumes 20 percent of your total oxygen and glucose stores. It functions best when arteries are kept clear, which is more likely to happen with exercise. Ultimately, genetics and lifestyle have a signifi-

Table 4.1 Functional Brain Categories and Associated Problems

Functional Category	Functions	Problems
Cognition	Memory.	Difficulty learning and retaining new information.
	Attention.	Poor concentration and easy distractibility.
	Decision making.	Illogical thinking; lack of planning skills; impaired judgment.
	Thought content.	Delusions.
Perception	Vision, hearing, taste, touch, and smell.	Hallucinations; illusions.
	Pain recognition.	Inability to sense pain.
	Ability to distinguish right and left.	Disorientation and confusion regarding locations.
Emotion	Ability to experience and express pleasure, displeasure, and loss appropriately.	Anhedonia, apathy; euphoria; inappropriate expression of emotions.
Behavior	Ability to act and respond appropriately to internal and external stimuli.	Aggression and agitation; slowed responses and movements.
	Body movements that are appropriate to and correlate with internal and external stimuli.	Repetitive or stereotyped behaviors; apraxia, echopraxia, abnormal gait.
Socialization	Ability to form cooperative and interdependent relationships with others.	Social withdrawal; awkward social behavior; inability to participate in recreational activities.

Sources: Heyada, 1996; Moller and Murphy, 1996.

cant impact on the aging process of the entire body, including the brain (Hedaya, 1996).

Functions of the Brain

The brain is the site of all integrative functions that govern our behavior, feelings, and thoughts. Major integrative functions include interpreting, analyzing, sorting, storing, and retrieving information about our internal and external environments. To aid comprehension, we can group brain functions into the following five categories: cognition, perception, emotion, behavior, and socialization. Within these five broad categories are the concepts of information processing, memory, sensation, motor activity, and interpersonal relationships. Table 4.1 summarizes these categories and concepts and lists associated problems.

Learning is the gathering of new knowledge, and memory is the retention of that knowledge for future use. Memory is not static but changes over time and involves a variety of brain systems. Two types of

memory exist: short-term memory and long-term memory. Short-term memory causes temporary changes in the function of neurons. It is only if the stimulation is strong and repetitive that long-term memory is activated. Long-term memory is further divided into two types: declarative and procedural. Declarative memory is memory for people and facts, is consciously accessible, and can be verbally expressed (can be declared). Procedural memory does not require conscious awareness and involves the memory of motor skills and procedures, such as riding a bicycle (Hedaya, 1996).

People with mental disorders may have noticeable problems in the form and content of their speech. When there is no apparent relationship between thoughts, the person is said to have **loose association.** A person appears to have **illogical thinking** when expressed ideas are inconsistent, irrational, or self-contradictory. Some people exhibit **tangential speech** when thoughts veer from the main idea and never get back to it. **Circumstantial speech** occurs when the person includes many unnecessary and insignificant details before arriving at the main idea. A person is said to have **pressured speech** when his or her speech is tense, strained, and difficult to interrupt.

Difficulties in cognition can cause errors in processing information from both the internal and the external environment. These errors result in symptoms such as poor concentration, lack of insight, illogical thinking, and delusions. Similarly, alterations in perceptual processes can lead to hallucinations and illusions relating to any of the five senses. When cognitive and perceptual functions are disturbed, emotions and affect can range from euphoria to severe depression, and behavior can range from slowed responses and movements to agitation or aggression. Some behaviors may appear confusing or even bizarre. Ultimately, socialization functions, such as the development of interpersonal relationships, are also impaired.

Neuroanatomy

To fully appreciate the complexity of mental disorders, it is important to have a basic understanding of neuroanatomy. Scientists are in the process of mapping the exact locations of specific brain functions. Box 4.1 describes several of the currently used brain imaging techniques helpful to this mapping.

The structure of the brain includes cells, nuclei, nerve tracts, hemispheres, and lobes. There are two types of *cells:* neurons and glial cells. Neurons consist of a cell body, dendrites, and an axon. The main function of the neuron is to receive and transmit stimuli using chemical and/or electrical energy. Glial cells are many times more numerous than neurons. Glial cells regulate groups of neurons by controlling the concentration of neurotransmitters and ions. They even release their own neurotransmitters, causing dramatic changes in nearby neurons. Neurons and glial cells are embedded in a matrix that contains growth factors, sugars, and proteins. *Nuclei* are dense collections of nerve cells with common functions. *Nerve tracts* are groups of nerve fibers carrying signals to and from the same area. The two main nerve tracts are the corpus callosum and the cingulum. The *corpus callosum* is a large body of nerve fibers that connects the left and right cerebral hemispheres and relays sensory information between the two. The *cingulum* is the main information highway of emotion. It integrates emotions with thinking in order to send a coherent message to the hypothalamus (Medina, 1996; Moller and Murphy, 1996).

Box 4.1

Brain Imaging Techniques

Positron Emission Tomography (PET)

Mapping via computer imaging that measures physiological processes in the brain such as blood flow, metabolic functions based on glucose utilization, density of neurotransmitters, location of neuroreceptors, and intricate brain circuitry.

Single Photon Emission Computerized Tomography (SPECT)

Measures the same physiological processes as PET but costs less and is more widely available; useful in monitoring the effects of medications on brain functions.

Neurometrics

Measures the electrophysiology of the brain, especially increased or decreased beta, alpha, theta, and delta waves.

Cerebral Blood Flow (CBF)

Measures the circulation of blood in a given brain region; blood flow to both gray matter and white matter can be determined.

Computer Electroencephalographic Tomography (CET)

Converts electrical signals into an electrical activity map of the brain; less accurate than PET but costs less and can be repeated without risk.

Magnetic Resonance Imaging (MRI)

Distinguishes gray and white matter in three dimensions; identifies structural abnormalities.

Magnetic Resonance Spectroscopy (MRS)

Expands MRI readings by adding radioactive tracers; identifies structural abnormalities in three dimensions as well as physiological abnormalities.

Cerebrum

The cerebrum, which constitutes 80% of the weight of the entire brain, consists of the two cerebral hemispheres, the cerebral cortex and its inner structures, and the deep structures of the basal ganglia. Each of the hemispheres has separate and unique functions.

Yet if one hemisphere is damaged, the other hemisphere seems to be able to take on some of its functions. The cerebral hemispheres are the sites of perceptual, cognitive, and higher motor functions, as well as emotion and memory.

Research indicates that hemispheric dysfunction is implicated in **alexithymia,** the inability to analyze, interpret, and name physical feelings and emotions (Hedaya, 1996). Many people with a variety of mental disorders experience this symptom and complain of feeling numb, both emotionally and physically. For example, people with alexithymia have difficulty sensing the presence of a hand on the arm or leg. A simple way to assess for this symptom is to ask them to put their hand on their leg. Then ask if they can feel their hand touching the leg and if their leg can feel the sensation of the hand. They will not be able to distinguish these sensations if they have alexithymia.

The outer portion of each hemisphere is called the *cortex*, which is divided into four lobes named for the bones of the skull under which they lie: frontal, temporal, parietal, and occipital. Each lobe has sensory, motor, and motivational synaptic relays and controls both sensory and motor processing and functioning. Damage to the lobes affects cognitive, perceptual, behavioral, and complex motor functions. Figure 4.1 shows the locations of the four cerebral lobes.

Frontal Lobe

The frontal lobe is the site of our ability to think, plan, and control movement. Specific functions include general motor ability and the motor aspects of spoken and written speech. The frontal lobe also regulates emotions and behavior and stability of the personality, and inhibits primitive emotional responses. Our ability to be motivated and follow through on plans is centered in this lobe. Another frontal lobe function is self-awareness, including our ability for self-evaluation and self-understanding, or *insight.*

Parietal Lobe

The parietal lobe is the site of the sensory functions of touch and temperature, and the perception of pain. Additional sensory functions include speech and the ability to recognize written words: to read the word "tree" and visualize a tree.

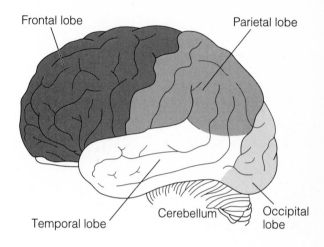

Figure 4.1 **The four lobes of the brain.**

A significant function of the parietal lobe is **proprioception,** the ability to know where our body is in time and space (position sense). An example of disordered proprioception frequently reported by people with mental disorders is the inability to see in three dimensions. This impairment may contribute to difficulty dressing, eating, and drinking in an organized manner. The parietal lobe also regulates the ability to evaluate muscular activity. This lobe may control a person's capacity to sit motionless for hours or to hold a single body part in one position for long periods of time. Another function of the parietal lobe is the ability to associate the memory of primary sensory experiences with more complex memories. Dysregulation of this function may result in repeating the same mistake over and over (Moller and Murphy, 1996).

Temporal Lobe

The temporal lobe is the site of the complex processes of memory, judgment, learning, and hearing. It also controls the production and understanding of speech, and is involved in the process of auditory hallucinations. It connects with the limbic system to allow for memory and the expression of emotions. Another temporal lobe function is gender identity, the sense of

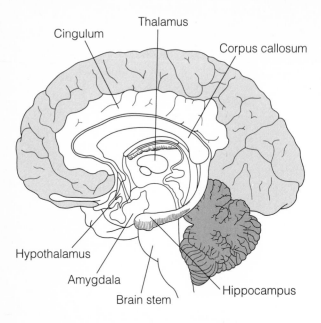

Figure 4.2 **Major structures of the limbic system.**

being female or male. It is important to distinguish gender identity from sexual identity or orientation, the site of which is deep inside the brain (Moller and Murphy, 1996).

Occipital Lobe

The occipital lobe is our visual center. It is responsible for sight and the ability to understand written words. It is also involved in producing visual hallucinations.

Limbic System

The limbic system is often referred to as "the emotional brain." Emotional responses such as anger, fear, anxiety, pleasure, sorrow, and sexual feelings are generated in the limbic system but are interpreted in the frontal lobe. Another function of the limbic system is the interpretation of our most basic and primitive sense: the sense of smell. The limbic system is thought to be the site of olfactory hallucinations. The ability to interpret sensations from the internal organs, referred to as visceral reflexes, also resides in this region (Hedaya, 1996).

The limbic system consists of portions of the frontal, parietal, and temporal lobes that form a con-

tinuous band of cortex in a ringlike formation around the top of the brain stem (Figure 4.2). Other structures of the limbic system are the amygdala and hippocampus. The *amygdala* coordinates the actions of the autonomic nervous system and the endocrine system and is involved in the control of emotions. When something scares or otherwise upsets us, the amygdala stamps that moment in memory. From then on, when something seems to resemble that original moment of distress, the amygdala recognizes the similarity and dictates our response in a few 100ths of a second, even before the stimulus reaches the cognitive centers of our brains. Dysfunction in the amygdala contributes to inappropriate rage and fear. The *hippocampus* is intricately involved in regulation of the immune system and in memory storage. Damage or incomplete formation of the hippocampus results in declarative memory impairment. People with hippocampal dysfunction appear to resist learning and may be perceived as lazy or unmotivated, when in fact they are unable to recall previously learned information.

Other limbic structures include the thalamus and hypothalamus. The *thalamus* enables us to have impressions of agreeableness or disagreeableness in response to sensations. It monitors sensory input and acts as a relay station in processing nearly all sensory and motor information coming from the spinal cord, brain stem, and cerebellum. The thalamus is thought to regulate levels of awareness and emotional aspects of sensory experiences by exerting a wide variety of effects on the cortex (Hedaya, 1996).

Thalamic dysfunction is involved in obsessive-compulsive disorder, schizophrenia, and the mood disorders, and contributes to the similarity in symptoms experienced by various people diagnosed with mental disorders. Dysfunction within the thalamus also makes it difficult for people to sense pain. A person with schizophrenia, for example, may experience flulike symptoms when there is actually a ruptured appendix.

The *hypothalamus* is a neuroendocrine (neurons which produce hormones) group of nuclei that is vital to homeostasis. As an integration center, the hypothalamus converts thinking and feeling into hormones, causing physical changes throughout the body via the autonomic nervous system. With the pituitary gland, the hypothalamus helps regulate the autonomic nervous system by assisting with the vital functions of water balance, blood pressure, sleep, appetite, temperature, and carbohydrate and fat metabolism.

Dysregulation can lead to excessive thirst and insatiable hunger. The hypothalamus may be involved in anorexia nervosa and bulimia nervosa. As one of the main concentration sites of the neurotransmitter dopamine, the hypothalamus is implicated in many of the common side effects of psychotropic medications that influence dopamine transmission (Hedaya, 1996).

Brain Stem

The brain stem, consisting of the midbrain, pons, and medulla, is the location of those functions vital to sustaining life. Such functions include the central processing of respiration, heart rate, balance, and blood pressure. The brain stem is also the home of the twelve cranial nerves, which carry sensory and motor information to and from higher brain regions. Two tiny structures, the locus ceruleus and the substantia nigra, produce norepinephrine and dopamine, respectively.

A network of neurons extending throughout the structures of the brain stem is known as the *reticular activating system* (RAS). The RAS controls both inhibitory and excitatory functions by receiving impulses from all over the body and relaying them to the cortex. It is the central structure in the brain responsible for arousal, wakefulness, consciousness, sleep regulation, and learning. It may influence whether our behavior is aggressive or passive. The relationship between RAS dysfunction and mental disorders is not well understood at this time.

Cerebellum

The cerebellum, which wraps around the brain stem, has a unique appearance and is composed of several lobes. The cerebellum helps coordinate the planning, timing, and patterning of skeletal muscle contractions during movement. It is the cerebellum that enables us to grasp a glass on the first try and walk in an upright manner. It maintains our posture and equilibrium by receiving input about balance from the inner ear. The cerebellum is responsible for the storage, retrieval, and use of procedural memory. Procedural memory impairments include difficulty performing tasks that are normally habitual, such as brushing teeth and getting dressed.

Table 4.2 summarizes the structures and functions of the brain and is a guide for the neuro-anatomical locations of dysfunctions.

Blood-Brain Barrier

Unlike capillaries throughout the rest of the body, brain capillary pores do not allow free movement of substances. Rather, the capillary endothelial cells use selective pinocytosis, the process by which these cells absorb various substances. There are two major functions of this blood-brain barrier. The first is to import critical nutrients, hormones, and drugs while exporting metabolic waste products. The second function is to protect the brain against the influx of toxins and other damaging substances, thus ensuring brain homeostasis.

Neurophysiology

We are all subject to fluctuations in brain chemistry. The structures of the brain depend on hundreds of chemicals—glucose, vitamins, minerals, amino acids, and neurotransmitters—to carry out their functions. As our brain chemistry fluctuates, we all experience episodic problems with speech patterns, memory recall, spontaneous decision making, and any or all of the other higher brain functions. In fact, during REM sleep, each of us experiences "symptoms" of mental illness. Box 4.2 describes what happens when we sleep. People who experience more severe disruptions in brain chemistry may exhibit symptoms of mental disorders.

Neurotransmission

Neurotransmission is the electrochemical process that allows nerve signals to pass from one cell to another at the synapse, the microscopic area where two neurons meet. As the impulse travels through the axon of a neuron, storage vesicles release neurotransmitters, which diffuse across the synapse and latch on to receptors. Receptors are docking sites on the dendrites of the second, or postsynaptic, nerve cell, and are specific to one neurotransmitter. Binding of the neurotransmitter to the receptor triggers the activation of the second cell. Once the transmitter completes its function, the receptor releases it back into the synapse. At this point, one of two things happens: the transmitter is deactivated by an enzyme or transporters take the transmitter back into the presynaptic terminal (reuptake). Transporters allow the body to recycle previously used transmitters so they do not

Table 4.2 **Major Brain Structures: Functions and Dysfunctions**

Structure	Functions	Effects of Dysfunction
Frontal lobe	Ability to think and plan	Difficulty with abstract thinking, attention, concentration; lack of motivation.
	Insight	Inability for self-evaluation.
	Stability of personality	Instability of personality.
	Inhibition of primitive emotional responses	Labile affect; irritability; impulsiveness; inappropriate behavior.
	Motor aspects of written speech	Unintelligible and illogical writing.
	Motor aspects of spoken speech	Words are garbled and difficult to understand.
Parietal lobe	Receiving and identifying sensory information	Inability to recognize sensations such as pain, touch, temperature; inability to sense pain from an uncomfortable body position.
	Memory association	Inability to learn from past.
	Proprioception	Inability to recognize the body in relation to the environment.
		Difficulty dressing, eating, etc. in an organized manner.
	Sensory speech	Inability to recognize spoken or written words.
Temporal lobe	Hearing	Auditory hallucinations.
	Complex memory	Memory impairment; difficulty learning.
	Emotion	Difficulty recognizing own emotions and controlling sexual and aggressive drives.
	Sexual identity	Confusion about masculinity and femininity.
	Production of speech	Types of aphasia.
	Analysis of speech	Difficulty attaching meaning to spoken words.
Occipital lobe	Vision	Visual hallucinations; loss of visual memory.
	Visual speech	Inability to understand the meaning of written words.
Limbic system	Regulation of emotional responses	Excessive emotional responses; inability to recognize own emotions; decreased ability of cognition to affect emotions.
	Interpretation of smell	Olfactory hallucinations; inability to interpret smell.
	Memory storage	Difficulty with declarative memory.
		Short-term and long-term memory problems; difficulty learning.
	Impressions of agreeableness or disagreeableness of sensations	Hypersensitivity or hyposensitivity to pain.
	Regulation of autonomic nervous system	Increased thirst; insatiable hunger.
Reticular activating system (RAS)	Receiving of impulses from entire body and relaying to cortex	Sedation and loss of consciousness; difficulty controlling aggression; may contribute to passivity.
Cerebellum	Coordination of skeletal muscles during movement	Difficulty learning motor skills; problems regulating the force and range of movements.
	Maintenance of equilibrium	Problems with balance.
	Maintenance of posture	Difficulty walking upright.

Box 4.2

How the Brain Goes Out of Its Mind

Every 80–90 minutes, during REM sleep, we become completely psychotic.

Experience	**Psychiatric Label**
We see things that are not there.	Hallucinations.
We believe things that could not possibly be true.	Delusions, magical thinking.
We become confused about times, places, and persons.	Disorientation.
Scenes simply appear and thoughts come unbidden.	Attention deficit.
We think we are awake even though we are doing and seeing impossible things.	Lack of insight
We experience wildly fluctuating emotions.	Labile affect.
We invent implausible narratives.	Confabulation, loose association.
We forget almost everything on awakening.	Amnesia.

This nocturnal madness is not only normal but probably essential to our health. Deprived of REM sleep, we become anxious and irritable, and have trouble concentrating. Understanding this normal delirium may help you become more empathetic with persons experiencing those same symptoms while awake.

Sources: Hobson 1996; LaBerge, Rheingold, 1990.

---

have to be replaced by biosynthesis (Blakely, 1996; Hayes, 1995; Thase and Howard, 1995). Figure 4.3 shows how neurotransmission occurs.

A number of factors may influence the process of neurotransmission. **Receptor antagonists** are substances that block receptor sites, thereby inhibiting or eliminating neurotransmission. **Receptor agonists** are substances other than the specific neurotransmitter that are capable of stimulating the receptor. Both antagonists and agonists can work strongly or weakly. Several alterations can occur during neurotransmission. Neurotransmitters may be deactivated or returned to the presynaptic terminal before they reach the receptors. The postsynaptic neuron can be temporarily deactivated so it fails to respond to the stimulus. Neurotransmitters can act together to enhance transmission of impulses while at other times they act as antagonists—with one neurotransmitter inhibiting the action of another. There are also molecules called phosphoproteins that serve as "on" and "off" switches along the pathway of neurotransmission. **Neuromodulators** are chemicals that alter the

threshold to the flow of information but do not necessarily alter the nature of the signal. They act as filters, allowing more or less information to be processed. As you can see, the process of neurotransmission is complicated with potential for errors at many points along the way (Ruden, 1997; Vanchieri, 1996). See Box 4.3 for factors influencing the rate of neurotransmission.

Neurotransmitters

Neurotransmitters act, as the word implies, to transmit signals from one neuron to another. They alter the frequency and intensity of the messages being sent. The greater the amount of neurotransmitters, the stronger the message. Neurons in different parts of the brain contain different neurotransmitters. Most neurons have numerous receptor types for a variety of neurotransmitters, enabling each neuron to receive many different signals. In addition, there are several types of receptor sites for each neurotransmitter. For

When a nerve impulse arrives at a presynaptic neuron, neurotransmitters are released from storage to carry the nerve impulse across the synapse to the next neuron.

Neurotransmitters attach to specific receptor sites on the postsynaptic neuron.

Receptors release the neurotransmitters back into the synapse. Many are taken back into the presynaptic neuron by transporters through a process called reuptake. Some of the neurotransmitters are deactivated by enzymes. In addition to reuptake, a fresh supply of neurotransmitters is made by and stored in the neuron.

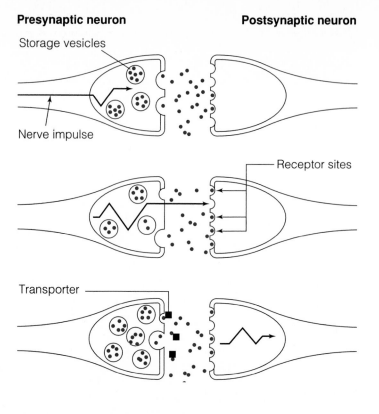

Figure 4.3 **Neurotransmission.**

Source: Adapted from material of Merrell Dow Pharmaceuticals.

example, there are 5 dopamine receptor types and 14 serotonin receptor types.

Neurotransmitters are separated into three categories: **biogenic amines, amino acids,** and **peptides.** It is difficult to fully appreciate the role of neurotransmitters; entire textbooks are devoted to each of them. Neurotransmitters do not operate in isolation. Much like a symphonic orchestra, they interact with each other and function as a group. It is believed that when dysfunctions occur with some neurotransmitters, others adapt and compensate for the dysfunction (Hayes, 1995). Table 4.3 on page 80 presents the basic functions and dysfunctions of the major neurotransmitters. You may want to review the principles of psychopharmacology in Chapter 8 after you read this section, as each category of medication affects one or more of the neurotransmitters.

Biogenic Amines

The biogenic amines are more often implicated in the psychobiology of mental disorders. There are six biogenic amine neurotransmitters: dopamine, serotonin, norepinephrine and epinephrine, acetylcholine, and histamine. They are synthesized in the neuron and are derived from two dietary amino acids: tyrosine and L-tryptophan.

Dopamine   Dopamine (DA) is considered the grandparent of neurotransmitters. It is a catecholamine from which norepinephrine and epinephrine are metabolized. An excess or deficit amount of DA affects the levels of these other neurotransmitters. DA greatly influences thought processing. It has been compared to the card catalog system in a library; as it is responsible for "sorting through" information and retrieving what is pertinent to the situation. Alterations in DA levels directly affect the ability of the frontal lobe to mediate abstract thinking. **Abstract thinking** is the ability to generalize information, make predictions, build on prior memory, and evaluate the consequences of decisions. In the absence of abstract thought, thinking becomes concrete. **Concrete thinking** is characterized by a focus on facts and details, a literal interpretation of messages, and an inability to

Box 4.3

Factors Influencing Rate of Neurotransmission

Speed Up Neurotransmission

- High level of precursors
- Increased synthesis of transmitters
- More transmitters in storage sites
- More transmitters released
- Greater number of receptors
- Slower reuptake process
- Fewer transmitters deactivated

Slow Down Neurotransmission

- Low level of precursors
- Decreased synthesis of transmitters
- Fewer transmitters in storage sites
- Fewer transmitters released
- Not enough receptors
- Faster reuptake process
- Too many transmitters deactivated

generalize. Concrete thinking is a significant problem in people with mental disorders because it results in impulsiveness, instant need gratification, egocentricity, and an inability to follow a multiple-stage command.

High levels of DA are reflected in sharper thinking, focused attention, and motivation to act and find what you need for survival. When you perceive that you need something, DA directs your motor system to move your body to get it. DA is also what makes you smile and feel alert and energetic. It drives you to seek pleasure and rewards and takes you on an emotional high. DA is the "gotta have it" neurotransmitter, the facilitator, and the motivator and as such is involved in most addictions from cigarettes to drug abuse to hypersexuality (Ruden, 1997).

Serotonin In contrast to DA, serotonin (5-HT) is the soother, the constrainer, and the anti-impulsive neurotransmitter. 5-HT acts to balance DA. It decreases your focus and flow of information and is what you need when you are feeling overwhelmed. 5-HT is the "got it" neurotransmitter, allowing you to stop a particular behavior when you have achieved what you need. For example, when you are hungry

DA drives you to search for food and 5-HT lets you know when you have had enough to eat. Without 5-HT you would be unable to stop eating once you found food (Ruden, 1997).

5-HT also facilitates social behavior by decreasing anxiety and increasing a sense of calmness. Abnormally low levels of 5-HT result in decreased impulse control, aggression, and violence.

Serotonin (5-HT) is quickly becoming the most widely researched neurotransmitter because of its broad range of functions. 5-HT tends to control the activity of other neurotransmitters and is the key player in all brain functions related to circadian rhythms. It is synthesized from the dietary amino acid tryptophan, most commonly found in milk.

A significant research finding relevant to mental health nursing is that isolation reduces 5-HT levels (Hedaya, 1996). This finding helps to explain some of the devastating effects of seclusion on many clients. The converse is also true. Spending time in the company of people who are trusted can raise 5-HT levels. Cocaine, alcohol, and nicotine are known to reduce 5-HT levels. Antidepressants are the primary drugs that affect 5-HT receptors.

Norepinephrine and Epinephrine Norepinephrine (NE) and epinephrine (E) are derived from dopamine and are the adrenaline of the brain. Although NE accounts for only 1% of all available neurotransmitter content, we are very sensitive to even the smallest fluctuations. NE and E function similarly to DA, with a role in regulation of mood, memory, cognition, energy, and appetite.

Acetylcholine Acetylcholine (ACH) is found in abundance in the brain and is the guardian angel of the parasympathetic nervous system. ACH continually strives to keep the sympathetic nervous system in check. DA and ACH function in relative balance. ACH is thought to greatly influence learning and memory; it may also be involved in mood and sleep disorders. Other effects include emotional regulation, social play, exploration, thermoregulation, water intake, and motor function.

Histamine Little is known about the functions of histamine as a neurotransmitter. We do know that histamine is involved in allergic reaction and may be involved in the medication side effects of sedation and hypotension. Recent research has suggested that histamine plays a role in sexual behavior.

Table 4.3 Neurotransmitters: Functions and Dysfunctions

Neurotransmitter	Functions	Effects of Excess	Effects of Deficit
Dopamine (DA)	Abstract thinking, decision making Ability to respond with reward-seeking behaviors Fine muscle movements Integration of thoughts and emotions Stimulation of hypothalamus to release hormones Increase in sex drive, facilitation of orgasm	Mild: Enhanced creativity and problem solving; ability to generalize situations; good spatial ability; premature ejaculation. Severe: Disorganized thinking, loose associations; disabling compulsions; tics; stereotypic behaviors.	Mild: Poor impulse control; poor spatial ability; inability to think abstractly; no joy, no anticipation of pleasure. Severe: Parkinson's disease; endocrine changes; movement disorders.
Norepinephine (NE) **Epinephrine (E)**	Alertness, ability to focus attention, ability to be oriented Necessary for learning and memory Primes nervous system for fight or flight	Hyperalertness; anxiety, panic. Paranoia. Loss of appetite Increased sensation-seeking behaviors.	Dullness, low energy. Depression.
Serotonin (5-HT)	Inhibition of activity; calmness, contentedness. Regulation of temperature and sleep cycle. Pain perception. Precursor to melatonin, which plays a role in circadian rhythms.	Sedation; decreased anxiety. Increased sleep. Decreased sex drive; decreased orgasms. Indecision. Craving for sweets and carbohydrates. If greatly increased, may have hallucinations.	Irritability, hostility; increased aggression. Decreased impulse control; increased suicidal tendencies. Insomnia. Increased sex drive.
Acetlycholine (ACH)	Preparation for action; stimulation of parasympathetic system. Emotional regulation. Social play, exploration. Control of muscle tone by balance with DA.	Self-consciousness, excessive inhibition; anxiety. Somatic complaints. Depression.	Lack of inhibition; euphoria. Poor short-term memory. Antisocial behaviors. Parkinson's disease.
GABA	Calmness, contentedness. Reduction of aggression.	Sedation. Impaired recent memory. Anticonvulsant.	Irritability. Lack of coordination. Seizures.

Amino Acids

The major excitatory amino acid neurotransmitters are glutamate (Gle) and aspartate. The major inhibitory amino acid neurotransmitters are glycine and GABA. Most amino acids can be made in the body.

Gamma Aminobutyric Acid   Gamma aminobutyric acid (GABA) is present in 30% of the synapses. GABA is the neurotransmitter that regulates anxiety and influences muscular coordination. Deficiencies can cause a high level of tension and anxiety as well as a lack of coordination. GABA may play a role in cognition, memory, and aggressive behavior. It is also one of the neurotransmitters involved in antianxiety-agent dependence. Antianxiety agents partially fill the receptor sites normally filled by GABA, and the normal production of GABA is reduced. Over time, the brain becomes reliant on the antianxiety agents to fill the receptor sites, and dependency results.

Peptides

Peptide neurotransmitters include substance P, neurotension, L-tryptophan (L-T), glycine, neuropeptide Y (NPY), and cholecystokinin (CCK). These neurotransmitters were discovered only recently and their functions are poorly understood. Since they are often found in the same neuron with other neurotransmitters, they may serve as modulators for other transmitters, the neuroendocrine system, and the autonomic system.

Other Neurotransmitters

In order for a substance to be classified as a neurotransmitter, it must be synthesized and stored in neurons, be released when stimulated, have specific receptor sites, and affect the rate of neurotransmission. New neurotransmitters are being discovered rapidly. Recent research suggests that nitrous oxide (laughing gas) and carbon monoxide are produced by neurons. These gases seem to carry signals over short distances and may in the future be classified as neurotransmitters (Hedaya, 1996).

Neurohormones

Hormones are chemical substances produced by cells within an organ or gland. Hormones are manufactured and stored in the cells. When the cells receive the appropriate signal, usually from the nervous system, they release an appropriate amount of the stored hormone into the circulatory system. Neurohormones are those hormones that act as neurotransmitters or modify the actions of neurotransmitters. The significant neurohormones are endorphin, DHEA, oxytocin, vasopressin, and PEA.

Endorphin

Endorphin is an opioid that we produce in the brain from a complex chain of amino acids. It plays a significant role in our ability to experience pleasure and it helps protect us from pain. Being touched and stroked by another person increases the amount of endorphin in our brain. Endorphin also increases when we smile and when we think positive thoughts. We may smile because we are experiencing a surge of endorphin or we may get a surge of endorphin when we smile.

DHEA

There is more DHEA (dehydroepiandrosterone) in our bodies than any other hormone. It could be called the parent of all hormones because most of our other hormones are derived from it. Although most of our DHEA is produced by the adrenals, our brain can make its own. DHEA improves cognition, protects the immune system, decreases cholesterol, promotes bone growth, and serves as an antidepressant. As the precursor of pheromones, it influences who we find attractive and who is attracted to us. DHEA serves as a natural aphrodisiac and increases in the brain during orgasm (Crenshaw, 1996).

Oxytocin

Oxytocin in secreted from the pituitary gland and travels to receptor sites in various parts of the brain as well as to the reproductive tract. It increases DA, 5-HT, estrogen, testosterone, prolactin, and vasopressin. Oxytocin promotes touching and is instrumental in the bonding between mates and between parents and children. It decreases cognition and impairs memory.

Vasopressin

Vasopressin balances oxytocin's influence. It improves cognition through enhancing attention and alertness while reducing emotional extremes. One benefit of vasopressin is its influence on how we think. It focuses us on the present moment and helps us pay attention to what we are doing. It is an antidote for both anxiety and depression.

Table 4.4 Causes of Brain Dysregulation

Cause	Source	Clinical Implications
Anatomical abnormalities	Trauma Brain tumors Problems in brain development	Difficulty in information processing and coping with daily life stresses
Lack of oxygen and/or glucose	Blood flow to brain slowed Lack of oxygen in blood Insufficient food intake	Symptoms of dementia, delirium, and schizophrenia
Alteration in electrolytes	Insufficient food intake Disordered electrolyte balance	Behavior may be stuporous or manic. Hallucinations and delusions may occur. Anxiety may be experienced.
Neurotransmitter dysfunction	Substance abuse Diets high in sugar and fat Genetic influence	Symptoms of depression, bipolar disorder, schizophrenia, and panic disorder. Difficulty in information processing and coping with daily life stressors.

PEA

PEA (phenylethylamine) is a natural form of amphetamine produced in our brain and fluctuates according to our thoughts, feelings, and experiences. It is believed that PEA is our "hormone of love," rising to high levels during romantic times in our lives and possibly involved in love at first sight. Low levels of PEA have been associated with depression and high levels may contribute to psychotic symptoms.

Psychonutrition

All phases of neurotransmission are affected by nutrition. Glucose is needed for neurotransmitter synthesis and secretion. Other necessary nutrients are amino acids, vitamins, minerals, and essential fatty acids. For example, B vitamins are necessary for synthesis of 5-HT and GABA, tryptophan is a precursor of 5-HT, choline is necessary for ACH synthesis, copper and tyrosine are needed for DA synthesis, carnitine promotes cognition, magnesium is involved in sleep, and vitamin C is needed to cope with stress (Hayes, 1995). As a nurse, you must be able to asses the client's nutritional status and dietary habits. Interventions may include supplemental vitamins and diet prescription.

Dysregulation

The ability to function and problem-solve in everyday life depends on how the brain functions and processes information. Dysregulation of the brain, regardless of the cause, results in disruption of the ability to process information. There are four main causes of brain dysregulation: anatomical abnormalities or damage, lack of oxygen and/or glucose, electrolyte imbalance, and neurotransmitter dysfunction (McCrane, 1996; Moller and Murphy, 1996). See Table 4.4 for specific examples of dysregulation. It is important that you understand the current information in biological psychiatry in order to respond to the client as a bio-psycho-social-spiritual being.

Key Concepts

Introduction

- Mental disorders are severe brain disorders that involve the brain, our hormones, our biochemistry, and our environment.

Development of the Brain

- Brain development results from constant interaction between genetic and environmental factors and occurs over three major developmental periods: organogenesis, rapid neuronal proliferation, and brain growth spurt.
- There are gender differences in brain anatomy, which may help explain gender-related differences in behavior.

Functions of the Brain

- The brain is the site of all integrative functions that govern our behavior, feelings, and thoughts.
- Declarative memory is memory relating to people and facts: the verbal expression of memory.
- Procedural memory is the memory of motor skills: the behavioral expression of memory.
- Loose association is thinking in which there is no apparent relationship between thoughts.
- Illogical thinking is characterized by inconsistent, irrational, or self-contradictory ideas.
- In tangential speech, thoughts veer from the main idea and never get back to it.
- In circumstantial speech, the person includes many unnecessary and insignificant details before arriving at the main idea.
- Pressured speech is tense, strained, and difficult to interrupt.

Neuroanatomy

- The main function of a neuron is to receive and transmit stimuli using electrochemical energy.
- Glial cells regulate groups of neurons by controlling the concentration of neurotransmitters and ions.
- Nuclei are dense collections of nerve cells with common functions.

- Nerve tracts are groups of nerve fibers carrying signals to and from the same area.
- The corpus callosum is a large body of nerve fibers connecting the left and right hemispheres.
- The cingulum integrates emotions with thinking to send a coherent message to the hypothalamus.
- The cerebral hemispheres are the sites of perceptual, cognitive, and higher motor functions, as well as emotion and memory.
- Alexithymia is the inability to analyze, interpret, and name physical feelings and emotions.
- The frontal lobe is the site of the ability to think and plan, control movement, and develop insight. It regulates the motor aspects of written and spoken speech, maintains the stability of the personality, inhibits primitive emotional responses, and regulates emotions and behavior.
- The parietal lobe is the site of receiving and identifying sensory information, memory association, proprioception, and sensory speech.
- The temporal lobe is the site of hearing, complex memory, emotions, sexual identity, and the production and understanding of speech.
- The occipital lobe is the site of vision and the ability to understand written words.
- The limbic system is the site of regulation of emotional responses, interpretation of smell, memory storage, and impressions of agreeableness or disagreeableness of sensations; it helps to regulate the autonomic nervous system.
- The reticular activating system (RAS) in the brain stem receives impulses from the entire body and relays them to the cortex.
- The cerebellum coordinates skeletal muscles during movement and maintains equilibrium and posture.
- The blood-brain barrier imports critical nutrients, exports metabolic waste products, and protects the brain against the influx of toxins.

Neurophysiology

- In neurotransmission, a cell releases neurotransmitters that diffuse across the synapse and activate the second cell by latching onto its receptors; after a transmitter fulfills its function, the receptor releases it back into the synapse, where it is either deactivated by an enzyme or transported back into the presynaptic terminal (reuptake).

- Receptor antagonists are substances that block receptor sites, thereby inhibiting neurotransmission.

- Receptor agonists are substances other than the receptor's specific neurotransmitter that are capable of stimulating the receptor.

- There are three categories of neurotransmitters: biogenic amines, amino acids, and peptides.

- Dopamine (DA) greatly influences thought processing, abstract thinking, muscular coordination, emotional responses, memory, and coping abilities; it makes you feel alert and energetic and takes you on an emotional high.

- Norepinephrine (NE) and epinephrine (E) play a role in mood, memory and cognitive functions, energy, and appetite.

- Serotonin (5-HT) is necessary for circadian rhythms and tends to control the activity of other neurotransmitters.

- Acetylcholine (ACH) is involved in the parasympathetic nervous system and has an effect on mood, sleep, and memory.

- Gamma aminobutyric acid (GABA) is an inhibitory neurotransmitter that is involved in neuromuscular coordination and in antianxiety-agent dependence.

- Endorphin is a neurohormone that has a significant role in the ability to experience pleasure.

- Most other hormones are derived from DHEA; DHEA improves cognition, protects the immune system, and serves as an antidepressant.

- Oxytocin promotes touching and is instrumental in the bonding process; it decreases cognition and impairs memory.

- Vasopressin improves cognition by enhancing attention and alertness.

- PEA is a natural form of amphetamine in our brain; low levels may contribute to depression and high levels may contribute to psychotic symptoms.

- All phases of neurotransmission are affected by nutrition.

- Dysregulation of the brain results in disruption of the ability to process information.

Review Questions

1. Because of his problems with procedural memory, you would expect Joe not to remember
   a. that you are his nurse.
   b. how to brush his teeth.
   c. his address and phone number.
   d. what he ate for breakfast.

2. Which of the following problems will Marc experience as the result of frontal lobe dysfunction?
   a. inability to see in three dimensions
   b. inability to understand what you are saying
   c. inability to follow through on plans
   d. inability to understand written words

3. Your client is experiencing auditory hallucinations. You know that this is most likely from a dysfunction in the
   a. occipital lobe.
   b. temporal lobe.
   c. parietal lobe.
   d. frontal lobe.

4. Asela says to you, "Where did you come from? Mars is in outer space. Do you work for the government? I like your shirt. When can I go home?" This is an example of
   a. loose association.
   b. tangential speech.
   c. circumstantial speech.
   d. concrete thinking.

5. Which of the following neurotransmitters tends to control the activity of the other neurotransmitters and is the key player in circadian rhythms?
   a. dopamine
   b. norepinephrine
   c. acetylcholine
   d. serotonin

References

Blakely, R. D. (1996). Norepinephrine and serotonin transporters. In S. J. Watson (Ed.), *Biology of Schizophrenia and Affective Disease* (pp. 49–81). Washington DC: APA Press.

Crenshaw, T. L. (1996). *The Alchemy of Love and Lust.* New York: GP Putnam's Sons.

Gur, R. C., et al. (1995). Sex differences in regional cerebral glucose metabolism during a resting state. *Science. 267*(5197), 528–531.

Hayes, A. (1995). Psychiatric nursing: What does biology have to do with it? *Arch Psychiatr Nurs. 9*(4), 216–224.

Hedaya, R. J. (1996). *Understanding Biological Psychiatry*. New York: WW Norton.

Hobson, J. A. (1996). How the brain goes out of its mind. *Harvard Mental Health Letter. 12*(8): 3–5.

LaBerge, S., Rheingold, H. (1990). *Exploring the World of Lucid Dreaming*. New York: Ballentine Books.

McCrane, S. H. (1996). The impact of the evolution of biological psychiatry on psychiatric nursing. *J Psychosoc Nurs. 34*(1), 38–46.

Medina, S. (1996). Genetic study of human behavior. *Harvard Mental Health Letter. 12*(10), 4–5.

Moller, M. D., & Murphy, M. F. (1996). *Recovering From Psychosis: A Wellness Approach*. Psych Rehab Nurses.

Ruden, R. A. (1997). *The Craving Brain*. New York: HarperCollins.

Thase, M. E., & Howard, R. H. (1995). Biological processes in depression. In E. E. Beckham & W. R. Weber (Eds.), *Handbook of Depression* (2nd ed.) (pp. 213–279). New York: Guilford Press.

Vanchieri, C. (1996, Winter). Tracing the intricacies of the dopamine pathway. *NARSAD Research Newsletter,* 1–3.

Skills for Clinical Practice

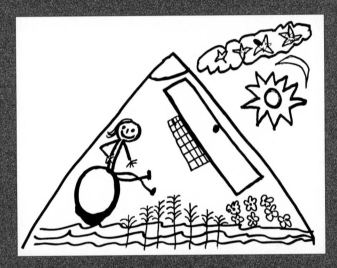

A SAFE PLACE: *I am sitting on a large rock founded in the tranquillity of the water, relaxed and happy, contented viewing the spacious beautiful world at its best. A large window of my soul to appreciate the beauty & wonder of it all. A large door—a passageway of choices; to open the door, to pursue and develop all my hopes and dreams.*

CHAPTER 5

Communicating and Teaching

Karen Lee Fontaine

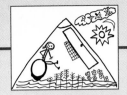

Objectives

After reading this chapter, you will be able to:

- Explain the significance of nonverbal communication.
- Discuss the characteristics of effective helpers.
- Describe effective communication techniques.
- Assess client areas of learning.
- Identify informal and formal teaching methods.

C ommunication is the foundation of interpersonal relationships and is a key factor in the nursing process. The purpose of communication is twofold: to give and receive information, and to make contact between people. As a student in mental health nursing, you use communication to assess clients and families as well as to implement your plan of care (giving and receiving information). Communication is also the means by which you initiate and establish relationships with clients (interpersonal contact). Clients use communication to share their feelings, express their thoughts, and tell you about their lives. Through interpersonal contact with you, clients and families learn more effective and adaptive ways of communicating with others.

The Nature of Communication

People often assume that communication is merely one person giving information to another person. However, communication is much more complex than the transfer of information. Communication takes place in the context of the people involved. To analyze communication, you must consider spoken words, paralanguage (sounds), the thinking process, emotions, nonverbal behavior, and the culture of the person who is sending the message. How the message is heard depends on the listening skills, analysis of the message, emotions, and culture of the person who is receiving the message. Figure 5.1 illustrates the process of communication.

Effective communicators analyze their own and others' communication in terms of the behavioral, affective, and cognitive messages implied in the transfer of information. *Behavioral analysis* considers how accompanying nonverbal actions modify or enhance the verbal message. *Affective analysis* includes understanding the emotions involved in the communication, which are imparted both verbally and nonverbally. *Cognitive analysis* involves comprehension of the stated words as well as the thinking process of the person communicating. The cognitive component is communicated verbally or in writing. Analysis of *paralanguage*, or sounds, provides additional information about the message that is being transmitted: the rate of speech, tone of voice, and loudness of the voice. Paralanguage also includes sounds that are not words, such as laughing, sobbing, snorting, and clicking of the tongue. You must also analyze how *culture* influences communication. Much of our communication is influenced by our cultural norms, for example, the use of personal space, acceptable body language, the amount of eye contact, and the types of paralanguage.

Nonverbal Communication

Because two-thirds of communication is considered to be nonverbal, it is critical that you observe, understand, and respond to the nonverbal cues of your clients. You must also be a "self-observer," paying attention to what messages you are communicating nonverbally. *Body language* includes your position, posture, and movements. Sitting face to face with a person will encourage more interaction than sitting side by side. Removing barriers between the two of you, such as desks or tables, will facilitate communication. Standing over a client who is sitting is a dominating or intimidating position and will often interfere with effective communication. A rigid body posture may express anger or fear, while a relaxed body posture expresses openness and a feeling of safety. Leaning back may convey a message of distance and withdrawal; learning forward indicates warmth and receptivity. People who sit with their arms and legs tightly crossed appear to be protecting themselves from some real or perceived danger. A person whose body seems to be pulling in on itself may be experiencing depression and low self-esteem. Body movements such as finger tapping, leg swinging, and nail biting may signal frustration, anxiety, anger, or embarrassment. Gestures such as pointing fingers, hands on hips, and shoulder shrugs are all aspects of communication.

Eye contact is extremely important in initiating, encouraging, and terminating communication. The listener usually maintains more eye contact than the speaker. Raised eyebrows may indicate interest, while frowning eyes may express disagreement. Suspicion is often communicated with narrowed eyes. Increased eye contact may be a cue that a person is anxious.

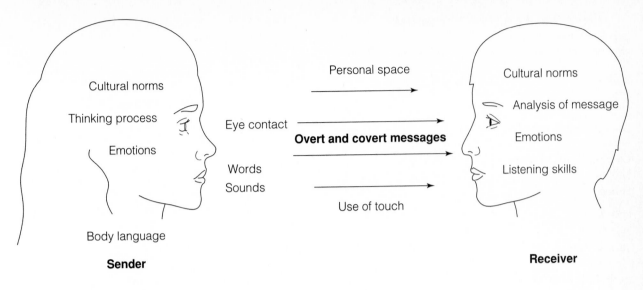

Figure 5.1 **The communication process.**

Minimal eye contact may be evidence of shyness, low self-esteem, or boredom with the interaction. Table 5.1 summarizes the forms of nonverbal communication.

Remember that different cultural and subcultural groups have varying patterns of nonverbal communication. Validate impressions and inferences with clients during the observing and interviewing processes. This is even more important when you and your client are from different cultural backgrounds. For example, in some cultures, minimal eye contact does not indicate low self-esteem or boredom but is considered polite and respectful.

Personal space and boundaries are culturally determined and may range anywhere from 2 inches to 2 feet (5–61 cm). In mental health nursing, it is essential to respect clients' boundaries and their need for personal space. This respect includes how closely you sit with clients, how much space you give them when walking together, and asking their permission before entering their room.

Touch is related to personal space and boundaries and is determined by cultural norms and previous experiences. In mental health nursing, the use of touch must be well thought out, so as to avoid misunderstandings. You must think about if, how, or when you might use touch with each client. It is usually better to ask people if you may touch their hands,

for example, than to make assumptions as to how comfortable they are with touch. Before touching others, ask yourself: What is the purpose of the touch? Is it appropriate? How might this person interpret the touch? With this kind of analysis, touch can be another form of nonverbal communication. The information in Table 5.2 gives clues to what might be the reasons behind certain cultural behaviors.

Listening

Failure to be heard and understood is painful. No one loses the need to communicate what it feels like in our own private world of experience. The importance of listening, as a part of communication, cannot be overestimated. Being listened to means that we are taken seriously, and the gift of someone else's attention and understanding makes us feel validated and valued. In opposition, not being listened to makes us feel ignored, unappreciated, cut off, and alone.

In order to listen well, we must interrupt our preoccupation with ourselves and enter into the experience of the other person. Successful communication occurs when you hear what people mean, not just what they say. Listening well is often silent but it is never passive. Listening means paying attention to what the person is saying, acknowledging feelings,

Table 5.1 Forms of Nonverbal Communication

Behavior	Possible Meaning
Standing	
At beginning or end of the interaction	Initiation or termination of the interaction
Over other person while talking	Intimidation or domination
Sitting	
Face to face	Interest
Side by side	Neutrality
Turned away	Termination of the interaction
At the edge of the chair	Anxiety or eagerness
Body Posture	
Relaxed	Friendliness, warmth
Rigid or tense	Fear or anger
Leaning back	Withdrawal, distance
Leaning forward	Interest, friendliness
Arms and/or legs tightly crossed	Self-protection, withdrawal
Shrinking in	Depression, low self-esteem
Turned away	Distance, withdrawal
Gestures	
Leg or foot shaking, finger tapping	Anxiety, frustration, anger
Fidgety, restless movements	Anxiety, embarrassment
Finger shaking, hands on hips	Authority, intimidation
Hiding hands	Shyness, insecurity
Fist-clenching	Anger, frustration
Wringing hands	Hopelessness, helplessness
Eyes	
Frequent eye contact	Interest, honesty
Minimal eye contact	Low self-esteem, shyness, boredom
Rapidly shifting eye contact	Confusion
Frequent blinking	Anxiety
Touch	
Touching arm or hand	Interest, concern

Sources: Collins, 1983; Navarra, Lipkowitz, and Navarra, 1990; Okun, 1987.

Table 5.2 Nonverbal Communication of Major Ethnic Groups in the United States

Group	Nonverbal Patterns
African	Touch is common with family, extended family members; close personal space.
Chinese	Not accustomed to being touched by strangers; avoid direct eye contact when listening; distant personal space.
Eastern Indian	Handshakes between men only; direct eye contact considered disrespectful.
Europeans	Eye contact acceptable; noncontact people; distant personal space; Southern countries have closer contact and touch.
Filipino	Touch is stressed; some may fear eye contact; if eye contact is established, maintain it.
Iraqi	Touch and embrace on arrival and departure.
Israeli	Touch is demonstrative.
Japanese	Handshakes acceptable; not accustomed to physical contact; distant personal space; direct eye contact shows lack of respect.
Mexican	Touch often used, especially between those of same sex; close personal space.
Native American	Periods of silence during communication shows respect; eye contact very limited; close personal space—no boundaries.
Saudi	Male may only touch females in family; handholding by men acceptable.

Sources: Nichols, 1995; Sieh and Brentin, 1997; Spector, 1996.

holding back on what you have to say, avoiding interruption, and controlling the urge to give advice. If you are rehearsing what you are going to say next when the other person is talking, you are not listening.

Better listening does not start with a set of techniques. It starts with making a sincere effort to pay attention to what is going on in the other person's experience. Listeners who pretend interest do not fool anyone for long–except, perhaps, themselves. Practice listening whenever your partner, family member, or friend speaks to you. Listen to them with the sole intention of understanding what that person is trying to express. Listen to yourself, get to know something about your own ways of communicating. Self-understanding will enable you to relate more effectively to other people (Nichols, 1995).

Levels of Messages

To understand consumers' experiences, you must listen to both overt and covert levels of the message being transmitted. *Overt messages* are conveyed by spoken words and are heard in the context of the person's feelings. Tone of voice, rate of speech, body posture, gestures, eye contact, and facial expression convey *covert messages,* which clarify or modify the overt message. An overt question like "What time are visiting hours?" may have different meanings depending on the covert messages that accompany it. It may be a simple request for information. If those words are spoken angrily and loudly or if body posture is visibly tense, the client may be trying to assume some degree of control in an environment in which he or she feels uncomfortably dependent. If those same words are spoken in a frightened tone of voice or if the eyes are dilated and the body quivering, the client may be terrified at being separated from loved ones or frightened about who will come to visit. Problems can arise not from a lack of technical communication skills but from an insensitivity to covert messages.

Communication Difficulties

In general, you will be more effective if you focus on listening and understanding clients' communication rather than trying to plan how you will respond. A common concern of nursing students is: What am I going to say next, and what is the client going to say then? Beginning students frequently focus on trying to say the "right thing" or use the "right technique" and may therefore appear either distant or over-supportive. More beneficial to clients is simply being yourself. As you become more comfortable with communication skills, saying the right thing will become secondary to listening and understanding.

Be aware of the pitfalls of being merely a polite listener, in which the listener goes through the motions of listening without truly hearing or understanding. Often seen in social interactions, this pattern can extend to nurse-client interactions. This may occur if you fear being regarded as inadequate or unintelligent. The polite listener is bored or impatient, and more interested in talking than in listening.

Nurses often assume that most of their communication has been listened to and understood by clients. However, feelings such as anxiety and anger may interfere with a client's ability to listen. Frequently ask yourself: Has the client listened to and understood what I have said? If you suspect that a client has not understood you, ask questions such as "Could you tell me what you heard me saying?" or "I'm not sure I said that very clearly. What did you hear?"

Nurses are taught to ask many questions during the history-taking and assessment processes. When this continues into the implementation phase, difficulties will usually develop. The nurse and client become simply questioner and questionee. The relationship becomes unequal because the questioner has the power to determine the course of the interaction. There is a tacit understanding that the questioner is the authority figure and the questionee must be submissive. A clue that too many questions are being asked is when clients give short answers or seldom take the initiative during interactions.

One of the most difficult aspects of communication is periods of silence. Students often feel uncomfortable with silence because of a belief that they should always have something therapeutic to say. With silent clients, the tendency among anxious students is to be excessively verbal. Silence has many meanings. Among them are:

- I am too tired to talk right now.
- I don't want to talk to you.
- I can't hear you; I'm listening to the voices.
- I don't know what you want from me.
- I'm lost and don't know what to say next.
- I don't know where this discussion is going.
- I would like to think about what was just said.
- I'm comfortable just being with you and not talking.

To respond appropriately, try to understand the reason for the client's silence. An observation such as "I've noticed that you have become very quiet. Could you tell me something about that quietness?" may encourage clients to share more.

Verbose clients may also pose problems. Students tend to be verbal with silent clients, but they tend to be passive with talkative ones. You may be reluctant to interrupt for fear of being thought disrespectful or feeling inadequate in the face of such unrelenting talk.

You may also feel a sense of relief that clients are finally talking to you. Some students mistakenly interpret clients' incessant verbalizing as evidence that the interactions are therapeutic. It is difficult to understand nonstop talk for more than 30 seconds. Interrupting will allow you to focus on the concerns being expressed and to convey a sense of involvement with the client's problems. Here are some examples of helpful interruptions:

- "You are bringing up a number of concerns. Could we discuss them one at a time?"
- "Let me interrupt you for a minute to make sure I understand what you are saying."
- "I don't want to stop you, but I need you to slow down so that I can understand better."

Characteristics of Caring Helpers

The ability to integrate the characteristics of caring helpers into nursing practice will increase growth and satisfaction for both you and your clients. These interpersonal qualities and skills are critical to the therapeutic relationship through which nursing interventions are implemented. Used in isolation from the nursing process, they become characteristics of a social rather than a professional relationship.

Nonjudgmental Approach

One characteristic of caring nurses is a nonjudgmental approach to clients. It may be impossible for you to be completely nonjudgmental about clients. You make cognitive judgments when you assess clients and formulate reasonable plans of care. Emotional judgments are evidenced by such statements as "I really like her" or "He frightens me." Clients are also judged within the social context of appropriate or inappropriate behavior. Spiritual judgments include moral approval or condemnation of another person. Cultural judgments include being critical of behaviors, beliefs, and values that are different from yours.

A nonjudgmental approach to clients means that you are not harshly critical of them. Develop sufficient self-awareness to identify pejorative thoughts and feelings about particular clients. With this insight, you can avoid acting on negative judgments. Nonjudgmental nurses allow clients to talk about thoughts and feelings, and they respect clients as responsible people capable of making their own decisions.

Acceptance

Acceptance of clients is another characteristic of caring nurses. Acceptance is affirming people as they are, and recognizing that clients have the right to emotional expression. Accepting nurses respect clients' thoughts and emotions and help them achieve self-understanding. As internal responses to one's perception of others and the environment, feelings are genuine and cannot be criticized, argued with, or denounced. To tell clients how they should or should not feel is to discount their past experiences, present state, and future potential. Being uncomfortable with one's own feelings often leads to discrediting the feelings of others.

Unless it is detrimental to the client or to others, accept client behavior. Certain behavior, such as masturbating in public, causes social embarrassment and discomfort to others and may later be a source of shame for the person. Protect clients by providing them with private space and time for this normal human activity. Set limits on activities that will lead to a client's complete exhaustion. Do not accept a client's violence toward self or others.

In determining whether or not a behavior is acceptable, first assess the probable consequences of the behavior. If you think it will be detrimental to the client or others, formulate a plan for intervention. Remember that if a client is incapable of changing behavior or chooses not to change it, physical force may be necessary. Ask the following questions during assessment: "Is this behavior detrimental, or is it just a source of irritation to me?" "Are the rules and regulations of the unit more important than the client's rights and dignity?" "Is this behavior dangerous enough to use physical force to stop it?" "Am I willing and able to use physical force to change the behavior?" The examples below illustrate this process.

Maria is a nurse in the emergency department. She is assigned to a client, Tom, whom the police have arrested for intoxication and disorderly conduct. He has been placed in a room designed to be safe for this type of client. When Maria enters the room, she finds Tom smoking a cigarette, which is against the rules of the department. When he ignores her requests to put out the cigarette, she attempts to take it away from him forcefully. Tom strikes out in anger, and Maria ends up with a facial cut that requires stitches.

Connie is a nurse on the psychiatric unit. She has been attempting to intervene with Roberta, a client who has become very angry with her roommate. When it is obvious that Roberta is losing control, Connie calls for help from other staff members, and they quickly formulate a plan for intervention. As Roberta picks up a chair and threatens her roommate, three staff members surround her and firmly take the chair away from her. She is then escorted to the quiet room, where two staff members remain with her until she has better control over her behavior.

It is apparent that Maria attempted to enforce the rules of the department without pausing to plan and prioritize. Since Tom was in a room by himself where there was no danger of fire, his smoking a cigarette did not constitute a fire hazard. Maria might have made the decision to remain with him while he finished his cigarette, to prevent any accidents with the smoking material. But using physical force to stop the behavior was inappropriate because the incident wasn't dangerous. If Maria was determined to stop Tom's behavior, she should have sought help and thought of a plan to accomplish this outcome.

In contrast, Connie identified that Roberta's behavior was unacceptable because there was the danger of her roommate's being injured. A plan was formulated and implemented so that no one on the unit was injured, and Roberta was given the opportunity to talk about the feelings underlying her unacceptable behavior.

Warmth

Another characteristic of caring nurses is warmth, the manner in which concern for and interest in clients is expressed. This does not mean that you should be effusive with clients or attempt to be their buddy. Warmth is primarily expressed nonverbally, by a positive demeanor, a friendly tone, and an engaging smile. Simply leaning forward and establishing eye contact are expressions of warmth, as is physical touch, as long as it is acceptable and not frightening to the client.

Empathy

Much has been written about empathy as a necessary characteristic of caring nurses. Empathy is the ability to see another's perception of the world. It is understanding how clients see themselves, what they are feeling, and what they are striving to become. Empa-thy is a two-step process of understanding and validating. The first step is careful consideration of the meaning of what clients are communicating and the feelings being expressed. The second step is communicating your understanding verbally so that clients are able to validate or correct your perceptions. Empathy can facilitate therapeutic collaboration and help clients experience and understand themselves more fully (Book, 1988; Williams, 1990).

Authenticity

To be a caring nurse means you rely on your authenticity—being genuinely and naturally yourself in therapeutic relationships. When you make a commitment to clients, you take on a professional role. This is different from "playing" the professional role, which makes a pretense of helping clients. When you are more concerned about how you appear than what you are and do, you erect a facade of helping and are incapable of being authentic with clients, peers, and supervisors.

Congruency

Nurses are genuine when their verbal and nonverbal behavior indicates congruency. Clients can quickly sense when you are incongruent, or saying one thing verbally and another thing nonverbally. Congruency is a necessary ingredient to building trust.

It is Steve's first day on the psychiatric unit as a nursing student. He is in the day room, interacting with a group of clients and two other students. He appears tense, with upright body posture, clenched hands, and a swinging foot. His voice is pitched higher than normal. One of the clients jokingly asks him, "What's the matter? Are you afraid of us crazies?" Steve quickly replies, "No, I'm not afraid. I like being here." The clients respond to him with looks of disbelief and change their focus to the other two students. Steve seeks out his instructor for help with this problem. The two of them discuss how his verbal and nonverbal communication did not match and the effect this incongruity had on the clients.

Several weeks later, Steve finds himself becoming increasingly frustrated with a client who has consistently refused to participate in any unit activities. This time he is able to be congruent and express his frustration directly to the client rather than trying to cover up his feelings.

Patience

It is essential that you have patience with consumers, to give them the opportunity to grow and develop. Patience is not passive waiting, but active listening and responding. By allowing them to grow according to their own timetables, patience gives clients room to feel, think, and plan what changes need to be made. You must also be patient with yourself. Look for opportunities to develop self-awareness and gain new knowledge. Moreover, recognize that professional competence is not simply a goal; it is a long-term process of learning and developing as a nurse.

Respect

Respect for clients is another characteristic of caring nurses. Respect includes consideration for clients, commitment to protecting them and others from harm, and confidence in their ability to participate actively in solving their own problems. Do not let the nurse-client relationship become a dependent, parent-child relationship.

Trustworthiness

Trustworthiness is a characteristic of caring nurses toward which all the preceding characteristics build. By using good interpersonal skills, you help clients attach to you emotionally, which in turn helps build trust. This therapeutic attachment is facilitated through the nursing process. When you are trustworthy, you are dependable and responsible. You adhere to time commitments, keep promises, and are consistent in your attitude. Clients learn they can rely on you. Trust is also built when you demonstrate your willingness to continue working with clients who show little progress.

When you are trustworthy, you respect the confidentiality of the nurse-client relationship. Clients need to have their privacy protected because of the stigma associated with mental disorders. Reassure clients that information will not go beyond the health care team. Because you and your clients may live in the same community, some clients may fear that people will learn they are receiving mental health care. To minimize this fear, emphasize the issue of confidentiality. (Confidentiality is covered further in Chapter 24.)

Distrust may develop when consumers are denied access to the information in their records. Consumers have the right to read their records; this right protects them by ensuring that all viewpoints, including their own, are represented. Sharing nursing notes can be beneficial in that further discussion can develop from your initial observations and interpretations. Every clinical agency has regulations for sharing record information with clients, and you must adhere to these rules.

Self-Disclosure

Trust develops when nurses offer appropriate self-disclosure. In order to establish trust and openness, beginning students often believe they should be no more than passive, nonjudgmental listeners. But trust cannot be achieved if you withhold your own thoughts and feelings. Only when relationships are open and active can real progress be made. Appropriate self-disclosure is always goal-directed and determined by the client's needs, not yours. Nurses frequently ask clients to talk about their feelings as a therapeutic intervention. For clients who have minimal interpersonal skills, however, it is equally important to teach them how to perceive other people's feelings and to validate this perception. Through your self-disclosure, clients can improve their interpersonal relationships. For clients, self-disclosure can lead to further self-exploration; they are often reassured that their feelings are real and shared by others.

Self-disclosure is not always appropriate. Clients who are acutely ill may not be able to see themselves as separate individuals from the staff. Self-disclosure in this situation may be a source of confusion because these clients may believe that you are talking about them. Self-disclosure about personal details is often inappropriate and should be avoided. If clients ask for information about your personal life, simply say you are uncomfortable sharing that information, and refocus the conversation on the client's issues.

Berta, a nursing student, is having a one-to-one session with Jim, her client of 2 weeks.

JIM: I notice you don't have a wedding band on. Does that mean you aren't married?

BERTA: That's right.

JIM: Do you have a boyfriend, or are you dating anyone right now?

BERTA: Jim, I'm not comfortable talking about my private life. We were just discussing your recent divorce. Could we go back to that topic, please?

JIM: I just want to know if you're available, that's all. I mean, maybe we could go out for dinner sometime after I get out of here.

BERTA: Jim, you know that our relationship is a professional one and is limited to my time here in the clinic with you. It is not possible to continue it after your discharge.

JIM: Well, I'm so lonesome since my wife left me, and you seem so nice and friendly.

BERTA: Let's talk about your loneliness and see if we can find more appropriate ways to deal with this problem.

Humor

Humor is a useful tool in effective nurse-client relationships. Some nurses erroneously consider humor to be "unprofessional." Healthful humor must be distinguished from harmful humor. Harmful humor ridicules other people by laughing *at* them. Humor is also potentially harmful if it is used to avoid resolving genuine problems. Healthful humor, on the other hand, is a way to elicit laughter. It occurs when you laugh *with* other people. Healthful humor is appropriate to the situation and protects a person's dignity. A good sense of humor is a mature coping mechanism and can help people adapt in difficult situations (Sieh and Brentin, 1997).

Humor creates and invites laughter; as such, it is a communication process. Humor is a cognitive communication that creates an affective response, such as delight or pleasure, followed by a behavioral response, such as smiling or laughing. Humor reduces anxiety and fear. It diffuses painful emotions, which the person cannot experience when laughing, and decreases stress and tension. Humor may also be a safety valve for the energy generated by anger. If people are able to look at an irritating situation and laugh rather than explode in anger, the energy is discharged in an adaptive manner (Sieh and Brentin, 1997).

There are cultural differences in expressing humor. All people laugh, and people of all cultures have a sense of humor. The greatest difference between cultural groups is the content of humor. For example, the Irish make jokes about drinking, whereas the Israelis do not. American humor tends to have sexual and aggressive themes, which are not present in Japanese humor. People from so-called pioneer countries, such as the United States, Australia, and Israel, express humor with exaggeration and tall tales; in contrast, British humor is understated and intellectual. Jews and Britons tell many jokes revolving around self-mockery (Robinson, 1991).

A client's sense of humor may be a diagnostic cue for you. Changes in patterns of laughter may indicate other difficulties in adaptation. Clients who are depressed retain a cognitive sense of humor, but they receive no pleasure and are unable to laugh. Clients who are in a manic phase find everything funny, but because of their lack of judgment, their humor can turn into sarcastic wit and be potentially harmful to others. Those experiencing suspicious thoughts cannot laugh about their situation and are so frightened that they view humor as evidence of a personal attack. Clients who have difficulty with abstract thinking have problems understanding jokes. The influence of alcohol or other drugs may reduce a person's inhibitions so that nearly all stimuli in the environment appear funny. In assessing clients, it is appropriate to ask, "What is your favorite joke?" Responses to this question will give you an indication of the client's sense of humor.

Techniques That Facilitate Effective Communication

Effective communication is not an inborn skill but rather a learned process. Many instructors have their nursing students write up their one-to-one interactions with clients—called process recordings—in order to analyze the communication process. This type of evaluation will help you understand yourself and your clients. The consistent use of analysis, along with input from peers and supervisors, will heighten your level of expertise. See Table 5.3 for an example of a process recording. Additional process recordings are found in Appendix E.

Questions can be either closed-ended or open-ended. *Closed-ended questions* can be answered with a yes, a no, or a simple fact. They are useful for finding out exact information or for helping a client focus on a topic more clearly. You will find that clients who are experiencing a high level of anxiety or disorganized thinking respond more easily to closed-ended questions. Examples are: "How long have you been married?" "Are you still living with your wife?" "Are you hearing voices right now?" *Open-ended questions* cannot be answered in a few short words. They are useful for increasing the client's participation in the interaction and for encouraging the client to continue the discussion. Examples are: "Would you tell me more about your relationship problems?" "How is that similar to your family when you were growing

■ *Table 5.3* Process Recording of Client Interview with Student Nurse

Student's name: Vickie

Client's name: Joe

Client profile: Joe, 42 years old, has a known history of schizophrenia, as does his mother and one brother. He came to the community mental health center saying that he had burrowed out from federal prison. He is unkempt. He says he does not brush his teeth "because I will choke on saliva. I choke whenever I swallow, but soon my surgery will fix that." He remains isolated from most people at the center. He often will not look at others. He shields his eyes and states, "You cannot see me because I am not real." Periodically he talks about being Sean Connery and says his brother is the younger Sean Connery.

Short-term goals for one-to-one interaction: One-to-one interaction occurs during activity time, which is being managed by the psychiatric technician today. The goal of the group and my goal is to work on improving Joe's self-esteem.

Student's Communication	Analysis of Student's Response	Client's Communication	Analysis of Client's Response
		Today I'm going to make another belt for my brother, who is a police officer.	*This is something Joe does well. Increases his self-esteem.*
I really like the belts you make. We have another task we should work on for awhile. We have paper and drawing pens. What would you think about drawing a picture today?	*Encouraging formulation of a plan. Self-esteem exercise might be beneficial to him.*		
		I don't know what to draw. (head down, loss of eye contact)	*Suspicious of my request. Loss of eye contact might mean mistrust or low self-esteem.*
Perhaps you could draw a picture of yourself.	*I want to try an exercise we were asked to do in one of our classes. My idea is to increase his self-esteem.*		
		(Joe goes and gets a sheet of paper and markers. He works on picture for 10 minutes.) Basic reproduction:	*Joe uses many symbols that I am not quite sure of (I later validated to get my answers). His picture is very detailed.*
Joe, can you tell me what this is on your face?	*Clarifying. I know there is a lot more to the picture than what I see, so I need to understand his perceptions.*		
		This is my beard where I haven't been able to shave. All of the techs are girls except for Allen, and Allen hasn't worked in a few days.	*Joe realizes that he needs/wants to shave, but because of personal beliefs he has refused to shave in front of female staff.*
(nodding) I understand.	*Accepting.*		

Table 5.3 continued

Student's Communication	Analysis of Student's Response	Client's Communication	Analysis of Client's Response
		I am Abraham Lincoln giving the Gettysburg address.	*Identifies his beard with the beard of Abraham Lincoln. Possibly delusion of grandeur.*
Could you explain about this to me? (I point to the black circle on his neck.)	*Clarifying.*		
		That hole causes me to choke when I eat. I can't swallow.	*Somatic delusion. This is a factor in his nutritional status because he believes he will choke if he swallows.*
How does that affect your eating?	*Exploring. I want to determine if this is the reason he is refusing to eat.*		
		If I eat sometimes I get choked, so I have to be sure and eat soft foods or liquids.	*His fear of choking could be related to a previous choking experience or have a totally different meaning altogether.*
Are you worried you will choke?	*Validating perception. I want to be sure we are talking about physically choking and not something more symbolic.*		
		I just have to be careful when I am chewing and I don't eat tough meat.	*Uses precautions because of his fear.*
What is this you're holding in your hands? (I point to his hands in the picture.)	*Clarifying. Time to move on past his fear of choking.*		
		Those are chains that are locked so I can't move my arms.	*He feels his hands are tied. This relates to what he told me last week about being awake while sleepwalking. Joe feels he can't do anything about his disease.*
How do you feel about that?	*Exploring.*		
		I'm a prisoner and I can't escape. I have tried so many times. (gazing at his hands, flat affect)	*Feels helpless and hopeless. Possibly after many failed attempts to get well?*
What do you think you can do when you feel this way?	*Encouraging formation of a plan of action. I want Joe to feel he has control.*		
		I can escape.	*Joe wants to somehow gain control but he needs direction in problem solving.*

continued ➤

■ *Table 5.3* **Process Recording of Client Interview with Student Nurse** *continued*

Student's Communication	Analysis of Student's Response	Client's Communication	Analysis of Client's Response
I'm sorry, could you tell me what you mean by "escape?"	*Clarifying.*		
		Free myself from these chains.	*Again, Joe wants control but lacks skills to problem-solve.*
What have you tried so far?	*Exploring solutions Joe has already tried; first step in problem-solving process.*		
		(Joe talks for 2 minutes about all the hospitals, "prisons," he has been in.) I just can't escape.	*Uses examples of situations in which he felt an external locus of control. Feels helpless.*
Have you thought about living in your own apartment?	*I'm not sure if this would be possible, but I want to open the door to other possible solutions. However, I jumped in with an answer too quickly. I should have let Joe identify other potential solutions.*		
		I wish I could live on my own.	*Focuses on my solution. This might be a positive start in problem solving for him.*
(Tech announces that activity time is up.) Joe, we have talked about some important issues today. You told me you want to escape your chains. Could we continue to talk about this in group today?	*Summarizing. I feel disappointed because I had just hit on target. We managed to get to the solution phase of problem solving, but no further. It's possible I got a late start and could have done this a lot sooner. I encourage Joe to continue talking in group, and hopefully he will continue with problem solving.*		
		(Nods his head.)	*Joe continues to feel hopeless.*

Source: Contributed by Vicki Manning, Purdue University Calumet.

up?" Use both open-ended and closed-ended questions during interactions, but use open-ended questions whenever possible or appropriate. If several closed-ended questions are asked in succession, the interaction takes on an atmosphere of cross-examination, and the client may become reluctant to continue.

Questions beginning with "What" are generally used to evoke facts. Examples are: "What kind of work do you do?" "What do you argue about?" Questions beginning with "How" lead to a discussion of feelings and may elicit a client's personal view of a situation. Examples are: "How did you feel when he gave you that ultimatum?" "How do you think your work should be supervised?" Questions beginning with "Could" allow the client to have some control over the interaction and are the most open-ended of questions. Examples are: "Could you give me an example of how he mistreats you?" "Could you tell me what is the most important problem to focus on today?" Questions beginning with "Why" lead to a discussion of reasons and often put clients on the defensive. "Why" questions do not typically help clients understand their situation more clearly but rather force them to explain and justify their behavior. Examples are: "Why did you skip group today?" and "Why did you say that to your husband?"

Effective communication techniques are those that communicate your listening, understanding, and caring. You must analyze the behavioral, affective, and cognitive components of communication in order to respond to overt and covert messages. Effective communication also encourages clients to examine feelings, explore problems in more depth, build on existing strengths, and develop new coping strategies. Table 5.4 provides examples of effective communication techniques.

Broad openings are open-ended questions or statements. The purpose of a broad opening is to acknowledge clients and to let them know you are listening and concerned about their interests. But the overuse of broad openings will force the relationship to remain on a superficial level.

Giving recognition is noting something that is occurring at the present moment for clients. It is a fairly superficial level of communication but indicates attention to and care for individuals.

Minimal encouragements are verbal and nonverbal reinforcers that indicate active listening to and interest in what clients are saying. They prompt clients to continue with what is being said.

Offering self is a way of informing clients of care and concern. It is used to offer emotional and moral support.

Accepting lets clients know you are comprehending their thoughts and feelings. It is one of the ways you express empathy.

Making observations moves the interaction to a deeper therapeutic level. It involves paying very close attention to the behavioral component of communication and connecting it to the affective and cognitive components. When communication is incongruous, you comment on the inconsistency and, with the client, explore the underlying meaning of the mixed messages. Clients who are experiencing disorganized thinking may be unable to take part in this process.

Validating perceptions gives clients an opportunity to validate or correct your understanding of what is being communicated. Using this technique will decrease confusion and affirm your genuine interest in understanding your clients.

Exploring helps clients feel free to talk and examine issues in more depth. As they organize their thoughts and focus on particular problems, their understanding of themselves and others increases.

Clarifying is useful when you are confused about clients' thoughts or feelings. It is appropriate to acknowledge your confusion and ask clients to rephrase what they just said.

Placing the event in time or *sequence* helps clients sort out what happened to them in what order. The goal is to help them understand the progression of events.

Focusing allows clients to stay with specifics and analyze problems without jumping from topic to topic. You may choose to focus on the main theme, to facilitate exploring the problem in more depth. Clients are often unaware of how they contributed to and participated in the development of their problems. By focusing on their feelings, thoughts, and behaviors, you pave the way for increased understanding and responsibility. Clients with disorganized thinking usually need help in staying focused.

Encouraging the formulation of a plan of action is the process of helping clients decide how they plan to proceed. In general, avoid telling clients what they should do. Instead, asking them what they will or might do will reinforce that they are in control of and responsible for themselves. If they are unable to formulate a plan of action, implement the problem-solving process. If clients are highly anxious or experiencing disorganized thinking, they may be unable to problem-solve or make appropriate judgments.

Suggesting collaboration is one technique of introducing the problem-solving process. It is an offer to help clients work through each step of the process and to brainstorm alternative solutions to their problems. Suggesting collaboration stresses the team effort of you and your client to develop more adaptive coping skills.

Restatement is the use of newer and fewer words to paraphrase the basic content of client messages. Restatement focuses on the cognitive component of communication and creates an opportunity to explore facts or reinforce something important clients have said.

Table 5.4 Effective Communication Techniques

Technique	Examples
Broad opening	"What would you like to work on today?" "What is one of the best things that happened to you this week?"
Giving recognition	"I notice you're wearing a new dress. You look very nice." "What a marvelous afghan that is going to be when you finish."
Minimal encouragement	"Go on." "Ummm." "Uh-huh."
Offering self	"I'll sit with you until it's time for your family session." "I have at least 30 minutes I can spend with you right now."
Accepting	"I can imagine how that might feel." "I'm with you on that [nodding]."
Making observations	"Mr. Robinson, you seem on edge. You are clenching your fist and grinding your teeth." "I'm puzzled. You're smiling, but you sound so resentful."
Validating perceptions	"This is what I heard you say. . . . Is that correct?" "It sounds like you are talking about sad feelings. Is that correct?"
Exploring	"How does your girlfriend feel about your being in the hospital?" "Tell me about what was happening at home just before you came in the hospital."
Clarifying	"Could you explain more about that to me?" "I'm having some difficulty. Could you help me understand?"
Placing the event in time or sequence	"Which came first . . . ?" "When did you first notice . . . ?"
Focusing	"Could we continue talking about you and your dad right now?" "Rather than talking about what your husband thinks, I would like to hear how you're feeling right now."
Encouraging the formulation of a plan of action	"What do you think you can do the next time you feel that way?" "How might you handle your anger in a nonthreatening way?"
Suggesting collaboration	"Perhaps together we can figure out . . . ." "Let's try using the problem-solving process that was presented in group yesterday."
Restatement	*Client:* Do you think going home will be difficult? *Nurse:* How difficult do you think going home will be?
Reflection	*Client:* I keep thinking about what all my friends are doing right now. *Nurse:* You're worried that they aren't missing you? *Client:* He laughed at me. My boss just sat there and laughed at me. I felt like such a fool. *Nurse:* You felt humiliated?
Summarizing	"So far we have talked about . . . ." "Our time is up. Let's see, we have discussed your family problems, their effect on your schoolwork, and your need to find a way to decrease family conflict."

Reflection involves understanding the affective component of communication and reflecting these feelings back to clients without repeating their exact words. Reflection helps clients focus on feelings and allows you to communicate empathy.

Summarizing is the systematic synthesis of important ideas discussed by clients during interactions. The goal is to help them explore significant content and emotional themes. Summarizing may also be used to move from one phase of the interaction to the next, to conclude the interaction, or to begin the interaction by reviewing the previous session.

See Table 5.5 for use of clarifying techniques when clients use unclear or nonspecific language.

Table 5.5 Unclear, Nonspecific Communication

Common Problem	Meaning	Verbal Example	Clarifying Technique
Deleting	Object of the verb is left out	"I'm afraid."	Inquire: "Afraid of what in particular?"
		"I'm really uncomfortable."	"What is making you uncomfortable?"
Unspecified verbs	Verbs in which the action needs to be more specific	"He really frustrates me."	Inquire: "How, exactly, does he frustrate you?"
		"They ignored me."	"In what way did they ignore you?"
Universal qualifiers	Words that generalize a few experiences to a multitude of experiences (all, every, never, always, nobody, only)	"I never do anything right."	Inquire: "Has there ever been a time that you did do something right?"
		"You always hurt me."	"Has there ever been a situation in which I haven't hurt you?"
Necessity and possibility	Statements that identify rules or limits to a person's behavior and that often indicate no choice (have to, must, can't, no one can, not possible, unable)	"I have to take care of other people."	Inquire: "What would happen if you didn't take care of other people?"
		"No one can get me out of this mess."	"What would happen if you got out of this mess?"
		"I can't do it."	"What stops you from doing it?"
		"It's not possible."	"What do you need?"
			"What will have to happen so it is possible?"

Techniques That Contribute to Ineffective Communication

Nurses who worry about what they are going to say next, who do not listen carefully, and who do not focus on trying to understand what clients are attempting to say are often ineffective communicators. Ineffective communication is also described as communication that avoids underlying feelings, remains on a superficial level, tells people what to do, or moralizes and expresses judgment. Table 5.6 provides examples of ineffective communication techniques.

Stereotypical comments indicate that you care little about the individual experiences of clients and are relying on folklore and proverbs to communicate.

Additional problems occur for clients whose thinking is concrete because many stereotypical comments rely on abstract understanding. Stereotypical comments are culture-specific and therefore make little sense to people with different cultural backgrounds.

Parroting is simply repeating back to clients the words they themselves have used. When you merely repeat what clients have said, the communication becomes circular, clients do not progress in understanding, and the interaction grinds to a halt.

Changing the topic occurs when you introduce topics that might be of interest to you but are not relevant to the client at that particular time. This technique can be a way of avoiding topics that make you uncomfortable. If you change the topic often, clients

Table 5.6 Ineffective Communication Techniques

Technique	Examples
Sterotypical comments	"What's the matter, cat got your tongue?" "Still waters run deep."
Parroting	*Client:* I'm so sad. *Nurse:* You're so sad.
Changing the topic	*Client:* I was so afraid I was going to have another panic attack. *Nurse:* What does your husband think about your panic attacks?
Disagreeing	"I don't see any reason for you to feel that way." "No, I think that is a silly response to your mother."
Challenging	"Is that a valid reason to become angry?" "You weren't really serious, were you?"
Requesting an explanation	"Why did you react that way?" "Why can't you just leave home?"
False reassurance	"Don't worry anymore." "I doubt that your mother will be angry about your failing math."
Belittling expressed feelings	"That was four years ago. It shouldn't bother you now." "You shouldn't feel that all men are bad." "It's wrong to even think of your mother like that."
Probing	"I'm here to listen. I can't help you if you won't tell me everything." "Tell me what secrets you keep from your wife."
Advising	"You sound worried. I think you'd better talk to your doctor or your rabbi." "I think you should divorce your husband."
Imposing values	*Client:* [With head down and low tone of voice.] I was going to go on the cruise, but my mother is coming to stay with me. *Nurse:* You must be looking forward to her arrival.
Double/multiple questions	"What makes you feel that you should stay? How would you get along if you left? Would you rent an apartment or move in with a friend?"

will begin to feel that what they are trying to say is not important. Clients may also change the topic if they are highly anxious about the topic being discussed or if their thinking is disorganized.

Disagreeing with clients' ideas and emotions denies them the right to think and feel as they do. Disagreeing provides clients with no opportunity to increase self-understanding.

Challenging clients forces them to defend themselves from what appears to be an attack by you. When you challenge clients, they are forced to offer reasons for their feelings, thoughts, or behaviors.

Requesting an explanation is similar to challenging and usually begins with "Why." The implication is that the client should not be behaving a certain way or experiencing a particular feeling.

False reassurance is another way of telling clients how to feel and ignoring their distress. They feel patronized when you act as if you know better and more than they do.

Belittling expressed feelings gives the message that you have not listened carefully, that you are ignoring the importance of their problems.

Probing occurs when you fail to respect clients' decisions regarding privacy of feelings and thoughts. Probing implicitly accuses them of keeping secrets and blames them for not progressing in treatment.

Advising occurs when you tell clients what to do, preventing them from exploring problems and using the problem-solving process to find solutions. Advising makes you, rather than the client, responsible for the outcome.

Imposing values is demanding that clients share your own biases and prejudices. It is preaching and moralizing rather than accurately understanding their values.

Double/multiple questions are ineffective because they tend to confuse clients. When asked a series of questions with no intervening opportunity to respond, clients may end up feeling bewildered or cross-examined.

Communicating Within Families and Groups

Nurses are involved with a variety of family systems, as well as informal and formal groups, in every clinical setting. Communication within families and communication within groups are presented together here because, for the most part, they are similar. To help people become more effective communicators, you must be able to analyze communication patterns.

The overall process to use in understanding family and group communication is as follows:

1. What do I see and hear? (Perception of nonverbal and verbal communication.)
2. How do the members feel? How do I feel? (Affective analysis.)
3. What does this mean? (Cognitive interpretation.)
4. Is my assessment correct? (Validation by asking others, gathering more information.)
5. How shall I respond? (Interventions based on your assessment.)

The significance of nonverbal communication must always be considered. When working with families or groups, ask yourself the following questions, and then interpret the significance of the answers:

- How closely together do people sit?
- Are some members physically isolated from others?
- Can each person see all the other members fairly easily?
- Do members look at the person who is speaking?
- Do members behave in a distracting manner while a person is speaking?
- How is touch used within the group?
- Are nonverbal behaviors directed toward a particular member or the entire group?

- How do facial expressions change throughout the interaction?
- What kind of gestures are used?
- Are there changes in voice tone?

Another consideration is the significance of verbal communication. Ask yourself the following questions, and interpret the significance of the answers:

- Is somebody refusing to talk?
- Who speaks to whom, about what, and when?
- Are there individuals who are speaking for others?
- Who interrupts others?
- Who is talkative?
- Who contributes little?
- Who asks questions?
- Who gives the answers?
- Who gives opinions?
- Who tries to clarify misunderstandings?
- Who initiates problem solving?
- If English is not the native language, how fluent are various family members?
- Are one or two members expected to interpret for others?

Affective expression between family and group members can be analyzed by answering these questions:

- To what extent is the communication of feelings encouraged?
- Are feelings expressed directly or indirectly?
- What happens when a member breaks the group's "rules" about expressing feelings?
- How much does the group encourage members to be sensitive to each other's feelings and to communicate this awareness?
- What are the feelings underlying the members' communication with one another?
- Who is helpful and friendly?

As a nurse, you help members improve their listening skills and their ability to be congruent in their communication by modeling and teaching effective communication. As they gain more adaptive skills, they will be better able to cope with individual, family, and group problems.

helpful in the process of examining your communication skills (Giles et al, 1994; Hummert, 1994).

Critical Thinking

Mary, a nursing student, has been assigned to care for Ifle, a 44-year-old client undergoing treatment on the psychiatric unit. Mary sits down close to Ifle, introduces herself, compliments Ifle on her appearance, and asks, "Are you doing okay today?' Ifle leans away from Mary, maintains a rigid posture, avoids eye contact, and nods her head yes. After several minutes of silence, Mary explains to Ifle that she has an hour that she can spend with her today. Following another long period of silence, Mary says, "I guess you're not in the mood to talk today, so I'll see you tomorrow." Mary leaves after spending 25 minutes with Ifle.

1. What actions by Mary demonstrated respect for Ifle?

2. What actions by Mary, if any, did not represent therapeutic communication skills and could decrease Ifle's confidence or trust in Mary?

3. Had you been Mary, how might you have interpreted Ifle's body language and silence during this first session?

4. How could Mary's interaction with Ifle been improved?

5. Why do you think Mary decided to leave after 25 minutes?

Suggested answers can be found in Appendix D.

Communicating with Older Adults

Older adults are sometimes the targets of patronizing speech such as slow speech, simple sentences, concrete vocabulary, and demeaning emotional tone. Some health care professionals even use baby talk especially with those elderly persons who live in nursing homes. Patronizing speech implies that there is a question regarding the competence of the older person; this communicates a lack of respect that undermines self-esteem and dignity.

Patronizing speech is the result of age-related stereotypes. Some of these negative beliefs are that older adults are feeble, egocentric, incompetent, and/or abrasive. It is important that you examine your beliefs about older people and how they communicate. You must also examine how you talk to older individuals. Asking for feedback from others is

Client and Family Education

Communication is the most important skill in the effective education of psychiatric consumers and their families. Good communication contributes to thorough assessment and accurate diagnosis of learning needs, and it is the major tool for implementing the teaching plan. You evaluate your teaching through verbal and (sometimes) written communication with your clients. Documentation is the written communication in records.

Education in the mental health care setting involves more than giving information to passive people. Education is an active process that is done *with* people, not *to* people. The steps of the nursing process are used in the educational process: assessing the learning needs, diagnosing the knowledge deficit with contributing factors, planning content, implementing the most effective methods of education, evaluating the effectiveness of the teaching, and documenting the entire process.

Assessment

The first step in the client/family teaching process is assessment. It is important that you understand their views of psychiatric disability. Clients and families often believe the cultural stereotypes—mental illness means being possessed by a demon, mental illness occurs only in people who are "bad," or families cause mental illness. Many clients may have been on several medications over a long period of time. You need to assess their knowledge base. Through assessment, determine what they have learned in previous contact with mental health professionals. If you have the erroneous view that psychiatrically disabled people cannot possibly understand their disorders, you will be surprised to learn how much they know.

Assessment also involves determining what consumers want and feel they need to know. Ask what they consider to be their most important problems at this time. Little progress will be made if you assume authority for prioritizing their problems. People are not likely to be open to learning about difficulties they consider unimportant; they will only learn material that is meaningful to them. You may need to help some individuals be specific if they have described their problems in vague terms.

> Max has been readmitted to the psychiatric unit because he stopped taking his medication 6 months ago. Ryan, his nurse, has determined that Max needs to learn why it is important to keep taking his medication. Max says the reason he doesn't do it is that his wife is always nagging him to take it. He believes if she would just leave him alone, he would not have a problem taking it. It is more important to Max to learn skills that will help him get along with and communicate better with his wife than to learn the facts about how his medication works.

Diagnosis

The nursing diagnosis most often used in client/family education is "knowledge deficit." When forming a nursing diagnosis, you must specify exactly what people need to learn and what the related factors may be. Examples are:

- *Knowledge deficit: lithium therapy* related to initiation of the drug.
- *Knowledge deficit: basic cooking skills* related to mother's doing all the cooking and her recent death.
- *Knowledge deficit: stress management* related to work stress that is contributing to high levels of anxiety and increased conflict at work.

Diagnosis also includes specifying what, if any, barriers exist that might hinder the teaching and learning process. Clients who are experiencing a great deal of anxiety have a very short attention span, an extremely narrowed perceptual field, and very little capacity to learn. Attempting to teach clients when they are in a manic phase, delusional, or experiencing hallucinations may not be practical. Disorganized thinking, obsessional thoughts, and other cognitive impairments make it very difficult for clients to learn. Those who are depressed and feel hopeless and helpless about the present and future may have no motivation to learn. Clients or family members who are angry and hostile need to find a way to manage their emotions before effective learning can take place. People who deny the reality of mental disorders will not be open to increasing their knowledge or improving their coping skills.

Planning

Preparing clients for as much self-care as possible in order to live in the least restrictive setting is both the focus and the goal of client/family teaching. Planning must be designed to meet the specific needs of the client and family. The educational plan should be directed not only toward increasing knowledge but also toward improved problem solving and more adaptive coping skills. Outcome criteria are developed in order to evaluate the behavioral, affective, and cognitive changes resulting from effective teaching and learning. Each chapter in Part III of this book includes a box describing client teaching.

To help people learn to cope with their current problems, emphasize the present: Change is possible only in the here and now. The past and future are also important, but only as perspectives on the present. Meanings attached to the past and expectations of the future influence present perceptions. But it is in the present that one evaluates the past, anticipates the future, and changes behavior. People who brood over past problems and pain without attending to the present are in danger of accepting the problems as permanent, with no hope for change. People who have dire future expectations and ignore the present potential for change will probably have their expectations fulfilled.

Implementation

Two of the most important skills you bring to client/family education are the ability to communicate clearly and the capacity to demonstrate warmth and caring. A humanistic approach has proven more successful than a technical approach in terms of client/family understanding and their willingness to participate in the process.

Family and friends often have questions about the disorder and want to know how they can best help. Including supportive others in education may improve the rehabilitative process because the living environment often affects the course of many mental disorders (Palmer-Erbs, 1996).

Education is both formal and informal. Examples of formal teaching are psychoeducational groups and audiovisual tools. The effectiveness of group education depends on a high level of skill on the part of the group leader. Consumers must be carefully assessed for appropriateness to the group. Those whose thinking is disorganized and those who are hyperactive, highly anxious, or hallucinating may not be appropriate for an educational group. One advantage of the group format is the ability to reach more people in a limited amount of time. Another advantage is that consumers interact with others who have similar problems and concerns. Sharing solutions to problems and coping behaviors can foster the learning process. The group should not have so many members that individuals have little opportunity to ask questions and provide answers. The best physical arrangement is a circle of chairs, to encourage a sense of connectedness.

Probably the most effective education format is the informal process. Every interaction you have with clients and their families is an opportunity to facilitate their learning. An example of informal teaching is when you discover a learning need and respond to it immediately. Examples are explaining the need for a new medication and helping a client control anger in response to an immediate situation.

General Areas of Learning

Client and family education may be the single most important factor in promoting healthy lifestyles. There are six general areas of learning to consider when implementing teaching plans. The first area relates to *knowledge of the mental disorder.* Clients and families who have struggled to live with psychiatric disabilities may be very knowledgeable in this area, in contrast to those who are experiencing disorders for the first time. Topics typically discussed are an explanation of the diagnosis, myths and folklore surrounding the disorder, goals of treatment, and the overall treatment plan. Clients and their families should also learn the signs and symptoms of relapse and know when to call the physician.

The second general area of learning is *medications.* Most clients and families are able to understand basic neurotransmission, which helps them understand how the medication works and why they need it. If they are caring for themselves, they should know when to take each medication and have a system for accurate administration at home. Teach them about the possible side effects and how to manage them. If there are any special precautions for a particular medication, emphasize them. Each chapter in Part Three includes a box describing medication teaching plans for specific clients. General medication teaching principles are covered in Chapter 8.

Some clients will need to learn activities relating to *managing ADLs.* They may never have had the opportunity to learn how to grocery shop, plan menus, prepare food, and do laundry. Some clients benefit from grooming groups, which reinforce basic hygiene, teach makeup and hair care, and help clients plan appropriate clothing, such as for job interviews and leisure activities. Some clients will need to learn how to use public transportation. Teach clients about available community resources for leisure activities, support groups, and religious expression.

Many clients and families need to learn the basics of *interpersonal communication.* They must be able to identify and express their own feelings and respect and listen to those of others. Family conferences and family therapy provide opportunities to help family members learn to communicate more effectively.

Clients often need to learn more effective skills for *coping with life,* including family, social, and vocational aspects. It is helpful if clients can identify how their illness has affected their lives and move on to a discussion of what the future might look like. Clients need to learn stress-avoidance and stress-management techniques, and how to manage any symptoms they may be experiencing. They often need to learn assertiveness skills and the problem-solving process. Some will need to develop a plan to avoid social isolation.

Another area of general learning is *community resources.* Types of programs are intermediate care facilities, partial-hospital programs, outpatient centers, respite care, transport resources, financial aid, pharmacies, and food programs. Self-help and support groups exist in most communities. Refer clients and their families to the National Alliance for the Mentally Ill, (800) 950-6264, or the National Mental Health Association, (800) 969-6642, for help in locating groups. Each chapter in Parts Three and Four includes a box with the names and addresses of support groups specific to each disorder or crisis situation.

The Problem-Solving Process

The most important process for clients and families to learn is how to solve problems. As they become increasingly skilled at problem solving, they will expand their coping skills and enhance the quality of their lives. In teaching the problem-solving process, focus on one problem at a time, and measure progress by observing small changes.

Box 5.1

Steps in Problem Identification

1. Client definition

   How would you describe the problem?

   For whom is this a problem? You? Family members? Employer? Community?

2. Significance of the problem

   When did this problem begin?

   What are the factors that cause this problem to continue?

3. Past and future influence

   What past events have influenced the current problem?

   What are your future expectations and hopes concerning this problem?

   What is the most you hope for when this problem is resolved?

   What is the least you will settle for to resolve this problem?

4. Concrete problem definition

   Is there more than one problem here?

   Which part of the overall problem is most important to deal with first?

Because all problems are connected, changes in one problem will cause changes in others. Remind people that in the past they have done their best to deal with problems, and that now new solutions may be found. Your role is to listen, observe, encourage, and evaluate. More effective coping behavior will be the ultimate result of the problem-solving process. But before the process can begin, you must help them identify their problem. Identification includes the person's definition of the problem, the significance of the problem, and the influence of the past and future. Box 5.1 describes the steps in problem identification.

Throughout the problem-solving process, it is extremely helpful to have clients keep a written list of all the ideas generated. The list can be modified as time goes on.

After problem identification has been completed, the steps of the problem-solving process consist of the following:

1. Identifying the solutions that have been attempted.

2. Listing alternative solutions.

3. Predicting the probable consequences of each alternative.

4. Choosing the best alternative to implement.

5. Implementing the chosen alternative in a real-life or practice situation.

6. Evaluating outcomes.

Box 5.2 lists sample questions for each step.

The first step is identifying what solutions have been tried thus far. The specifics of the attempts, how the attempts were implemented, and what occurred as a result must all be clarified. Because the problem continues to exist, these solutions were not effective, so they should be either modified or discarded.

The second step is having the client list alternative ways of solving the problem. Frequently, the client will have only one or two ideas. You can propose brainstorming sessions to increase creativity in problem solving. All possible solutions, even those that are unrealistic or absurd, are written down. Thinking of absurd solutions often opens the mind to other creative, realistic solutions to the problem. Finally, after the client has listed all his or her ideas for solving the problem, you can add your own suggestions.

The third step is predicting the probable consequences of each alternative, which helps clients anticipate outcomes of behavior. After thorough discussion, you and your client go on to the fourth step: choosing the best alternative to implement. Do not make this decision for clients; doing so would undermine the process by placing them in a childlike, dependent position. Using action-oriented terms, develop the selected solution further, as concretely and specifically as possible. At the same time, formulate measurable outcomes to use in evaluating the process.

The fifth step is implementing the proposed solution in either a practice or a real-life situation. Clients must be allowed to make mistakes during this step. If you rescue them, you are giving the message that they are incapable of taking charge of their lives.

Evaluation is the sixth step in the problem-solving process. Review the outcomes, and determine the degree of success or failure in achieving them. Suc-

Box 5.2

Steps in the Problem-Solving Process

1. Identify attempted solutions

   What have you done to try to solve the problem thus far?

   How exactly did you do this?

   What happened when you tried this?

2. List alternatives

   What other ideas do you think you could try?

   What might be some absurd solutions to this problem?

   What else might be effective?

   Have you thought about . . . ?

3. Predict consequences

   What might happen if you tried the first idea?

   Is there anything else that might happen?

   What might happen if you tried the second idea (etc.)?

4. Choose the best alternative

   Which alternative seems like the best decision at this time?

   What specific behaviors are you going to try with this alternative?

   Specifically, how will things be different if you are successful?

5. Implement the alternative

   With whom are you going to attempt this solution?

   When are you going to practice this new behavior?

   Is there anything you need from me to help you try this out?

6. Evaluate

   What was the result of your attempted solution?

   Were your expectations met successfully?

   Is there anything that needs to be modified?

   If you were not successful, what other alternative idea from the list could you try?

cessfully achieving an outcome means that the solution was effective and that it can continue to be implemented. Failing to achieve an outcome means you and your client need to analyze how and why the solution was ineffective. Then return to step 4, and either select a new solution or modify the old one.

As clients experience the steps of the problem-solving process, they increase their skills, which then can be applied to other problematic areas of life. With an improved ability to make and assume responsibility for decisions, they develop an internal locus of control, leading to competence and self-esteem.

When clients are acutely ill and unable to think logically, the problem-solving process is not an appropriate intervention. The interaction below illustrates the problem-solving process in action with a nurse and client.

> Beth, a 25-year-old graduate student, has been seeing Miyuki, a nurse therapist, for several months. Beth has been in a long-term relationship with a married man who has been physically and emotionally abusive to her.
>
> BETH: It's really time now to end the relationship. I've known for a long time that it's not good for me to stay with Todd. I just don't know how to do it.
>
> MIYUKI: What have you tried to do so far in ending the relationship?
>
> BETH: In the past two years, I've told Todd several times that I don't want to see him any more. Then he doesn't call me for a month and I start to miss him, so I give in when he finally calls me.
>
> MIYUKI: So, when you say no to Todd, he punishes you by not calling, with the end result that he manipulates you into going back to him.
>
> BETH: Yes, I guess that's what happens. What's really unbelievable is that I don't even like him very much anymore. What I really miss is the sex after a while. So I just give in because of the sex.
>
> MIYUKI: If you really want to end this relationship, how might you go about doing it differently since just telling him hasn't seemed to work?
>
> BETH: All my friends have been telling me to dump Todd. I guess I could tell some of them that I'm finally going to do it.

MIYUKI: What might happen if you did that?

BETH: Well, when I would be tempted to go back to Todd, I could call them up for some moral support not to go back. I guess I would have to tell them ahead of time that's what I'd want them to do.

MIYUKI: Are there some friends who would be better than others to depend on in this situation?

BETH: I think Carmela and Grace would be the best. They would try and help me, but they also wouldn't make me feel like a fool if I failed again. Leslie and Eva would just yell at me and be very critical.

MIYUKI: What else might help you break up with Todd?

BETH: I suppose I could try and do things with different friends. I always sit at home waiting for Todd to call me. I haven't gone out much with my friends in a long time.

MIYUKI: How would that help you not go back to Todd?

BETH: At least I wouldn't be so lonesome. Maybe it's the loneliness as much as the sex that makes me go back to him.

MIYUKI: What are some of the things that might get in the way of your staying away from Todd?

BETH: He has told me for years that no one else would want me because I'm fat and ugly and the only thing I'm good for is sex. I guess I really believe that after hearing it for so long. What if no one else will ever love me for the rest of my life?

MIYUKI: It's understandable how you believe what he has told you. Men who are abusive undermine their victim's self-esteem to prevent the victim from leaving. It seems to me that is another aspect of the problem we should also try to solve. Let's finish discussing the loneliness and friends issues first, and then move on to your self-esteem issue.

Evaluation

Client and family education is effective if the outcome criteria are met. The only way to discover what people have learned is through evaluation. Evaluation must be measurable; that is, people must be able to

---

Box 5.3

Problems in Client Education

Assessment

Teaching material was not meaningful to the client.

Diagnosis

Barriers to learning were not identified.

Planning

Areas of learning were stated in vague terms.

Outcome criteria were vague and unmeasurable.

The focus remained on the past rather than on present problems.

Implementation

Communication skills were ineffective.

The nurse displayed a distant, uncaring attitude toward the client.

The family and significant others were not included.

The teaching methods and tools were not appropriate for the client.

Evaluation

Areas of learning were no longer appropriate for the client's circumstances.

---

hear or see evidence that they did or did not meet the outcome criteria. If criteria were not met, look for where the problem might be. The difficulty could be in any of the steps of the nursing process. Box 5.3 describes common problems that prevent meeting the outcome criteria. Use this box as a guide for locating problems in education. Revise your teaching according to evidence from the evaluation.

Evaluation can be done in a number of ways. You can have people verbalize attitudes, values, feelings, and facts. Written tests may be appropriate for cognitive information. Interpersonal skill achievement can be evaluated by role playing. Psychomotor skill achievement can be evaluated by having the learner demonstrate the skill for you. This final step of the nursing process is critical to effective education.

Documentation

Documentation is an important step in the process of education. Communication between all members of the multidisciplinary team is essential to the effectiveness of the process. Much of that communication is through documentation. Documentation also provides legal protection for the staff. The rule is the same as with any other nursing activity: If it is not written down in the chart, it did not happen.

Documentation should include areas of learning, what has been taught, client/family response to the teaching, degree of success in meeting the outcome criteria, and what further areas of teaching are required. Any one of a number of forms may be used to document education, including narrative notes and teaching flow sheets. It is your responsibility to document all phases of client education in which you are involved.

Key Concepts

Introduction

- Communication is the foundation of interpersonal relationships and is a key factor in the nursing process.

The Nature of Communication

- To analyze communication you must consider spoken words, paralanguage, the thinking process, emotions, nonverbal behavior, and the culture of the person sending the message.

- Nonverbal communication includes body language, eye contact, personal space, and the use of touch.

- Listening means paying attention to what the person is saying, acknowledging feelings, holding back on what you have to say, avoiding interruption, and controlling the urge to give advice.

- Characteristics of effective helpers include a nonjudgmental approach, acceptance, warmth, empathy, authenticity, congruency, patience, trustworthiness, self-disclosure, and humor.

- Closed-ended questions determine specific information and may be helpful to clients experiencing high levels of anxiety or disorganized thinking. If these are overused, however, the interaction takes on an atmosphere of cross-examination.

- Open-ended questions help increase the client's participation in the interaction and encourage the client to continue the discussion.

- Techniques that facilitate effective communication include broad openings, giving recognition, minimal encouragements, offering self, accepting, making observations, validating perceptions, exploring, clarifying, placing the event in time or sequence, focusing, encouraging the formulation of a plan of action, suggesting collaboration, restatement, reflection, and summarizing.

- Techniques that contribute to ineffective communication include stereotypical comments, parroting, changing the topic, disagreeing, challenging, requesting an explanation, false reassurance, belittling expressed feelings, probing, advising, imposing values, and double/multiple questions.

- Understanding family and group communication includes the perception of communication, affective and cognitive interpretation, validation, and interventions.

- The interpretation of nonverbal communication, verbal communication, and affective expression will enable you to help families and groups become more effective communicators.

- Patronizing speech with older adults is the result of age-related stereotypes and implies that the older adult is incompetent and without dignity.

Client and Family Education

- Communication is the most important skill in effective education.

- Assessing areas of learning includes the client's and family's view of mental illness, knowledge of medications, and what they want and need to know.

- You must diagnose any barriers to learning such as anxiety, manic behavior, delusions, hallucinations, disorganized thinking, obsessional thoughts, depression, anger, hostility, and denial of the mental disorder.

- The goal of teaching is to prepare clients and families for as much self-care as possible in order to live in the least restrictive setting.

- The six general areas of learning are knowledge of the mental disorder, medications, managing ADLs, interpersonal communication, coping with life, and community resources.

- The steps of the problem-solving process are identifying the problem, identifying attempted solutions, listing alternative solutions, predicting consequences, choosing the best alternative, implementing the alternative, and evaluating the outcome.

- Client/family education is effective if the outcome criteria are met.

- All steps of the education process must be documented in the client's record.

Review Questions

1. You have observed that, while talking to you, Al's body is rigid and he has been shaking his foot and clenching his fists. Al may be experiencing

   a. low self-esteem.

   b. anger.

   c. anxiety.

   d. fear.

2. Identify which of the following questions is the best example of the communication technique of placing an event in time or sequence.

   a. How do your parents feel about your new boyfriend?

   b. Could you explain more about that to me?

   c. When did you first notice that your wife seemed frustrated?

   d. It sounds like you're feeling hopeless—is that correct?

3. Your client has asked you what she should do about her job. You reply, "I think you should quit your job because it is just too stressful." This is an ineffective communication technique for which reason?

   a. It demands an explanation from the client.

   b. It disagrees with the client.

   c. It belittles the client's feelings.

   d. It tells the client what to do.

4. Being listened to makes each of us feel validated because it means the listener is

   a. hearing the words we are saying.

   b. taking us seriously.

   c. ignoring all other people.

   d. making assumptions about who we are.

5. Which is the second step in the problem-solving process?

   a. identifying the problem

   b. listing alternative solutions

   c. identifying attempted solutions

   d. predicting consequences

References

Collins, M. (1983). *Communication in Health Care* (2nd ed.). St. Louis, MO: Mosby.

Giles, H, et al. (1994). Talking age and aging talk. In M. L. Hummert, J. M. Wiemann, & J. F. Nussbaum. (Eds.). *Interpersonal Communication in Older Adulthood* (pp. 130–161). Thousand Oaks, CA: Sage.

Hummert, M. L. (1994). Stereotypes of the elderly and patronizing speech. In M. L. Hummert, J. M. Wiemann, & J. F. Nussbaum (Eds.). *Interpersonal Communication in Older Adulthood* (pp. 162–184). Thousand Oaks, CA: Sage.

Navarra, T., Lipkowitz, M. A., & Navarra, J. G. (1990). *Therapeutic Communication*. Slack.

Nichols, M. P. (1995). *The Lost Art of Listening*. New York: Guilford Press.

Okun, B. F. (1987). *Effective Helping* (3rd ed.). Belmont, CA: Brooks/Cole.

Palmer-Erbs, V. (1996). A breath of fresh air in a turbulent health-care environment. *J Psychosoc Nurs, 34*(9), 16–21.

Robinson, V. M. (1991). *Humor and the Health Professions* (2nd ed.). Thorofare, NJ: Slack.

Sieh., A. & Brentin, L. K. (1997). *The Nurse Communicates*. Philadelphia: Saunders.

Spector, R. E. (1996). *Cultural Diversity in Health and Illness*. Norwalk, CT: Appleton & Lange.

Common Clinical Problems

Mary Moller
Karen Lee Fontaine

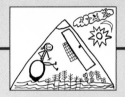

Objectives

After reading this chapter, you will be able to:

- Identify problems that are symptomatic of a number of mental disorders.
- Intervene with clients who are experiencing hallucinations, delusions, self-mutilating behavior, and aggression.

Key Terms

delusion
hallucination
illusion
psychosis
self-mutilation

During your clinical rotation in mental health nursing, you will encounter certain common problems. These problems occur in a variety of settings, including inpatient units, residential care programs, outpatient settings, and the home. Not necessarily related to a specific disorder, these problems may be symptoms of a number of mental disorders. Violence against one's self, such as self-mutilation, and violence against others are two problems needing immediate intervention. Hallucinations and delusions often accompany **psychosis,** a state in which a person is unable to comprehend reality and has difficulty commuicating and relating to others. Hallucinations may trigger violent episodes if voices command the person to hurt their self or others. Delusions may lead to dangerous situations such as jumping from high places because of the belief that one can fly. (A residual phase of the illness often follows the active phase and is characterized by less severe symptoms.)

Clients Experiencing Hallucinations

A **hallucination** is the occurrence of a sight, sound, touch, smell, or taste without any external stimulus to the corresponding sensory organ. The experience is real to the person. Perceptual changes are often an early symptom in mental disorders. **Illusions** are simply one or more of your five senses playing tricks on you. They are a sensory misperception of environmental stimuli. An example is looking at a cord on the floor and thinking you are seeing a snake. A common illusion is seeing heat rising from highway pavement and believing there is a large pool of water on the pavement.

Although hallucinations are most commonly associated with schizophrenic disorders, only 70% of clients with schizophrenia experience them. Hallucinations also occur in the manic phase of bipolar disorder, severe depression, substance dependence, and substance withdrawal. Hallucinations represent a complex interaction between brain physiology, environmental stimuli, and the person's perception of the world. Studies have shown that 90% of people who experience hallucinations also experience delusions (Moller, Rice, and Murphy, 1998).

Auditory hallucinations, which account for 70% of hallucinations, are thought to be caused by dysfunction in the language centers of the cerebral cortex, located in the temporal lobes of the brain. These sounds can fluctuate from a simple noise or voice, to a voice talking about the client, to a voice talking about what the client is thinking, to complete conversations between two or more people. The majority of people say the hallucinations are distressing to them. The voices may make derogatory remarks and try to get them to do or say something that is potentially harmful to themselves or others (Buccheri et al, 1996).

Visual hallucinations are thought to be caused by dysfunction in the occipital lobes of the brain. They can fluctuate from flashes of light or geometric figures, to cartoon figures, to elaborate and complex scenes or visions. Visual hallucinations are often accompanied by auditory hallucinations.

Gustatory and *olfactory hallucinations* typically consist of putrid, foul, and rancid tastes or smells of a repulsive nature. *Tactile hallucinations* involve the sense of touch. People may verbalize feeling electrical sensations coming from the ground or inanimate objects. *Kinesthetic hallucinations* involve the feeling of body processes such as blood pulsing through the veins, food digesting, or urine forming. These types of hallucinations are typically associated with organic changes such as those that occur in a stroke, brain tumor, seizures, substance dependence, and substance withdrawal (Moller, Rice, and Murphy, 1998).

A *command hallucination* is a special type of auditory hallucination that is potentially dangerous. Occasionally, the command can be to do something useful, such as calling the doctor. More typically, the voice orders the person to do something that is frightening and may cause harm, such as cutting off a body part or striking out at someone. Fear from command hallucinations can also cause dangerous behavior, such as jumping out a window to escape a person who is trying to intervene.

Hallucinations are as real to the person having them as your dreams are to you. They are symptoms that need to be assessed in the same manner as any other symptoms. Left unattended, hallucinations will continue and may escalate. Talking about one's hallucinations is a reassuring and self-validating experience. Such a discussion can take place only in an atmosphere of genuine interest and concern.

Ask yourself: How can I tell if my client is actually experiencing hallucinations? Behaviors often perceived as inappropriate may be a response to hallucinations. These behaviors include inappropriate laughter, conversations with an unseen person, difficulty paying attention to the task at hand, and a slow verbal response. In the case of severe hallucinations, the person may be unable to respond to anything in the external environment. See Table 6.1 for assessment cues that a client may be hallucinating.

Hallucinations serve as a useful indicator in the ongoing assessment of a client's level of functioning. It is important to identify hallucinations as a *symptom* of psychosis. Consider them problems to be solved. They can interfere with ADLs to the point of complete withdrawal, depending on the level of intrusiveness. Hallucinations also fluctuate in levels of intensity and are related to the level of anxiety the person is experiencing. In the residual phase of a mental disorder, the hallucinations are at level I or II and are described as chronic hallucinations. In level I, the client experiences a moderate level of anxiety, and the hallucination is comforting. If the anxiety does not escalate, the hallucination is within conscious control. As anxiety becomes severe, level II hallucinations become condemning. There is less control over the experience, and the person may withdraw from others to avoid embarrassment from the symptom.

In the active, or psychotic, phase of a mental disorder, hallucinations are at level III or IV and are described as acute hallucinations. The client is disoriented and confused and may not be able to tell you about the experience. Level III hallucinations are accompanied by severe anxiety, and the hallucination has become controlling. The person gives in to the experience and may feel lonely if the hallucination stops. Level IV hallucinations are accompanied by panic-level anxiety, and the hallucination is conquering. There may be command hallucinations with a potential for danger, and the person may be filled with terror. Table 6.2 describes the four levels of intensity of hallucinations in more detail.

Intervening with clients experiencing hallucinations requires patience and the ability to spend time with them. Clients consistently report the following four interventions to be most helpful during the acute phase of hallucinations:

1. Having someone with them.
2. Hearing a real person talk.

Table 6.1 Hallucinations and Client Behaviors

Sense	Observable Client Behaviors
Auditory	■ Moving eyes back and forth as if looking for someone ■ Listening intently to a person who is not speaking ■ Engaging in conversation with an invisible person
Visual	■ Suddenly appearing startled, frightened, or terrified by another person or object or by no apparent stimulus ■ Suddenly running into another room
Olfactory	■ Wrinkling nose as if smelling something horrible ■ Smelling parts of the body ■ Smelling the air while walking toward another person ■ Responding to an odor with terror
Gustatory	■ Spitting out food or beverage ■ Refusing to eat, drink, or take medications
Tactile	■ Slapping self as if putting out a fire ■ Trying to brush invisible things, like bugs, off the body ■ Jumping up and down on the floor as if avoiding pain or other stimuli to feet
Kinesthetic	■ Verbalizing and/or obsessing about body processes ■ Refusing to complete a task that may require a part of the body the client believes is not working

Source: Moller, Rice, and Murphy, 1998.

3. Being able to see the person who is talking.
4. Being touched.

It is crucial that you not leave clients alone during this intense and often frightening experience. When you talk to them, you may need to talk slightly louder than usual, but use very short and simple phrases. Maintain friendly eye contact, and use their preferred name. If the hallucinations are being caused by

Table 6.2 Hallucinations: Levels of Intensity

Level	Characteristics	Behaviors
I: Comforting Moderate level of anxiety. Hallucination is generally of a pleasant nature.	Client experiences intense emotions such as anxiety, loneliness, guilt, and fear and tries to focus on comforting thoughts to relieve anxiety; recognizes that thoughts and sensory experiences are within conscious control if the anxiety is managed. Residual phase; nonpsychotic.	Grinning or laughter that seems inappropriate; moving lips without emitting any sounds; rapid eye movements; slowed verbal responses as if preoccupied; silent and preoccupied.
II: Condemning Severe level of anxiety. Hallucination generally becomes repulsive.	Sensory experience of any of the identified senses is repulsive and frightening; client begins to feel a loss of control and may attempt to distance self from the perceived source; may feel embarrassed by the sensory experience and withdraw from others. Residual phase; nonpsychotic.	Increased autonomic nervous system signs of anxiety such as increased heart rate, respiration, and blood pressure; attention span begins to narrow; preoccupation with sensory experience; loss of ability to differentiate hallucination from reality.
III: Controlling Severe level of anxiety. Hallucination becomes omnipotent.	Client gives up trying to combat the experience and gives in to it; content of hallucination may become appealing; client may experience loneliness if sensory experience ends. Active phase; psychotic.	Directions given by the hallucination will be followed rather than objected to; difficulty relating to others; attention span of only a few seconds or minutes; physical symptoms of severe anxiety such as perspiring, tremors, inability to follow directions.
IV: Conquering Panic level of anxiety. Hallucination generally becomes elaborate and interwoven with delusions.	Sensory experiences may become threatening if client doesn't follow commands; hallucinations may last for hours or days if there is no therapeutic intervention. Active phase; psychotic.	Terror-stricken behavior such as panic; strong potential for suicide or homicide; physical activity that reflects content of hallucination such as violence, agitation, withdrawal, or catatonia; inability to respond to complex directions; inability to respond to more than one person.

abnormalities in the temporal lobes, clients may not be able to hear you but will see that your mouth is moving and have a sense that you are real. Perceiving that someone real is talking and calling them by name validates that they are alive. Even if they may not be able to respond to you, they are aware of your presence. Touch may be helpful at this time. Proceed slowly and tell the client that you are about to touch him and where this touch will occur. Sometimes it is helpful to extend your hand toward the client and ask him to grab hold. In this way, you can serve as an anchor and improve his sense of reality. Ask the client to describe what is happening. Talking about the hallucination gives the person permission not to continue to try and hide the experience. Look around the immediate area and identify any possible environmental triggers. Objects that are reflective or cause glare, such as television screens, photographs behind glass, and fluorescent lights, can contribute to visual hallucinations. Encourage the person to describe feelings related to the hallucinations. If asked, simply point out that you are not experiencing the hallucination. Do not argue about what is or is not occurring. The client is usually seeking validation and may be grateful to learn that you are not experiencing the same phenomenon (Moller, Rice, and Murphy, 1996).

Clients experiencing hallucinations have no voluntary control over the neurobiologic dysfunction that is causing the hallucinations. Hallucinations cannot be simply willed or talked away. Isolating clients during this time of sensory confusion often exacerbates the hallucinations. Remain nearby, because having a real person to talk and listen to will help them return to reality. People who experience ongoing hallucinations can be assisted to accept and cope with their hallucinations. These strategies involve focusing, reducing anxiety, and distraction. See Box 6.1 for self-help strategies.

Clients Experiencing Delusions

Delusions are false beliefs that cannot be changed by logical reasoning or evidence; they result from misunderstanding reality. These ideas are firmly sustained in spite of what everyone else thinks and evidence to the contrary. It is important to realize that a delusion does not always last. It may be fixed in the person's mind only for a few weeks or months. Many clients have reported relief when they realized the belief was a delusion and not a reality.

When there is an extensively developed central delusional theme from which conclusions are deduced, the delusions are called *systematized*. Delusions can be a single thought, or they can pervade the person's entire cognitive process. Of people experiencing delusions, 90% have concurrent hallucinations. Delusions are believed to be caused by dysfunction in the information-processing circuits within and between the brain's two hemispheres. If one of the functions of the brain is to make order out of chaos, these strange thoughts may serve a purpose. As with hallucinations, the severity of delusions can be a valuable indicator in monitoring the course of a mental disorder.

There are a number of delusional types. *Grandiosity*, also known as *delusions of grandeur*, is an exaggerated sense of importance or self-worth. It is often accompanied by beliefs of magical thinking. *Delusions of persecution* involve beliefs that someone is trying to harm them and, therefore, any personal failures in life are the fault of these harmful others. *Delusions of control* occur when the person believes that feelings, impulses, thoughts, or actions are not one's

Box 6.1

Hallucinations and Self-Help Strategies

Self-monitor.

- Keep a journal of when each hallucination occurred and what was happening at the time.
- Develop a list of what makes a hallucination better or worse.

Read aloud/talk with someone.

- Speaking may reduce the loudness, clarity, and duration of auditory hallucinations.
- Reality orientation may reduce fear associated with hallucinations.

Increase physiological arousal level.

- Walking or jogging may distract from hallucinations.
- Doing housework or yard work may distract from hallucinations.

Decrease physiological arousal level.

- Listening to music or a relaxation tape with headphones decreases anxiety and shifts attention away from hallucination.
- Wearing earplugs may decrease environmental triggers.

Talk back to/ignore the voices.

- Responding to the voices may make them go away.
- Saying "stop and go away" aloud is a thought-stopping technique to reduce auditory hallucinations.
- Naming environmental objects aloud may block the auditory input of the voices.

Participate in structured activities.

- Hallucinations decrease in situations with more structure such as playing games, participating in groups, etc.

Sources: Buccheri et al, 1996; Frederick and Cotanch, 1995.

own but are being imposed by some external force. *Religious delusions* involve false beliefs with religious or spiritual themes. *Erotomanic delusions* are beliefs that a person, usually someone famous and of higher status, is in love with her/him. *Somatic delusions* occur when people believe something abnormal and dangerous is happening to their bodies. *Ideas of reference* are remarks or actions by someone else that in no way refer to the person but that are interpreted as related to her or him. *Thought broadcasting* occurs when people believe that their thoughts can be heard by others. *Thought withdrawal* is the belief that others are able to remove thoughts from one's mind. *Thought insertion* is the belief that others are able to put thoughts into one's mind. Chapter 12 presents clinical examples of the different types of delusions.

Religious ideas that may appear to be delusional in one culture may be commonly held in another. It is important that you be able to distinguish religious beliefs and experiences from delusional psychotic symptoms (Lukoff, Lu, and Turner, 1995). Psychotic episodes:

- are more intense than usual experiences in their religious community
- are often terrifying for the person
- involve obsessional preoccupation with the delusion
- are associated with deterioration of self-care and social skills
- often involve special messages from religious figures

Clients cope with delusions in several ways. Some adapt by simply learning to live with them, some deny their presence, and others want to understand and manage them when they occur. Guidelines for intervening with clients experiencing delusions are given in Box 6.2.

Clients Who Self-Mutilate

Self-mutilation is the deliberate destruction of body tissue without conscious intent of suicide. Other terms used to describe self-mutilation include deliberate self-harm, self-injurious behavior, and aggression against the self. Self-mutilative behavior may occur once or sporadically, or it may become repetitive. The behavior occurs in an estimated 24–40% of mental health clients. It is a symptom associated with child-

Box 6.2

Intervening with Clients Experiencing Delusions

Provide opportunity to discuss delusion.

- Delusions are often very frightening.
- Provide comfort and reassurance.
- Refocus conversation to another topic after listening to delusion.
- Assist client to identify situations where it is socially unacceptable to discuss delusions.

Monitor delusions for content.

- Identify beliefs that may be self-harmful or harmful to others.
- Protect the client and others from behaviors that might be harmful.
- Encourage client to verbalize delusions to caregivers before acting on them.

If asked, simply point out that the delusion is not your experience.

- Always present reality, but do it gently, without implying the client is wrong.
- Do not reason, argue, or challenge the delusion.
- Do not attempt to logically explain the delusion; only the client understands the logic behind the delusion.

Identify triggers of the delusion.

- Focus on the underlying feelings; unexpressed feelings can trigger delusions.
- Assist client to avoid or eliminate stressors that precipitate delusions.

Identify coping techniques.

- Reinforce and focus on reality by talking about real events and people.
- Plan recreational, diversional activities that require attention and skill.

Sources: Klebanoff and Smith, 1997; Moller and Murphy, 1996.

hood sexual abuse, borderline personality disorder, eating disorders, cognitive impairment disorders, obsessive-compulsive disorder, posttraumatic stress disorder, dissociative identity disorder, and mental retardation. Self-mutilation may occur in response to delusions, command hallucinations, and substance abuse or dependence (Romans, 1995; Torem, 1995).

Self-injury takes many forms. The most common forms are superficial to moderate self-mutilation behaviors, including skin cutting, skin carving (words, designs, symbols), skin burning, severe skin scratching, needle sticking, self-hitting, tearing out hair, inserting dangerous objects into the vagina or rectum, ingesting sharp objects, bone breaking, and interfering with wound healing. Occasionally, serious acts of self-mutilation occur, such as eye enucleation, castration, and amputation of fingers, toes, or limbs. People who self-mutilate often use multiple methods of self-harm. Stereotypic self-mutilation occurs in fixed patterns that are often rhythmic, such as head banging and finger biting. This behavior occurs most often in people who are institutionalized for mental retardation (Connors, 1996; Torem, 1995). Box 6.3 describes the stages of self-mutilation. Biological studies have found that the neurotransmitters dopamine (DA) and serotonin (5-HT) influence self-mutilative behavior. Both DA and 5-HT dysfunction are related to impulsive and aggressive behaviors. Dysphoria may be lessened as endorphins are released in response to the physical pain (Faye, 1995). The behavior is generally impulsive, and the onset is often linked to a stressful situation. As one client described her experience: "I thought I needed to be punished, that I was bad. I'd cut myself and get relief. I got relief from seeing my own blood; it was like my feelings were flowing out." Some of the many meanings of or reasons for self-mutilation are:

- ending a dissociative experience
- reorienting from flashbacks
- re-enactment of childhood trauma
- reconnecting to a feeling of being real and alive
- seeking distraction from emotional pain
- releasing tension or anger
- punishing oneself
- requesting nurturance
- feeling powerful and in control
- manipulating others

It is very important to establish a trusting relationship with clients who self-mutilate. They have probably experienced much criticism and little understanding regarding their self-injurious behavior. Vic-

Box 6.3

Stages of Self-Mutilation

Stage 1: Precipitating Event
- This may include events such as the loss of a significant relationship or the perception or threat of an imminent loss.

Stage 2: Intensification of Feelings
- Unpleasant feelings such as anxiety, anger, helplessness, hopelessness, emptiness, and despair increase to high levels.

Stage 3: Attempts to Cope
- Client tries to delay the act of self-inflicted violence.

Stage 4: Action
- Client "gives in" to internal demand to self-mutilate.
- Acts of self-mutilation occur in private; unless medical attention is required, the behavior is often not discovered.

Stage 5: Aftermath
- Client may experience feelings of relief from tension or feelings of shame, guilt, or sense of failure.

Sources: Faye, 1995; Torem, 1995.

tims often have been told that they should just stop the behavior and have been scolded for not being competent enough. Under these conditions, the failure to stop the self-harm leads to even greater shame and concealment. They respond best to a nonjudgmental and accepting attitude, a caring approach, and the setting of limits to minimize the potential for physical injury. It is also understandable that staff members may react with frustration and even guilt when clients choose to harm themselves despite well-planned interventions and a caring approach (Loughrey, 1997).

There are three basic goals in helping clients manage their self-harmful behavior. The first goal is to encourage communication about self-injury, since clients are often secretive and shameful about the behavior. Supportive listening may help them communicate and thus feel less isolated. The second goal is to improve the related quality of life, such as through reducing their shame and isolation, decreasing their self-criticism, and ensuring that they receive adequate medical attention. Your ability to respond without blame or shame may help clients begin the process of self-healing. The third goal is to diminish or extinguish the use of self-mutilation as a coping tool. As clients grow in their understanding of their own experiences, they will improve their ability to manage, live with, or cease their behavior. Box 6.4 describes appropriate nursing activities when intervening with people who self-mutilate. Finding alternatives to self-harm behaviors is a critical step for people who wish to stop hurting themselves. Sometimes this means learning new skills in the areas of problem solving, or in relaxation and anxiety reduction. Box 6.5 lists non-injurious alternatives clients may wish to consider.

Clients Who Are Aggressive

Physical aggression and destruction of property are among the most severe and frightening client behaviors. Violence is often directed at family members in the home and may result in physical injuries. Other persons attacked by clients include friends and acquaintances, health care professionals, or other clients in health care settings. The best predictor of future violence in a client is a history of violent behavior. Physical assault is an increasing problem, but it is important to recognize that most clients are not violent. It is believed that the increase in violence is related to increased substance abuse by people with mental disorders. Tardiff (1997) describes the relationship of violence to substance use:

- direct effect of the substance on the brain—especially crack cocaine, which is associated with irritability, impulsiveness, and paranoid delusional thinking

- exposure to a dangerous environment, such as drug dealing and crack houses

- activities, such as robbery and prostitution, through which money is obtained for drugs

Violence may also be a consequence of poor frustration tolerance, ineffective individual coping, impulsivity, and real or imagined threats to the person's territory, body space, or life. In residential and day

---

Box 6.4

Behavior Management: Self-Harm

Identify the functions of the behavior.

- In a nonjudgmental manner, ask "How does this help you?" or "What does this do for you?" This will increase clients' self-understanding and decrease feelings of shame.

Identify the triggers.

- Have clients keep a journal describing the stressors preceding the behavior, situations in which the behavior occurs, and the effect on others.

Use behavioral contracts.

- Contracts focus on the fact that clients are responsible for their own behavior and they have to live with the consequences of their behavior.

- Contracts include a clear understanding of treatment goals and mutual expectations of behavioral change.

Sources: McCloskey and Bulechek, 1996; Torem, 1995.

---

programs and inpatient settings, aggression and violence have been related to staff provocation. Violence occurs at a higher rate in settings where staff have an authoritarian or controlling approach to clients. Telling clients what they can or cannot do, detaining them against their will, and forcing them to take medication contribute to staff-client conflicts. When these actions are used with people who are used to controlling their environment through aggression and violence, one can predict an escalation of violent behavior (Harris and Morrison, 1995).

Aggression affects every person in the environment in which it occurs. A violent client may be injured directly from the aggressive behavior or during the restraining procedure. Other clients and staff members may be accidentally injured. Out-of-control behavior frightens everyone, and violence disrupts the residential, program, or unit morale.

Seclusion and restraints are traditional methods for controlling violent clients. However, because these procedures require physical force (called a *take*

Box 6.5

Alternatives to Self-Mutilation

Non-harmful Symbolic Enactments

- Draw the "blood" or "cuts" on paper.
- "Injure" a toy or stuffed animal.
- Make marks with red marker or crayon on your skin.

Physical Awareness

- Breathe slowly and mentally scan each part of the body.
- Stroke your arm or leg, place ice on your skin, snap a rubber band on your wrist.

Distraction

- Promise yourself to wait 5–10 minutes before self-injuring.
- Read a book, watch a video, go to a movie.

Interpersonal Contact

- Call a friend; talk about the impulse toward self-harm.
- Call a support group member.

Physical Activity, Tension Reduction

- Exercise, dance, play a physical game.

Art and Writing Activities

- Draw the feeling or the memory.
- Write about your feelings; write a letter to a significant person.

Expressive Anger Activities

- Pound a tennis racket on a bed; pound pillows.
- Break old dishes or glasses in safe ways; throw ice cubes; smash aluminum cans.

Sources: Connors, 1996; Torem, 1995.

---

down), which increases the risk of injury, there are ethical concerns. (For further information on seclusion and restraints, see Chapter 7.) Use of physical force with clients reinforces their perception that violence is a valid method of gaining control. It also reinforces the client's self-image as a tough person and increases the likelihood of future violent confrontations. Unfortunately, these methods do not teach clients coping skills to help them avoid using aggression in the future. Because clients often view restraints as punishment, this method fosters distrust of, and malice toward, staff members (Harris and Morrison, 1995).

At this time, no medication has been approved specifically for the treatment of aggression. Antipsychotic drugs, the most commonly used medications, are given primarily for their sedative effects. They may be effective over time for those clients who are aggressive in response to the active phase of their mental disorder. Sedatives and antianxiety agents may help those who do not respond to other measures designed to reduce aggression.

Telling people what they can do is more effective than stating what is not allowed. "Put the chair by the table" may work better than, "Don't pick that chair up." Telling people what they cannot do may set up power struggles. Losing control can be equally frightening to clients as to staff. Another approach is to give clients choices. "There are two quieter places you may go to: your room or the deck. Which one would you like?" Each time a choice is given, the person will pause and consider the option. Each pause decreases the amount of energy behind the anger. Giving choices also helps people to feel they have some control in the situation (Ferguson and Smith, 1996; Maier, 1996). See Box 6.6 for nursing activities directed at anger control assistance.

Talking down is another effective approach. The immediate goal is to gain some time and help the person regain self-control. People who are under the influence of alcohol or drugs are not appropriate for this intervention. The first step is to set the stage. This means you should know what your route of escape would be or that help is immediately available. Making certain that you have their attention, use a soft assertive voice and short sentences in a nonthreatening manner. Do not overreact or talk too much. Avoid using threatening body language such as clenched fists, hands on hips, or arms crossed. Keep a nearby but safe distance and do not physically touch the person. If the client says "Get away from me!", move away in a slow manner that is respectful of their communication but not a sign of fear.

Box 6.6

Anger Control Assistance

Anticipate potentially aggressive situations.

- Limit access to frustrating situation until client is able to express self appropriately.
- Monitor the potential for inappropriate aggression.
- Remove potential weapons.

Intervene before the behavior escalates to out-of-control aggression.

- Assist client in identifying the source of anger.
- Identify the function that anger, frustration, and rage serve for the client.
- Establish expectation that client can control the behavior.
- Provide physical outlets for expression of anger or tension.

- Help client identify the benefits of expressing anger in an adaptive, nonviolent way.
- Identify consequences of inappropriate expression of anger.
- Instruct on use of calming measures such as deep breaths and self-controlled time outs.

Teach nonviolent coping strategies.

- Do this at a time when the client is not angry or tense.
- Help client plan strategies to prevent inappropriate expression of anger (time outs, counting backwards from 100 by 3s).
- Help client develop appropriate methods to express feelings (assertiveness, "I" feeling statements).
- Roleplay potentially frustrating situations.

Sources: Klebanoff and Smith, 1997; McCloskey and Bulechek, 1996.

The second step is the actual talking down. For the time being, agree with what the client is saying. Avoid arguing so that you do not get stuck on the content of the client's communication. At this point it does not matter if all nurses are uncaring, whether you should go jump in the lake, or who your ancestors are. None of that matters. What matters is that you de-escalate the person by not arguing and not giving the person a reason to continue to be angry. Continue to speak in a soft voice and give the person choices. If all else fails and you are in a setting with adequate staff, a take down may be the last option (Klebanoff and Smith, 1997; Maier, 1996). See Chapter 7 for take down measures and the use of restraints.

Key Concepts

Introduction

- Common clinical problems, such a hallucinations, delusions, self-mutilating behavior, and aggression, are symptoms of a number of mental disorders.

Clients Experiencing Hallucinations

- A hallucination is the occurrence of a sight, sound, touch, smell, or taste without any external stimulus to the corresponding sensory organ. The experience is real to the person.

- An illusion is a sensory misperception of a real environmental stimulus.

- Auditory hallucinations are caused by dysfunction in the language centers of the cerebral cortex, located in the temporal lobes.

- Visual hallucinations are caused by dysfunction in the occipital lobes.

- Gustatory, olfactory, tactile, and kinesthetic hallucinations are associated with organic changes such as those that occur in a stroke, a brain tumor, seizures, substance dependence, and substance withdrawal.

- A command hallucination is potentially dangerous because the voice may order the person to cause harm to self or others.

- Illusions are misperceptions of actual environmental stimuli.

- Left unattended, hallucinations will continue and may escalate.

- Cues that a client is hallucinating include inappropriate laughter, conversations with an unseen person, difficulty paying attention to the task at hand, and a slow verbal response.

- If the hallucinations are severe, the person may be unable to respond to anything in the environment.

- Hallucinations can serve as an indicator in the course of a mental disorder.

- The levels of intensity of the hallucination correspond to levels of anxiety.

- Level I hallucinations are accompanied by moderate anxiety, and the hallucination is comforting. If the anxiety does not escalate, the hallucination is within conscious control.

- Level II hallucinations are accompanied by severe anxiety, and the hallucination becomes condemning. There is less control over the experience, and the person may withdraw from others to avoid embarrassment.

- Level III hallucinations are accompanied by severe anxiety, and the hallucination is controlling. The person gives in to the experience and may feel lonely if the hallucination stops.

- Level IV hallucinations are accompanied by panic-level anxiety, and the hallucination is conquering. There may be command hallucinations with a potential for danger, and the person may be filled with terror.

- Clients report that it is most helpful to have someone with them, to hear a real person talk, to see the person who is talking, and to be touched while they are experiencing hallucinations.

- Self-help strategies include self-monitoring, reading aloud/talking with someone; increasing or decreasing physiological arousal level, talking back to or ignoring the voices, and participating in structured activities.

Clients Experiencing Delusions

- Delusions are false beliefs that cannot be changed by logical reasoning or evidence. They may have a central theme and be systematized or may extend to many areas and be nonsystematized.

- Types of delusions are grandeur; persecution; control; religious; erotomanic; somatic; ideas of reference; and thought broadcasting, withdrawal, and insertion.

- Intervening with clients experiencing delusions includes providing the opportunity to discuss the delusions, monitoring for content, pointing out your different experience, identifying triggers, and identifying coping techniques.

Clients Who Self-Mutilate

- Self-mutilation is the deliberate destruction of body tissue without conscious intent of suicide. It is a symptom that is associated with many mental disorders.

- The most common forms of self-mutilation are superficial to moderate behaviors.

- DA and 5-HT dysfunction and the release of endorphins may influence self-mutilative behavior.

- Some of the many meanings of or reasons for self-mutilation are ending dissociation, reorienting from flashbacks, re-enactment of childhood trauma, reconnecting to feeling real, seeking distraction from emotional pain, releasing tension or anger, punishing the self, requesting nurturance, feeling powerful, and manipulating others.

- Stages of self-mutilation are precipitating event, intensification of feelings, attempts to cope, action, and aftermath.

- Goals in helping clients manage their behavior are to encourage communication, improve the quality of life, and diminish or extinguish the use of self-mutilation.

- Help clients identify the functions and the triggers to self-mutilate; develop behavioral contracts to help clients regain control.

- Alternatives to self-harm include symbolic enactments, physical awareness, distraction, interpersonal contact, physical activity, art and writing activities, and expressive anger activities.

Clients Who Are Aggressive

- The best predictor of future violence in a client is a history of violent behavior.

- The increase in violence is related to increased substance abuse; factors include the direct effect of the drug on the brain, exposure to dangerous environments, and illegal activities to obtain drugs.

- Violence occurs at higher rates in settings where staff have an authoritarian or controlling approach to clients.

- Seclusion and restraints may be used to manage an aggressive client, but these can lead to further injury and do not teach the client coping skills for avoiding aggression in the future.

- Sedatives and antianxiety agents may be helpful in managing aggressive clients.

- Telling clients what they can do, giving them choices, and talking them down are appropriate interventions for the client who is aggressive.

- Anger control assistance includes anticipating potentially aggressive situations, intervening before behavior is out of control, and teaching nonviolent coping strategies.

Review Questions

1. You notice that your client is sitting by herself and moving her eyes back and forth as if looking for someone. This behavior indicates that you must assess for the presence of

    a. delusions.

    b. hallucinations.

    c. illusions.

    d. anxiety.

2. A self-help strategy for the person experiencing hallucinations is

    a. listening to music with headphones.

    b. sitting in a quiet room.

    c. thinking about the meaning of the hallucination.

    d. taking an extra dose of medication.

3. As a nurse you should monitor the content of clients' delusions. The rationale is to

    a. point out reality.

    b. eliminate stressors.

    c. identify harmful beliefs.

    d. reassure that the belief is not real.

4. Alternatives to self-mutilation include

    a. reading aloud to drown out the voices.

    b. marking the skin with a red marker.

    c. pointing out that the behavior is unusual.

    d. putting the person in seclusion.

5. Use of physical force with clients reinforces that

    a. violence is a valid method of gaining control.

    b. the staff is in control, not the clients.

    c. anger is an inappropriate feeling.

    d. clients can control their own behavior.

References

Buccheri, R., et al. (1996). Auditory hallucinations in schizophrenia. *J Psychosoc Nurs, 34*(2), 12–25.

Connors, R. (1996). Self-injury in trauma survivors. *Am J Orthopsychiatry, 66*(2), 197–206.

Faye, P. (1995). Addictive characteristics of the behavior of self-mutilation. *J Psychosoc Nurs, 33*(6), 36–39.

Ferguson, J. S., & Smith, A. (1996). Aggressive behvior on an inpatient geriatric unit. *J Psychosoc Nurs, 34*(3), 27–32.

Frederick, J. , & Cotanch, P. (1995). Self-help techniques for auditory hallucinations in schizophrenia. *Issues Ment Health Nurs, 16*(3): 213–224.

Harris, D., & Morrison, E. (1995). Managing violence without coercion. *Arch Psychiatr Nurs, 9*(4), 203–210.

Klebanoff, N. A., & Smith, N. M. (1997). *Behavioral Management in Home Care*. Philadelphia: Lippincott.

Loughrey, L., et al. (1997). Patient self-mutilation: When nursing becomes a nightmare. *J Psychosoc Nurs, 35*(4), 30–34.

Lukoff, D., Lu, F. G., & Turner, R. (1995). Cultural considerations in the assessment and treatment of religious and spiritual problems. *Psychiatr Clin North Am, 18*(3), 467–485.

Maier, G. Y. (1996). Managing threatening behavior. *J Psychosoc Nurs, 34*(6), 25–30.

McCloskey, J. C., & Bulechek, G. M. (1996). *Nursing Interventions Classification (NIC)* (2nd ed.). St. Louis, MO: Mosby.

Moller, M. D., Rice, M. J., & Murphy, M. F. (1998). *Psychiatric Protocals for Family Nurse Practitioners*. Philadelphia: Saunders.

Romans, S. E., et al. (1995). Sexual abuse in childhood and deliberate self-harm. *Am J Psychiatry, 152*(9), 1336–1342.

Tardiff, K., et al. (1997). Violence by patients admitted to a private psychiatric hospital. *Am J Psychiatry, 154*(1), 88–93.

Torem, M. S. (1995). A practical approach in the treatment of self-inflicted violence. *J Holistic Nurs, 13*(1), 37–52.

CHAPTER 7

Treatment Modalities

Leslie Rittenmeyer
Karen Lee Fontaine

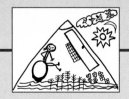

Objectives

After reading this chapter, you will be able to:

- Identify the various professional roles in the mental health care setting.
- Identify the principles of milieu, individual, group, and family therapy in the clinical setting.
- Provide basic care for clients experiencing seclusion, restraints, or electroconvulsive therapy.

*I*deas about where and how treatment is rendered to clients in need of mental health care have changed drastically during the past four decades. Prior to the 1960s, most clients with mental disorders were institutionalized in long-term care facilities, some never leaving the institution in their lifetime. In 1955, the U.S. government established a commission to create a comprehensive plan for meeting the population's mental health care needs. In 1963, Congress passed an act that was the beginning of the community mental health movement. This act was based on the philosophy that individuals would receive better care if they remained in the local communities they knew and were not separated from their families and friends. The general plan was a complete array of community-based services available to all people seeking mental health care. Each community mental health center was expected to provide five basic services: inpatient care, outpatient care, emergency care, partial hospitalization, and consultation and education to the community. In addition to mental health centers, the plan included after-care programs, halfway houses, and foster care.

The vision was a noble one, but by the 1990s it was clear that the system fell far short of the original goals. Programs such as individual or relationship therapy, employee assistance, crisis intervention, stress reduction, and grief therapy are usually available to people who can pay at least a minimal fee. Unfortunately, services for those who are psychiatrically disabled are often disorganized and poorly funded. People who are persistently mentally ill are often unable to cope with the complex public system of care. When one's thoughts are disorganized, it is difficult and frustrating to try to locate appropriate help. Because they have been ill for years, and often unable to work, they frequently have extremely limited financial resources. As a result, they may be homeless, live in shelters, or have rooms in cheap boarding hotels. At times they may be brought to the acute care setting by caseworkers or the police. After being stabilized by medication, they are discharged back into the community, only to begin the vicious cycle over again. If they are a danger to themselves or others, they may be referred or court-ordered to a public long-term care facility. There is usually a waiting list for these facilities, and there is often inadequate funding for quality care. Following long-term treatment, clients are once again discharged back into the community.

You will meet mentally ill clients in a variety of clinical settings—in emergency rooms, in the general hospital, in homes, and in shelters. Even if psychiatric nursing is not your specialty, there are standards of care that all nurses are expected to provide. You must be able to relate to these clients in a therapeutic manner and foster a caring relationship. You must familiarize yourself with a wide variety of community resources so that you can provide the appropriate referrals.

Mental Health Care Professionals

Many different professional groups provide services to clients experiencing mental health problems. All are educated according to the philosophical and theoretical beliefs of their particular discipline, which gives them specific skills. In reality, the functions and responsibilities of the various professionals often overlap.

Nurses

Nurses assume a wide variety of roles within the mental health care system. Specific roles are determined by educational level and specialized preparation. Advanced practice nurses with a doctorate or master's degree in mental health nursing are found in all settings, from private practices to community centers to acute care hospitals. These nurses are well educated in individual and group therapy and may have taken advanced preparation in such other areas as family therapy, sex therapy, and/or substance abuse therapy. Nurses with a bachelor's or associate degree are most often employed by inpatient or partial-hospitalization facilities.

Nurses gather assessment data for the purpose of diagnosing, planning, implementing, and evaluating care. Because they spend more time with clients than any other staff members do, they often have the most information about a client's day-to-day level of functioning. With this knowledge base, nurses act as the liaison between other members of the multidisciplinary team.

Nursing also assumes responsibility for the physiological integrity of clients. Aside from psychiatrists, nurses are the only other members of the team who have the education and skill to perform physiological assessments. While other team members may not understand the significance of physical problems, nurses are expected to identify potential or actual problems and follow up with the appropriate action.

Client education about health is another area of expertise nurses bring to the psychiatric setting. Empowering clients with knowledge about their illness and prescribed treatments is very important. You will find information on medication teaching specific to each of the mental disorders in the appropriate chapters.

Psychiatrists

Psychiatrists are physicians who have completed a residency program in psychiatry. They are able to admit clients to the inpatient setting and order the necessary diagnostic and laboratory tests. They are responsible for diagnosing mental disorders and prescribing medications and other somatic therapies. Some are well educated in psychotherapy, and others focus more heavily on the biochemical causes of mental illness. Subspecialities include psychiatrists who work with children and adolescents, those who work with older adults, and those who work with special types of problems such as eating disorders, substance abuse, and crisis situations.

Psychologists

Psychologists practice in all areas of the mental health care system. People with a bachelor's degree in psychology are frequently hired as mental health technicians in inpatient and residential settings. Those with a master's degree in psychology are often employed in community mental health centers. Those with a doctorate in psychology (clinical psychologists) usually maintain a private practice or contract their services to an agency.

Most clinical psychologists are educated in psychotherapy and conduct individual, couple, family, and group sessions. One of the characteristics that distinguishes them from other professionals is their expertise in psychological testing. Psychologists administer and interpret all psychological tests that aid in the diagnosis and treatment of clients.

Psychiatric Social Workers

Psychiatric social workers have earned a master's degree in social work. They are found on inpatient units, in community mental health centers, and in private practice. Many states require the presence of a psychiatric social worker to perform social histories and arrange placement for clients. These trained professionals are the best informed about referral resources for clients. Many are educated in psychotherapy and provide individual, couple, family, and group sessions. People with a bachelor's degree in social work may be hired as mental health technicians for inpatients or as case managers for outpatients.

Occupational Therapists

Occupational therapists have either a bachelor's or a master's degree in occupational therapy. Usually employed on inpatient units or in partial-hospitalization programs, they are responsible for providing activities that help clients increase their attention span, improve their motor skills, expand their socialization skills, and improve their ability to perform ADLs. Through goal-directed activities, occupational therapists create situations in which clients can feel a sense of accomplishment.

Recreational Therapists

Recreational therapists usually have a bachelor's degree. They are responsible for providing group diversional activities that allow clients to engage in appropriate social and physical functions on inpatient units or in partial-hospitalization programs.

Specialists

The mental health care system often includes therapists with specialized expertise. These specialists may be skilled in the use of dance, art, music, and play to help clients communicate their thoughts, feelings, and needs in creative ways. Pastoral counselors and healers from various cultural and religious groups are also part of the multidisciplinary team in many clinical settings.

Collaboration

The current challenge to all mental health care professionals is to learn how to collaborate in order to ensure the best possible care for all clients. We must

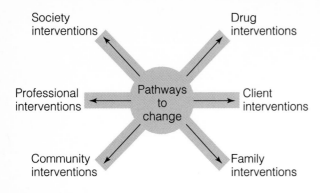

Figure 7.1 **Pathways to change.**

give up our "What's in it for me?" attitude. It is necessary to develop cooperative relationships based on trust, communication, and commitment to quality care. Building on each other's ideas and goals will help all of us develop new strategies for mental health care delivery.

Nurses also collaborate with consumers of mental health care. Nurses help clients acquire new knowledge and skills for basic living, learning, and working in the community and in developing new resources for success. Consumers must be treated with dignity and respect. They have the same needs, aspirations, rights, and responsibilities as other people. They have the right to access the opportunities and supports everyone needs as well as a variety of mental health services. Collaboration involves people who have mental illnesses, their family members, and professionals, all of whom are working together to improve quality of life and achieve the highest level of functioning (Rogers, 1996).

Mental Health Care Consumers

For decades, people with mental disorders were shut away in psychiatric institutions and effectively barred from demanding better treatment while their families were blamed and shamed into silence. That is now changing. People with mental disorders and their families are fighting for civil rights protection and more government services. According to the National Institute of Mental Health, one in three adult Americans meets the criteria for a mental disorder at some point during his or her lifetime. Consumers are children, adolescents, adults, and older adults, and they come from all segments of society. They need a wide variety of services: individual therapy, crisis intervention, family therapy, group therapy, residential services, short-term or long-term inpatient services, rehabilitative services, partial-hospitalization programs, and home care programs. Figure 7.1 illustrates the various pathways to healing for clients.

Increasingly, psychiatric nurses are supporting consumer-sensitive health care goals and programs. Mental health care should be consumer-centered, based on and responsive to the needs of the consumers rather than of the mental health system or the needs of the professionals. Consumers have the right to the fullest possible control over their own lives and should be actively involved in treatment planning decisions, including selecting the services and therapies they want and need, the setting of care, and who will provide the care. Consumers have the right to humane treatment; to personal privacy; to be free from excessive medication, physical restraint, and isolation; to exercise the right to refuse treatment; and to be free from retaliation (Schauer, 1995). Box 7.1 provides a list of mental health care consumers' rights, as established by Congress.

A variety of treatment options are available to consumers. The choice may be dictated by the setting of care, as in milieu therapy, or by the people involved, as in family therapy. Consumers often participate in several therapies during the course of their mental disorder. The rest of this chapter describes the more common treatment modalities.

Managed Care

The theory behind managed care is effective collaboration with nursing, medicine, home care, ambulatory care, and administration. The goals are to increase appropriate use of resources, encourage collaborative team practice, facilitate continuity of care, and decrease length of need for services in order to promote quality and cost-effective outcomes. Case managers are currently employed in almost every imaginable health care setting, including acute care hospitals, rehabilitation facilities, community centers, outpatient clinics, and home care. Case managers are responsible for a number of activities. First, they *identify clients,* determining whose needs are congruent with the available services and resources. At times they may increase access to services through outreach to difficult-to-reach people such as those who are homeless or noncompliant. At other times they may limit services by ensuring that only those who are eligible will receive services. Once case managers identify clients, they must *assess individual needs and strengths.* Case managers work with other providers to determine the best way to meet those needs and support skills and strengths. This planning determines *linkage,* the next step in treatment. The case manager links clients to available services by helping them meet the qualifying criteria. If services are inaccessible, case managers may *broker* for services, that is, they create access to services. They also serve as *advocates* when they negotiate with agencies and policy makers in an effort to gain resources for consumers. *Coordination* ensures that providers deliver service in a consistent manner. Almost all case managers also provide *direct care* in the form of a therapeutic relationship, supportive psychotherapy, and crisis response (American Psychiatric Association, 1997; Krul, 1997).

Treatment Settings

Consumers of mental health services may receive their care in a variety of settings. These settings vary with regard to the types of services offered; the amount of support, structure, and restrictiveness; and the hours of operation.

Supportive housing is a program used for consumers who do not live with their families and who would benefit from some degree of assistance in self-care and self-management. These programs can increase social and vocational functioning, improve quality of life, and decrease homelessness and rehospitalization. See Box 7.2 for descriptions of the types of residential facilities.

Psychosocial clubhouses are therapeutic communities where staff function as administrators whose role is to encourage decision making and socialization by the "members" of the club. Club activities focus on recreational, vocational, and residential functions. The approach is transitional, with individuals gradually assuming more responsibility and privileges.

Box 7.1

Mental Health Care Consumers' Rights

1. Right to appropriate treatment supportive of a person's personal liberty.
2. Right to an individualized, written treatment plan and its appropriate periodic review and reassessment.
3. Right to ongoing participation in the treatment plan and a reasonable explanation of the plan.
4. Right not to receive treatment, except in an emergency situation.
5. Right not to participate in experimentation without informed, voluntary, written consent.
6. Right to freedom from restraint or seclusion.
7. Right to a humane treatment environment.
8. Right to confidentiality of records.
9. Right of access to one's mental health care records.
10. Right of access to telephone, mail, and visitors.
11. Right to be informed of these rights.
12. Right to assert grievances based on the infringement of these rights.
13. Right of access to a qualified advocate to protect these rights.
14. Right to exercise these rights without reprisal.
15. Right to referral to other mental health services on discharge.

Source: Adapted from Mental Health Systems Act Report, 1980.

Medication clinics are part of a more comprehensive program. They are helpful to clients who cannot manage their medications on their own. Nurses administer medications as well as monitor for side effects. Client education is a major focus of these clinics.

Day treatment programs are used to provide ongoing supportive care and are usually not time-limited. They provide structure and programs to help prevent relapse and to improve social and vocational functioning. They may also provide family therapy.

Box 7.2

Types of Residential Facilities

Transitional Halfway Houses
- Provide room and board until suitable housing is available

Long-Term Group Residences
- On-site staff
- Appropriate for psychiatrically disabled person
- Indefinite length of stay

Cooperative Apartments
- No on-site staff
- Staff make regular visits to assist residents

Intensive-Care or Crisis Community Residences
- Used to help prevent hospitalization or shorten length of hospitalization
- On-site nursing staff and counseling staff

Foster or Family Care
- In private homes
- Close supervision of foster family to assure a therapeutic environment

Nursing Homes
- Appropriate for some geriatric or medically disabled consumers
- Activity programs and psychiatric supervision

There is a gradual introduction to the type of structured activities encountered in a full day of employment. Clients may be employed part-time while in the program. Day treatment programs have low staff-to-client ratios and minimal or no nursing staff.

Day hospitalization can be used as an alternative to inpatient care or following a brief hospitalization. The advantage over inpatient care is less disruption of the person's life and treatment in a less restrictive environment. The person should not be at risk of harming self or others and should be able to cooperate minimally in treatment. The day hospital is staffed similarly to the staffing of the day shift on an acute inpatient unit.

Residential crisis services is a new alternative to hospitalization. Consumers include adolescents with psychiatric problems, people in an acute psychiatric emergency resulting from a life crisis, or other individuals with acute psychiatric episodes. The residential crisis service offers a respite from their current living situation, which may be stressful or unsatisfactory, and provides intensive treatment in a program that utilizes medications, milieu therapy, and other forms of therapy.

Treatment in *hospitals* has the advantage of providing a safe, structured, and supervised environment, lowering the stress on both consumers and family members. Stays have been reduced to three to eight days. Hospitalization allows the heath care team to closely monitor the level of symptoms and reactions to treatments. Hospitalization is indicated for those people who are considered at risk of harm to themselves or others, and for people who are unable to care for themselves because of severely disorganized thinking, delusions, or hallucinations.

There remains a small group of clients who require *long-term hospitalization* for their own safety as well as for the protection of family and community. These individuals profit most from treatment programs that emphasize highly structured behavioral interventions such as a token economy, point systems, and skills training that can improve their level of functioning.

Crisis Response Services

In the traditional mental health system, the hospital is used to stabilize acute illness, but staff may have limited ability to help clients adapt to the real world on discharge. Psychiatrically disabled clients often cannot or will not follow up with services at a clinic, resulting in relapse into acute illness. Family or police bring them to the emergency department, where they are admitted to the acute care setting. This perpetuates the cycle of crisis–rehospitalization–discharge–crisis. Some people go into crisis because they are unable to understand their everyday problems and are unable to participate in a complex treatment plan. Some are unable to access their own care because the services are limited, expensive, and often inconvenient. Some go into crisis due to lack of housing, an absence of a social group, or relapse with drugs or alcohol. These problems result in feelings of shame, humiliation, and guilt. One person in crisis has an impact on the lives of others in the community—friends, family, neighbors, coworkers, and passersby. Those around the individual in crisis can be fearful, rejecting, or even hostile.

Many acutely mentally ill people can be evaluated, treated, and stabilized by bringing therapists directly to clients in crisis. Mobile emergency treatment services bridge the gap between inpatient, outpatient, and family-based care. Some clients are too anxious, fearful, agitated, or depressed to come into traditional treatment settings. Visiting clients in their own environment helps the professional maximize clients' home and community resources. Emergency services need to be available when clients' coping skills are overwhelmed or when mental illness worsens and clients begin to experience dangerous symptoms (Zealberg and Santos, 1996).

Mobile crisis services are staffed by interdisciplinary teams of psychiatrists, nurses, social workers, psychologists, and counselors. The team is available 24 hours a day, 365 days a year. The mobile team may be called to private homes, group homes, shelters, hotels, street corners, malls, public buildings, recreational areas, police stations, or anywhere in the entire community. In the majority of requests for mobile assistance, professionals are at little, if any, risk. However, if the situation is potentially dangerous—an assaultive person, one who is suicidal, or a homicidal person with a weapon—the team members attempt to calm and support the client over the phone before or during their ride to the client's location. In this type of situation the police are always asked to accompany the treatment team. The client must be informed that the police will be coming along and that the police will leave once everything is under good control. If clients are not manageable in the community setting, the team will bring them into the hospital (Zealberg and Santos, 1996). See Box 7.3 for intervention guidelines.

Milieu Therapy

In its earliest conception, *milieu* was a word that described a scientifically planned community. Research efforts focused on defining the types of environments that would be most therapeutic for specifically diagnosed psychiatric clients. The work of Cummings and Cummings (1962) suggested that the environment (milieu) itself might be a strong force in bringing about changes in client behavior.

Kraft (1966) defined the idea of milieu more precisely as a therapeutic community in which the entire social structure of the unit or residence is designed to be part of the helping process. Kraft's idea of a therapeutic community emphasized the social and interpersonal interactions that become the therapeutic tools influencing change in client behavior. This view differed somewhat from the pure idea of milieu therapy, in which the emphasis was on "manipulation" of the environment to effect therapeutic change.

Box 7.3

Intervention Guidelines for Mobile Crisis Services

Control Behavior
- Use the approach that is least restrictive but that maximizes safety for everyone.
- Make sure you are not alone, especially in a closed-in area.
- Remain calm and be observant as you approach the client.
- Remove items that could become harmful, such as ties, necklaces, pens, and pencils. Stop about 6 feet away.
- Introduce yourself and address client by last name. Ask permission to use client's first name.
- If you do not feel endangered, ask whether client will shake hands with you.
- Explain procedures using simple, ordinary language, e.g., "I need to check your blood pressure."

Assess Quickly
- Rule out a potentially life-threatening process that could be causing client's psychiatric signs and symptoms, such as hypoglycemia, head injury, or neurological illness.
- Look for Med-Alert bracelet, signs of injury.

Treat Specifically
- Psychotic and agitated behavior must be treated vigorously.
- Appropriate medication will decrease violent symptoms and rapidly decrease the danger to self and others.

Sources: Drake, 1996; Zealberg and Santos, 1996.

Milieu therapy has certain basic goals, whether the setting is a group home, a community center, a day program, or an inpatient unit. These goals include an emphasis on clients as responsible people, group and social interaction, clients' rights to choose and participate in a variety of treatments, and informality of relationships with health care professionals.

Characteristics of the Therapeutic Milieu

Clear Communication

Communication between all people in the milieu is open, honest, and appropriate. Clients are encouraged to express their thoughts and feelings without retaliation, and staff members have a responsibility to hear what clients are saying without feeling threatened. Communication skills are role-modeled by staff members, helping clients learn the positive effects of therapeutic communication. Respect for the dignity of each person in the milieu is emphasized through the communication process.

Providing a Safe Environment

Policies, procedures, and rules of the residence, center, or unit are designed to ensure the safety of all members of the therapeutic milieu. All members of the community are informed of the rules. Structures and controls are provided for clients who are confused, anxious, suicidal, homicidal, or out of control to assure their safety as well as the safety of those around them.

Providing an Activity Schedule with Therapeutic Goals

In short-term acute care settings, clients will usually be at different levels of functioning. In most therapeutic communities, clients will be assigned to specific groups for activities. This assignment usually depends on the client's level of functioning at the time of admission and is changed as the client's level of functioning improves. Level of functioning can be determined by asking questions such as:

- Does the client have some insight into the illness? Little insight? No insight?
- How well does the client understand the goals of treatment? Well? Only slightly? Not at all?
- Is the client in contact with reality?
- How motivated is the client?

It is common to see high-functioning groups, moderate-functioning groups, and low-functioning groups in the same setting. Activities are then planned to meet the individual needs, interests, and skills of clients in that group.

Group activities are balanced to provide clients with different types of experiences. We all need balance between work, sleep, and play—a fact that is frequently overlooked in the psychiatric setting. Even a well-functioning person would have difficulty with 6 hours of intense therapy in one day. Therefore, the activity schedule is varied, with daily therapeutic community meetings, group therapy, ADL training, some type of physical activity such as sports or movement therapy, art therapy, play therapy, medication teaching and other educational groups, reality orientation groups, periods of rest and relaxation, time for one-to-one interactions, free time, and mealtime.

Providing a Support Network

Clients will begin to feel a sense of support from the therapeutic community or milieu. Through the process of group therapy and other support groups, clients begin to feel a sense of commonality with other clients. Clients often value treatment that helps them feel some control over crisis and a sense of social connectedness. One of the greatest benefits of the therapeutic community is that it is one of the few places where clients may feel safe, secure, and supported.

Because in many settings nurses spend more time with clients than do any other staff members, they often have the most influence on the effectiveness of the milieu. As a nurse, you can help establish the milieu as an open, confirming, and dignified place for people to be ill and to get well. Individuals who are psychiatrically disabled have problems relating to others. When clients have been conditioned to a life of loneliness and stigma, you may find it takes a great deal of time to establish the trusting relationship necessary for successful treatment. As nurses, we are healers, and through the milieu we create an atmosphere of nurturance and protection that removes the pressure to "cure" and allows the sometimes slow process of healing to take place.

Individual Psychotherapy

Individual psychotherapy is a reciprocal agreement between client and therapist to enter into a therapeutic relationship. It is performed by a variety of health care professionals such as advanced practice nurses, psychiatrists, psychologists, and psychiatric social workers. The goals of psychotherapy are to help clients clarify perceptions; identify feelings; make connections between thoughts, feelings, and events; and gain insight. The process can also help clients develop better coping strategies such as problem solving, stress reduction, and crisis management. For some, it is an opportunity to feel supported in their struggle to overcome symptoms or interpersonal problems. Some individual therapies deal with specific issues, such as sex therapy or eating disorders. Certain therapies are short-term and the goals are met relatively quickly. Others are long-term because they deal with deep-rooted anxieties or problems. There are many different models of individual psychotherapy—for example, cognitive therapy, intrapersonal therapy, humanistic therapy, and existential therapy—as well as models that combine several approaches.

Group Therapy

Group therapy is a beneficial experience in which people with psychologic, cognitive, or behavioral dysfunctions are helped through a process of change by the group and group leaders. Groups can be held in an inpatient unit, an outpatient clinic, a community mental health center, or a variety of other settings. There are three types of groups: task, education, and supportive/therapeutic. *Task groups* are designed to carry out a particular type of task and are product-oriented. The emphasis is on problem solving and decision making. In the clinical setting, a task group might plan and prepare a community meal. *Education groups* teach members about a specific topic. An example is a medication teaching group. *Supportive/therapeutic groups* provide support to the members as they work through their problems. The group helps members identify feelings and behaviors they wish to change. The supportive/therapeutic group provides a safe environment for people to work out their particular problems through sharing experiences with other members. An example is a group working toward building self-esteem.

Yalom (1995) identified mechanisms of change within a group and called them curative factors of group therapy. These factors provide a rationale for a variety of group interventions. Table 7.1 lists and describes the curative factors.

Nurses function as group therapists in many different settings, establishing the type of group that is appropriate for the desired outcomes. Groups may be led by a single nurse leader, or the leadership may be shared by two cotherapists. Some of the important tasks of the group leader include encouraging members to remain in the group, helping the group develop a sense of cohesiveness, and establishing a code of behavior and norms with the group. Nurses perform these tasks through two basic roles: technical expert and role model. Nurses function as *technical experts* by using their experience and leadership position to help the group establish norms for behavior. Nurses function as *role models* by setting examples for the types of behavior that support the healthy functioning of the group.

Family Therapy

In family therapy, the family system is treated as a unit, and the focus is on family dynamics. The goal is to help families cope and improve their communication and interpersonal skills. Families strive to maintain balance and harmony. When change affects this balanced state, families must use their internal and external resources to adapt. Healthy families seem to adapt more efficiently than dysfunctional families. Change is so frightening or alien to some families that they invest their energies in maintaining the status quo. The result is that they seem more interested in enabling the illness of one of its members than in supporting changes that will improve health.

Family therapy is a specialized area of study. Becoming a family therapist requires extensive preparation. This is not to say that nurses in the mental health care system will not intervene with families at all. It is very likely that nurses in both inpatient and outpatient settings will have a great deal of contact with the families of their clients. Family members are usually not in formal family therapy and only have contact with the nurse who assumes the responsibility of working with the family and client.

When nurses work with families informally, they assess for a number of factors, including:

- relationships between individual members of the family
- roles assumed by various members of the family
- family communication patterns

Table 7.1 Curative Factors of Group Therapy

Factor	Description
Installation of hope	As clients observe other members farther along in the therapeutic process, they begin to feel a sense of hope for themselves.
Universality	Through interaction with other group members, clients realize they are not alone in their problems or pain.
Imparting of information	Teaching and suggestions usually come from the group leader but may also be generated by the group members.
Altruism	Through the group process, clients recognize that they have something to give to the other group members.
Corrective recapitulation of the primary family group	Many clients have a history of dysfunctional family relationships. The therapy group is often like a family, and clients can learn more functional patterns of communication, interaction, and behavior.
Development of socializing techniques	Development of social skills takes place in groups. Group members give feedback about maladaptive social behavior. Clients learn more appropriate ways of socializing with others.
Imitative behavior	Clients often model their behavior after the leader or other group members. This trial process enables them to discover what behaviors work well for them as individuals.
Interpersonal learning	Through the group process, clients learn the positive benefits of good interpersonal relationships. Emotional healing takes place through this process.
Existential factors	The group provides opportunities for clients to explore the meaning of their life and their place in the world.
Catharsis	Clients learn how to express their own feelings in a goal-directed way, speak openly about what is bothering them, and express strong feelings about other members in a responsible way.
Group cohesiveness	Cohesiveness occurs when members feel a sense of belonging.

Sources: Adapted from Ballinger and Yalom, 1995; Yalom, 1995.

- achievement of the developmental tasks of the family
- normal coping strategies used by the family
- family support systems
- sociocultural norms and values of the family

Family therapy is indicated when the nurse or family determines that the family system is impaired because of the presence of a psychosocial problem or mental disorder in one or more family members. All family members must feel that they are part of the problem-solving and decision-making processes and that their personal welfare is always considered.

Behavioral Therapy

Behavioral therapy is based on the principle that all behavior has specific consequences. Behavior is changed by conditioning: a process of reinforcement, punishment, and extinction. Consequences that lead to an increase in a particular behavior are referred to as *reinforcement*. Positive reinforcement is providing a reward for the desired behavior. Negative reinforcement is the removal of a negative stimulus to increase the chances that the desired behavior will occur. Consequences that lead to a decrease in undesirable behavior are referred to as *punishment*. Positive punishment is the addition of a negative consequence if the undesirable behavior occurs. Negative punishment is the removal of a positive reward if the undesirable behavior occurs. *Extinction* refers to the progressive weakening of an undesirable behavior through repeated nonreinforcement of the behavior.

Most behavioral therapists believe that reinforcement procedures are more desirable than punishment procedures. There is no doubt that punishment is effective and is sometimes necessary when the behavior is dangerous. But behavior that is changed through reinforcement is a more desirable clinical outcome than behavior changed through punishment.

Behavior therapy is not a set of techniques that are followed for every client. Rather, the plan is tailored to the person's assets, deficits, values, culture, and environmental resources. Clients are expected to be active participants, and therapists design learning experiences designed to modify maladpative behavior patterns.

Intervention focuses on changing those behaviors that have the most detrimental effect on the client. The nurse takes an active role in the process of helping clients identify learned behaviors that can be changed. There must be a plan, which is made clear to everyone working with the client, that identifies the goals of treatment and the behavioral consequences. Reinforcement is used to effect change, and if punishment procedures are necessary, clients are consistently assured that painful responses are reversible. As with many of the other therapies, nurses are in an ideal position to evaluate client response to treatment. Because they spend a great deal of time with clients, nurses can see developing patterns of behavioral change.

Somatic Therapies

Seclusion

Seclusion is used when it is essential to protect the client or others from harm and is considered an emergency intervention. Seclusion is the process of confining a client to a single room in which he or she is alone but carefully observed by members of the staff. Staff members must be careful not to use seclusion to retaliate against clients for inappropriate but harmless behaviors. Box 7.4 lists the reasons for implementing seclusion, the benefits of seclusion, and contraindications to seclusion.

Once the decision has been made to use seclusion, a staff member is designated as the team leader, who will also talk to the client. Another staff member is a

---

Box 7.4

Seclusion

Reasons for Implementing Seclusion

- Clients have lost control, are exhibiting destructive behavior, and do not respond to verbal command or physical contact.
- Clients are overstimulated by the environment and need time out to regain internal control.
- Clients ask to go to seclusion while attempting to take control of their own behavior.
- Clients have agreed by contract to seclusion as a consequence of certain behaviors.

Benefits of Seclusion

- Through containment, the client is at less risk to self or others.
- Through isolation, the client is relieved of the need to relate to others.
- Seclusion gives the client time to master a small, contained world.
- Through decreased sensory input, the client is allowed a respite from the many sensory stimuli in the environment.

Contraindications to Seclusion

- Clients who are medically unstable and need close observation.
- Clients who are at high risk for suicide and need one-to-one observation.

Sources: Cashin, 1996; Morales and Duphorne, 1995.

---

monitor. This person is a nonparticipant who can troubleshoot, observe, and give feedback to the staff. A separate staff member manages the other clients on the unit, whose anxiety may escalate as they observe the process.

The group leader and support staff then proceed toward the client without hesitation. This show of force may be enough to prevent the client from exhibiting out-of-control behavior. The leader tells the client the reason seclusion is necessary, and then asks the client to walk to the seclusion room accompanied by staff members. Aggression is always controlled with the least restrictive means possible. If the client refuses to walk to the seclusion room, staff members

Table 7.2 Nursing Care for Clients in Seclusion

Nursing Diagnosis	Interventions
Feeding self-care deficit	Provide food at mealtimes. Offer fluids every 2 hours. Document intake.
Toileting self-care deficit	Offer use of bathroom every 2 hours or as necessary. Document use of bathroom.
Bathing/hygiene self-care deficit	Provide opportunities for washing of hands and face. Provide opportunities for brushing teeth. Document.
High risk for violence	Observe client through audiovisual monitoring system or through window every 5–10 minutes. Remove all dangerous objects from room. Use medication as ordered to help client regain control. Provide opportunities for brief one-to-one contact. Restrain client if behavior becomes violent. Document observations.

will bring the client to the floor and restrain each limb at the joint. Staff are trained in take-down procedures so that neither clients nor staff will be injured. It is important that you know the state statutes regarding seclusion, since they vary from state to state. As students, the best way you can help is to remain with the other clients who may be frightened (Cashin, 1996). Table 7.2 describes nursing care for clients in seclusion.

Physical Restraint

The most restrictive measure to control aggressive behavior is the use of four-point restraints and seclusion. These external controls, which usually involve the use of force, often create strong negative feelings for both clients and staff. Use of physical force with clients reinforces their perception that violence is a valid method of gaining control. Clients describe the experience as frightening, confusing, depressing, degrading, dehumanizing, and inducing anger, guilt, and loss of self-esteem. Because clients often view restraints as punishment, this method fosters distrust of, and malice toward, staff members. They should be the *last* option used to control behavior (Smith, 1995).

Clients come to a mental health setting expecting help, not hurt. You, as a nurse, are taught to use therapeutic skills when interacting with clients, not to humiliate or punish them. The time of entry into the mental health system is an appropriate time to find out what helps clients to calm down. For example, music might be soothing to one client but irritating to another. Observe for early signs and symptoms of increasing anxiety or agitation. Telling clients what

they can do is more effective than stating what is not allowed. "You may smoke your cigarette outside" may work better than, "Put that cigarette out, you know the rules." Telling people what they cannot do may set up power struggles. Losing control can be equally frightening to clients as to staff. Another approach is to give clients choices. "Do you want to try a relaxation tape or would you like me to do the relaxation exercise with you?" Giving choices helps people feel they have some control in the situation. See Chapter 6 for other interventions for clients who are aggressive.

The use of physical restraint is sometimes necessary, but restraints must always be used judiciously. Clients' legal rights must be considered, as well as state mental health codes. Restraints should be considered only if clients are a danger to themselves or others, if they are in danger of complete physical exhaustion, and when other means of control are not effective. When clients are in restraints they must be treated as intensive care clients, with close attention by one staff member to provide reality orientation, comfort measures, and reassurance that they are not being punished. Clients must be told as often as necessary what they must do or not do to be released from restraints. Restraints should be used for the shortest possible period of time. Appropriate medications aimed at decreasing anxiety can lessen threatening behavior. Document the care you provide to restrained clients. Documentation should include even the simplest interventions, such as reorienting, as well as the frequency of your reassessment (Morales and Duphorne, 1995). Table 7.3 describes nursing care for clients in restraints.

Table 7.3 Nursing Care for Clients in Restraints

Nursing Diagnosis	Interventions
Impaired physical mobility	Release restraints every 2 hours and do range of motion exercises. Take to bathroom or offer urinal or bedpan. Provide food at mealtimes, and offer fluids every 2 hours. Provide hygiene measures. Document interventions.
High risk for injury	Pad restraints and check circulation. Release restraints every 2 hours and check circulation. Check vital signs every hour. Document interventions.
Situational low self-esteem	Reassure client that restraints will be removed when client is able to regain control. Allow client to express feelings. Provide privacy. Communicate a plan to remove the restraints.
High risk for violence	Observe client through audiovisual monitoring system or through window every 5–10 minutes. Use medication as ordered to help client regain control. Provide opportunities for brief one-to-one contact. Document observations.

Electroconvulsive Therapy

Electroconvulsive therapy (ECT) produces a deliberate, artificially induced grand mal seizure of the brain. This affects a wide range of neurotransmitters and neurohormones, increases slow wave activity, reduces regional cerebral blood flow and glucose metabolism, and increases the blood-brain permeability.

The most common indications for ECT are major depressive disorder and bipolar I disorder, depressed. It is indicated for clients in the following situations (Prudic et al, 1996; Fitzsimons, 1995):

- failure to respond to medications
- severe symptoms, such as severe psychosis or dangerously suicidal or homicidal behaviors
- adverse reactions to psychotropic medications
- medical conditions, such as heart disease or glaucoma, that could be worsened by psychotropic medications
- previous successful response to ECT
- client preference

ECT is sometimes employed in the treatment of people with schizophrenia. It is primarily used in clients experiencing catatonia, those who have predominate affective symptoms, those who have had a previous successful response to ECT, and those who do not respond to medications. ECT is an effective treatment for depression in the elderly but it is generally underused. ECT is safe in all trimesters of pregnancy and may be less harmful to the fetus than psychotropic medications.

Before a client is given ECT, a complete history is taken, along with physical and neurological exams. There are several contraindications for ECT: brain tumor, recent cerebral vascular accident (CVA), subdural hematoma, recent myocardial infarction (MI), congestive heart failure, angina pectoris, retinal detachment, and acute or chronic respiratory disease (Fitzsimons, 1995).

The client should ingest nothing by mouth for at least 8 hours prior to the treatment. Thirty minutes prior to the treatment, the client is given 1 mg atropine sulfate IM to control secretions and to prevent bradycardia, which sometimes occurs with ECT. A short-acting barbiturate or etomidate is administered intravenously as anesthesia. Succinylcoline chloride (Anectine) is injected to induce muscle relaxation and prevent the full-body muscular response to the grand mal seizure. Electrodes are placed on either one side of the temple or on both sides, through which the current is delivered. Side effects are more severe or persistent with the use of bilateral as opposed to right unilateral electrode placement. The client usually awakens 10–15 minutes after the procedure. Table 7.4 describes nursing care for clients receiving ECT.

Memory is often affected by ECT—both memory of past events and newly learned information. Within 6–9 months, the ability to learn new material returns to normal. Memory for past events also returns, except for the days prior to and during the course of

■ *Table 7.4* **Nursing Care for Clients Receiving ECT**

Nursing Diagnosis	Interventions
Knowledge deficit	Teach client and family about treatment and side effects. Allow client and family time to verbalize their understanding of the procedure. Document teaching.
Anxiety	Stay with client before and after treatment.
Altered thought processes	Reassure client that amnesia and confusion are reversible. Reorient client as needed.

ECT treatment (Sobin et al, 1995). The development of magnetic stimulation therapy (MST) is underway. Some severely depressed clients may respond to magnetic stimulation of their brain's left prefrontal cortex in much the same way that they respond to ECT. In MST an electromagnetic coil induces a current in the brain. This current has a more specific target in the brain and is not affected by skull thickness (Fitzsimons and Mayer, 1995).

Psychosocial Nursing Interventions

Social Skills Training

Individuals who are psychiatrically disabled often benefit from social skills training. Such training is provided over an extended period of time, perhaps even longer than a year. Teaching strategies include instruction, feedback, social reinforcement, modeling, behavioral rehearsal, and evaluation. Clients learn to interact appropriately with strangers, family members, friends, and at work or school. The nurse teaches clients conversational skills such as initiating conversations, asking questions, making appropriate self-disclosures, and ending conversations gracefully. Clients often need to learn assertive behaviors that allow them to stand up for their rights, act in their own best interest, and express positive feelings about others. They may need to learn conflict resolution skills, which involves learning negotiation skills so that conflicts with others can be worked out in a satisfactory manner.

Physical Exercise

Physical exercise is a useful intervention to decrease anxiety and depression. Exercise enhances mental functioning, mood, and general well-being. To be most effective, exercise should be aerobic and last at least 20 minutes. It may be difficult for people suffering from depression to summon the energy to exercise. They often say, "I'll exercise when I feel better." An appropriate response on your part would be, "You'll feel better when you exercise." Often people are more consistent if they have an exercise partner, perhaps a friend or family member.

Self-Help Groups

As a nurse, you frequently refer clients to self-help groups, which are very important for consumers of mental health care. The characteristics of self-help groups include:

- Clients define own needs.
- Members have equal power.
- Groups are autonomous from mental health professionals.
- Attendance is totally voluntary.
- People are respected as people, not thought of as clinical diagnoses.
- Groups may be responsive to a special population such as bilingual, disabled, or those defined by racial, gender, or sexual identity.

Self-help groups function to educate community members, to help friends and family support the individual, and to act as a crisis support, a source of referrals, and an advocate to help people get their needs met through the health care system. Because people who are psychiatrically disabled often have a very restricted social network or are even socially isolated, the interpersonal contact of self-help groups is vitally important. These groups contribute to an increased self-esteem, a sense of identity, increased dignity, and improved self-responsibility.

Psychoeducation

An important part of rehabilitation is psychoeducation for clients, family, and friends. Knowledge about the disorder and treatment helps family members provide for the needs of the client, develop their own coping strategies, and develop a collaborative relationship with professionals. Psychoeducation includes information about the etiology, treatment, and prognosis of the mental disorder. Clients and families are taught stressors associated with relapse, setting of realistic expectations, stress management, communication skills, and problem-solving skills. When families' educational needs are met, they have an increased ability to cope, understand, and deal with their loved one's illness.

Key Concepts

Introduction

- In spite of the 1963 congressional act, services for the severely and persistently mentally ill are often disorganized and poorly funded.

Mental Health Care Professionals

- Many different professional groups provide services to clients. The functions and responsibilities of the various professionals often overlap.

- Nurses with advanced degrees work in settings from private practices to community centers to acute care hospitals. Nurses with basic degrees are most often employed by inpatient or partial-hospitalization facilities.

- Nurses use the nursing process in providing care to clients. They also act as liaisons between other members of the multidisciplinary team, assume responsibility for the physiological integrity of clients, and implement client education about health.

- Psychiatrists are physicians who admit clients to inpatient settings, order diagnostic tests, and prescribe medications and other somatic therapies.

- Psychologists specialize in the administration and interpretation of psychological tests and conduct individual, couple, family, and group sessions.

- Psychiatric social workers are the most knowledgeable professionals about referral resources for clients. Many are also educated in psychotherapy.

- Occupational therapists provide clients with those types of activities that help increase their attention span, improve their motor skills, expand their socialization skills, and improve their ability to perform ADLs.

- Recreational therapists provide healthy diversional activities in groups.

- Therapists with specialized expertise include those educated in the use of dance, art, music, and play to help clients communicate their thoughts, feelings, and needs in creative ways.

- Nurses collaborate with consumers, family members, and other professionals, all of whom are working together to help clients improve their quality of life and achieve the highest level of functioning.

Mental Health Care Consumers

- Consumers of mental health care come from all segments of society and are in need of a wide variety of services. Consumers must participate in the selection of services and therapies, the setting of care, and the selection of the care provider.

Managed Care

- Case managers identify clients, assess individual needs and strengths, provide linkage, broker for services, serve as advocates, coordinate service, and provide direct care.

- Treatment settings include supportive housing, psychosocial clubhouses, medication clinics, day treatment programs, day hospitalization, residential crisis services, acute care hospitals, and long-term hospitals.

- Mobile crisis services evaluate, treat, and stabilize clients by bringing therapists directly to people in crisis.

Milieu Therapy

- Milieu refers to the therapeutic community in which the entire social structure of the unit or residence is designed to be part of the helping process. The goals are to provide a physically and emotionally safe environment, to provide activities that orient and socialize clients, and to provide opportunities for learning and healing.

Individual Psychotherapy

- The goals of individual psychotherapy are to help clients gain insight; clarify perceptions; identify feelings; make connections between thoughts, feelings, and events; and develop better coping strategies such as problem solving, stress reduction, and crisis management.

Group Therapy

- There are three types of groups. Task groups are designed to carry out a particular type of task, education groups teach members about a specific topic, and supportive/therapeutic groups provide support to members as they work through their problems.

- The curative factors of group therapy are the installation of hope, universality, the imparting of information, altruism, the corrective recapitulation of the primary family group, the development of socializing techniques, imitative behavior, interpersonal learning, existential factors, catharsis, and group cohesiveness.

Family Therapy

- Family therapy is indicated when the nurse determines that the family system is impaired because of the presence of a psychosocial problem or mental disorder in one or more family members. Intervention focuses on helping families cope and improve their communication and interpersonal skills.

Behavioral Therapy

- Behavioral therapy is based on the principle that all behavior has specific consequences. Behavior is changed through the process of conditioning, which includes reinforcement, punishment, and extinction.

Somatic Therapies

- Somatic therapies include seclusion, restraints, and electroconvulsive therapy (ECT).

- Seclusion is used when it is essential to protect the client or others from harm. It is the process of confining a client to a single room in which he or she is alone but carefully observed by members of the staff.

- Restraints should be considered only if clients are a danger to themselves or others, or if they are in danger of complete physical exhaustion. Clients' legal rights must be considered, as well as state mental health codes. This should be the last option used to control behavior.

- Depression is the most common indication for ECT. It may also be used with older adult clients, pregnant women, or those with manic symptoms. Contraindications include brain tumor, recent CVA, subdural hematoma, recent MI, congestive heart failure, angina pectoris, retinal detachment, and acute or chronic respiratory disease.

Psychosocial Nursing Intervention

- Social skills training teaches clients conversational skills, assertive behaviors, and conflict-resolution skills.

- Physical exercise decreases anxiety and depression.

- Self-help groups contribute to increased self-esteem, a sense of identity, increased dignity, and improved self-responsibility.

- Psychoeducation teaches clients and families how to meet needs, develop coping strategies, communicate clearly, and solve problems effectively.

Review Questions

1. The concept of "therapeutic community" is related to which of the following treatment modalities?

   a. Group therapy

   b. Milieu therapy

   c. Family therapy

   d. Behavioral therapy

2. Which of the following is a benefit of seclusion?

   a. The client is relieved of the need to relate to others.

   b. The unit can be managed with fewer staff.

   c. Clients are encouraged to communicate with others.

   d. Clients are forced to be responsible for themselves.

3. You are providing social skills training to a group of residents in your home. Which of the following topics would you include?

    a. Physical exercise decreases anxiety and depression.

    b. All members of the group have equal power.

    c. How to study and modify family dynamics.

    d. How to initiate and end conversations.

4. For the client who is in restraints, how often should the restraints be released?

    a. every 15 minutes

    b. every 2 hours

    c. every 4 hours

    d. only when the client is in complete control

5. For which of the following people would ECT be contraindicated?

    a. a pregnant woman

    b. an elderly person

    c. a person with a recent MI

    d. a person with cancer

References

American Psychiatric Association. (1997). Practice guidelines for the treatment of patients with schizophrenia. *Am J Psychiatry, 154*(Suppl. 4), 1–63.

Ballinger, B., & Yalom, I. D. (1995). Group therapy in practice. In B. Bongar & L. E. Beutler (Eds.), *Comprehensive Textbook of Psychotherapy* (pp.189–204). Oxford, England: Oxford Univ. Press.

Cashin, A. (1996). Seclusion: The quest to determine effectiveness. *J Psychosoc Nurs, 34*(11), 17–21.

Cummings, J., & Cummings, E. (1962). *Ego and Milieu.* Atherton Press.

Drake, R. D. (1996, August 8). What is assertive community treatment? *Harvard Mental Health Letter, 10*(8): 8.

Fitzsimons, L. (1995). Electroconvulsive therapy: What nurses need to know. *J Psychosoc Nurs, 33*(12), 14–17.

Fitzsimons, L., & Mayer, R. L. (1995). Soaring beyond the cuckoo's nest: Health care reform and ECT. *J Psychosoc Nurs, 33*(12), 10–13.

Kraft, A. (1966). The therapeutic community. In S. Arieti (Ed.), *American Handbook of Psychiatry: Vol. 2.* New York: Basic Books.

Krul, R. (1997). Nurses as case managers. *Nurs Spectrum, 10*(4), 11.

Mental Health System Act Report. Amendment to Senate Bill 1179. 1980 (Sept. 23). No. 96-980.

Morales, E., Duphorne, P. L. (1995). Least restrictive measures. *J Psychosoc Nurs, 33*(10), 13–16.

Prudic, J. et al. (1996). Resistance to antidepressant medications and short-term clinical response to ECT. *Am J Psychiatry, 153*(8), 985–992.

Rogers, S. (1996). National clearinghouse serves mental health consumer movement. *J Psychosoc Nurs, 34*(9), 22–25.

Schauer, C. (1995). Special report: Protection and advocacy: What nurses need to know. *Arch Psychiatr Nurs, 9*(5), 233–239.

Smith, S. B. (1995). Restraints. *J Psychosoc Nurs, 33*(7), 23–28.

Sobin, C., et al. (1995). Predictors of retrograde amnesia following ECT. *Am J Psychiatry, 152*(7), 995–1001.

Yalom, I. D. (1995). *The Theory and Practice of Group Psychotherapy* (4th ed.). New York: Basic Books.

Zealberg, J. J., & Santos, A. B. (1996). *Comprehensive Emergency Mental Health Care.* New York: WW Norton.

CHAPTER 8

Psycho-pharmacology

Karen G. Vincent-Pounds

Objectives

After reading this chapter, you will be able to:

- Describe the physiological and therapeutic effects of psychotropic medications.
- Discuss the side effects and toxic effects of psychotropic medications.
- Discuss the use of psychotropic medications with special populations.
- Describe the process of client medication teaching.

*I*n the past several decades, attention has turned to research on brain dysfunction and neurotransmitter imbalances and their relationship to mental illness. The discovery of new medications to treat mental disorders occurs almost monthly. This new frontier of psychiatric thought, research, and treatment greatly affects nursing practice. Before proceeding, you may want to review neurobiology in Chapter 4. Additional information about medications is found in each of the disorders chapters in Part Three.

Psychotropic medications are medications that affect cognitive function, emotions, and behavior. They are categorized into four groups: antipsychotic, antidepressant, antianxiety, and mood-stabilizing medications. They may be used alone or in combination with one another.

Antipsychotic Medications

Physiological Effects

Characteristics of severe mental illness are classified as positive and negative. To make sense of this, you must understand that positive does not mean good and negative does not mean bad. Rather, positive characteristics are added behaviors that are not normally seen in mentally healthy adults, such as hallucinations, delusions, or loose association. Positive characteristics are thought to result from an excess of dopamine (DA) or from hypersensitive DA receptors and are usually responsive to medication. Negative characteristics are the absence of behaviors that are normally seen in mentally healthy adults, such as social withdrawal, minimal self-care, concrete thinking, and flat affect. Until recently, negative characteristics have been less responsive to treatment with antipsychotic medications. Antipsychotic medications act by blocking the overreactive DA receptors or by decreasing the amount of available DA (Zimbroff et al, 1997). See Chapter 12 for further description of positive and negative characteristics.

Therapeutic Effects

The therapeutic purpose of antipsychotic medications is to decrease as many of the psychotic symptoms as possible. This action allows clients to assume more control over their lives. With reduced symptoms, they can participate more effectively in other forms of treatment.

Conventional antipsychotic medications are generally more successful at relieving the positive symptoms of mental illness than the negative ones. It may take 2–4 weeks to see clinical improvement from these medications. Although no evidence suggests the superiority of any one conventional antipsychotic agent, some people respond better to one drug than another. Choosing which medication to use with individual clients also depends on its side effects. For example, one client may respond well to haloperidol but have dangerous episodes of hypotension, while another client may do well on haloperidol with little or no side effects. Approximately 15–30% of clients are resistant to conventional antipsychotic medication. Half of the people will get one or more side effects and, in response, many will discontinue their medication (Tollefson et al, 1997).

New-generation or atypical antipsychotic medications decrease both positive and negative symptoms of mental illness. Negative symptoms impose great suffering on people by interfering with their psychosocial functioning. Atypical agents are characterized by:

- effectiveness in eliminating the negative as well as the positive symptoms
- effectiveness for many people who are not responsive to conventional agents
- effectiveness for people who also experience depressive symptoms
- a significantly lower incidence of EPS effects, which increases compliance

These drugs affect all of the DA receptors, many of the 5-HT receptors, and the histimine receptors. Studies have shown these medications to be effective and safe in long-term treatment of mental illness.

Initially, clients take or receive their medication in divided doses, 2–4 times a day, which decreases the occurrence of side effects. It usually takes 1–4 weeks before the client shows a significant response to the medication. Once the client's symptoms are under control, the dosage may be changed to once a day. Once maintenance on a particular drug is established, the client is kept on the lowest possible dosage to minimize the risk of developing tardive dyskinesia, a

Table 8.1 **Antipsychotic Medications**

Class	Generic Name	Trade Name	Adult Dosage (mg/day)
Atypical antipsychotics	clozapine	Clozaril	300–900
	olanzapine	Zyprexa	5–20
	quetiapine	Seroquel	150–750
	risperidone	Risperdal	4–16
	sertindole	Serlect	12–24
Phenothiazines	acetophenazine	Tindal	40–120
	chlorpromazine	Thorazine	30–800
	fluphenazine	Prolixin, Permitil	1–40
	mesoridazine	Serentil	75–300
	perphenazine	Trilafon	8–64
	thioridazine	Mellaril	150–800
	trifluoperazine	Stelazine, Suptazine	15–20
	triflupromazine	Vesprin	60–150
Thioxanthenes	chlorprothixene	Taractan	75–600
	thiothixene	Navane	6–120
Butyrophenones	haloperidol	Haldol	1–50
Dibenzoxazepine	loxapine	Loxitane	10–160
Dihydroindolone	molindone	Moban	15–225
Diphenylbatylperidine	pimozide	Orap	1–10

permanent movement disorder resulting from long-term treatment with antipsychotic medication (Zimbroff et al, 1997). The potency of an antipsychotic medication has an important bearing on its side effects. *Potency* is the power to produce the desired effects per milligram of the medication. For example, Thorazine (chlorpromazine) is a low-potency medication; therefore, it takes more of this medication to create the desired effect. Haldol (haloperidol) is an example of a high-potency medication; the effective dosage is small compared to low-potency medications.

Table 8.1 lists the various antipsychotic medications. The dosage range indicates the potency of each medication.

Side Effects

The most common side effects of conventional antipsychotic medications include anticholinergic effects, photosensitivity, and extrapyramidal side effects (EPS) (see Table 8.2 and Table 8.3). Smooth body movements depend on a critical ratio of DA to ACH in the brain. When medications block DA receptors, they lower this ratio, and extrapyramidal side effects occur. *Dystonia* has an abrupt onset, with frightening muscle spasms in the head and neck. Oculogyric crisis and laryngospasm are terms used to describe acute dystonic reaction in specific body regions. These reactions usually occur within the first 5 days of therapy or when dosage is significantly increased. Episodes are more likely to occur during the afternoon and evening than during the night and morning. Males and younger people are at higher risk for dystonia (Mazurek and Rosebush, 1996).

Parkinsonism is evidenced in clients' stooped posture and shuffling gait. Their faces resemble masks, and they may drool. They experience tremors and pill-rolling motions of the thumb and fingers at rest. This reaction is likely to begin within the first 30 days of treatment and occurs throughout the use of the medication. *Akathisia* is the inability to sit or stand still, along with a feeling of anxiety. This side effect usually

Table 8.2 Side Effects of Conventional Antipsychotics and Counteracting Measures

Side Effect	What This Means . . .	Measures
Akathisia	Feeling restless or jittery Needing to fidget, pace around	Beta blocker Inderal (propranolol)
Dystonia	Sudden muscle spasm Oculogyric crisis Laryngospasm	Benadryl (diphenhydramine) Cogentin (benztropine)
Parkinsonism	Tremor, stiffness, stooped posture, shuffling gait Akinesia—feeling slowed down	Cogentin (benztropine) Symmetrel (amantadine) Akineton (biperiden) Kemadrin (procyclidine) Benadryl (diphenhydramine)
Neuroleptic malignant syndrome	Muscle rigidity Hyperpyrexia Hypertension Confusion, delirium	Supportive measures Discontinue antipsychotic medication May give muscle relaxants
Tardive dyskinesia	Involuntary movements of face and body Swallowing problems	Goal is prevention Reduce dose of antipsychotic medication
Anticholinergic physical effects	Dry mouth Blurry vision Trouble urinating Constipation	Medications as below Teach client to rinse mouth with water, chew sugarless candy/gum, drink 6–8 glasses of fluid each day Teach client to eat bulky foods
Anticholinergic mental effects	Memory difficulties Confusion	Akineton (biperiden) Cogentin (benztropine) Artane (trihexyphenidyl) Kemadrin (procyclidine) Symmetrel (amantadine)
Weight gain	Up to 40% of clients gain weight	Teach client to decrease caloric intake, exercise daily
Sexual difficulties	Loss of sexual desire Loss of erection or ejaculation Anorgasmia	Try different antipsychotic medication Discuss problem with client and partner

Table 8.3 Medications for EPS

Class	Generic Name	Trade Name	Adult Dosage (mg/day)
Anticholinergic	amantadine	Symmetrel	100–300
	benztropine	Cogentin	1–6
	biperiden	Akineton	2–8
	diphenhydramine	Benadryl	50–300
	ethopropacine	Parsidol	50–200
	orphenadrine	Disipal, Norlex	50–300
	procyclidine	Kemadrin	5–30
	trihexyphenidyl	Artane	6–10
Specialized agents	bromocriptine	Parlodel	5–50
	dantrolene	Dantrium	60–600
	propranolol	Inderal	30–120

begins within the first 60 days of treatment and persists as long as the client is on medication. This side effect is extremely distressing to people and is a frequent cause of medication noncompliance. It is less responsive to treatment than are parkinsonism and dystonia. A number of medications may be used to lessen the EPS effects of the conventional antipsychotics. These medications reduce ACH, thereby restoring the DA-ACH ratio (Kapur and Remington, 1996).

Neuroleptic malignant syndrome (NMS) is a potentially fatal extrapyramidal symptom. It affects 1–2% of clients who take conventional antipsychotic medication. The risk is higher when clients are on two or more of these medications. Symptoms of NMS develop suddenly and include muscle rigidity and respiratory problems. Hyperpyrexia ranges from 101F to 107F (38C–41.6C). During the next 2–3 days, clients develop tachycardia, hypertension, respiratory problems, confusion, and delirium. The mortality rate with NMS is 14–30%; it is estimated that 1000–4000 people die every year. There is no specific treatment for NMS other than supportive measures and discontinuation of the medication. Parlodel (bromocriptine) may be of some help in halting the DA blockage. Muscle relaxants may lessen the rigidity (American Psychiatric Association, 1997; Keltner, 1997a).

Tardive dyskinesia occurs in 20–25% of clients who take conventional antipsychotic medications for over 2 years. Females and older people are at higher risk for tardive dyskinesia. Many of the cases are mild, but the disorder can be socially disfiguring. Symptoms include frowning, blinking, grimacing, puckering, blowing, smacking, licking, chewing, tongue protrusion, and spastic facial distortions. Abnormal movements of the arms and legs include rapid, purposeless, irregular movements; tremors; and foot tapping. Body symptoms include dramatic movements of the neck and shoulders and rocking, twisting pelvic gyrations and thrusts. Because tardive dyskinesia is often irreversible, the goal is prevention. If symptoms begin to appear, the medication is reduced or the person is switched to a newer antipsychotic medication (American Psychiatric Association, 1997).

Because of the side effects, many people do not like the way their bodies feel when taking conventional antipsychotic medication. Interference with sexual functioning is fairly common. One out of every 3–4 clients experiences one or more of the following problems: decreased sex drive, decreased ability to orgasm, difficulty with erections, delayed ejaculation, or orgasm without ejaculation. These side effects are less likely to occur with high-potency, low-dose medications. Almost half report weight gain. Anticholinergic side effects are unpleasant and can occur in 15–50% of people treated with these drugs. Identifying and managing side effects may help people stay on the medication and maintain a higher level of functioning, thus avoiding acute hospitalization.

Some people will stop taking their medication and relapse, while others relapse first and, as a result of their symptoms, stop taking their medication (Crenshaw and Goldberg, 1996).

Among the atypical antipsychotics, Clozaril (clozapine) has the most significant side effect in that about 1% of those taking this drug develop agranulocytosis. This carries a 40% fatality rate, usually from an overwhelming infection. Monitoring WBCs weekly for the first six months, and then every other week, is required to administer this drug safely. It is desirable that the WBCs stay above 3500 cells/cm. Other side effects of atypical antipsychotic medications include sedation, weight gain, hypersalivation, nervousness, headache, and dizziness. All of these agents appear to be relatively free of EPS (Keltner, 1997b).

Toxicity and Overdose

The primary symptom of overdose is CNS depression, which may extend to the point of coma. Other symptoms include agitation and restlessness, seizures, fever, EPS, arrhythmias, and hypotension. Caring for a client who has overdosed includes monitoring vital signs, especially of cardiac function; maintaining a patent airway; and gastric lavage. Antiparkinsonian medications may be given for EPS. Valium (diazepam) may be given for seizures.

Administration

Administration of antipsychotic medications is oral, in liquid or pill form, or by injection. Long-acting injectable medications such as Prolixin (fluphenazine) decanoate and Haldol (haloperidol) decanoate are often used to treat clients with schizophrenia. These medications are administered IM once every 3–4 weeks, a helpful regimen for clients who have difficulty remembering to take medications daily.

Antidepressant Medications

Physiological Effects

The neurotransmitters involved in depression are dopamine (DA), serotonin (5-HT), norepinephrine (NE), and acetylcholine (ACH). It is believed that during a depressive episode, there is a functional deficiency of these neurotransmitters or hyposensitive receptors. Antidepressant medications increase the amount of available neurotransmitters by inhibiting neurotransmitter reuptake, by inhibiting monoamine oxidase (MAO), or by blocking certain receptors (Thase and Howland, 1995).

Therapeutic Effects

Antidepressant medications can be classified as older generation agents, the multicyclics and monoamine oxidase inhibitors (MAOIs); and the new generation agents, the selective serotonin reuptake inhibitors (SSRIs) and the serotonin-norepinephrine reuptake inhibitors (SNRIs). The new generation medications have dramatically changed the treatment of depression, with more effective action and fewer side effects. Because depressions are heterogeneous in terms of which neurotransmitters are depleted, different people respond differently to various antidepressants. At times, a period of trial and error is necessary to determine which medication is most effective. The therapeutic purpose of antidepressants is to decrease as many of the depressive symptoms as possible, thereby enabling clients to participate more effectively in other forms of treatment. Maintenance continues until clients are free of symptoms for 4 months to 1 year. Then the drugs are slowly discontinued.

Antidepressants do not cause dependence, tolerance, addiction, or withdrawal. It takes an average of 10–14 days for the beginning effect of most antidepressants, and the full effect may not be apparent for 4–6 weeks. Approximately 30% of clients do not respond after a trial of 4–6 weeks. At that point, the physician may try a different antidepressant or augment with other medications. Table 8.4 lists the antidepressant medications. A significant number of clients improve when 600 mg of lithium is added to the antidepressant treatment. Other clients improve when triiodothyronine (T_3) is administered daily. For clients who are delusional or severely agitated, antipsychotic medication may be indicated (Mulsant et al, 1997).

Side Effects

Both multicyclics and MAOIs may have anticholinergic effects such as dry mouth, blurred vision, urinary retention, and constipation. CNS effects include

Table 8.4 Antidepressant Medications

Class	Generic Name	Trade Name	Adult Dosage (mg/day)
Aminoketone	bupropion	Wellbutrin	100–450
Selective serotonin reuptake inhibitor (SSRI)	fluoxetine	Prozac	20–80
	fluvoxamine	Luvox	50–300
	mirtzazpine	Remeron	5–60
	paroxetine	Paxil	50–200
	sertraline	Zoloft	50–200
Serotonin-norepinephrine inhibitor (SNRI)	venlafaxine	Effexor	75–375
	nefazodone	Serzone	200–600
Tricyclic	amitriptyline	Elavil, Endep	50–300
	amoxapine	Asendin	50–400
	clomipramine	Anafranil	75–250
	desipramine	Norpramin, Petrofrane	50–300
	doxepin	Adapin, Sinequan	50–300
	imipramine	Tofranil	50–300
	nortriptyline	Aventyl, Pamelor	30–125
	protriptyline	Vivactil	10–60
	trimipramine	Surmontil	50–300
Tetracyclic	maprotiline	Ludiomil	50–225
	mirtazapine	Remeron	15–45
Phenylpiperazine	trazodone	Desyrel	50–600
MAOI	isocarboxazid	Marplan	10–30
	phenelzine	Nardil	45–90
	tranylcypromine	Parnate	30–60

drowsiness, lethargy, insomnia, and restlessness. Orthostatic hypotension and tachycardia may occur in the early phases of treatment. The best known side effects are sexual dysfunctions and weight gain. Men and women may experience desire disorders and painful intercourse. Women may have orgasmic problems and decreased lubrication. Men may have difficulty with erections and inhibited ejaculation. Medications with the least sexual side effects and the least weight gain (0–10 pounds) are Norpramin (desipramine) and Pamelor (nortriptyline). Those with the most significant sexual side effects and the greatest weight gain (5–40 pounds) include Elavil (amitriptyline), Adapin (doxepin), and Anafranil (clomipramine).

The SSRIs and SNRIs have fewer anticholinergic effects, fewer cardiac effects, fewer sexual problems, less sedation, and less weight gain. Rapid ejaculation may improve when taking SSRIs (Crenshaw and Goldberg, 1996). Box 8.1 lists the side effects of antidepressant medications.

MAOIs decrease the amount of monoamine oxidase in the liver, which breaks down the essential amino acids tyramine and tryptophan. If a person eats food that is rich in these substances while taking an MAOI, he or she risks a hypertensive crisis. The first sign of a hypertensive crisis is a sudden and severe headache, followed by neck stiffness, nausea, vomiting, sweating, and tachycardia. Death can result

Box 8.1

Side Effects of Antidepressant Medications

Anticholinergic Effects

Dry mouth, blurred vision, urinary retention, constipation

CNS Effects

Drowsiness, weakness and lethargy, insomnia, tremor of hands

Cardiovascular Effects

Orthostatic hypotension, tachycardia

Photosensitivity

Severe sunburn after 30–60 minutes of exposure

Sexual Effects

Erectile dysfunction, ejaculatory dysfunction, nonorgasmic response

Other Effects

Weight gain, weight loss with Prozac (fluoxetine) and Zoloft (sertraline), hypertensive crisis with MAOIs

Box 8.2

Food to Avoid with MAOIs

Absolutely Restricted

Aged cheeses; aged and cured meats; improperly stored or spoiled meat, fish, or poultry; banana peel; broad bean pods; sauerkraut; soy sauce and other soy condiments; draft beer.

Consume in Moderation

Red or white wine (no more than two 4-oz glasses per day); bottled or canned beer, including non-alcoholic (no more than two 12-oz servings per day).

Source: Gardner, 1996.

from circulatory collapse or intracranial bleeding. Box 8.2 lists the foods and medications clients must avoid while taking a MAOI. Sexual side effects of MAOIs include desire problems, erection difficulties, orgasmic problems, and slower ejaculation.

The SSRIs and SNRIs increase the availablity of 5-HT, which relieves depression but can also cause the hyperserotonergic state known as the serotonin syndrome (SS). This syndrome is more likely to occur when these agents are used in combination with MAOIs. Serotonin syndrome develops very quickly and is characterized by:

- mental changes such as agitation, confusion, hypomania
- altered muscle tone such as hyperreflexia, rigidity, twitching, tremor
- autonomic changes such as hyper- or hypotension; tachycardia, diaphoresis
- CNS changes such as discoordination, coma, seizures
- hyperthermia with temperatures as high as 101F to 107F (30C to 41.6C)

Treatment of SS is supportive, which includes controlling hyperthermia with antipyretics and cooling devices. Muscle rigidity and twitching can be treated with Klonopin (clonazepam), Cogentin (benztropine), and Ativan (lorazepam). Anticonvulsants are used for seizures (Keltner, 1997a).

Toxicity and Overdose

Symptoms of toxicity include confusion, disturbed concentration, agitation, irritability, hallucinations, seizures, dilated pupils, delirium, hypotension or hypertension, hyperactive reflexes, tachycardia, arrhythmia, respiratory depression, coma, kidney failure, and cardiac arrest. Caring for a client who has overdosed includes monitoring vital signs, especially of cardiac function, and maintaining a patent airway. Vomiting is induced if the client is alert, while gastric lavage is initiated for the client who is stuporous. Following this procedure, activated charcoal may be administered to minimize absorption. Antilirium (physostigmine) 1–3 mg may be given IV to counter-

Critical Thinking

Mrs. Salazar is a 67-year-old client who is being placed on Prozac (flouxetine hydrocholoride), a selective serotonin reuptake inhibitor (SSRI), for depression. The nurse teaches Mrs. Salazar and her daughter that:

- they may not notice an improvement in Mrs. Salazar's depression for 2–4 weeks.

- side effects such as dry mouth, blurred vision, insomnia, rapid heart beat, or sexual dysfunction can occur.

- Prozac can cause significant weight gain and hypertension. The nurse advises Mrs. Salazar to reduce her salt intake and maintain a low-calorie, low-fat diet.

- toxicity to the drug is uncommon, but can occur; therefore, confusion, irritability, or seizures should be reported to the physician immediately.

Upon completion of teaching Mrs. Salazar and her daughter about the drug, the nurse turns and leaves the room.

1. How would you explain the actions of a serotonin reuptake inhibitor to Mrs. Salazar and her daughter?

2. How will Mrs. Salazar know if the SSRI is being effective?

3. Based on your understanding of these drugs, evaluate the nurse's teaching session with Mrs. Salazar and her daughter.

4. What aspects of teaching should be different for Mrs. Salazar than for younger clients on the same drug?

5. What is the best explanation for including Mrs. Salazar's daughter in the teaching session?

Suggested answers can be found in Appendix D.

act the toxic effects. Valium (diazepam) may be administered for seizures and vasopressors or lidocaine for cardiovascular effects (Glod, 1996).

If MAOIs and other antidepressants are administered together, serious reactions may occur. Symptoms include hyperthermia, severe agitation, delirium, and coma. Seven to 14 days should elapse between the use of MAOIs and other antidepressants.

Administration

Administration of antidepressant medications is oral. It usually takes 2–4 weeks to reach therapeutic levels, at which point the client is able to notice a reduction in symptoms. Other people may actually see changes in energy and mood before the client experiences an improvement. It is important to educate clients about this fact so that they do not become frustrated and stop taking the medication before it becomes effective.

For further information on antidepressant medications, therapeutic blood levels, and associated client teaching, see Chapter 11.

Antianxiety Medications

Physiological Effects

Benzodiazepine antianxiety medications act on the limbic system and the reticular activating system (RAS). They produce a calming effect by potentiating the effects of gamma aminobutyric acid (GABA), one of the inhibitory neurotransmitters. CNS depression can range from mild sedation to coma. Other physiological effects include skeletal muscle relaxation and anticonvulsant properties. Azaspirone antianxiety medications do not bind at GABA receptors but rather balance 5-HT activity by stimulating the 5-HT receptors. These medications do not tranquilize and sedate and may have mild antidepressant effects. Typically, it takes 1–2 weeks for the level of anxiety to decrease (Crenshaw and Goldberg, 1996).

Therapeutic Effects

Although antianxiety medications will not eliminate all the symptoms of anxiety, they will decrease the level of anxiety, thereby enabling clients to function

Table 8.5 Antianxiety Medications

Class	Generic Name	Trade Name	Adult Dosage (mg/day)
Benzodiazepines	alprazolam	Xanax	0.75–4.0
	chlordiazepoxide	Librium	15–100
	clonazepam	Klonopin	5–20
	clorazepate	Tranxene	15–60
	diazepam	Valium	6–40
	halazepam	Paxipam	60–160
	hydroxyzine	Atarax, Vistaril	200–400
	lorazepam	Ativan	4–12
	oxazepam	Serax	30–120
	prazepam	Centrax	10–60
Azaspirones	buspirone	BuSpar	15–60
Metathizanone	chlormezanone	Trancopal	300–800

more effectively. These medications are used for anxiety symptoms, anxiety disorders, acute alcohol withdrawal, and convulsive disorders. For specific information about which medications are most effective for the various anxiety disorders, see Chapter 9.

Individual benzodiazepines differ in potency, speed in crossing the blood-brain barrier, and degree of receptor binding. High-potency and short-acting benzodiazepines include Xanax (alprazolam), Ativan (lorazepam), Paxipam (halazepam), and Serax (oxazepam). Low-potency and long-acting benzodiazepines include Tranxene (clorazepate), Valium (diazepam), and Librium (chlordiazepoxide). Table 8.5 lists the various antianxiety medications.

Side Effects

Side effects of benzodiazepines are primarily related to the general sedative effects and include drowsiness, fatigue, dizziness, and psychomotor impairment. Sedation usually disappears within 1–2 weeks of treatment. These medications potentiate the effects of alcohol on the CNS, leading to severe CNS depression. When administered intravenously, there is a potential for cardiovascular collapse and respiratory depression. There is a potential for abuse in vulnerable client populations. Benzodiazepines may improve

sexual aversion, vaginismus, and rapid ejaculation. They may also cause erection problems.

BuSpar (buspirone) has no potential for dependence and does not potentiate the effects of alcohol on the CNS. It is the drug of choice for clients who are prone to substance abuse or for those who require long-term treatment with antianxiety medications. Its side effects include drowsiness, dizziness, headache, and nervousness. This drug does not affect sex drive or arousal; in fact, sexual desire is often enhanced. It may improve delayed ejaculation and may worsen rapid ejaculation (Crenshaw and Goldberg, 1996).

Box 8.3 lists the side effects of antianxiety medications.

Toxicity and Overdose

Symptoms of toxicity include euphoria, relaxation, slurred speech, disorientation, unsteady gait, and impaired judgment. Symptoms of overdose include respiratory depression, cold and clammy skin, hypotension, weak and rapid pulse, dilated pupils, and coma. Caring for a client who has overdosed includes monitoring vital signs, especially of cardiac function, and maintaining a patent airway. If the client is alert, vomiting is induced, while gastric lavage is initiated for the client who is stuporous. Following this procedure, activated charcoal may be administered to minimize absorption. Forced diuresis may increase elimination of the medication (Saltzman, Green, and Badaracco, 1995).

Administration

All the antianxiety medications may be taken orally. Antacids interfere with the absorption of these medications and should not be taken until several hours later. Atarax and Vistaril (hydroxyzine) may also be administered IM. Librium (chlordiazepoxide), Valium (diazepam), and Ativan (lorazepam) may be administered IM and IV.

Benzodiazepines should not be discontinued abruptly because of the risk of withdrawal symptoms, which include seizures, abdominal and other muscular cramps, vomiting, and insomnia. These medications must be gradually reduced very carefully.

Mood-Stabilizing Medications

Physiological Effects

The mood stabilizers include a small group of diverse medications that are useful in stabilizing clients' affect. Lithium is the best known and most often prescribed mood stabilizer. In recent years, several anticonvulsant medications have been added to this category: Tegretol (carbamazepine), Depakene and Depakote (valproate), and Klonopin (clonazepam). Calcium channel blockers (Calan and Isoptin) are increasingly being used with success in manic disorders either alone or in combination with other mood stabilizers.

The specific action of these medications is unclear. In the body, lithium substitutes for sodium, calcium, potassium, and magnesium. It also interacts with DA, NE, and 5-HT and it seems to have an effect on the G proteins associated with receptors. Like antidepressants, lithium normalizes REM sleep abnormalities which are present in the mood disorders. It is thought that carbamazepine reduces the rate of impulse transmission and that valproate increases levels of the inhibitory neurotransmitter GABA. Increasing GABA activity seems to have an antimanic, anitpanic, and antianxiety effect. Manic episodes may be

---

Box 8.3

Side Effects of Antianxiety Medications

CNS Effects

Drowsiness, fatigue, dizziness, headache, paradoxical excitement (benzodiazepines), psychomotor impairment; potentiates other CNS depressants (benzodiazepines)

Cardiovascular Effects with IV Use

Hypotension, cardiovascular collapse

Respiratory Effects with IV Use

Respiratory depression

Other Effects

Dependence (benzodiazepines)

---

triggered by persistent low-level stimulation of the brain, referred to as "kindling." The anticonvulsants may be effective in that they block this persistent stimulation. Clients with an acute manic episode have been found to have increased levels of intracellular calcium, which decrease when lithium is administered. Calcium channel blockers have been found to also be effective in the treatment of bipolar disorder and seem to work best in people who also respond to lithium (Hedaya, 1996; Masters, 1996).

Therapeutic Effects

For clients with problems such as bipolar disorder, major depression, schizoaffective disorder, treatment-resistant schizophrenia, alcohol withdrawal, and other problems concerning the regulation of mood, mood-stabilizing medications have been found to be helpful.

The antimanic effectiveness of lithium is 60–70%; some people seem to be resistant to it and others cannot tolerate the side effects. Because it takes 1–3 weeks to control symptoms, antipsychotic medications or benzodiazepines are given initially for more immediate relief. Lithium reduces the frequency, duration, and intensity of both manic and depressive episodes and is the drug of choice for long-term treatment of bipolar disorder.

Table 8.6 Mood-Stabilizing Medications

Class	Generic Name	Trade Name	Adult Dosage (mg/day)
Lithium	lithium carbonate	Eskalith, Lithane, Lithobid	900–2400, acute 300–1200, maintenance
	lithium citrate	Cibalith-S	900–2400, acute 300–1200, maintenance
Anticonvulsants	carbamazepine	Tegretol	200–1400
	valproate	Depakene, Depakote	750
	clonazepam	Klonopin	1.5–20
Calcium channel blockers	verapamil	Calan, Isoptin	120–360

Tegretol (carbamazepine) has a favorable response rate in about 60% of clients and is most often used with persons who are unable to take lithium. If given in combination, it may also increase the effectiveness of lithium. Depakene and Depakote (valproate) have a 57% response rate. They may make a person who is lithium-resistant responsive to it. Valproate may be especially useful in rapid cycling bipolar disorder and in treating the mood disorders associated with organic sydromes. Klonopin (clonazepam) is a benzodiazepine that is also an anticonvulsant. Its use is typically in addition to lithium, the combination of which lengthens the periods of remission. It has a more rapid onset than the other anticonvulsants, which may take 2–3 weeks to be effective. Calan and Isoptin (verapamil) are calcium channel blockers that seem to work best in people who also respond to lithium (Masters, 1996).

Table 8.6 lists the mood-stabilizing medications.

Side Effects

The early side effects of lithium often disappear after 4 weeks. These side effects include lack of spontaneity, memory problems, difficulty concentrating, nausea, vomiting, diarrhea, and hand tremors. Weight gain and a worsening of acne often persist throughout treatment. The side effects of Tegretol (carbamazepine) are primarily related to the CNS and include drowsiness, dizziness, blurred or double vision, ataxia (unsteady or staggered gait), and nystagmus (involuntary rolling of the eyes). They often disappear over time and are less likely to occur when dosage is gradually increased. Women taking oral contraceptives may experience breakthough bleeding and may also have false-positive pregnancy tests. Likewise, the side effects of Depakene and Depakote (valproate) tend to occur early in treatment and include sedation, tremor, ataxia, and gastrointestinal effects. Weight gain tends to persist throughout treatment, and clients may stop taking their medication as a result. Side effects of calcium channel blockers include nausea, constipation, dry mouth, bradycardia, and hypotension (Hedaya, 1996; Masters, 1996). Box 8.4 lists the side effects of mood-stabilizing medications.

Toxicity and Overdose

There is a fine line between therapeutic levels and toxic levels of lithium. Older people are more susceptible to lithium toxicity. Causes of toxicity include excessive intake (deliberate or accidental) and reduced excretion of lithium (resulting from kidney disease and low salt intake). Box 8.5 lists the signs of lithium toxicity. Caring for a client who is toxic includes monitoring vital signs, maintaining a patent airway, and administering intravenous fluids (adding NaCl if hyponatremic). Severe toxicity is treated with hemodialysis (Hedaya, 1996). Symptoms of toxicity with Tegretol (carbamazepine) include seizures, hypotension, arrhythmia, respiratory depression, and coma. Depakene/Depakote (valproate) overdose can cause severe coma and death. There is no specific treatment other than monitoring vital signs, main-

Box 8.4

Side Effects of Mood Stabilizers/Anticonvulsants

Carbamazepine

CNS Effects

Drowsiness, dizziness, blurred or double vision, ataxia, nystagmus

Gastrointestinal Effects

Transient nausea

Valproate

CNS Effects

Sedation, mild tremor, ataxia

Gastrointestinal Effects

Nausea, vomiting, diarrhea, loss of appetite

Other Effects

Weight gain

Box 8.5

Signs of Lithium Toxicity

Mild (serum level about 1.5 mEq/L)

- Slight apathy, lethargy, drowsiness
- Decreased concentration
- Mild muscular weakness, slight muscle twitching
- Coarse hand tremors
- Mild ataxia

Moderate (serum level about 1.5–2.5 mEq/L)

- Severe diarrhea
- Nausea and vomiting
- Mild to moderate ataxia
- Moderate apathy, lethargy, drowsiness
- Slurred speech
- Tinnitus (ringing in the ears)
- Blurred vision
- Irregular tremor
- Muscle weakness

Severe (serum level above 2.5 mEq/L)

- Nystagmus
- Dysarthria (speech difficulty due to impairment of the tongue)
- Deep tendon hyperreflexia
- Visual or tactile hallucinations
- Oliguria or anuria
- Confusion
- Seizures
- Coma or death

taining a patent airway, and decreasing absorption by the use of activated charcoal. Narcan (naloxone) may be used to reverse the coma (Masters, 1996).

Administration

The administration of lithium is oral, in capsule or liquid form. There is some speculation that the liquid form is absorbed more quickly and is therefore more beneficial when initiating the medication. Some capsules are in slow-release or controlled-release forms. Lithium is usually administered in divided doses, and the ultimate dosage is determined by the reduction of symptoms and blood lithium levels.

Both carbamazepine and valproate are available in tablet and liquid forms. They are given in divided doses, beginning with low dosage and a gradual increase. The ultimate dosage is determined by the reduction of symptoms, blood levels, and side effects. Calcium channel blockers are increased gradually over several days, during which clients are monitored for hypotension and bradycardia (Masters, 1996). For further information on mood-stabilizing medications and associated client teaching, see Chapter 11.

Special Populations and Psychopharmacological Treatment

Certain groups of clients present a challenge to nurses when psychotropic medications are part of their treatment. These groups include older adults, pregnant women, children, medically complex clients, those who are psychiatrically disabled, and culturally diverse clients.

Older Adults

The physiological changes of aging affect the use of psychotropic medications. Absorption of medication is influenced by a decrease in gastric emptying time, a reduction in blood flow to the gastrointestinal system, and a decrease in GI motility. Once through the gastrointestinal system, most psychotropic medications bind to albumin. Albumin levels decrease with aging, and there is more free-floating medication in the bloodstream, thereby contributing to increased sedation in older adults. At the same time, adipose fat tissue increases by 10–50% over the age of 65. Medications such as the long-acting benzodiazepines, which are stored in fat tissue, are thus available for longer periods of time. Changes in liver metabolism contribute to slower metabolism of medications, which prolongs elimination and leads to increased toxicity. The renal filtration rate may decrease by 50% by age 70, which also contributes to increased toxicity. Aging reduces the amount of NE, 5-HT, DA, ACH, and GABA in the central nervous system, leading to increased receptor sensitivity. The result is a change in responsiveness to medications (Brown and Lempa, 1997).

Older adults are more sensitive than younger adults to the side effects of antipsychotic medications. Increased sedation may lead to confusion and agitation. Orthostatic hypotension increases the risk of falls and fractures. Older people are likely to have more severe EPS, especially a higher risk of tardive dyskinesia. Those drugs that have high potency and low dosage are particularly successful in small doses.

Older adults are also more sensitive to antidepressant side effects. The anticholinergic effects may increase symptoms of prostatic hypertrophy, blurred vision, and constipation. The new generation of antidepressants, the SSRIs and SNRIs, are especially useful for treating depression in older people. The response time between initiation of the medication and relief of depressive symptoms is much shorter than with multicyclic antidepressants. The most commonly used are Prozac (fluoxetine) for those people experiencing psychomotor retardation, and Zoloft (sertraline) for those experiencing anxiety.

The most common side effect of the MAOIs is orthostatic hypotension. The dietary restrictions of MAOIs often preclude their use by older adults (Hedaya, 1996). See Chapter 11 for more detail on the use of antidepressant medication with older adults.

Because the metabolism of antianxiety medications slows with aging, medications that are metabolized quickly are more frequently prescribed. Older clients are more sensitive to the side effects of sedation, which may contribute to confusion and agitation. Other effects in older adults include unsteadiness, slowed reaction time, increased forgetfulness, and decreased concentration. Table 8.7 lists the medications preferred for older adults.

Pregnancy

The benefits and dangers of the use of antidepressants must be carefully considered for women who are pregnant, breastfeeding, or trying to conceive. Multicyclic antidepressants and SSRIs do not have any significant increase in birth defects. MAOIs may cause birth defects and contribute to complications during delivery. Lithium should be avoided during the first trimester of pregnancy. The atypical antipsychotics do not appear to cause birth defects. However, it is recommended that the dose is lowered as much as possible a few days before birth to avoid withdrawal syndrome in the infant. Women should be discouraged from breastfeeding while they are taking psychotropic medications because these medications pass into breast milk (Blumenthal, 1996).

Children

Children tend to have a faster absorption rate compared to adults. Children also metabolize medications more quickly than adults. This increased efficiency in absorption and metabolism indicates that it is more appropriate to administer smaller multiple doses through the day rather than larger, less frequent doses. Dosages for children are based on the child's tolerance of side effects. Other considerations include effects on growth retardation, school performance problems, lower cognitive test scores, and reproductive risks that extend beyond treatment (Unis, 1993).

Medically Complex Clients

Medically complex clients are those who have an underlying medical problem with or without a preexisting psychiatric disorder. For instance, the development of delirium or acute confusional states occurs in some 80% of hospitalized clients (Inouye and Charpentier, 1996). The cause may be environmental (ICU

Table 8.7 Medications for Older Adults

Class	Generic Name	Trade Name	Older Adult Dosage (mg/day)
Antipsychotic	fluphenazine	Prolixin, Permitil	0.25–6.0
	haloperidol	Haldol	0.25–6.0
	risperidone	Risperdal	4–16
	thiothixene	Navane	4–20
	trifluoperazine	Stelazine, Suptazine	4–20
Antidepressant	desipramine	Norpramin, Petrofrane	25–150
	nortriptyline	Aventyl, Pamelor	10–35
	phenelzine	Nardil	7.5–30.0
	tranylcypromine	Parnate	10–40
	venlafaxine	Effexor	75–375
Antianxiety	alprazolam	Xanax	0.125–2.0
	lorazepam	Ativan	0.5–4.0
	oxazepam	Serax	10–60

psychosis), medication toxicity, or underlying pathophysiology of the illness. The essential part of diagnosis and treatment of these clients is determining the underlying cause of the symptoms. If the cause is medical, such as pneumonia, Parkinson's disease, or undiagnosed infections, then treating the underlying disorder will eliminate the psychiatric symptoms. Depression may result from hyperthyroidism, hypothyroidism, diabetes, or AIDS. It may also be caused by medications such as antihypertensives, antiarthritics, sedatives, and cardiovascular medications.

Recent studies have shown that medical clients who have depressive symptoms may respond better to Ritalin (methylphenidate) than to traditional antidepressants (Gomez and Gomez, 1994). Both drugs are used for short duration and usually within the time frame of improvement in the medical condition.

Clients with chronic illnesses may suffer from major depression. The treatment of choice is a trial of antidepressant therapy. Clients with a history of cardiac problems may be more difficult to treat with antidepressants because these medications may trigger further arrhythmias.

Clients with both a medical illness and psychiatric symptoms must be monitored for multidrug interactions. Americans over the age of 64 use 30% of the prescription drugs sold, along with an unknown number of over-the-counter (OTC) medications (Hedaya, 1996). These data point to the problem of polypharmacy, especially in the older adult population—but more important, to the increased likelihood of multidrug interaction, which is potentially life-threatening. Assess the functional level and baseline cognitive abilities of clients to determine whether they are able to learn or retain information about their medications. Obtain a complete listing of the medications. Do not simply ask what medications clients are taking; have them bring in medications and describe their administration. Consult a pharmacist to determine whether any drug may interact adversely with others.

Psychiatrically Disabled Clients

Despite advances in medical science, some clients remain psychiatrically disabled. The symptoms these clients suffer from are usually debilitating and interfere dramatically with their ability to function in daily life. Their capacity to learn or retain new information is often impaired. Assessing cognitive skills is important in designing appropriate teaching strategies. Determine what medications have been effective in the past and how well the client was able to remain on the medication. Identifying supportive people in the client's environment, as well as community resources, can be helpful for medication compliance.

Culturally Diverse Clients

Ethnopharmacology is a topic investigated in the past decade. Researchers are examining the benefits of drug treatment and determining levels that produce drug toxicity, and have found that these are not the same for all groups of people. High metabolism of a medication may contribute to ineffective treatment, while a low metabolic rate may increase side effects or lead to toxicity. For example, Asians tend to be slower metabolizers of medications, whereas African Americans demonstrate a faster metabolism. Recognizing the ethnic differences in response to drugs promotes giving culturally competent care.

Cultural assessment should be taken prior to negotiating a treatment plan that includes medication. This assessment should identify client beliefs about the causes of mental illness, home remedies, spiritual treatments, and attitudes toward health care professionals. Personal beliefs about medication will influence compliance. For example, if the client believes taking medicine is a sign of weakness, he or she may not take it at all. Those who believe in the "magic" of medication may take extra pills, thinking that more is better. If English is not the client's native language, it may be necessary to have a translator help with medication teaching.

Nursing Interventions

The accompanying box lists the nursing interventions classifications (NIC) that are appropriate for medication management and client/family education (McCloskey and Bulechek, 1996).

Physiological: Complex:
Drug Management

Medication Management
Part of psychiatric nursing is the administration and management of psychotropic drugs. Proper medication management can often make a tremendous dif-

ference in a consumer's life. Adult clients have many of their own ideas about medications and do have the right to refuse treatment. The word "noncompliance" has negative connotations such as disobeying or being defiant. However, it is still the commonly used term among health care professionals. It is up to us, as nurses, to ensure that compliance means mutually agreed upon goals and outcomes rather than simply clients obeying orders. It is not just people with mental disorders that struggle with this issue. People with diabetes, hypertension, chronic lung disease, and others have compliance problems also. If we are to understand people's refusal to take medications, we have to find out their reasons, which are many and often intermixed. Compliance problems can be roughly divided into three categories: errors due to the illness, side effects, and lack of education (Crane, Kirby, and Kooperman, 1996; Francell, 1994).

A common error due to one's mental disorder is believing that one is not ill. Awareness of illness, or insight, seems to be affected by both biological and psychological factors. Arguing or threatening clients is useless. Saying something like, "If you don't take your meds, you'll end up in the hospital" has a blaming sound to it. It may be better to say, "Most of the time, if a person stops their meds, they end up in the hospital." Threatening clients is unethical and is heard in such statements as, "If you don't take your meds, you cannot have your cigarettes today." Forgetfulness or memory loss may be other errors related to a mental disorder. You need to plan strategies for helping these clients to remember to take their medications.

Intolerance of side effects is another factor in noncompliance. When a side effect becomes severe, it is no longer a side effect; it becomes the primary effect of the medication. The more severe the side effect, the more people cannot feel the positive effect of the drug. See Box 8.6 on ways to manage side effects. As new drugs are developed with reduced side effects and increased effectiveness, clients will be able to manage their medications more easily.

The third reason for noncompliance is errors due to lack of education. This includes reasons such as stopping the drug because they feel better, not knowing what the medication is for, enjoying the "highs" of mania, and the public stigma of mental illness.

Nursing Interventions Classification

MEDICATION ADMINISTRATION

DOMAIN: Physiological: Complex

Class: *Drug Management*

    Interventions: *Medication Management:* Facilitation of safe and effective use of prescription and over-the-counter drugs

Class: *Thermoregulation*

    Interventions: *Temperature Regulation:* Attaining and/or maintaining body temperature within a normal range

DOMAIN: Behavioral

Class: *Patient Education*

    Interventions: *Teaching:* Prescribed Medication: Preparing a patient to safely take prescribed medications and monitor for their effects

Source: McCloskey and Bulechek, 1996.

Box 8.6

Managing Side Effects of Medication

Dry Mouth

- Chew sugarless gum/suck hard candy
- Maintain good mouth hygiene
- Use artificial saliva preparation

Urinary Retention

- Mild—turn on running water while attempting to urinate
- Severe—bethanacol 10–30 mg, 3–4 times a day

Constipation

- Natural laxatives—bulk in foods, increase fluid intake
- Bulk laxatives—Metamucil, Surfak, Colace
- Stimulating laxatives—milk of magnesia, Dulcolax, Senekot

Nausea

- Take medication at mealtime or bedtime

Weight Gain

- Monitor weight
- Control intake
- Exercise

Drowsiness

- Take medication at bedtime
- Increase morning caffeine intake

Orthostatic Hypotension, Dizziness

- Get up slowly from a lying or sitting position
- Use support hose and perform calf-muscle exercises
- Monitor blood pressure regularly

Hand Tremor

- Take medication with food
- Inderal (propranolol)

Physiological: Complex: Thermoregulation

Temperature Regulation

When thinking about heat exhaustion or heat stroke, we generally imagine those at risk to be people with chronic medical problems, especially older individuals. However, many psychotropic medications make clients more susceptible to heat-related illnesses. Table 8.8 lists the medications and drugs that increase the risk. Other factors increasing the risk for heat exhaustion or heat stroke are obesity, self-care deficits, inadequate living conditions, and difficulty in recognizing signs and symptoms of heat-related illnesses. You can help clients plan ahead by providing written and verbal information about the increased risk for heat stroke. Clients should be taught to maintain an adequate fluid intake while avoiding caffeinated drinks, which tend to increase heart rate. During the day, clients can plan to spend time in an air-conditioned building such as a library, a mall, mental health centers, or cooling centers. Cool baths or showers and loose light clothing are also beneficial (Batscha, 1997).

Behavioral: Patient Education

Teaching: Prescribed Medication

Successful treatment depends to a great extent on clients' understanding of the treatment and their participation in making the best treatment decisions for themselves. Medication teaching is an important consideration for any client taking psychotropic medications. Clients and families must be actively involved in either individual or group teaching sessions.

Client and Family Participation

Consumers of mental health care have the right to make decisions about taking medications. As a nurse, your role is to help clients and families understand how to make such decisions. Some of the influences on this decision-making process are:

- the media (magazine articles, newspaper and television reports)

Table 8.8 Medications/Drugs and Heat-Related Illnesses

Medication/Drug	Increased Risk Through:
Antipsychotics	Altered sweat production, impaired temperature regulation, impaired thirst recognition, weight gain
Anticholinergics	Altered sweat production
Tricyclics	Altered sweat production, weight gain
SSRIs	Increased heat production, inhibited heat loss
MAOIs	Weight gain
Lithium	Increased heat production, inhibited heat loss, fluid loss through increased urination
Beta blockers	Dehydration through increased sweating
Smoking	Respiratory conditions such as asthma or emphysema impair oxygen exchange, which inhibits heat loss
Alcohol	Excess fluid loss through increased urination
Stimulants	Increased metabolic requirements

Sources: Auerbach, Fleisher, and Knochel, 1993; Batscha, 1997.

- client's and family's relationships with health care professionals; the freedom to ask questions or the fear of disapproval
- the severity of the illness and symptoms
- the positive and negative personal experiences clients have had with medications
- the convenience of taking the medication as it fits into the person's lifestyle
- group support and suggestions for managing side effects

Other influences that affect the decision include the number of medications prescribed, health benefits, financial concerns, and social support systems available in the community.

An important topic for discussion is that of side effects. Most repeat hospitalizations occur because clients stop taking their medications in response to disturbing side effects such as weight gain and sexual dysfunction. They may need help in reporting their concerns and fears so they can be more active mental health care consumers.

Teach clients the purpose of their medications, how to take them (timing, with food or alone, actions to take if doses are missed), potential side effects, and when to call the doctor. Combine verbal and written instructions. Use pictures for those clients who are unable to read English. Box 8.7 describes general client teaching for all medications. Each of the disorders chapters in Part Three includes a box on client teaching for specific medications.

Medication Teaching Groups

Medication teaching groups are successful with most clients. Talking with others and helping others with similar disabilities provides emotional support and reinforces medication information. The groups use role playing, audiovisual tools, lectures, and discussion. Crane, Kirgy, and Kooperman (1996) describe the various functions of medication groups:

- providing information about medications
- helping clients discuss and manage fears about medications
- increasing client understanding of mental disorders and the role of medications
- expanding client participation in the treatment planning process
- helping clients become accountable for their decision making

Family Support

To achieve the best outcome, family members and/or significant others must be viewed as potential allies and resources for rehabilitation. In one study, clients with schizophrenia were assigned to one of four groups, each of which included medication treatment: medication treatment only, social skills training group, family education group, and social skills training plus family education group. There was a 41%

Box 8.7

Medication Teaching

- Carry at all times a card or other identification listing the names of the medications you are taking.
- Do not take nonprescription medication without approval from your doctor.
- If you experience drowsiness or dizziness, do not drive or operate dangerous machinery.
- Do not drink alcohol or use other drugs.
- Limit your intake of caffeine.
- Do not stop taking the medication abruptly; this might produce withdrawal symptoms.
- If weight gain becomes a problem, increase your exercise and decrease your caloric intake.

---

relapse rate for those only receiving medication treatment. Those receiving social skills training or family education relapsed at a rate of 20%. Those who received social skills training and family education experienced no relapse at all (Armstrong, 1993).

Family members can be a significant support to the client and can, when educated, help with symptom monitoring, decision making regarding medications, and avoiding relapses. Families are a significant resource for the care and long-term management of their relatives if they are given practical support and information. Begin teaching family members with your initial contact with them. Help them express their feelings about living with the person who has the disorder. Identify the strengths the family brings to the living situation. Support the family in developing ways to maintain the client at the highest level of functioning.

Family education is accomplished in both individual and group sessions. The functions of medication groups, as described above, also apply to the family. Each family member must weigh the costs and benefits of any and all medication. Support their right to participate in these treatment decisions by functioning as a client advocate in the clinical setting.

Key Concepts

Introduction

- Psychotropic medications affect cognitive function, emotions, and behavior. They are categorized into four groups: antipsychotic, antidepressant, antianxiety, and mood-stabilizing medications.

Antipsychotic Medications

- Conventional antipsychotic medications are more effective in diminishing the positive characteristics (hallucinations, delusions, loose association, inappropriate affect) than in diminishing the negative characteristics (withdrawal, minimal self-care, concrete thinking, flat affect) of severe mental illness. Atypical antipsychotic agents decrease both positive and negative symptoms.

- By reducing symptoms, medication enables clients to assume more control over their lives and participate more effectively in other forms of treatment.

- It usually takes 1–4 weeks before the client shows a significant response to antipsychotic medication.

- Extrapyramidal side effects (EPS) are caused by an imbalance of DA and ACH and are more frequently associated with high-potency medications. Atypical antipsychotics have the lowest incidence of EPS.

- Types of EPS include dystonia, pseudoparkinsonism, akathisia, neuroleptic malignant syndrome (NMS), and tardive dyskinesia.

- Side effects such as sedation, orthostatic hypotension, weight gain, and sexual dysfunction cause a high percentage of clients to stop taking their medication.

- The primary symptom of overdose is CNS depression; other symptoms are agitation, seizures, fever, EPS, arrhythmias, and hypotension.

Antidepressant Medications

- Antidepressant medications increase the amount of available neurotransmitters by inhibiting reuptake, inhibiting monoamine oxidase (MAO), or blocking receptors.

- It often takes 2–4 weeks before the client begins to show clinical improvement. To prevent relapse, medications are continued for 4–5 months after recovery from depression.

- Side effects of antidepressants include anticholinergic effects, CNS effects, and cardiovascular effects.

- If a person eats food rich in tyramine and tryptophan while taking an MAOI (MAO inhibitor), he or she risks a hypertensive crisis, which may be fatal.

- Symptoms of toxicity include severe CNS changes, cardiovascular changes, respiratory depression, and possible death.

Antianxiety Medications

- Benzodiazepines potentiate the effects of GABA in the limbic system and the reticular activating system.

- Azaspirones attach to 5-HT and DA receptors.

- Side effects of benzodiazepines include sedation, potentiation of the effects of alcohol, and chemical dependence.

- BuSpar (buspirone) is the drug of choice for clients who are prone to substance abuse or those who require long-term treatment.

- Symptoms of toxicity are primarily CNS effects. Symptoms of overdose include respiratory depression, cold and clammy skin, hypotension, weak and rapid pulse, dilated pupils, and coma.

- All the antianxiety medications may be taken orally. Atarax and Vistaril may also be administered IM. Librium, Valium, and Ativan may be administered IM and IV.

- Benzodiazepines should not be discontinued abruptly because of the risk of severe withdrawal symptoms.

Mood-Stabilizing Medications

- Mood-stabilizing medications include lithium, Tegretol, Depakene, Depakote, Klonopin, Calan, and Isoptin.

- Mood stabilizers are effective for clients with bipolar disorder, major depression, schizoaffective disorder, treatment-resistant schizophrenia, alcohol withdrawal, and other problems concerning the regulation of mood. They are most effective as antimanic medications.

- The early side effects of lithium disappear after 4 weeks, except for weight gain and a worsening of acne.

- There is a fine line between therapeutic levels and toxic levels of lithium. Older people are more susceptible to toxicity.

- Toxicity with Tegretol and Depakene/Depakote can cause coma and even death.

Special Population and Psychopharmacological Treatment

- Older adults must be carefully monitored because aging affects the absorption and metabolism of medications. Decreased albumin levels and a decreased renal filtration rate lead to higher levels of medication in the blood. Aging reduces the amount of neurotransmitters in the CNS.

- Older adults are more sensitive than younger adults to the side effects of many medications. Increased sedation may lead to confusion and agitation. Orthostatic hypotension increases the risk of falls and fractures.

- Older adult clients are more likely to have severe EPS and anticholinergic side effects.

- The benefits and dangers of psychotropic drugs must be carefully considered for women who are pregnant, breastfeeding, or trying to conceive.

- Children absorb and metabolize medications more quickly than adults and should be given smaller multiple doses throughout the day.

- Medically complex clients who experience medical problems and psychiatric symptoms must be assessed for the underlying cause, such as environmental causes, medication toxicity, or underlying pathophysiology of the illness.

- Clients must be assessed for multidrug interactions; many people take several medications at once.

Nursing Interventions

- Compliance problems are often related to errors due to the illness, side effects, and lack of education.

- Variables that influence a client's decision whether or not to take medication include the media, relationships with health care professionals, severity of the illness, personal experiences, group support and suggestions, the number of medications, health benefits, financial concerns, and social support systems in the community.

- Clients must be taught the purpose of their medications, how to take them, potential side effects, and situations in which to call the physician.

- Medication teaching groups provide information, help manage fears, increase understanding of mental disorders and the role of medications, expand client participation in treatment planning, and help clients become accountable for decision making.

- To achieve the best possible outcome, families and significant others must be included in medication teaching.

Review Questions

1. Which of the following meals would be most appropriate for a client who is taking an MAOI for depression?
   a. poached chicken, rice, green beans
   b. sweet and sour chicken on soy sauce rice
   c. pizza with aged cheddar cheese
   d. cured ham and scalloped potatoes

2. Your client is experiencing parkinsonism side effects of antipsychotic medication. Which of the following agents will be ordered to counteract these effects?
   a. Paxil (paroxetine)
   b. Ativan (lorazepam)
   c. Clozaril (clozapine)
   d. Benadryl (diphenhydramine)

3. Which of the following medications will decrease both positive and negative characteristics of schizophrenia?
   a. Thorazine (chlorpromazine)
   b. Serlect (sertindole)
   c. Haldol (haloperidol)
   d. Mellaril (thioridazine)

4. Your client who is taking Haldol (haloperidol) suddenly develops severe muscle spasms in his head and neck. How would you describe this reaction in your documentation?
   a. akathisia
   b. tardive dyskinesia
   c. acute dystonic reaction
   d. neuroleptic malignant syndrome

5. When a client begins antidepressant therapy, within what time frame can he or she expect to feel better?
   a. 2–3 days
   b. 1 week
   c. 2–4 weeks
   d. 4–6 weeks

References

American Psychiatric Association. (1997). Practice guidelines for the treatment of patients with schizophrenia. *Am J Psychiatry, 154*(Suppl. 4), 1–63.

Armstrong, H. E. (1993). Review of psychosocial treatments for schizophrenia. In D. L. Dunner (Ed.), *Current Psychiatric Therapy.* (pp. 183–188). Philadelphia, PA: Saunders.

Auerbach, P. S., Fleisher, G. R., & Knochel, J. P. (1993). Heatstroke: Be ready for summer. *Patient Care, 27*(9): 52–62.

Batscha, C. L. (1997). Heat stroke: Keeping your clients cool in the summer. *J Psychosoc Nurs, 35*(7), 12–17.

Blumenthal, S. J. (1996). Women and depression. *The Decade of the Brain, 7*(3), 1–4.

Brown, A., & Lempa, M. (1997). Late life depression. *NARSAD Newsletter, 12*(3): 10–15.

Crane, K., Kirby, B., & Kooperman, D. (1996). Patient compliance for psychotropic medications. *J Psychosoc Nurs, 34*(1), 8–15.

Crenshaw, T. L., & Goldberg, J. P. (1996). *Sexual Pharmacology.* New York: W W Norton.

Francell, E. G. (1994). Medication: The foundation of recovery. *Innovations & Research, 3*(4), 31–40.

Gardner, D. et al. (1996). The making of a user-friendly MAOI diet. *J Clin Psychiatry, 57*(3): 99–104.

Glod, C. A. (1996). Recent advances in the pharmacotherapy of major depression. *Arch Psychiatr Nurs, 10*(6): 355–364.

Gomez, G., & Gomez, E. (1994). The use of psychotropic drugs to treat anxiety in the elderly. *J Psychosoc Nurs, 32*(12), 30–34.

Hedaya, R. J. (1996). *Understanding Biological Psychiatry.* New York: W W Norton.

Inouye, S. K., & Charpentier, P. A. (1996). Precipitating factors for delirium in the hospitalized elderly person. *JAMA, 275*(11), 852–857.

Kapur, S., & Remington, G. (1996). Serotonin-dopamine interaction and its relevance to schizophrenia. *Am J Psychiatry, 153*(4), 466–476.

Keltner, N. L. (1997a). Catastrophic consequences secondary to psychotropic drugs, Part 1. *J Psychosoc Nurs, 35*(4), 41–45.

Keltner, N. L. (1997b). Catastrophic consequences secondary to psychotropic drugs, Part 2. *J Psychosoc Nurs, 35*(5), 48–50.

Masters, J. C. (1996). When lithium does not help. *Geriatr Nurs, 17*(2), 75–78.

Mazurek, M. F., & Rosebush, P. I. (1996). Circadian pattern of acute, neuroleptic-induced dystonic reactions. *Am J Psychiatry, 153*(5), 708–711.

McCloskey, J. C., & Bulechek, G. M. (1996). *Nursing Interventions Classification (NIC)* (2nd ed.). St. Louis, MO: Mosby.

Mulsant, B. H. et al. (1997). Low use of neuroleptic drugs in the treatment of psychotic major depression. *Am J Psychiatry, 154*(4), 559–562.

Saltzman, C., Green, A., & Gadaracco, M. A. (1995, July). *Essential Psychopharmacology.* Symposium presented in 6th Summer Seminars for Mental Health Professionals, Harvard Medical School, Div. Cont. Ed. and the Mass. Mental Health Center, Div. Psychiatry.

Thase, M. E., & Howland, R. H. (1995). Biological processes in depression. In E. E. Beckham & W. R. Leber (Eds.), *Handbook of Depression* (2nd ed.) (pp. 213–279). New York: Guilford Publications.

Tollefson, G. D. et al. (1997). Olanzapine versus haloperidol in the treatment of schizophrenia and schizoaffective and schizophreniform disorders. *Am J Psychiatry, 154*(4), 457–465.

Unis, A. S. (1993). Safety of psychotropic agents in treatment of child and adolescent disorders. In D. L. Dunner (Ed.), *Current Psychiatric Therapy* (pp. 440–445). Philadelphia: Saunders.

Zimbroff, D. L. et al. (1997). Controlled, dose-response study of sertindole and haloperidol in the treatment of schizophrenia. *Am J Psychiatry. 154*(6), 782–791.

VISIT OUR WEBSITE!
www.awnursing.com

PART III

Mental Disorders

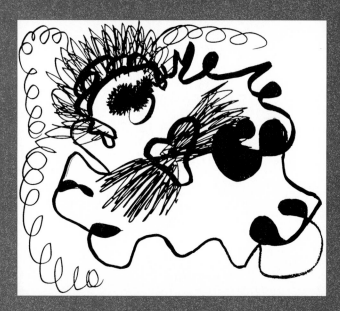

HOW I SEE MY ILLNESS: *I am transformed into this Monster, full of fire which is exploding in my head and heart. When the fire explodes, I am engulfed in a world where my boundaries disintegrate and I am lost & locked in a place of bottomless black pits.*

CHAPTER 9

Anxiety Disorders

Karen Lee Fontaine

Objectives

After reading this chapter, you will be able to:

- Formulate examples of conscious and unconscious attempts to manage anxiety.
- Distinguish between the different characteristics of the various anxiety disorders.
- Differentiate concomitant disorders from the primary anxiety disorder.
- Describe the alterations in neurobiology occurring in the anxiety disorders.
- Apply the nursing process when intervening with clients experiencing anxiety disorders.

Key Terms

agoraphobia
anxiety
body dysmorphic disorder
compulsions
conversion disorder
coping mechanisms
defense mechanisms
depersonalization disorder
dissociative amnesia
dissociative disorders
dissociative fugue
dissociative identity disorder (DID)
generalized anxiety disorder (GAD)
hypochondriasis
obsessions
obsessive-compulsive disorder (OCD)
pain disorder
panic attack
panic disorder
phobic disorders
posttraumatic stress disorder (PTSD)
secondary gains
somatoform disorders
somatization disorder

Anxiety is an uncomfortable feeling that occurs in response to the fear of being hurt or losing something valued. Some professionals distinguish between fear and anxiety. When this distinction is made, fear is a feeling that arises from a concrete, real danger, whereas anxiety is a feeling that arises from an ambiguous, unspecific cause or that is disproportionate to the danger. Believing that it makes no difference whether the danger is real or not, in this book we use the terms interchangeably because the sensations feel identical in the body.

Anxiety is a common human emotion. Like other people, you probably are anxious about certain aspects of your life. When you began the study of nursing, you were introduced to a new and foreign subculture, that of health care professionals and institutions. Your first few days in the clinical setting were likely highly anxious times, as you were uncertain about your skills and insecure in your role as a nursing student. As your skills increased and your professional role became more comfortable, your level of anxiety decreased. Now, as you begin your experience in mental health nursing, your anxiety once again increases as you struggle with new skills and new professional roles. You are probably skeptical of your ability to intervene with clients and are uncertain about what is expected of you in this role. Some of you not only have to adapt to the health care subculture but also are adapting to a different larger culture because of geographical relocation or becoming part of a more culturally diverse group of people. Since anxiety interferes with learning, for both you and clients, finding effective coping mechanisms is necessary for optimal education.

In addition to understanding the meaning of anxiety, it is important to know its process and characteristics, as well as the defenses against anxiety. Consciously and unconsciously, people try to protect themselves from the emotional pain of anxiety. Conscious attempts are referred to as **coping mechanisms,** which may be effective or ineffective. Ineffective coping mechanisms may be such things as becoming involved in physical fights, abusing substances, social withdrawal, or being unable to focus on the situation.

People often effectively use physical activity—walking, jogging, competitive sports, swimming, strenuous housecleaning—to counteract the tension associated with anxiety. Effective cognitive coping behavior includes realistically reviewing strengths and limitations, determining short- and long-term goals (both individual and family), and formulating a plan of action to confront the anxiety-producing situation. Effective affective coping behavior may include expressing emotions (laughter, words, tears) or seeking support from family, friends, or professionals. Stress-reduction techniques may also be used, such as meditation, progressive relaxation, visualization, and biofeedback. Effective coping mechanisms contribute to a person's sense of competence and self-esteem.

Unconscious attempts to manage anxiety are referred to as **defense mechanisms**. They often prevent people from being sensitive to anxiety and therefore interfere with self-awareness. When they allow for gratification in acceptable ways, defense mechanisms may be adaptive; however, when the anxiety is not reduced to manageable levels, the defenses become maladaptive. (See Chapter 1 for examples of defense mechanisms.)

The consistent use of certain defenses leads to the development of personality traits and characteristic behaviors. How a person manages anxiety and which defense mechanisms are used are more behaviorally formative than the source of the anxiety. Consider the basic human need to be loved and cared for by another person. The anxiety produced by fear of the loss of love may result in a variety of behaviors. One person may be driven to constantly look for love and affirmation by engaging in frequent one-night sexual encounters. Another person may seek out and develop a warm, intimate relationship. A third person may be so frightened of not finding love and so fearful of rejection that he or she avoids relationships to decrease the anxiety. The management of defenses can become so time-consuming that little energy remains for other aspects of living. The consistent use of particular and fixed responses to anxiety leads to the development of the anxiety disorders discussed in this chapter.

It is estimated that 23 million adults suffer from anxiety disorders, making these disorders the single largest mental health problem in the United States. Only 25% receive psychiatric intervention; the remaining 75% use other health care services or go untreated. Without relief, anxiety disorders can dramatically reduce productivity and significantly diminish the quality of life (Brown and Lempa, 1996). Clients with varying levels of anxiety are found in all types of clinical facilities, from community clinics to medical-surgical settings to intensive care units. In a person who has the added stress of an acute or chronic physical illness, the anxiety disorder may be especially pronounced. Box 9.1 lists the categories and different types of disorders presented in this chapter.

Knowledge Base

This section describes the various disorders that develop in response to anxiety. At times it may be difficult to determine which disorder the person is experiencing, as the symptoms often cut across the various disorders. This should not be a great problem for you since your focus, as a nurse, is on clients' responses to their illnesses.

Generalized Anxiety Disorder

Generalized anxiety disorder (GAD) is a chronic disorder characterized by persistent anxiety but without phobias or panic attacks. Affecting more than 5% of the population, it usually begins in the late teens to early twenties. It can be triggered by stress or come out of nowhere. Most sufferers worry excessively about everyday concerns such as whether or not the boss thinks they are doing a good job, or how they are going to pay the bills. In more severe cases, a victim may become preoccupied with catastrophic thoughts and visions. Other symptoms include overall fatigue, muscular tension, and restlessness. This unremitting stress and tension can suppress the immune system, which makes one more susceptible to disease (Sands, 1996).

Panic Disorder

Panic attack is the highest level of anxiety, characterized by disorganized thinking, feelings of terror and helplessness, and nonpurposeful behavior. It may occur in a variety of anxiety disorders. In this intense experience, people believe they are about to die, lose control, or "go crazy." See Table 9.1 for symptoms of the panic level of anxiety. Some studies suggest that occasional panic attacks occur in 35% of the U.S. population. These episodes are usually associated with public speaking, interpersonal conflict, exams, or other situations of high stress (Brown and Lempa, 1996; Pfaelzer and Ellison, 1996).

Box 9.1

Categories and Types of Disorders

Anxiety Disorders

- Generalized Anxiety Disorder
- Panic Disorder: with or without agoraphobia
- Obsessive-Compulsive Disorder
- Phobic Disorders: Specific, Social, Agoraphobia
- Posttraumatic Stress Disorder
- Acute Stress Disorder

Dissociative Disorders

- Dissociative Amnesia
- Dissociative Fugue
- Depersonalization Disorder
- Dissociative Identity Disorder

Somatoform Disorders

- Somatization Disorder
- Conversion Disorder
- Pain Disorder
- Hypochondriasis
- Body Dysmorphic Disorder

Panic disorder, which is diagnosed when there are recurrent panic attacks, may occur with or without agoraphobia and usually develops in early adult life. It affects more than 1.5 million Americans. Typically, the onset of panic attacks is sudden and unexpected, with intense symptoms lasting from a few minutes to an hour. The episodes involve intense fear and a premonition of doom, which is accompanied by shortness of breath, hyperventilation, choking sensations, dizziness, tingling, trembling, sweating, chest pain, tachycardia, and heart palpitations. The disorder is often chronic or recurrent and may progress to include avoidance and phobic behaviors. Many people develop severely restricted lifestyles and limitations in role functioning, both of which result in a chaotic family system (Pfaelzer and Ellison, 1996; Sherbourne, Wells, and Judd, 1996; Wakefield and Pallister, 1997).

Table 9.1 Physiological Characteristics According to Levels of Anxiety

Anxiety Level	Physiological Response
Absence	Normal respirations
	Normal heart rate
	Normal blood pressure
	Normal gastrointestinal function
	Relaxed muscle tone
Mild	Occasional shortness of breath
	Slightly elevated heart rate and blood pressure
	Mild gastric symptoms such as "butterflies" in the stomach
	Facial twitches, trembling lips
Moderate	Frequent shortness of breath
	Increased heart rate, possible premature contractions
	Elevated blood pressure
	Dry mouth, upset stomach, anorexia, diarrhea, or constipation
	Body trembling, fearful facial expression, tense muscles, restlessness, exaggerated startle response, inability to relax, difficulty falling asleep
Panic	Shortness of breath, choking or smothering sensation, sweating
	Hypotension, dizziness, chest pain or pressure, palpitations, chills or hot flashes
	Nausea
	Agitation, poor motor coordination, involuntary movements, entire body trembling, facial expression of terror
	Feeling of losing control, fear of dying

A variation of panic disorder is nocturnal panic. Panic attacks awaken the person and usually occur within 1–4 hours after falling asleep, usually during non-REM sleep. No one knows the cause of nocturnal panic, although some believe it may be related to sleep apnea. Panic is further discussed later in the chapter along with agoraphobia, since the two disorders often occur together.

Dowoyne has been experiencing panic attacks for the past 6 months. He feels very stressed at work because his new boss is "riding everyone." His girlfriend was recently fired by the same boss. He describes his panic attacks as a combination of dizziness, trembling, sweating, gasping for breath, and severe pounding of his heart. When the panic subsides, he feels exhausted, as if he had survived a traumatic experience. It has become very stressful for him to commute to work on the train because he fears having an attack in front of everyone. Dowoyne is seriously considering changing jobs so he won't have to take the train.

Obsessive-Compulsive Disorder

Obsessions are unwanted, repetitive thoughts that lead to feelings of fear or guilt, such as the thought of killing someone or of being contaminated with germs. **Compulsions** are behaviors or thoughts used to decrease the fear or guilt associated with obsessions. Behaviors might involve hoarding objects or frequent washing of hands. Cognitive compulsions, or thoughts, might be silently counting or repeatedly thinking a sequence of words. When obsessive-compulsive thoughts and behaviors dominate a person's life, the person is described as having **obsessive-compulsive disorder (OCD)**. OCD affects approximately 2% of the U.S. population, or 1 million adolescents and 3 million adults. Onset usually occurs during the early twenties, but it may occur as late as age 50 and as early as age 5. An equal percentage of women and men are affected (Brown and Lempa, 1996; Stein et al, 1997). The degree of interference in the lives of OCD sufferers can range from slight to incapacitating. Rapoport (1989) describes the severity in terms of time involved in the compulsive behavior:

- mild: less than 1 hour a day
- moderate: 1–3 hours a day
- severe: 3–8 hours a day
- extreme: nearly constant

Some people believe that OCD is really a spectrum disorder, that is, not one disorder but several that exhibit repetitive, unwanted behavior. These disorders include compulsive shopping, compulsive gambling, substance abuse, nail biting, hair pulling, autism, anorexia and bulimia, somatization disorders, paraphilias, stuttering, and tic disorders. The validity of this hypothesis has not yet been tested (Hedaya, 1996).

Behavioral Characteristics

Almost all people have experienced a mild form of obsessive-compulsive behavior known as *folie du doute,* consisting of thoughts of uncertainty and compulsions to check a previous behavior. Some common forms are setting the alarm clock and checking it before being able to sleep, turning off an appliance and then returning to make sure it was off, and locking the door and then checking to be sure it is locked. People are bothered by uncertainty and have such thoughts as "Are you sure you locked the door?" There is a feeling of subjective compulsion: "You better check to make sure you locked the door." But there is often a resistance to the compulsion: "You don't have to check the door because you know you locked it." The obsessive thoughts continue and anxiety increases until the compulsive behavior is performed.

> Jeanine's mother always worried that the house would be set on fire if she forgot to unplug the iron. Now an adult, Jeanine always checks three times that she unplugged the iron before she leaves the laundry room. Her obsessive thoughts focus on the house burning down with her two children in it. Returning to check the iron reduces her fear to manageable levels. If she resists the urge to perform the compulsion, her anxiety mounts until she is forced to check the iron.

People with OCD often display consuming, and at times bizarre, behavior. OCD sufferers describe their behavior as being forced from within. They say, "I have to. I don't *want* to, but I *have* to." Of the women, 90% are compulsive cleaners who have an unreasonable fear of contamination and avoid contact with anything thought to be unclean. They may spend many hours each day washing themselves and cleaning their environment. Cleaning rituals and avoidance of contamination decrease their anxiety and reestablish some sense of safety and control. With increased public awareness of AIDS, one-third of people with OCD now cite the fear of AIDS to explain their washing behavior.

Male OCD sufferers are more likely to experience compulsive checking behavior, which is often associated with "magical" thinking. They hope to prevent an imagined future disaster by compulsive checking, even though they may recognize it to be irrational.

Children with OCD may appear to have learning disabilities when the compelling need to count or check interferes with homework and testing. Other examples of obsessive behavior are arranging and rearranging objects, counting, hoarding, seeking order and precision, and repeating activities such as going in and out of a doorway. The ritualistic behavior may become so severe that the person may not be able to work or socialize. Professional help may not be sought until the individual is unable to meet basic needs, or when the family can no longer tolerate the symptoms (Yonkers and Gurguis, 1995). See Box 9.2 for types of obsessions and compulsions.

> Two years after Betty had moved in, her two-bedroom condo was so cluttered with junk mail, newspapers, unfinished craft projects, old clothes, and broken gadgets that the only spot to sit was on one side of the bed. When Betty finally asked a friend for help, he spent 14 hours throwing out her junk—which she reclaimed from the dumpster as soon as he left. She feared that something dreadful would happen if she threw those things away.

> Jay feels a drop in his eye as he looks up while passing a building and cannot dismiss the thought that someone with AIDS has spit out of a window. To reassure himself, he proceeds to knock on the door of every office on that side of the building, asking if anyone there has spit out the window.

Affective Characteristics

People with OCD often experience a great deal of shame about their uncontrollable and irrational behavior, and they may try to hide it. They may be consumed with fears of being discovered. OCD sufferers respond to anxiety by feeling tense, inadequate, and ineffective. To alleviate the anxiety, control is all-important. They fear that if they do not act on their compulsion, something terrible will happen. Thus, in most cases, compulsions serve to temporarily reduce anxiety. But the behavior itself can create further anxiety. The affective distress may range from mild anxiety to almost constant anxiety about thoughts and behaviors. Obsessive-compulsive people often experience hopelessness that their situation will never improve. They may also develop phobias when faced with situations in which they can no longer maintain control (Yonkers and Gurguis, 1995).

Box 9.2

Types of Obsessions and Compulsions

Obsessions: unwanted, repetitive thoughts

- Fear of dirt, germs, contamination
- Fear of something dreadful happening
- Constant doubting
- Somatic concerns
- Aggressive and/or sexual thoughts
- Religious ideation

Compulsions: behaviors or thoughts used to decrease fear or guilt associated with obsessions

- Grooming, such as washing hands, showering, bathing, brushing teeth
- Cleaning personal space
- Repeating movements, such as going in and out of doorways, getting in and out of chairs, touching objects
- Checking, such as doors, locks, appliances, written work
- Counting silently or out loud
- Hoarding
- Frequent confession (of anything)
- The need to ask others for reassurance
- The need to have objects in fixed positions

Cognitive Characteristics

Traditionally, it has been thought that OCD is ego-dystonic because many sufferers feel tormented by their symptoms. These people recognize the senselessness of much of their behavior and want to resist it. The drive to engage in the behavior is overpowering, however, and they often feel extreme distress about their actions. A smaller number have limited recognition of their behavior, and a few are unable to see their behavior as senseless.

The most common preoccupations involve dirt; safety; and violent, sexual, or blasphemous thoughts. There may be magical thinking, false beliefs, superstitions, or religious ideation, the content of which is culturally determined. OCD sufferers are consumed with constant doubts, which leads to difficulty with concentration and mental exhaustion. They doubt everything related to their particular compulsion and cannot be reassured by what they see, feel, smell, touch, or taste. They say, "No matter how hard I try, I cannot get these thoughts out of my mind."

> Shane will not go into public places because he fears he will have intolerable sexual thoughts or falsely accuse someone of committing a crime.

> Ramona's persistent urge to shout out an obscenity or blasphemy in church can be suppressed only by counting slowly backward from 100 to one.

Phobic Disorders

Like OCD, *phobic disorders* are behavioral patterns that develop as a defense against anxiety. Other features common to these disorders include fear of losing control, fear of appearing inadequate, defense against threats to self-esteem, and perfectionistic standards of behavior.

Almost all people try to avoid physical dangers. If this avoidance is generalized to situations other than realistic danger, it is called a *phobia*. It is estimated that 20–45% of the general population have some mild form of phobic behavior. However, phobic disorders occur in only 5–15% of the population (Brown and Lempa, 1996). There are many phobic disorders, but they all have four features in common:

1. They are an *unreasonable* behavioral response, both to the sufferer and to observers.
2. The fears are *persistent*.
3. The sufferer demonstrates *avoidance behavior*.
4. This behavior may become *disabling* to the sufferer.

Although the feared object or situation may or may not be symbolic of the underlying anxiety, the *primary fear* in all phobic disorders is the fear of losing control.

A *specific phobia* is a fear of only one object or situation; it can arise after a single unpleasant experience. The most common phobias are of old dangers such as closed spaces, heights, snakes, and spiders. Very seldom are people phobic about current dangers such as guns, knives, and speeding cars. Phobias usually begin early in life and are experienced as often by men as by women. People with specific phobias experience anticipatory anxiety; that is, they become anxious even thinking about the feared object or situation. A specific phobia is not disabling unless the feared object or situation cannot be avoided.

> Since Carlos was bitten by a rattlesnake 5 years ago, he has developed a specific phobia of snakes. Normally, his phobia causes no disability because he lives in a large urban area. However, the phobia has prevented him from participating in certain leisure activities such as hiking and camping.

> Janelle has a specific phobia of being in an elevator with other people. Her phobia is mildly disabling because she must use the stairs almost all the time. Her vocational opportunities are somewhat limited because she is unable to work on the upper floors of a high-rise office building.

Social phobias are fears of social situations. They may take many forms, such as stage fright, fears of public speaking, using public bathrooms, eating in public, being observed at work, and being in crowds of people. All these fears focus on losing control, which may result in being embarrassed or ridiculed. The degree to which the person is disabled depends on how easily the social situation can be avoided.

> Asela has a social phobia about using a public bathroom when others are present in the facility. As a result, her trips outside her home are limited in time to the extent of her bladder capacity.

Agoraphobia, the most common and serious phobic disorder, is a fear of being away from home and of being alone in public places when assistance might be needed. A person with agoraphobia will avoid groups of people, whether on busy streets or in crowded stores, on public transportation or at town beaches, at concerts or in movie houses. Places where the person might become trapped, such as in tunnels or on elevators, are also sometimes avoided.

Of people diagnosed with agoraphobia, 70–85% are women. Three theories have tried to explain the high incidence of agoraphobia in women. One theory suggests that men and women have agoraphobia in equal numbers. The disorder is undetectable in most men, however, because socialization discourages them from expressing anxious feelings and teaches them to cope with anxiety through other means. Another theory says that the statistics reflect a real difference between the sexes—that socialization has taught men to "tough out" their fears and women to avoid their fears. The third theory suggests that endocrine

changes in women make them more susceptible than men to anxiety (Yonkers and Gurguis, 1995).

Agoraphobia is often triggered by severe stress. Moving, changing jobs, relationship problems, or the death of a loved one may precipitate it. The two peak times for the onset are between ages 15 and 20 and then again between ages 30 and 40. Some people may experience a brief period of agoraphobia, which then disappears, never to recur. If it persists for more than a year, the disorder tends to be chronic, with periods of partial remission and relapse (Hedaya, 1996).

Behavioral Characteristics

The dominant behavioral characteristic of people with phobic disorders is avoidance. Fearing loss of control, they avoid the phobic object or situation that increases their level of anxiety. If the person demonstrates minor rechecking or ritualistic behavior, avoidance may take on an obsessive-compulsive aspect. Even when they know their fears are irrational, they still try to avoid the object or situation. If it cannot be avoided easily, the behavior may interfere with overall functioning and even lifestyle.

People who suffer from disabling agoraphobia are excessively dependent because their avoidance behavior dominates all activities. They may even be so panic-stricken outside the home that they become housebound.

> Edith, who lives in a large urban area, developed agoraphobia 10 years ago during a time of severe marital distress. In the beginning, she merely avoided large crowds of people. She then began to fear leaving her neighborhood. Five years ago, she became housebound and experienced panic attacks if she attempted to leave her home. Two years ago, her phobia progressed to the point that she cannot leave her living room couch. She now needs a great deal of assistance in the activities of daily living. Her husband and a cleaning woman provide for her basic needs. She is alert and continues to manage all the household finances and any other activities that can be accomplished from her couch.

Affective Characteristics

For people suffering from phobic disorders, fear predominates. Mainly, there is fear of the object or situation. There are also fear of exposure, which could result in being laughed at and humiliated, and fear of being abandoned during a phobic episode.

When confronted with the feared object or situation, phobic people feel panic, which may include a feeling of impending doom. Panic in itself is often accompanied by additional fears, such as losing control, causing a scene, collapsing, having a heart attack, dying, losing one's memory, and going crazy. Having once experienced an unexpected attack of panic, they begin to fear the attack will happen again. Because these attacks are so terrifying, the fear of another attack becomes the major stress in their lives. This *fear of fear,* which is extreme anticipatory anxiety, may become the dominant affective experience, particularly for people with agoraphobia (Brown and Lempa, 1996).

Cognitive Characteristics

The behavioral and affective characteristics of people with phobic disorders are ego-dystonic. Although sufferers recognize that their responses are unreasonable and their thoughts irrational, they are unable to explain them or rid themselves of them. They are consumed with thoughts of anticipatory anxiety and have negative expectations of the future. Phobic people develop low self-esteem and describe themselves as inadequate and as failures. They believe they are in great need of support and encouragement from others. They begin to define themselves as helpless and dependent and often despair of ever getting better. They may even begin to believe they are mentally ill and fear ending up in an institution for the rest of their lives.

In an attempt to localize anxiety, phobic people often use defenses that allow them to remain relatively free of anxiety as long as the feared object or situation is avoided. Defenses—such as repression, displacement, symbolization, and avoidance—can also keep the original source of anxiety out of conscious awareness. In agoraphobia, however, defense mechanisms are not adequate to keep anxiety out of conscious awareness. People with agoraphobia live in terror of future panic attacks, and anticipatory anxiety is a constant state.

> Ever since he has been married, Mike has been emotionally abusive to Velda, telling her what a worthless wife, a terrible housekeeper, and an unimaginative lover she is. Velda has now developed a phobic fear of dirt, germs, and contamination. This phobia so dominates her life that whenever Mike comes home, she immediately scrubs the floor where he has walked because "you can't tell where he has been or what dirt or germs he is bringing in on his shoes."

Because the anxiety caused by Mike's abuse and his threats to abandon her was too painful to confront, *repression* was used to force her fears out of conscious awareness. Since repression is never completely successful by itself, the anxiety became *displaced* from her inadequacies in the relationship and transferred to dirt, germs, and contamination. Constant cleaning then became *symbolic* of her fears and threatened self-esteem, over which she had more control than her husband's behavior.

Posttraumatic Stress Disorder

People exposed to dangerous and life-threatening situations may develop **posttraumatic stress disorder (PTSD)**. PTSD is described as acute when the symptoms begin shortly after the traumatic experience and chronic when the symptoms appear months or years later. Any time a trauma occurs, the potential to develop PTSD exists. In severe trauma, a person confronts extreme helplessness and terror in the face of possible annihilation. Ordinary coping behaviors are ineffective, action is of no avail, and the person can neither resist nor escape. For example, rape, child sexual abuse, and battering involve the use of force by the perpetrator. Whether it is a sudden shock or a repetitive torment, the stress of the assault is inescapable and the end result is often PTSD. It is important to understand that PTSD sufferers are normal people who have experienced such abnormal events as physical or sexual assault, hostage situations, natural disasters, and military combat (Reeves and Ellison, 1996). (Chapters 18, 19, and 20 discuss rape, domestic violence, and sexual abuse.)

Traumatic events may result in two categories of symptoms: undercontrol and overcontrol. Those with undercontrol relive the event and are diagnosed as having PTSD. Those with overcontrol experience denial and amnesia and are diagnosed as having one of the dissociative disorders. Thus, PTSD and the dissociative disorders have similar precipitating causes.

Behavioral Characteristics

People with PTSD often exhibit a hyperalertness resulting from their need to constantly search the environment for danger. Increasing anxiety can cause unpredictably aggressive or bizarre behavior. PTSD sufferers may resort to abusing drugs or alcohol in an effort to decrease this anticipatory anxiety. They may also behave as if the original trauma were actually recurring. Thus, they may try to defend themselves against a past enemy who is perceived to be in the present. Triggering events create a continuous cycle of reminders. Examples are the anniversary of the crime or event; holidays and family events, especially if a perpetrator is involved; tastes, touches, and smells; and media coverage such as articles, talk shows, and movies. Many of these people develop a phobic avoidance of the triggers that remind them of the original trauma. Avoidance may become so all-encompassing that a socially isolated lifestyle develops (Shalev et al, 1996).

> Holly was robbed and beaten at gunpoint on a Sunday evening as she put her car in her garage. A few days later, she tried to return to work. "I tried to walk to the corner to take the bus and was so terrified to walk just half a block for fear I would be assaulted again. When I came home from work, I was terrified again to walk the half block and I cried all the way home. I was afraid to come out of the house after that and would ask family and friends to come and get me when I had to go somewhere. I felt like a prisoner."

Affective Characteristics

People suffering from PTSD experience chronic tension. They are often irritable and feel edgy, jittery, tense, and restless. They often experience labile affective responses to the environment. Anxiety is frequent and ranges from moderate anxiety to panic. When triggers remind them of the original trauma, the original feelings are experienced with the same intensity.

Guilt is another common affective characteristic of PTSD. When the traumatic event entailed the death of others, the guilt stems from the person's having survived when others did not. In addition, if the person is a war veteran, he may feel guilty about the acts he was forced to commit to survive the combat experience (Foa, Riggs, and Gershuny, 1995).

In addition to anxiety, tension, irritability, aggression, and guilt, there can be a numbing of other emotions. Often people with PTSD discover they can no longer appreciate previously enjoyed activities. Feeling detached from others, they are unable to be intimate or tender. Obviously, this difficulty contributes to relationship problems.

Cognitive Characteristics

A sudden, life-threatening trauma often causes people to re-evaluate themselves and their experiences. In the face of imminent death, the fantasy of personal immortality is exploded. Confrontation with severe injury or death results in long-lasting changes in a person's thinking patterns.

Memory may be affected by trauma. Memory of the traumatic event may be erased by amnesia, which may vary from a few minutes to months or even years. Some may have intermittent memories about the trauma that range from quick flashes to entire recollections of the event. Although this experience is distressing, it may be tolerable if the memories are infrequent. In contrast to amnesia, some people experience memories that return in the form of unpredictable and uncontrollable flashbacks. These memories can be so intrusive and persistent that people become obsessed by them. Recurring nightmares, in which the person re-experiences the event, are also common. A person may become preoccupied with thoughts of the trauma recurring. All these cognitive changes contribute to the development of an external locus of control, and PTSD sufferers feel themselves to be at the mercy of the environment.

> Jeanmarc, 35 years old, has a home decorating business. Three months ago he was stabbed in the back by a client while working in her home. The attack was unprovoked and Jeanmarc did not attempt to defend himself for fear of hurting the woman and thus ending up in prison. His attacker lives in his neighborhood and is now out on bail. He states that since the incident he has been preoccupied with death. His sleep has deteriorated to 2–3 hours a night and he has terrible nightmares. Other symptoms include decreased appetite, a 20-pound weight loss, decreased concentration, listlessness, decreased sex drive, headaches, and diarrhea. Prior to the event, he lived by himself in an apartment. Since the attack he moved in with his sister and her three children. His relationships with both his sister and his girlfriend are strained due to his recurrent symptoms.

Another cognitive characteristic that may accompany PTSD is self-devaluation. For some, the sense of self is shattered, while for others it is not allowed to develop at all. Repetitive childhood trauma interferes with the developmental organization of the personality. Being treated like an object results in feelings of dehumanization. A rape survivor may be influenced by cultural myths and begin to believe she was responsible for the act of violence committed against her. Survivors of disasters often feel guilty, believing that other, more capable people deserved to live more than they. Upon returning from Vietnam, many veterans were assailed by society's reproach and indifference. This devaluation became a part of the self-image of many veterans (Bremner et al, 1996).

Acute Stress Disorder

Some people who are exposed to an extreme traumatic stressor develop acute stress disorder. During or shortly after the trauma, these individuals may feel numb and emotionally nonresponsive, have a decreased awareness of their environment, and may experience amnesia for part or all of the event. Like PTSD sufferers, they often experience recurrent images and flashbacks, which contribute to the avoidance of stimuli that remind them of the trauma. These events cause significant distress and impair activities of daily living. Acute stress disorder begins within a month of the traumatic event, lasts at least 2 days, and goes away within 4 weeks. If symptoms persist beyond 4 weeks, the person is given the diagnosis of PTSD.

Dissociative Disorders

Dissociative disorders are characterized by an alteration in conscious awareness of behavior, affect, thoughts, and memories, and an alteration in identity, particularly in the consistency of personality. The alteration in identity may be identity loss or the presence of more than one identity. Regardless of the type of dissociative disorder, all sufferers at times demonstrate behavior totally different from their usual behavior. Dissociative disorders are often precipitated by a traumatic event.

Dissociative amnesia, memory loss not caused by an organic problem, is usually related to a traumatic event. The most common type is *localized amnesia,* in which memory loss occurs for a specific time related to the trauma. *Selective amnesia* is localized for a specific time, with partial memory of events during that time. The least common types of psychogenic amnesia are *generalized amnesia,* a complete loss of memory of one's past, and *continuous amnesia,* in which memory loss begins at a particular point in time and continues to the present.

Yuki's firstborn child died of sudden infant death syndrome 3 months ago. Although she remembers arriving in the emergency department with her baby, she continues to have no memory of finding him in his crib, calling the paramedics, or hearing the doctor telling her that her baby was dead.

Dissociative fugue is a rare dissociative disorder in which people, while either maintaining their identity or adopting a new identity, wander or take unexpected trips. The disorder is often precipitated by acute stress. The episode may last several hours or several days. During the fugue state, these people may appear either normal or disoriented and confused; they usually behave in ways inconsistent with their normal personality and values. The fugue state often ends abruptly, and there is either partial or complete amnesia for that period. Both dissociative amnesia and dissociative fugue are most commonly seen during war and in the aftermath of disasters. **Depersonalization disorder** is characterized by persistent or recurrent feelings of being detached from one's body or thoughts. People describe feeling like robots, being an outside observer of their bodies or thoughts, or feeling like they are living in a dream. They remain oriented to reality in that they know they are not really robots or living in a dream. The incidence and prevalence of this disorder are unknown, as it is one of the least-studied dissociative conditions. It usually begins in adolescence and is often not responsive to either therapy or medication (Simeon et al, 1997).

Dissociative identity disorder (DID), formerly multiple personality disorder, is the most severe form of dissociative disorders. This diagnosis is given when at least two personalities exist in the same person. Each personality, or "alter," is integrated and complex; that is, each has its own memory, value structure, behavioral pattern, and primary affective expression. The host personality, which is the original personality, has at best only a partial awareness of the other alters. People with DID suffer from an alteration in conscious awareness of their total being.

Recent reports agree that the origin of DID is severe, sadistic, often sexual, child abuse. The abusive incidents are repeated over time and inconsistently alternate with expressions of care and concern from the abuser. For example, abused children basically live in two separate worlds: the daylight world, where they play, have friends, and go to school; and the nighttime world, where all the trauma occurs (Ellason and Ross, 1997; Kluft, 1996). DID is used as a model to illustrate the characteristics of all the dissociative disorders. Because symptoms fluctuate with DID, the specific characteristics exhibited change according to experiences and the degree of stress at any given time.

Behavioral Characteristics

Children are unable to protect themselves adequately from violent abuse by adults. Unpredictable and often cruel, these adults at times protect and nurture and at times torment and torture. The children feel confusion, anxiety, helplessness, and rage. To survive, the host personality usually behaves passively, trying to placate the abuser. Thoughts and feelings that conflict with passivity are dissociated from the host personality, and new personalities develop around all the dissociated thoughts and feelings.

Each personality has its own behavioral characteristics, sometimes completely opposite from those of any of the other personalities. Behavior intolerable in one personality may be expressed when a different personality is in control. One personality may use drugs; one may never use drugs. One may be a prostitute; one may be a faithful spouse. One may be an executive; one may be a parent. One may continually attempt suicide; one may abort suicide attempts. Physically, one may be blind and one may have no physical sensations. One may have hypochondriasis, one may have bulimia, and one may never be ill. Current research is focusing on the power of the mind to actually change physiology, since different personalities demonstrate dramatic differences in brain-wave patterns. Apparently, the brain is able to even alter the immune system so that one personality has extreme allergies while another has no allergies (Riley, 1995).

Affective Characteristics

The host personality, who has no awareness or limited awareness of the other personalities, experiences bewilderment and fear about "lost" time. When others report what was said and done during the time another personality was dominant, the host personality often feels anxiety. As many as 60% of people with DID experience panic attacks (Evans and Sullivan, 1995).

The personalities of a person with DID can be grouped into three categories according to dominant affect and behavior. Some personalities symbolize the *victim self*. They are pleasant in affect and passive in behavior. Another group is the *aggressive self*. They

tend to dominate during periods of stress. One personality may physically express anger, another may be suicidal, and another may be sexually aggressive. The third group of personalities, the *protective self* (sometimes called the *inner self-helper*), are rational and calm and have the most awareness of the other personalities. One of these may have total memory for all the others. The personalities of this group manage new external danger as well as protect against internal helplessness and despair (Riley, 1995). Table 9.2 summarizes the DID personality categories.

Efrain has been working for several years with Judith in outpatient therapy. Over a period of time he has been introduced to the following personalities within her "family" system:

Judith—35 years old, married, one son; very traditional, good housekeeper, attends church regularly, dresses in a careful and "proper" manner; good at art, draws with right hand. Role in the "family" is to be responsible.

Little Judy—4–5 years old; gentle, shy, playful; likes to draw "pretty" pictures, draws with her left hand. Role in the "family" is to serve as a distraction when there is too much pain and fear.

Mary—a teenager; assertive and outgoing; does not attend church, doesn't like housework, prefers to wear blue jeans and t-shirts; very knowledgeable about drugs; assumes large gaps of missing time are related to drug use. Role in the "family" is the 'party animal,' able to have fun and play with peers.

Sue—15 years old; has a chip-on-the-shoulder, I-don't-care attitude; out only at night; likes "pretty clothes"; sees self as totally separate from "family"; plans to use men as she has been used. Role in the "family" is to try to understand sexuality, express anger for entire family.

Gail—powerful and wise personality; knows all the personalities and is known by all the others; position of trust in the family. Role in the "family" is as a spiritual guide to everyone.

Sometimes Judith would find herself at one of Mary's parties, wearing blue jeans and a sweatshirt; at times Mary would find herself sitting in church wearing a dress; both Judith and Mary were horrified by these experiences.

Table 9.2 Categories of DID Personalities

Category	Characteristics/Purpose
Victim-Self Personalities	
Host	Often unaware of the others; feels powerless.
Children	Stay at given ages; contain memories and affect of childhood trauma; may be autistic.
Handicapped	May be blind, deaf, paralyzed.
Aggressive-Self Personalities	
Persecutor	Has a great deal of energy; may try to harm or kill the others.
Promiscuous	Expresses forbidden urges that are often sexual.
Substance abusers	Addiction limited to these personalities.
Protective-Self Personalities	
Protector	Counterbalance to persecutor; protects the person from internal and external danger.
Inner self-helper	Emotionally stable; can provide information about how the personalities work.
Memory tracer	Has most of the memory for the entire life history.
Cross-gender	In women, these personalities tend to be protectors; in men, they tend to be "good mother" figures.
Administrator	Often this is the personality who earns a living; may be a very competent professional.
Special skills	Skills may be related to work, artistic endeavors, or athletic activities.

Cognitive Characteristics

Periods of amnesia are characteristic of people with DID. Since the host personality has, at best, only partial awareness of the others, the host has no memory of the times when other personalities dominated. In some instances, the amnesia is not readily apparent because the host personality has learned to use confabulation (imaginary memory) to cope with the "lost" time. Different personalities may learn different skills, and the skills may not be transferable between personalities. See Box 9.3 for signs of DID in children and adolescents.

The personalities often complain about unidentified people trying to influence them or control their minds. A high percentage of people with DID describe hearing voices in their heads. With these two characteristics, it is not surprising that these individuals may be misdiagnosed as having schizophrenia (Evans and Sullivan, 1995).

> One day, Judith began to cry and tell her therapist how frightened she becomes at times because she hears voices arguing with each other. One voice (Mary) keeps talking about killing Judith and giving very detailed descriptions of how she is going to accomplish this. Another voice (Gail) argues back with all the reasons Judith should not be harmed. Judith reports that, at times, the argument becomes very loud and disruptive, and she feels like she is "going crazy."

In DID, the defense mechanisms of repression and dissociation are used to manage the anxiety, rage, and helplessness the child experiences in response to severe abuse. The only way for these people to survive the pain of the trauma is to eliminate it from conscious awareness. Dissociation is accomplished by self-hypnosis, which correlates with the onset of the abuse. This soon becomes the dominant method of managing severe stress, and people with DID are able to quickly and spontaneously enter hypnotic trances. What is a life-saving process in childhood becomes a self-destructive tool in adulthood.

Somatoform Disorders

The *somatoform disorders*—somatization, conversion, pain disorder, hypochondriasis, and body dysmorphic disorder—all involve physical symptoms for which no underlying organic basis exists. People diagnosed with a **somatization disorder** have multiple physical complaints involving a variety of body systems. This is a chronic disorder that usually begins in the teenage years and is identified more often in women than in men. Men may express symptoms of the disorder less dramatically, or perhaps physicians have been less likely to perceive men as having multiple unexplained somatic symptoms. A **conversion disorder,** characterized by sensorimotor symptoms, can

Box 9.3

Signs of Dissociative Identity Disorder in Children and Adolescents

Extreme inconsistencies in abilities and performance

- May vary from day to day, month to month.
- Performance depends on which personality is out and on age and developmental level.
- Teacher may suspect Attention Deficit Disorder.
- Marked variation in preferred food/clothing.
- Choice of friends changes repeatedly.

Tantrums or destructive behaviors

- Child may not remember these tantrums afterward.

Denial of behavior observed by others

- Adults may interpret denial as lying.
- "Angry" personality acts out, disappears, leaves bewildered "good" child to take punishment.

Excessive daytime "spacey" behaviors, sleep disturbances

- Parents/teachers see this as extreme inattention.
- Some personalities may be only "out" at night.

Forgetting that does not make sense to others

- Forgets how to get home from school, activities from day before; often says "You didn't tell me that."
- Poor learning from experience.

Regressive behavior

- Younger personalities.

Sources: Riley, 1995; Shirar, 1996.

appear at any age but typically begins and ends abruptly. It is usually precipitated by a severe trauma such as war. Sensory symptoms range from paresthesia and anesthesia to blindness and deafness. Motor symptoms range from tics to seizures to paralysis. A person with a conversion disorder has only one symptom, whereas a person with a somatization disorder has several. Pain that cannot be explained organically is the primary symptom of a **pain disorder.** Unconscious conflict and anxiety are believed to be the basis for the pain. People with **hypochondriasis** believe they have a serious disease involving one or several body systems, despite all medical evidence to the contrary. Or, they are terrified of contracting certain diseases. These people are extremely sensitive to internal sensations, which they misinterpret as evidence of disease. This disorder usually begins in mid-life or late in life and affects women and men equally (Cantor, 1996).

Body dysmorphic disorder is a preoccupation with an imagined or slight defect in physical appearance. The most common concerns involve the face—facial skin, nose, and hair. As with those suffering from eating disorders, there is a lot of concern with bodily appearance. The disorder is probably related to OCD in that their thoughts are intrusive and they compulsively check their body appearance. They may avoid social and work activities because of embarrassment leading to social isolation. They experience feelings of low self-esteem, shame, and worthlessness, which may lead to suicidal thoughts and attempts (Allen and Edwards, 1997; Brawman-Mintzer, 1995).

Conversion disorders are rare, but the other somatoform disorders are frequently seen in community settings, health care offices, and acute care units. These three disorders account for a large portion of the medical expense in the United States. It is estimated that 4–18% of all physician visits are made by the "worried well." People with these disorders truly suffer, however; they must not be discounted as malingerers or manipulators. As a nurse, you can often provide a long-term caring relationship, which may be the most important intervention in preventing needless tests, medications, and surgeries. When people with somatoform disorders feel no one is listening to or caring for them, they often go from one health care professional to another, duplicating tests and medical interventions. By being knowledgeable and sensitive, you can protect these clients by maintaining them within one health care system (Cantor, 1996).

Behavioral Characteristics

Typically, clients experiencing somatoform disorders purchase many OTC medications to reduce their symptoms or pain. Inadvertent drug abuse may result when medications are prescribed for long periods by a variety of physicians. Dependence on pain relievers or antianxiety agents is a common complication of these disorders.

These clients frequently discuss their symptoms and disease processes. Many adapt their behavior patterns and lifestyle to the disorder. Adaptation can range from a minor restriction of activities to the role of a complete invalid.

In the past year, Dorothy has been seen by eight health care providers, including her family physician, a cardiologist, an internist, an orthopedist, a chiropractor, a proctologist, and a cancer diagnostician. After extensive and repeated testing, no evidence of organic disease was found. Dorothy continues to complain about the incompetence of these people and is in the process of finding new health care providers.

Affective Characteristics

The primary gain in somatoform disorders is the reduction of conflict and anxiety. People with these disorders are usually unable to express anger directly out of fear of abandonment and loss of love. They actively avoid situations where others will become angry with them. As a result, there is an unconscious use of physical symptoms to manage the anxiety caused by conflicting issues (Cantor, 1996).

When they fail to get relief from the physical symptoms, these clients experience more anxiety. It may be manifested by obsessions about the physical illness, depression, or phobic avoidance of activities associated with the spread of disease.

Some people with conversion disorders exhibit *la belle indifference,* a relative lack of concern for their physical symptoms. People showing a sudden onset of symptoms, even severe ones like paralysis or blindness, sometimes seem nonchalant about their condition. This reaction usually occurs in people who do not want to be noticed by others. But others with conversion disorders may be very verbal about their distress over the sudden appearance of symptoms. This reaction is more likely to occur in people with a high need for attention and sympathy.

Cognitive Characteristics

Somatoform disorder sufferers are obsessively interested in bodily processes and diseases. Almost all their attention is focused on the discomfort they are experiencing. So obsessed are they with their bodies that they are constantly aware of very small physical changes and discomforts that would go unnoticed by others. In hypochondriasis, these changes are regarded as concrete evidence of an active disease process.

Jesus is convinced that he has AIDS in spite of all negative diagnostic tests. He is not reassured by the fact that he is at low risk because of having been in a monogamous relationship for 20 years, has never used IV drugs, and has never had a blood transfusion. He is hyperalert to all slight variations in bodily function and regards these normal variations as evidence of AIDS.

Denial is the major defense mechanism in clients with somatoform disorders. Initially, these clients deny the source of anxiety and conflict, and the energy is transformed into physical complaints. Along with physical symptoms is a denial that there could be any psychological component to the physical symptoms. If confronted with the possibility of a psychological cause, clients often change health care providers in an effort to maintain their system of denial. Rarely will they follow through on referrals for psychotherapy.

Social Characteristics of Anxiety Disorders

OCD is a devastating illness that alters the lives of both clients and their family members. OCD symptoms are all-encompassing and involve family members and the home itself. Relationships are often strained and at times destroyed. Family members find themselves manipulated into enabling behavior in order to keep the peace and often end up bitter and resentful. Nearly all affected children involve their parents, and sometimes siblings, in their rituals (Cooper, 1996).

The impact of agoraphobia on the family system is usually severe and may cause considerable disruption to family patterns of behavior. People with agoraphobia are often unable to leave the home, which means they cannot be employed outside the home, cannot go out with friends, and cannot attend their children's school or sports activities. Thus, though appearing weak, they actually have a great deal of power to control family and friends through their dependency and helplessness.

Advantages from or rewards for being ill are referred to as **secondary gains.** The secondary gains of agoraphobia are the relinquishing of responsibilities, the satisfying of dependency needs that cannot be met directly, and the power to control others. Weakness as a form of control cannot work without another's cooperation. The secondary gains for the partner may be in fulfilling nurturing needs or being the main support of the family (Cantor, 1996). Family members of people with PTSD have a great deal of anxiety. One of the defenses for coping with the traumatic event is the numbing of emotions, or emotional anesthesia. Because of the PTSD sufferer's feelings of detachment, alienation, and doubts about an ability to trust and love, interpersonal relationships are strained to the limit. Loss of the ability to communicate feelings makes relationship problems inevitable. Outbursts of anger and aggression further alienate family and friends.

The media are a contributing factor in somatoform disorders. Magazines, radio, and television bombard us with advertisements for "cures" for every imaginable physical problem. In addition, there has recently been an emphasis on staying healthy—an emphasis that, at times, seems like a morbid preoccupation with death. Another form of the somatoform disorders is an obsessive, unrealistic fear of contracting HIV, the virus that causes AIDS. AIDS centers across the country report an increase in calls from low-risk people who are terrified they may have AIDS. With such intense media attention, it is hardly surprising that people become obsessed with bodily processes (Sherbourne, Wells, and Judd, 1996).

Any one of the somatoform disorders may completely disrupt a person's life. Sufferers may need to change their vocation to one more adaptable to their physical symptoms. Others may be unable to work in any capacity, either inside or outside the home. The chronic nature of these disorders often places a severe financial and emotional strain on the family. Physician, diagnostic, and hospital expenses may place the family in debt. The emotional drain on both client and family leads to increased stress and interpersonal conflict, especially when there is no physical improvement. This increased level of conflict contributes to the continuation of the disorder, and a vicious cycle is established.

Culture-Specific Characteristics

While anxiety may be a universal emotion, the context in which it is experienced, the meaning it is given, and the responses to it are strongly influenced by cultural beliefs and practices. Cross-cultural studies have found significant differences in the expression of anxiety. These include differences in the type of specific fears as well as the associated behavioral, affective, and cognitive characteristics. See Table 9.3 for culture-bound syndromes related to anxiety.

Physiological Characteristics of Anxiety Disorders

Healthy people can usually adapt to anxiety for brief periods of time. However, when the cause is unknown, the intensity severe, or the duration chronic, normal physiological mechanisms no longer function efficiently.

In mild anxiety, people experience an agreeable, perhaps even a pleasant, increase in tension. They may also experience a twitch in the eyelid, trembling lips, occasional shortness of breath, and mild gastric symptoms.

As anxiety increases to the moderate level, the survival response of fight or flight begins. Starting in the cerebral cortex, this response is mediated through the body's nervous system and endocrine system. The sympathetic nervous system and the response of the adrenal glands lead to changes throughout the body. Heart rate increases and blood pressure rises to send more blood to the muscles. There may be frequent episodes of shortness of breath. The pupils dilate, the person may sweat, and the hands may feel cold and clammy. Some body trembling, a fearful facial expression, tense muscles, restlessness, and an exaggerated startle response may all be noticeable. There is an increased blood glucose level due to increased glycogenolysis. The moderately anxious person may verbalize subjective experiences such as a dry mouth, upset stomach, anorexia, tension headache, stiff neck, fatigue, inability to relax, and difficulty falling asleep. There may also be urinary urgency and frequency as well as either diarrhea or constipation. Sexual dysfunction may include painful intercourse, erectile disorder, orgasmic difficulties, lack of satisfaction, or a decrease in sexual desire.

When anxiety continues to the panic level, the body becomes so stressed it can neither adapt effectively nor organize for fight or flight. At this level of anxiety, the person is helpless to care for or defend the self. As blood returns to the major organs from the muscles, the person may become pale. Hypotension, which causes the person to feel faint, may also occur. Other signs are a quavering voice, agitation, poor motor coordination, involuntary movements, and body trembling. The facial expression is one of terror, with dilated pupils. A person feeling panic may complain of dizziness, lightheadedness, a sense of unreality, and, at times, nausea. Some of the most frightening symptoms of the panic level of anxiety are

Table 9.3 Culture-Bound Syndromes

Type	Culture	Symptoms
Dissociative States		
Amok	Malaysia	Brooding, followed by homicidal frenzy, followed by amnesia; other cultures have terms describing similar symptoms. *DSM-IV* diagnoses: Dissociative State; Impulse Control Disorder.
Falling out/Blacking out	Southern US, Caribbean	Sudden collapse, eyes open but unable to see; may be aware of surroundings but feel helpless to move. *DSM-IV* diagnosis: Acute Stress Disorder.
Latah	Malaysia	Hypersensitivity to sudden fright; echopraxia, echolalia, dissociative or trance-like behavior. *DSM-IV* diagnosis: Attention Disorder.
Pibloktog	Eskimo	Abrupt episodes of extreme excitement and irrational behavior, followed by seizures and transient coma, followed by amnesia; in contrast to amok, this occurs primarily in women and violence is often not displayed. *DSM-IV* diagnosis: Psychogenic Fugue.
Grisi siknis	Nicaragua, Honduras	Mainly in young women; believe being attacked by devils; running is most distinctive feature; may be aggressive. Similar to pibloktog. *DSM-IV* diagnosis: Psychogenic Fugue.
Shin-byung	Korea	Anxiety, somatic complaints, later followed by dissociation; attributed to possession by ancestral spirits. *DSM-IV* diagnosis: Atypical Dissociative Disorder.
Anxiety States		
Ataque de nervios	Latin America	Shaking, palpitations, flushing, shouting/striking out, convulsive movements, sometimes amnesia; commonly precipitated by upsetting events. *DSM-IV* diagnosis: Panic Attacks.
Dhat	Asia	Symptoms associated with ejaculation, often during dreams; extreme anxiety, hypochondriasis, fear of depletion of physical and mental energy. *DSM-IV* diagnosis: Somatoform Disorder.
Koro	Southeast Asia	Believe penis is retracting into body and that this will end in death; extreme anxiety; often occurs in epidemics. *DSM-IV* diagnoses: Panic Attack, Somatoform Disorder.
Kayak angst	Eskimo, Greenland	Intense anxiety associated with fear of drowning when going out to sea in a kayak; disorientation, social impairment. *DSM-IV* diagnosis: Panic Disorder.
Taijin kyofusho	Japan	Intense anxiety about body/body parts/body functions; more frequent among the young. *DSM-IV* diagnosis: Social Phobia.
Somatoform States		
Brain fag	Africa	Predominant complaint is fatigue; mostly male students in response to stress of schooling; pain/pressure in head and neck; decreased concentration. *DSM-IV* diagnosis: Mood Disorder.
Shenjing shuairuo	China	Physical and mental exhaustion, decreased concentration, memory loss, insomnia, loss of appetite, irritability. *DSM-IV* diagnosis: Major Depression.

Sources: Cantor, 1996; Kirmayer, Young, and Hayton, 1995; Levine and Gaw, 1995.

chest pain or pressure, palpitations, shortness of breath, and a choking or smothering sensation (Hedaya, 1996). Each person tends to experience the physiological sensations in a pattern that repeats itself with every episode of anxiety. Some people are primarily aware of internal organ reactions, whereas others primarily exhibit symptoms of muscular tension. Still others experience both visceral and muscular responses.

A number of medical conditions may cause secondary anxiety or produce symptoms mimicking panic. These conditions are hypoglycemia, hyperthyroidism, hypoparathyroidism, Cushing's syndrome, pheochromocytoma, pernicious anemia, hypoxia, hyperventilation, audiovestibular system disturbance, paroxysmal atrial tachycardia, caffeinism, and withdrawal from alcohol or benzodiazepines. People with panic disorder, including agoraphobia, have a significantly higher incidence of mitral valve prolapse (MVP) than the general population: 57% compared to 5–7%. The exact relationship between MVP and panic is unclear. The symptoms of MVP—particularly tachycardia, palpitations, and shortness of breath—are similar to the symptoms of panic levels of anxiety. People predisposed to panic attacks often interpret the sensations of MVP as increased anxiety. The interpretation or expectation then evokes panic. Individuals with panic disorder frequently have significantly higher cholesterol levels compared to control groups. It is thought that chronic anxiety, like stress, increases blood cholesterol (Wakefield and Pallister, 1997). People with somatization disorders have multiple physical symptoms involving a variety of body systems. These symptoms may be vague and undefined, and they do not follow a particular disease pattern. Pain is the primary symptom in pain disorder. The pain is severe and prolonged and usually does not follow the nerve-conduction pathways of the body. Conversion disorder symptoms can occur in any of the sensory or motor systems of the body. The person may become suddenly blind or deaf. Loss of speech may range from persistent laryngitis to total muteness. Body parts may tingle or feel numb. Motor symptoms range from spasms or tics to paralysis of hands, arms, or legs.

In hypochondriasis, symptoms may be limited to one or several body systems. The most frequent symptoms appear in the head and neck. These include dizziness, loss of hearing, hearing one's own heartbeat, a lump in the throat, and chronic coughing. Symptoms in the abdomen and chest are common, including indigestion, bowel disorders, palpitations, skipped or rapid heartbeats, and pain in the left side of the chest. Some people may also have skin discomfort, insomnia, and sexual problems (Cantor, 1996).

Concomitant Disorders

There is a high correlation between anxiety disorders and substance abuse. As many as 50–60% of those who abuse substances also have one of the anxiety disorders. Typically, severe anxiety precedes the onset of the substance abuse, although for some the abuse precedes the anxiety. Believing that alcohol decreases anxiety, people with anxiety disorders often self-medicate in an effort to feel better. In fact, alcohol actually increases anxiety. The combination of increased anxiety, addiction, and continued self-medication contributes to an ever-increasing self-destructive cycle (Brown and Lempa, 1996).

Frequently, depression follows the onset of an anxiety disorder. It is thought that depression and anxiety disorders share a common biological predisposition, which may be activated by stress. The depression, which may range from mild to severe, may be a response to feelings of loss of control, hopelessness, helplessness, decreased self-esteem, and severe restrictions on lifestyle. Suicide can be a lethal complication. Of those suffering from panic attacks, 20% make suicide attempts (Hedaya, 1996; Hollifield et al, 1997).

Causative Theories

No single theory can adequately explain the cause and maintenance of the anxiety disorders. They are best understood as a complex interaction of many theories.

Neurobiological Theory

It appears that some component of anxiety runs in families, although the exact role of genetic predisposition is unknown at this time. Illustrating this point, the rate of panic disorder in families is 20%, compared to 4% in the general population. Some believe anxious individuals have an overly responsive autonomic nervous system related to a dysfunction of serotonin (5-HT) and norepinephrine (NE) neurotransmission. A hyperactive autonomic nervous system may be responsible for the characteristics of panic levels of anxiety. Research is continuing in the following areas: a deficiency in certain receptors, causing surges of NE; CNS abnormalities, particularly in the locus coeruleus of the pons, which inhibit the ability to moderate sensory input; and an increased sensitivity to carbon dioxide, leading to rapid breathing and sensations of suffocation. Panic attacks often occur in areas such as restaurants, elevators, cars, and planes, where there is an increased concentration of people and carbon dioxide (CO_2). Fresh air has a CO_2 level of 300 parts per million (ppm). In cars the CO_2 level reaches 750 ppm and as high as 900 ppm in elevators and planes. As CO_2 increases in the brain, neurons in the brain stem activate and send signals to the locus coeruleus, which increases the release of NE, leading to the fight-or-flight response. Stimulants that alter NE transmission (including caffeine, cocaine, amphetamines) can precipitate panic attacks. It is believed that some biological vulnerability is present, which—when combined with certain psychological, social, and environmental events—leads to the development of panic disorder (Hedaya, 1996; Perna et al, 1996).

Social phobia may be associated with decreased dopamine (DA) transmission related to a reduced number of DA synapses. The enhancement of DA transmission leads to increased activity, novelty seeking, and exploratory behavior, all of which are the opposite of symptoms of social phobia (Tiihonen, 1997).

Research in obsessive-compulsive disorder is now focusing on genetic factors. In this disorder, children and adults experience identical symptoms, whereas in most of the other mental disorders, children's symptoms are quite different from those of adults. In addition, 50% of adults with OCD state that their symptoms began when they were children; only 5% of adults with other mental disorders report childhood onset. In 39% of women with OCD who also have children, the onset of the disorder occurred during pregnancy. Of OCD sufferers, 20% have a first-degree relative with the same problem. Father-son combinations are the most common in these families. It is unlikely that the behavior is learned within the family, given the high level of secrecy. In addition, children and parents may have very different rituals; for example, the parent may engage in checking rituals, whereas the child may engage in washing rituals (Pauls, 1995; Rapoport, 1989).

Increased activity in the frontal lobes and basal ganglia has been demonstrated through PET scans, which measure glucose metabolism in different areas of the brain. PET scans provide some evidence of neurological deficit in some individuals suffering from OCD. The abnormality apparently lies in a pathway that links the frontal lobes of the cerebral cortex with the basal ganglia. Heightened activity in the cortex may reflect obsessional thinking, while compulsions may originate in the basal ganglia where body movements are planned and executed (Eisenberg, 1995; Greenberg et al, 1997). There appear to be biological changes in PTSD that illustrate the influence of psychological events on neurobiology. When high levels of adrenaline and other stress hormones are circulating, memory traces are deeply imprinted. These are then reactivated as if the traumatic event were actually occurring. Traumatic nightmares can occur in stages of sleep in which people do not ordinarily dream. Thus, traumatic memories appear to be based in altered neurophysiological organization (Reeves and Ellison, 1996).

Intrapersonal Theory

Intrapersonal theorists view anxiety disorders as a reaction to anticipated future danger based on past experiences such as separation, loss of love, and guilt. The resulting anxiety is pushed out of conscious awareness by the use of repression, projection, displacement, or symbolization. As stress increases, the defenses become increasingly inefficient, symptoms develop, and the person engages in repeated self-defeating behavior.

People suffering from anxiety disorders often have an external locus of control. They regard life events as out of their control, occurring by luck, chance, or fate. When stressful events occur, they attribute the feeling of anxiety not to themselves but to external sources, which then can be phobically avoided.

In dissociative disorders, stressful life events are disowned and kept out of conscious awareness by amnesia. For example, a young girl who is abused physically and sexually by her father remains dependent on her family system. The perpetrator is a trusted parent, and the other parent is incapable of protecting or rescuing her from the situation. The trauma of abuse leaves the child terrified, depressed, angry, and filled with shame and guilt. Dissociating the abuse and denying the events enable the child to remain in the family with the least amount of pain.

Anxiety is viewed as a major component of the somatoform disorders. The original source of the anxiety is unrecognized, and the discomfort is experienced as physical symptoms or disorders. Somatoform disorders may also be unconscious expressions of anger in those unable to communicate such feelings directly. Because physical distress provides an acceptable excuse for avoiding certain activities and situations, people may unconsciously use physical limitations to rationalize their inadequacies (Cantor, 1996).

Interpersonal Theory

Interpersonal theorists believe people with anxiety disorders become anxious when they sense or fear disapproval from significant others. They may feel trapped in unpleasant circumstances, believing they are unable to leave the situation. Fearing abandonment, they are unable to behave assertively during conflict. Thus, the anxiety experienced during interpersonal conflict is displaced onto the immediate surroundings, thereby allowing them to deny the interpersonal problem. Obsessive-compulsive or phobic behavior protects the self and the relationship during interactions with significant others.

Interpersonal theories focus on the secondary gains for people suffering from somatoform disorders. For those with a high degree of dependency, physical symptoms may receive a great deal of attention and support from significant others. The sympathy and nurturing these people receive may be a major factor in maintaining the disorders. The attention from others may be viewed as seeking reassurance of care and love or, since sick or weak people are often in a position of power, as an unconscious attempt to gain power and control.

Cognitive Theory

Cognitive theorists believe symptoms develop from ideas and thoughts. On the basis of limited events, people with anxiety disorders magnify the significance of the past and overgeneralize to the future. They become preoccupied with impending disaster and self-defeating statements. These cognitive expectations then determine reactions to and behavior in various situations (Wakefield and Pallister, 1997). Cognitive theory explains phobic disorders in a three-part sequence: (1) Phobic people have negative thoughts that increase anxiety and actually precede the feeling of fear in the phobic situation. Phobic people also have irrational thinking and unrealistic expectations

about what might occur if the phobic situation is encountered. (2) These anticipatory thoughts and feelings enhance the physiological arousal level even before the phobic situation is encountered. (3) The physiological arousal level is misinterpreted. Although thought to be caused by an external object or situation, the arousal is caused by the negative thoughts and irrational expectations. This mislabeling of feelings causes phobic people to displace the feelings onto objects or situations that can be avoided (Cantor, 1996).

Learning Theory

Phobias may be learned from significant others. If a child observes a parent experiencing anxiety in certain situations, the child may learn that anxiety is the appropriate response. For example, if the mother has a phobic avoidance of elevators, the child soon learns to fear entering an elevator. A child can also learn parental fears through information given by the parent. A father may talk about the dangers of going outside when it is dark, and the child may develop agoraphobia during the nighttime (Pollack et al, 1996). People who develop dissociative disorders often consider themselves passive and helpless. They are fearful of others' anger and aggressive behavior. Unable to behave assertively or aggressively, they learn to cope by escaping or avoiding the anxiety-producing situations. Thus, they learn to avoid pain through amnesia or the development of dissociative identities.

Behavioral Theory

Closely related to learning theory is the behavioral theory of how phobic disorders develop. Behavioral theorists believe phobias are conditioned, learned responses. Classical conditioning occurs when a stimulus results in anxiety or pain. The person then develops a fear of that particular stimulus. An example is a person who fears all dogs after being bitten by one dog. The learning component of behavioral theory states that the avoidance of the phobic object or situation is negatively reinforced by a decrease in anxiety. Because the person experiences less anxiety when avoiding the object or situation, avoidance becomes a habitual response.

Behavioral theorists view OCD as learned responses to anticipatory anxiety. It is thought that these individuals always expect bad things to happen and worry constantly. The compulsive behaviors and thoughts are maladaptive attempts to reduce anxiety.

According to behavioral theory, the somatoform disorders are learned somatic responses. It is thought that these individuals are unable to deal directly with stress and habitually respond to stress with physical sensations or symptoms.

Feminist Theory

Feminist theory has been used to explain the disproportionate number of women who experience agoraphobia. These theorists believe women have been reinforced to behave dependently, passively, and submissively. This behavior often results in adult women who are unable to assume responsibility for themselves and who view themselves as incompetent and helpless. Often, the symptoms are reinforced by family members who also have been socialized to expect women to be helpless and dependent. Thus, the pattern of withdrawal can continue until the woman is completely homebound (Yonkers and Gurguis, 1995).

Psychopharmacological Interventions

Medications are often used on a short-term basis to help people manage anxiety disorders. Table 9.4 summarizes these medications.

In GAD, the therapeutic goal in using antianxiety agents is to limit unpleasant symptoms to help the person return to a high level of functioning. A non-benzodiazepine antianxiety agent, BuSpar (buspirone), is more effective than the benzodiazepines in managing GAD. BuSpar blocks 5-HT receptors and causes minimal sedation. This medication is better than the benzodiazepines for the addiction-prone person because dosage increases result in a general sense of feeling ill. In addition, BuSpar reacts only minimally with alcohol, since it interacts very little with other CNS depressants. However, clients should be cautioned not to expect an immediate effect (Brown and Lempa, 1996).

Because anxiety may be related to a dysregulation of 5-HT and NE, tricyclic antidepressants have been used in the medical treatment of GAD. Tofranil (imipramine) has been found to be the most effective medication in this group.

Several types of medications may be used to treat panic disorders and agoraphobia. Xanax (alprazolam) may significantly reduce panic attacks after 6–8 weeks of treatment. However, the addictive properties and strong withdrawal effects limit the use of this medication. BuSpar (buspirone) appears to be an effective treatment without addictive properties and strong withdrawal effects. The tricyclic antidepressant Tofranil (imipramine) and the MAOI Nardil (phenelzine) seem to prevent panic attacks. Clients must usually take these medications for 8 weeks before the therapeutic effect is noticeable. The antianxiety properties of antidepressants reduce anxiety and improve the secondary depression resulting from panic disorders and agoraphobia. SSRIs produce fewer cardiac effects than other antidepressants. This reduces the chances that clients think they are experiencing panic attacks when in reality it is the side effects of the medication (Brown and Lempa, 1996; Pfaelzer and Ellison, 1996).

Social phobias severe enough to interfere with occupational functioning may be treated with a beta-blocker, either Inderal (propranolol) or Tenormin (atenolol). Beta-blockers are particularly effective in situations where cardiovascular symptoms of anxiety are disruptive to the individual. Because they do not cross the blood-brain barrier, beta-blockers have no effect on neurotransmission, nor do they produce loss of fine motor control (Katzelnick, 1995).

The following serotonin reuptake inhibitors (SSRIs) are often effective in the treatment of OCD: Prozac (fluoxetine), Zoloft (sertraline), Luvox (fluvoxamine), and Paxil (paroxetine). Of people suffering from OCD, 70–80% respond to these medications (OCD—Part II, 1995).

Probably the most useful drugs for people with PTSD are the antidepressants, which not only relieve depression but improve sleep and suppress intrusive thoughts, jumpiness, and explosive anger. SSRIs are prescribed most often. Inderal (propranolol) and Tenormin (atenolol), beta-blockers, may reduce the restlessness and anxiety by depressing the sympathetic nervous system.

See Table 9.4 for a summary of medications used for the anxiety disorders. You are encouraged to review Chapter 8 for more in-depth information on these medications.

Multidisciplinary Interventions

Medications play an important role in medical interventions, but intrapersonal and interpersonal aspects must also be treated. Clients and their families need to cope with various aspects of anxiety, learn to take

Table 9.4 Medications Commonly Used to Treat Anxiety Disorders

Generic Name	Trade Name	Disorders
Antianxiety Agents		
buspirone	BuSpar	GAD, panic disorder, agoraphobia, PTSD
alprazolam	Xanax	Panic disorder, PTSD
Tricyclic Antidepressants		
imipramine	Tofranil	GAD, panic disorder, agoraphobia
SSRIs		
fluoxetine	Prozac	Panic disorder, OCD, body dysmorphic disorder
fluvoxamine	Luvox	
paroxetine	Paxil	
sertraline	Zoloft	
MAOIs		
phenelzine	Nardil	Panic disorder, agoraphobia
Beta-Blockers		
atenolol	Tenormin	Social phobia (given before the event), PTSD
propranolol	Inderal	

control of their lives, and manage family stress. All of these are accomplished through a blending of techniques and the use of individual, family, and group psychotherapy.

The most effective behavioral intervention technique is *exposure and response prevention*. Clients are exposed, in reality or in their mind, to feared situations or objects and try to refrain from or delay their usual phobic or ritualistic response. Gradually, the unwanted response disappears. *Stress inoculation training* involves rehearsing other coping skills and testing these skills under stressful situations. While this process provides fairly immediate relief from anxiety, it must be practiced over a period of time for long-term effect.

> Florean has a strong fear of contamination. Whenever she touches any surface that she thinks might be contaminated, she washes her hands for 5 minutes. With the help of her therapist, Florean has planned a program in which she will touch a wastebasket several times and stop herself from washing her hands until 1 minute has passed. The goal is to refrain from hand washing for longer and longer periods of time. After that goal has been reached, Florean will work on reducing the length of time she spends washing her hands until the behavior is largely under her control.

Individual psychotherapy and *hypnosis* are used to uncover the abuse and trauma of DID. Nonverbal therapies such as play therapy, art therapy, and occupational therapy, and journal writing are also extensively used. One goal is to help the client discover that the various personalities are real and distinct but are not separate individuals. The client learns that all the personalities belong to each other and that they are all parts of the same person and same body. Hypnosis helps the personalities come to know each other, communicate with each other, and share skills.

Medication Teaching

Clients with Anxiety Disorders

Antidepressants

The effect of medications may not be felt for up to 18 weeks.

Use a sunscreen and wear protective clothing to prevent sunburn.

Rise slowly from a sitting or lying position to prevent a sudden drop in blood pressure.

Report any GI symptoms to your doctor such as nausea, vomiting, diarrhea or loose stools, and weight loss.

Report any increased anxiety or restlessness to your doctor.

Men sometimes experience erectile problems or ejaculatory difficulty, and women sometimes experience problems with orgasm. If any of these occurs, discuss with your doctor.

This medication decreases the seizure threshold, making you more prone to have a seizure. Because alcohol and some drugs also lower the seizure threshold, do not use these substances while taking this medication.

Abrupt discontinuation of this medication can lead to serious withdrawal reactions such as fever and rebound worsening of anxiety disorder symptoms.

Antianxiety Agents

The effect of the medication may not be felt for 7–10 days.

Report any restlessness or spastic movements to your doctor.

Do not use alcohol or any drugs that depress the central nervous system. Taken in combination, they can be fatal.

Do not stop taking the medication abruptly. Severe withdrawal reactions may occur such as anxiety, depression, insomnia, vomiting, sweating, convulsions, and delirium.

Beta-Blockers

Take medication with meals to decrease the potential for GI upset.

Report any of the following to your doctor: slow heart rate, dizziness, confusion, shortness of breath.

If you are diabetic, monitor your blood glucose levels closely.

The Nursing Process

Assessment

Assess the client using the knowledge base provided in this chapter. Because of the shame and secrecy surrounding anxiety disorders, clients may not reveal symptoms unless you ask direct, specific questions. An organized scheme of focused assessment ensures that all areas—behavioral, affective, cognitive, and social characteristics—are assessed. As always, assessment questions must be modified to the individual client's cognitive, developmental, educational, and language abilities. See the Focused Nursing Assessment tables on the following pages.

You will see the majority of clients suffering from anxiety disorders in community settings, clinics, physicians' offices, emergency departments, and medical-surgical units. Because these clients often have complicated and detailed medical histories, careful physiological assessment is necessary. Remember that, at any given time, a client with an anxiety disorder may develop an organic illness. Thus, continual physiological assessment is a necessary component of your nursing care.

The physiological assessment must differentiate anxiety responses from various organic conditions that have similar symptoms. The most common conditions are hypoglycemia, hyperthyroidism, hypoparathyroidism, pheochromocytoma, and MVP. Similar symptoms may also occur during withdrawal from barbiturates and antianxiety agents and with the use of cocaine. High levels of caffeine, amphetamines, theophyllines, beta-agonists, steroids, and decongestants may also be initially confused with anxiety disorders. Anxiety will frequently be seen as another symptom in people who have been diagnosed with schizophrenia, a mood disorder, or an eating disorder.

Children and child personalities can be assessed through verbal interaction, nonverbal observations, and parental or teacher reports. Young children may not have the language skills to describe their thoughts and feelings, but they are often able to communicate through play, sand trays, and art. Nonverbal assessments should be consistent with the child's developmental level.

Diagnosis

The next step in the nursing process is to analyze and synthesize the assessment data to form nursing diagnoses. You must consider the client's level of anxiety as well as the behavioral, affective, cognitive, and physiological responses to the anxiety. Other considerations are the client's self-evaluation, degree of insight, positive coping behavior, defense mechanisms, and the family/friendship systems. See the Nursing Diagnoses box.

Outcome Identification

Once you have established diagnoses, you and the client mutually identify goals for change. Client outcomes are specific behavioral measures by which you, the client, and significant others determine progress toward these goals. The following are examples of outcomes that may be pertinent to those with anxiety disorders:

- verbalize feeling less anxious
- verbalize less tension and restlessness
- experience fewer episodes of panic
- report less time in obsessive-compulsive behaviors
- verbalize less shame about the disorder
- develop effective coping behaviors
- utilize support systems when anxious
- report fewer dissociative episodes
- verbalize fewer somatic complaints

See also the Critical Pathway for a Client with Panic Disorder: Outpatient Treatment on pages 194–195.

Nursing Interventions

Nursing diagnoses give direction for the development of goals and outcome criteria, which help focus your nursing care. If possible, involve the client in developing the plan of care. If the client wants something quite different from what you expect, the nursing care plan will not be appropriate; in fact, it will likely be sabotaged by the client. The overall goal is to help the client improve the response to anxiety and develop more constructive behavior to manage anxiety. The

Nursing Diagnoses

Clients with Anxiety Disorders

Anxiety, mild, related to threat to self-concept due to fear of being out of control.

Ineffective breathing pattern related to choking or smothering sensations, shortness of breath, and hyperventilation associated with the panic level of anxiety.

Sensory-perceptual alteration related to decreased perceptual field during panic level of anxiety.

Alteration in thought processes related to difficulty in concentrating and concrete thinking during panic level of anxiety.

Ineffective individual coping related to being consumed with obsessive and/or compulsive behavior.

Alteration in family process related to detachment and inability to express feelings, or to struggle for power and control.

Fear related to confrontation with feared object or situation.

Powerlessness related to lifestyle of helplessness.

Sleep pattern disturbance related to recurrent nightmares.

Social isolation related to fear of leaving neighborhood or home or to physical symptoms and disability.

High risk for violence, self-directed or directed at others, related to inability to verbalize feelings or poor impulse control.

Spiritual distress related to a view of the world and people as threatening following a severe traumatic event.

box on page 196 provides an overview of the nursing interventions classifications (NIC) for people with anxiety, dissociative, or somatoform disorders.

Behavioral: Psychological Comfort Promotion

Anxiety Reduction

Clients who are extremely anxious or in a panic state of anxiety respond best to a calm, direct approach. Stay with clients to promote safety and reduce fear. Provide reassurance that you will stay with them and

Text continues on page 196

Focused Nursing Assessment

CLIENTS WITH ANXIETY DISORDERS

Behavior Assessment	*Affective Assessment*	*Cognitive Assessment*	*Social Assessment*

Obsessive-Compulsive Disorder

What kinds of objects or situations do you feel a need to check or recheck frequently?	Describe how you experience the feeling of anxiety.	Describe the qualities you like about yourself. Describe the qualities you do not like about yourself.	In what way do habits or thoughts get in the way of work? Social life? Personal life?
How much time during a day do you spend on checking activities?	What happens to you when you feel out of control in situations?	What are your thoughts about your compulsive behavior?	Describe situations in which you feel close to and warm with your family members.
Describe any movements you are forced to repeat.	Describe your relationships with significant others.	Would you like to decrease the need for your compulsive behavior?	In what ways do you feel dependent on your family?
What kinds of things do you count, silently or out loud?	How do these others relate to you?	How much time a day do you spend doubting what you have done?	
	What are your greatest fears in life?	What are the fears you worry about every day?	

Phobic Disorders

What situations or objects do you try to avoid in life?	What are your greatest fears in life?	Do you dislike being controlled by your fears?	Who is able to support you in avoiding your feared situations or objects?
Describe what you do to avoid these situations or objects.	Do you fear others laughing at you? Being humiliated? Being abandoned by others? Being alone in an unfamiliar situation?	What does the future look like for you?	Describe how family living patterns have changed around your fears.
To what degree do these fears interfere with your daily routines?		Describe the qualities you like about yourself. Describe the qualities you do not like about yourself.	Under what circumstances are you able to socialize with friends?
Are your social or work activities limited to a prescribed geographic area?	What feelings do you experience when you are confronted with the situation or object that you fear?	How much support do you need from others to cope with life?	
How often and in what circumstances are you able to leave home?	What else happens to you at this time?	How helpless and dependent on others do you feel?	
	To what degree do you fear having future panic attacks?		

Posttraumatic Stress Disorder

Under what circumstances do you experience outbursts of aggressive behavior?	How much time during a day do you feel tense or irritable?	Describe difficulties you have had with concentration.	In what ways do your family members and friends tell you that you are distant or cold in your relationships with them?
In what ways have you been re-experiencing the original trauma?	Have you been experiencing panic attacks?	Describe difficulties you have had with your memory.	Describe your communication patterns with family members and friends.
In what ways do you attempt to avoid situations or activities that may remind you of the original trauma?	Describe the guilt you have been experiencing in relation to the original trauma.	How often, in a day, do you have recurrent thoughts about the original trauma? Do you feel you have control over these thoughts?	

Behavior Assessment	Affective Assessment	Cognitive Assessment	Social Assessment

Posttraumatic Stress Disorder *continued*

Behavior Assessment	Affective Assessment	Cognitive Assessment	Social Assessment
How frequently do you participate in social activities? Have you had any employment difficulties since the original trauma?	What types of activities do you enjoy doing? What are sources of pleasure for you in your life? Describe relationships in which you feel emotionally close to other people.	Describe any nightmares you have. Describe the qualities you like about yourself. Describe the qualities you do not like about yourself.	Describe what happens when you lose control of your anger. How is violence handled within your family system? Are you divorced, or have you been threatened with divorce?

Dissociative Identity Disorder*

Behavior Assessment	Affective Assessment	Cognitive Assessment	Social Assessment
Does the client have widely varying behavior patterns, such as at times being submissive and quiet and at other times loud and outspoken? Does the client have different styles of dressing that correspond to a change in behavior? Are vocational or leisure skills inconsistent; that is, are these skills apparent at some times and not at other times?	Does the client experience anxiety about "lost" time? In what ways is the client passive and submissive? In what ways is the client angry and aggressive?	Describe the frequency of amnesic periods. Under what circumstances does this amnesia seem to appear? Are there times when the client can remember specific events and other times when there is amnesia for the same events?	Do family members describe the client as having different personalities? How has the family tried to manage the situation thus far? Is there a known history of child abuse for the client? Describe the client's relationship to his or her parents as a child.

Somatoform Disorders

Behavior Assessment	Affective Assessment	Cognitive Assessment	Social Assessment
What OTC medications are you currently taking? How effective are they? What prescription medications are you currently taking? How effective are they? What medications have you taken in the past? What results were obtained with them? Who have you consulted professionally for your illness in the past 5 years? What diagnostic procedures have been performed? What surgeries have you had in your lifetime?	In what situations do you experience feelings of anger? In what situations do you experience feelings of anxiety? In what way do you share your feelings with others? How do you respond when others become angry with you?	How often, in a day, are you aware of your physical symptoms? How aware are you of bodily sensations? Do you believe you have a serious illness? Has this illness been confirmed by a health care professional? Describe your level of concern for your physical health.	How is your family managing with your illness? Who is supportive to you in this illness? Who cares for you when you are unable to care for yourself? How has your illness affected the family's financial situation?

*Since the client is unaware of changes in personalities, the assessment data are based on your observations and family reporting.

Critical Pathway for a Client with Panic Disorder: Outpatient Treatment

Expected length of treatment 8 weeks	Date _____ Weeks 1–2	Date _____ Weeks 3–6	Date _____ Weeks 7–8
Weekly outcomes	Client will: ▪ Identify initial goals for therapy. ▪ Contract for ongoing treatment. ▪ Participate in treatment plan. ▪ Begin to identify sources of anxiety/panic.	Client will: ▪ Identify ongoing goals for therapy. ▪ Maintain contract for ongoing therapy. ▪ Participate in treatment plan. ▪ Identify strategies to manage anxiety and panic.	Client will describe ongoing strategies to manage panic disorder. Client will demonstrate ability to cope with ongoing feelings of panic. Client will describe strategies to cope with an inability to cope with stressors.
Assessments, tests, and treatments	Psychosocial assessment to include mental status, mood, affect, behavior, and communication. Assist client to explore factors that precipitate panic attacks.	Psychosocial assessment. Assess recent history of anxiety and panic attacks. Explore contributing factors. Discuss effectiveness of cognitive restructuring strategies.	Psychosocial assessment. Assess recent history of anxiety and panic attacks. Explore contributing factors. Discuss effectiveness of cognitive restructuring strategies.
Knowledge deficit	Orient client to therapy program. Assess learning needs of client. Review initial plan of care. Assess understanding of teaching. Discuss the etiology and management of anxiety and panic disorders. Discuss the physical symptoms of panic and the importance of understanding the meaning of anxiety and panic disorders. Instruct client to maintain journal of anxiety and panic attacks.	Review therapy program and treatment objectives. Review journal of recent panic attacks. Assist client to identify the early signs of anxiety and panic attacks. Discuss strategies to cope with early signs and symptoms of panic attacks, including talking or activity. Discuss additional strategies to cope with panic attacks including expressing anger, positive self-talk, or guided imagery. Teach principles of cognitive restructuring and practice during session. Teach relaxation techniques and practice during session. Discuss use of exercise to alleviate anxiety/panic. Assist client to explore problem-solving strategies. Assess understanding of teaching.	Review plan of care. Review principles of cognitive restructuring. Assess understanding of teaching.

	Date _____ Weeks 1–2 *continued*	Date _____ Weeks 3–6 *continued*	Date _____ Weeks 7–8 *continued*
Diet	Nutritional assessment. Encourage well-balanced diet from all food groups. Contract with client to avoid stimulants.	Encourage a well-balanced diet from all food groups. Encourage the avoidance of stimulants.	Encourage a well-balanced diet from all food groups. Encourage the avoidance of stimulants.
Activity	Discuss the importance of regular aerobic exercise. Contract for regular exercise program. Sleep pattern assessment. Discuss strategies to provide sleep-enhancing atmosphere for 45 min prior to sleep.	Review ability to begin and continue exercise program. Maintain contract for regular exercise programs. Encourage client to practice relaxation response. Discuss effectiveness of sleep-enhancing strategies.	Review ability to continue exercise program. Maintain contract for regular exercise programs. Discuss effectiveness of sleep-enhancing strategies.
Psychosocial	Approach with nonjudgmental and accepting manner. Observe and monitor behavior. Assist client to understand relationship of unexpressed feelings to anxiety and panic experience. Encourage client to express feelings, thoughts, ideas, and beliefs.	Approach with nonjudgmental and accepting manner. Observe and monitor behavior. Encourage client to express feelings, thoughts, ideas, and beliefs. Provide positive feedback for efforts to incorporate coping strategies into daily life. Assist client to understand relationship of feelings to panic. Assist client to realistically identify strengths and limitations. Explore ways of reframing limitations in a positive manner. Assist client to practice and implement effective coping strategies. Assist client to identify potentially stressful situations and role-play coping strategies.	Approach with nonjudgmental and accepting manner. Encourage client to review strategies to manage anxiety and panic.
Medications	Identify target symptoms.	Assess target symptoms. Assess need for medications and refer as indicated. Routine meds as ordered.	Assess target symptoms. Routine meds as ordered.
Consults and discharge plan	Family assessment. Establishment objectives of therapy with client.	Review with client progress toward therapy objectives.	Review with client progress toward therapy objectives. Make appropriate referrals to support groups.

Nursing Interventions Classification

CLIENTS WITH ANXIETY, DISSOCIATIVE, OR SOMATOFORM DISORDERS

DOMAIN: Behavioral

Class: *Psychological Comfort Promotion*

Interventions: *Anxiety Reduction:* Minimizing apprehension, dread, foreboding, or uneasiness related to an unidentified source of anticipated danger.

Calming Technique: Reducing anxiety in patient experiencing acute distress.

Class: *Coping Assistance*

Interventions: *Emotional Support:* Provision of reassurance, acceptance, and encouragement during times of stress.

Security Enhancement: Intensifying a patient's sense of physical and psychological safety.

Spiritual Support: Assisting the patient to feel balance and connection with a greater power.

Support System Enhancement: Facilitation of support to patient by family, friends, and community.

Class: *Cognitive Therapy*

Interventions: *Cognitive Restructuring:* Challenging a patient to alter distorted thought patterns and view self and the world more realistically.

Class: *Communication Enhancement*

Interventions: *Socialization Enhancement:* Facilitation of another person's ability to interact with others.

DOMAIN: Family

Class: *Life Span Care*

Interventions: *Family Integrity Promotion:* Promotion of family cohesion and unity.

DOMAIN: Physiological: Basic

Class: *Nutrition Support*

Interventions: *Nutritional Counseling:* Use of an interactive helping process focusing on the need for diet modification.

Class: *Activity and Exercise Management*

Interventions: *Exercise Promotion:* Facilitation of regular physical exercise to maintain or advance to a higher level of fitness and health.

Source: McCloskey, J. C., & Bulechek. G. M., 1996.

---

that this attack will go away. Speak slowly in a gentle voice and use short simple sentences, as highly anxious people have great difficulty focusing or concentrating. Examples are: "I will stay," "Sit down," or "I will help." Loosen any tight clothing to ease the sensation of choking. Tell clients to take slow, deep breaths, and breathe with the client to demonstrate and to gradually slow down the breathing. Direct them to imagine inhaling and exhaling through the soles of the feet. During a panic attack, people feel disconnected from the environment and this imagery helps people feel grounded and therefore safer. If possible, move to a quieter room in the home, clinic, or hospital.

Clients who have a phobia experience anxiety when confronted with the feared object or situation. Help them express the fears which interfere with their lives while presenting a nonjudgmental attitude. Encourage clients to search for, confront, and relieve the source of the original anxiety. Together, you can rehearse various coping behaviors that increase their sense of control. They may picture the event step-by-step, picture themselves coping effectively, and practice relaxation techniques during this process. This visualization helps them move in the direction of their expectations. Visualizing effective coping reinforces their self-image as a person capable of dealing with fear, while relaxation training reduces the physical sensations that provoke anxiety and panic.

Distraction techniques are also useful tools because they allow the person to remain in control when experiencing moderate levels of anxiety. Examples of distraction techniques are listening to music, reading a book, talking to a close friend, and playing a game. Positive imagery allows the person to focus away from the anxiety-producing stimulus and onto a positive image that feels safe. Examples are picturing sitting quietly on a beach, being held by a trusted person, and playing with a pet. Counting backward by threes also provides a distraction from the sensations of anxiety.

Many anxiety-disordered clients find *journal keeping* extremely helpful. Making entries one or several times a day is a useful way to keep track of thoughts, feelings, and memories. This self-monitoring technique helps them identify events preceding, during, and after anxiety occurs. They are encouraged to write down effective coping strategies that they will be able to refer to during a future time of anxiety. For clients with OCD, journal keeping often helps them begin to identify anxiety cues and to initiate anxiety-reducing techniques before the anxiety becomes overwhelming. Clients with DID might find journal keeping to be less threatening than sharing the same details verbally with you. Talking about the abuse is usually a later step. Because several personalities often write, the journal becomes one way the personalities can communicate and cooperate with one another. Some DID units have a journal group in which clients talk about self-discovery through writing.

Clients who have a somatization disorder benefit from set limits on the amount of time they talk about their physical complaints. Encourage them to recognize and discuss their fears rather than to somaticize their feelings. Avoid implying that physical symptoms are imaginary because anxiety would increase if the client did not feel believed.

Calming Technique

Calming techniques such as muscle relaxation and deep breathing are useful for managing the psychophysiological dimensions of anxiety. The goal is to provide clients with a skill response so that they can experience anxiety without feeling overwhelmed. In addition to focusing on and relaxing specific muscle groups, teach clients to take a deep breath through the nose, hold the breath for a count of three, and then exhale while silently saying the word "relax." Even fairly young children can be taught this technique.

Other calming techniques you can teach clients involve changing their sensory experiences or getting involved in activities. Some people like to take a walk or read a book, others like to hold on to a pillow or rub a worry stone, and others find that talking to a friend or singing a song calms them down. They can say positive affirmations aloud such as: "I am calm and happy," "My breathing is slow and even," "I am very relaxed."

Behavioral: Coping Assistance

Emotional Support

Clients need reassurance and encouragement during times of stress. Assist clients in distinguishing between feelings such as anxiety, frustration, guilt, and hostility. Discuss ways to express feelings appropriately in order to provide more effective options for managing them. Help clients recognize that suppressing feelings requires energy, which is depleting. If clients fear that direct verbal expression of negative feelings leads to rejection from others, suggest they problem-solve to find safe physical outlets for their negative feelings, such as exercise, working out in the gym, or pounding clay.

Clients who have a lifestyle of helplessness feel powerless in many areas of their lives. Do not force them into situations they cannot handle, but instead support their defenses as long as necessary to protect themselves. Do not try to reason away helpless behavior, since helplessness serves to control anxiety. Provide only as much assistance as is needed to help them gradually gain control over their lives. Explore beliefs that support a helpless mode of behavior, taking into consideration cultural values and patterns. Identify secondary gains such as decreased responsibility and increased dependency, and problem-solve ways to meet needs in a more adaptive fashion. As clients gain insight, they will be better able to modify their behavior.

Clients who experience compulsive or ritualistic behavior need support and encouragement in managing their daily lives. Often clients are aware that their behavior is pointless but are unable to make changes in these activities. Help clients problem-solve ways in which they can modify their environment and personal schedules so that rituals can be included into daily routine. Safety measures may need to be implemented, such as plenty of dry towels and hand lotion for those who compulsively wash their hands. Explore the relationship between obsessive behavior and anxiety reduction, and problem-solve to find other behaviors that are more effective in managing anxiety. One such behavior may be daily schedule planning, which helps people feel in control of what happens to them. Clients who are obsessed with work and routines need help planning and scheduling hobbies and pleasurable activities during leisure time.

Security Enhancement

Some people experience a moderate level of anxiety in response to fears of being out of control. You can begin to help by having clients identify one anxiety-producing situation. Problem solving will be more effective when it is focused on a manageable single situation. Discuss clients' thoughts regarding control issues as well as their negative anticipatory thoughts. Teach them to redefine the sensations of anxiety as sensations of excitement, since they will be less disabled if their expectations are positive. Help them analyze their fears of losing control and make the connection between these fears and their increased anxiety. Talk over the possibility of the potential loss of control in this specific situation in order to differentiate between fantasy and the reality of the fear. Review how anxiety has been handled in the past and what behaviors were most effective. Teach relaxation techniques and explain that one cannot be relaxed and anxious at the same time. These skills will facilitate clients' sense of control over anxiety and life events.

Spiritual Support

People who experience severe traumatic events often suffer from spiritual distress because the world has become threatening. Explore clients' perceived lack of control over life events. Encourage them to search for meaning in the trauma to further their reestablishing a purpose in life. To increase their feelings of connectedness to others, help them identify interpersonal support systems. Be available to listen to their feelings; this allows them to vent rather than suppress their emotions. If appropriate, refer them to a religious counselor of their choice and support their use of meditation, prayer, or other religious traditions and rituals.

Support System Enhancement

Support systems are an essential component of managing anxiety disorders. Group therapy and self-help support groups are often effective treatment approaches, particularly for clients with phobic disorders and PTSD. Groups of people with similar problems provide an environment where each person can establish trust and share with others. In group therapy, more significant improvement is often seen than in individual therapy. Within the group, members are able to identify with others' feelings of anger, fear, guilt, and isolation. This identification increases the participation of, and resulting support for, each person. Support groups are very helpful for family members. Information they receive about the disorders helps them understand that the client is not to blame for the problem. In addition, groups focus on stress management, the problem-solving process, adaptive coping measures, and ways to mobilize other resources. See the Self-Help Groups at the end of this chapter for these community resources.

Behavioral: Cognitive Therapy

Cognitive Restructuring

Cognitive intervention techniques concentrate on teaching people to change their maladaptive beliefs, self-statements, and phobic imagery that contribute to anxiety disorders. In guided self-dialogue, clients are taught to think certain thoughts before acting, such as "I will get on the elevator and go to the second floor successfully." In a technique known as thought stopping, they are taught to say "stop" to obsessional thoughts. Some clients work in changing irrational ways of thinking, such as "Thinking is the same as acting" or "There is a right and wrong in every situation."

Clients who worry a great deal can be taught to control their worrying thoughts. The process begins with identifying the thoughts, which are often so automatic that they are no longer aware of them. They can then choose to either counter the thoughts, or challenge the thoughts. Countering the thoughts involves distraction, which prevents the buildup of anxiety. This might be engaging in a vigorous physical activity or mental activity such as reciting poetry. Some people find that refocusing and concentrating on some aspect in the environment, such as counting the number of items on a shelf, is helpful. Challenging the thoughts is a process of identifying which thoughts are unrealistic, exaggerated, and catastrophic. Examples are: "Yesterday was terrible; today is likely to be awful too," "I stammered during my speech so I have ruined my daughter's wedding and she won't forgive me," and "My son is late—he's had an accident." These thoughts can be transformed into: "Yesterday was terrible; no, parts of it were good and although parts were uncomfortable, I coped." "I stammered during my speech, this is not the end of the world. Many people get nervous when speaking in public," and "My son is late; maybe he got held up in traffic."

Behavioral: Communication Enhancement

Socialization Enhancement

Clients may have relationship difficulties and will benefit from social skills training. In a group setting, they can learn how to be less self-absorbed, pay attention to others' feelings and thoughts, and be considerate of others. People who have learned to behave passively and dependently often benefit from assertiveness training. Others have had limited practice with communication skills and need to be taught appropriate ways to communicate. They are encouraged to express their feelings directly and say what they mean. Both assertiveness and communication skills are best learned within a group format to allow for practice and feedback.

Family: Life Span Care

Family Integrity Promotion

Relationship or family therapy is appropriate in many cases. Family members may need help defining and clarifying their relationships. Some fear losing themselves in a close relationship, so they interact with distance and alienation. Others get caught in a pattern of excessive dependency and must discover how this type of helplessness actually establishes a position of power within the family. Often, family members have secondary gains that meet individual needs such as nurturing or control but that interfere with the growth and development of the family system. They must understand how the illness may, in fact, perpetuate existing family dynamics. They must learn how to restore and maintain balance without the presence of an anxiety disorder. Family members often need help labeling feelings and sharing them with one

another. You can teach the use of "I" language to express thoughts and feelings, such as "I think . . ." or "I feel. . . ." "I" statements help people assume responsibility for their own feelings rather than blaming others with "you" statements, such as "You make me feel . . ." or "You never do anything right."

Physiological: Basic: Nutrition Support

Nutritional Counseling

Nutritional interventions include teaching clients about balanced diets, how to shop wisely, and how to cook simple meals. Because caffeine, chocolate, and alcohol may increase anxiety, strongly encourage them to stay away from these substances. L-tryptophan (TRY) is an amino acid that is essential for the production of both 5-HT and niacin. If clients increase their intake of niacin, TRY will be forced to produce more 5-HT. Available in time-release capsules, it should not be taken by those suffering from peptic ulcer, liver impairment, diabetes, or gout. Vitamin B_6 is necessary for the conversion of TRY to 5-HT. It is important for clients to recognize that vitamin B_6 is depleted from the body by the use of antidepressants, birth control pills, and antihypertensive agents. Clients may need to supplement their vitamin B_6 intake in these cases (Cantor, 1996).

Physiological: Basic: Activity and Exercise Management

Exercise Promotion

Exercise has an overall relaxing effect on the body and may be used to manage anxiety. Discuss with clients the benefits of exercise and design a program that fits their lifestyle. Assist clients to prepare and maintain a progress graph/chart to motivate their adherence to the exercise program.

Evaluation

The final step of the nursing process, evaluation, is the basis for modifying the plan of care. This is accomplished by you and the client after determining whether the expected outcomes have been met. If they have, you determine whether the diagnosis is resolved and the client is coping effectively. If the problem is only partially resolved, develop new outcome criteria. When you and the client determine that none of the expected outcomes has been met, use the problem-solving process to determine the cause. It may be that not enough time has elapsed or that outcomes were inappropriate or too long-term. If the outcomes are valid, evaluate the interventions. Perhaps the interventions were inappropriate or not individualized for the particular person, or perhaps they were not consistently implemented. When the difficulty in the nursing process is identified, modify your care on the basis of the evaluation to ensure the client's healthier adaptation to anxiety.

■ *Clinical Interactions*

A Client with Obsessive-Compulsive Disorder

Detra, age 23, lives with her parents and has recently become obsessed with thoughts of her parents' deaths. She has developed several compulsions to manage the associated anxiety. When walking outside, she must never step on a crack in the sidewalk, and she silently repeats to herself over and over again: "Step on a crack, break your mother's back." She also fears that if she does not keep the house clean enough, her parents will get sick and die. She usually spends at least 8 hours a day cleaning their two-bedroom apartment. She insists the windows and doors remain closed to prevent contamination and allows no one into the apartment other than immediate family members. Lately, she has begun to use a magnifying glass to see if she has missed cleaning any fingerprints off the tables and chairs. In the interaction, you will see evidence of:

- ego-dystonic feelings about the obsession
- a desire to resist the obsession
- shame about her uncontrollable behavior
- temporary relief of anxiety by compulsive behavior

NURSE: It sounds like you have a lot of worries.
DETRA: Yeah.
NURSE: Your mother said you worry about the family a lot. Is that true?

DETRA: Yeah.
NURSE: Are you worried about your parents right now?
DETRA: No, not if I don't think about it.
NURSE: Well, when you're worried about your parents, does anything help?
DETRA: Yeah. [Pauses, looks embarrassed.] It's really stupid. I clean the apartment over and over all day long.
NURSE: You are constantly cleaning. Does that help?
DETRA: Sort of, but it's stupid.
NURSE: What do you mean, stupid?
DETRA: Just stupid. I wish I could quit thinking about it.
NURSE: Do you have other worries you wish you could quit thinking about?
DETRA: Yeah.
NURSE: Tell me about one of your other worries that you think is kind of stupid.
DETRA: I worry about dirt and germs coming in through the windows and doors.
NURSE: Do you do anything when you have these worries?
DETRA: I go around the apartment and keep checking that all the windows and doors are sealed. I search to see if there is any way germs can get in.
NURSE: When you check the windows and doors, that helps your worry about germs?
DETRA: Yeah. That's stupid, isn't it?
NURSE: Well, it sounds like you have a problem, but I don't think you're stupid. ■

Self-Help Groups

Clients with Anxiety Disorders

Anxiety Disorders Association of America
6000 Executive Boulevard, Suite 200
Rockville, MD 20852

CHANGE: Free From Fears
2915 Providence Road
Charlotte, NC 28211
(704) 365–0140

MPD Dignity
P.O. Box 4367
Boulder, CO 80306

Multiple Personality Clinic, Rush University
Rush North Shore Medical Center
9600 Gross Point Road
Skokie, IL 60076

Obsessive Compulsive Foundation, Inc.
P.O. Box 70
Milford, CT 06460-0070
(203) 874-3843

Obsessive Compulsive Information Center
Department of Psychiatry
University of Wisconsin Center for Health Sciences
1600 Highland Avenue
Madison, WI 53792

Phobia Society of America
133 Rollins Avenue, Suite 4B
Rockville, MD 20852
(301) 231–9350

Veteran Outreach Program
Disabled American Veterans
807 Maine Avenue, SW
Washington, DC 20024
www.v-o-p.org

Key Concepts

Introduction

- Coping mechanisms are conscious attempts to control anxiety, which, if effective, contribute to a person's sense of competence and self-esteem.

- Defense mechanisms are unconscious attempts to manage anxiety, attempts that may or may not be successful.

Knowledge Base

- Generalized anxiety disorder (GAD) is a chronic disorder characterized by persistent anxiety without phobias or panic attacks.

- Panic attacks, the highest level of anxiety, are characterized by disorganized thinking, feelings of terror and helplessness, and nonpurposeful behavior.

- Panic disorder is a progressive anxiety disorder characterized by sudden and unexpected panic attacks. It may or may not be accompanied by agoraphobia.

- Obsessive-compulsive disorder (OCD) is characterized by unwanted, repetitive thoughts and behaviors.

- People with phobic disorders suffer from persistent, unreasonable fears that result in avoidance behavior, which is often disabling. When confronted with the feared object or situation, the person panics.

- Agoraphobia is characterized by fear of being away from home and of being alone in public places when assistance might be needed.

- The major defense mechanisms present in phobias are repression, displacement, symbolization, and avoidance.

- Posttraumatic stress disorder (PTSD) is characterized by a constant anticipation of danger and a phobic avoidance of triggers that remind the person of the original trauma. Other characteristics include irritability, aggression, and flashbacks.

- Acute stress disorder is a short-term response to an extreme trauma. If it persists longer than one month, the client is given the diagnosis of PTSD.

- Dissociative disorders are characterized by an alteration in conscious awareness of behavior, affect, thoughts, and memories, and an alteration in identity, particularly in the consistency of personality.

- People with a dissociative disorder block the thoughts and feelings associated with a severe trauma from conscious awareness. This may take the form of amnesia, fugue, depersonalization, or identity disorder (DID).

- The somatoform disorders involve physical symptoms for which no organic basis exists. Denial is used to transform anxiety into physical symptoms. The disorders include somatization disorder, conversion disorder, pain disorder, hypochondriasis, and body dysmorphic disorder.

- People with anxiety disorders may have a profound effect on their family systems. They may control their family through dependency and helplessness or though detachment and emotional distance. Secondary gains may perpetuate the disorder.

- The meaning of anxiety and the responses to it are strongly influenced by cultural beliefs and practices.

- Signs of mild anxiety include an agreeable increase in tension, occasional twitches or shortness of breath, and mild gastric symptoms.

- Signs of moderate anxiety include increased heart rate and blood pressure, shortness of breath, sweating, trembling, restlessness, fatigue, tension headache, and stiff neck.

- Signs of panic include hypotension, agitation, poor motor coordination, nonpurposeful behavior, dizziness, chest pain, palpitations, a choking sensation, and a feeling of terror.

- There is a high correlation between anxiety disorders and substance abuse, depression, and suicide.

- Many factors contribute to the development of anxiety disorders. These include altered neurobiology, inefficient defense mechanisms, problems with interpersonal relationships, cognitive expectations, learned avoidance responses, and rigid gender-role expectations.

- A variety of antianxiety agents and antidepressants may be used for treatment, along with individual, family, and group psychotherapy.

Nursing Process

- You will be assessing the majority of clients with anxiety disorders in community settings, clinics, offices, emergency departments, and medical-surgical units.

- Most of the nursing diagnoses in this chapter apply to many individuals regardless of the specific medical diagnostic category. It is through understanding the issues and problems most significant for each client that care plans are developed and implemented.

- Techniques for reducing anxiety include muscle relaxation, deep breathing, physical exercise, and distraction techniques.

- Stay with the person experiencing a panic state and speak slowly in short, simple sentences.

- Journal keeping is an effective way for clients to keep track of their thoughts, feelings, and memories.

- Calming techniques include deep breathing, muscle relaxation, changing sensory experiences, doing activities, and positive affirmations.

- Help clients identify secondary gains and find more adaptive ways to meet those needs.

- Aid clients in the search for meaning in life, connecting with others, and developing a support system.

- Cognitive interventions include guided self-dialogue, thought stopping, and changing irrational ways of thinking.

- Many clients benefit from social skills training, assertiveness training, and communication skills training.

- Relationship or family therapy is appropriate in many cases, as the entire family system suffers from the effects of anxiety disorders.

- Nutritional interventions include teaching clients to increase their intake of niacin and vitamin B_6, which are necessary for the production of 5-HT.

- The nursing process is dynamic, and an evaluation of outcomes leads to further assessment and modification of the plan of care.

Review Questions

1. Your client is taking Tofranil (imipramine) for treatment of his panic disorder. Which of the following statements would be included in your teaching plan?

   a. Do not drink alcohol because both alcohol and Tofranil lower the seizure threshold.

   b. Do not drink alcohol because both alcohol and Tofranil cause CNS depression.

   c. If you are diabetic, you must closely monitor your blood glucose levels while taking Tofranil.

   d. You will not feel the effect of this medication for 4–6 days.

2. Pam is experiencing the panic level of anxiety. What is the most appropriate nursing intervention?

   a. Leave her alone so she can get control of herself.

   b. Stay with her to reassure her of her safety.

   c. Have her join a group of people so she will feel better.

   d. Put her in a waist restraint until she calms down.

3. Maureen is experiencing severe agoraphobia. She and Dick have been married for 25 years and have no children. Which one of the following interventions would be appropriate during family therapy?

   a. Protect her from the need to make multiple decisions.

   b. Modify their schedules so her rituals are not interrupted.

   c. Explore how her perfectionism is uncomfortable for her husband.

   d. Identify her secondary gains such as decreased responsibility and increased dependency.

4. Which of the following assessment questions would be best to ask a client with obsessive-compulsive disorder?

   a. Do you dislike being controlled by your fears?

   b. How much time during a day do you spend on checking activities?

   c. In what ways have you been re-experiencing the original trauma?

   d. How aware are you of bodily sensations?

5. Which of the following interventions is part of cognitive restructuring?

   a. mapping all the known personalities

   b. providing information about the disorder

   c. challenging thoughts that are unrealistic and exaggerated

   d. encouraging clients to express their thoughts and feelings directly

References

Allen, M., & Edwards, D. M. (1997). The broken mirror. *Treatment Today, 9(2)*, 8–9.

Brawman-Mintzer, O. (1995). Body dysmorphic disorder in patients with anxiety disorders and major depression. *Am J Psychiatry, 152*(11), 1665–1667.

Bremner, J. D., et al. (1996). Chronic PTSD in Vietnam combat veterans. *Am J Psychiatry, 153*(3), 369–375.

Brown, A., & Lempa, M. (1996, Fall/Winter). The prevalance of anxiety disorders. *NARSAD Research Newsletter*, 13–18.

Cantor, D. (1996). *Phantom Illness*. Boston: Houghton Mifflin.

Cooper, M. (1996). Obsessive-compulsive disorder: Effects on family members. *Am J Orthopsychiatry, 66*(2), 296–304.

Eisenberg, L. (1995). The social construction of the human brain. *Am J Psychiatry, 152*(11), 1563–1575.

Ellason, J. W., & Ross, C. A. (1997). Two-year follow-up of inpatients with dissociative identity disorder. *Am J Psychiatry, 154*(6), 832–839.

Evans, K., & Sullivan, J. M. (1995). *Treating Addicted Survivors of Trauma*. New York: Guilford Press.

Foa, E. B., Riggs, D. S., & Gershuny, B. S. (1995). Arousal, numbing, and intrusion. *Am J Psychiatry, 152*(1), 116–120.

Greenberg, B. D., et al. (1997). Effect of prefrontal repetitive transcranial magnetic stimulation in obsessive-compulsive disorder. *Am J Psychiatry, 154*(6), 867–869.

Hedaya, R. J. (1996). *Understanding Biological Psychiatry*. New York: Norton.

Hollifield, M., et al. (1997). Panic disorder and quality of life. *Am J Psychiatry, 154*(6), 766–772.

Katzelnick, D. J. (1995). Sertraline for social phobia. *Am J Psychiatry, 152*(9), 1368–1371.

Kirmayer, L. J., Young, A., & Hayton, B. C. (1995). The cultural context of anxiety disorders. *Psychiatr Clin North Am, 18*(3), 503–522.

Kluft, R. P. (1996). Treating the traumatic memories of patients with dissociative identity disorder. *Am J Psychiatry, 153* (Suppl. 7), 103–110.

Levine, R. E., & Gaw, A. C. (1995). Culture-bound syndromes. *Psychiatr Clin North Am, 18*(3), 523–550.

McCloskey, J. C., & Bulechek, G. M. (1996). *Nursing Interventions Classification (NIC), 2nd ed*. St. Louis: Mosby.

OCD—Part II. (1995). *Harvard Mental Health Letter*, 6, 12 , 1–3.

Pauls, D. L. (1995). A family study of obsessive-compulsive disorder. *Am J Psychiatry, 152*(1), 76–84.

Perna, G., et al. (1996). Family history of panic disorder and hypersensitivity to CO_2 in patients with panic disorder. *Am J Psychiatry, 153*(8), 1060–1065.

Pfaelzer, C., & Ellison, J. M. (1996). Panic disorder. In J. M. Ellison (Ed.), *Integrative Treatment of Anxiety Disorders* (pp. 53–76). American Psychiatric Press.

Pollack, M. H., et al. (1996). Relationship of childhood anxiety to adult panic disorder. *Am J Psychiatry, 153*(3), 376–381.

Rapoport, J. L. (1989). *The Boy Who Couldn't Stop Washing*. Washington, D.C.: Dutton.

Reeves, P., & Ellison, J. M. (1996). Posttraumatic stress disorder. In J. M. Ellison (Ed.), *Integrative Treatment of Anxiety Disorders* (pp. 135–152). American Psychiatric Press.

Riley, E. (1995). I am what I am: Inpatient treatment for people with dissociative identity disorder. *Capsules & Comments in Psych Nurs, 2*(2), 94–103.

Sands, B. F. (1996). Generalized anxiety disorder, social phobia, and performance anxiety. In J. M. Ellison (Ed.), *Integrative Treatment of Anxiety Disorders* (pp. 1–51). American Psychiatric Press.

Shalev, A., et al. (1996). Predictors of PTSD in injured trauma survivors. *Am J Psychiatry, 153*(2), 219–225.

Sherbourne, C. D., Wells, K. B., & Judd, L. L. (1996). Functioning and well-being of patients with panic disorder. *Am J Psychiatry, 153*(2), 213–218.

Shirar, L. (1996). *Dissociative Children*. New York: Norton.

Simeon, D., et al. (1997). Feeling unreal: 30 cases of DSM-III-R depersonalization disorder. *Am J Psychiatry, 154*(8), 1107–1113.

Stein, M. B., et al. (1997). Obsessive-compulsive disorder in the community. *Am J Psychiatry, 154*(8), 1120–1126.

Tiihonen, J. (1997). Dopamine reuptake site densitites in patients with social phobia. *Am J Psychiatry, 154*(2), 239–242.

Wakefield, M., & Pallister, R. (1997). Cognitive-behavioral approaches to panic disorder. *J Psychosoc Nurs, 35*(3), 12–20.

Yonkers, K. A., & Gurguis, G. (1995). Gender differences in the prevalence and expression of anxiety disorders. In M. V. Seeman (Ed.), *Gender and Psychopathology* (pp. 113–130). American Psychiatric Press.

CHAPTER 10

Eating Disorders

Karen Lee Fontaine

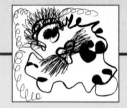

Objectives

After reading this chapter, you will be able to:

- Discuss the causative theories of eating disorders.
- Assess clients from physical, psychological, and sociocultural perspectives.
- Plan overall goals in the care of eating-disordered clients.
- Individualize standard interventions to specific clients.
- Evaluate and modify the plan of care for clients with eating disorders.

Key Terms

anorexia nervosa
bulimia nervosa
dichotomous thinking
ego-dystonic behavior
ego-syntonic behavior
ideas of reference
magnification
overgeneralization
personalization
Russell's sign
selective abstraction
superstitious thinking

Anorexia nervosa and bulimia nervosa are not single diseases but syndromes with multiple predisposing factors and a variety of characteristics. Although the most obvious symptom is the eating problem, these disorders are not simply a matter of eating too much or too little. It is because of the complex interaction of biological, psychological, developmental, familial, and sociocultural factors that certain people develop eating disorders.

There is no clear-cut distinction between the two disorders, and they have many features in common. The traditional division of anorexia and bulimia is still appropriate until more is known about eating disorders. Body weight may be a significant distinguishing characteristic; people with anorexia are severely underweight and people with bulimia are at normal or near-normal weight. About 50% of normal-weight people with bulimia have a history of anorexia and low body weight. In addition, 47% of those with anorexia exhibit bulimic behaviors. Thus, the two disorders can occur in the same person, or the person can revert from one disorder to the other. There are far more similarities than differences between anorexia and bulimia (Beumont, 1995; Keel and Mitchell, 1997). However, to help you understand the differences, the disorders have been separated in this chapter.

People with **anorexia nervosa** lose weight by dramatically decreasing their food intake and sharply increasing their amount of physical exercise. Individuals with **bulimia nervosa** develop cycles of binge eating followed by purging. The severity of the disorder is determined by the frequency of the binge/purge cycles.

The bulimic pattern is different from binge eating in the obese population. The obese who overeat tend to follow one of two patterns, neither of which includes purging the body after excessive food intake. The first pattern is overeating in response to losing control over a weight-loss diet. Although these people lose weight in weight-control programs, they regain it after going off the diet. The second pattern is overeating because of the enjoyment of food. Seldom attempting to diet, these people have no sense of loss of control. They are more accepting of their body size and understand it to be the result of their enjoyment of eating (Stunkard and Sobal, 1995).

Determining the incidence of anorexia and bulimia is difficult because of the variety of definitions that exist. Certainly, the frequency of these disorders has been increasing, but the increase may be partly due to increased reporting. Estimates are that eating disorders affect 8–20% of the population, with 85–90% of sufferers being female. The disorders usually develop during adolescence: age 13–17 for anorexia and age 17–23 for bulimia. The age of onset has been dropping in recent years, and we now see children as young as age 7 with anorexia. The disorders appear to begin at developmental milestones such as the beginning of puberty, starting or finishing high school, starting college, becoming self-supportive, or marrying (Hedaya, 1996; Fairburn et al, 1996; Keel and Mitchell, 1997).

You will encounter people with eating disorders in a number of clinical settings. In schools, camps, community health care settings, pediatric units, medical-surgical units, and intensive care units, you must be aware of the characteristics of eating disorders so you can provide prompt attention to those in need. More young women 15–24 years old die from anorexia than all other causes combined. They have a suicide rate that is much higher than the general population. With a mortality rate as high as 22%, it is extremely risky to underestimate the seriousness of eating disorders (Owen and Fullerton, 1995; Sullivan, 1995).

Knowledge Base: Obesity

Obesity is the most common form of malnourishment in the United States. It is estimated that one out of five Americans is overweight and that 10% of the population is more than 35% above ideal body weight, or obese. Since the mental health of obese people is comparable to that of the general population, obesity is not considered a mental disorder. The only similarity between obesity and anorexia and bulimia is dissatisfaction with body size and shape. Therefore, a brief overview is presented here, and you are encouraged to consult other resources for a more comprehensive description.

Obesity is thought to result from a variety of combinations of psychosocial and physiological factors. There is no universal cause and therefore no single treatment approach. There are many ways of becoming and staying obese.

A variety of psychosocial factors may contribute to the development and maintenance of obesity. Eating habits are primarily learned patterns of behavior in response to both hunger (a physiological sensation) and appetite (social and psychological cues). Some people manage negative feelings—such as anxiety, anger, and loneliness—by overeating. Others may view eating as a reward. These patterns may have been learned in childhood if parents used food as a way to decrease stress or reward good behavior. Because social events are frequently associated with food, some people make a connection between pleasure and eating—a connection that may predispose them to overeating. Because of the high level of prejudice against obese people in America, the social consequences of being overweight can be severe (Stunkard and Sobal, 1995).

Many researchers believe physiological factors are more significant than psychosocial factors. Recently, a gene for obesity, *ob*, and its protein product, leptin, were discovered. Leptin is produced in fat cells and travels to the brain, where it decreases appetite and increases metabolic rate. There is evidence that most cases of human obesity result from a defect in the brain's response to leptin.

In both obese and nonobese people, the amount of body fat seems to be precisely regulated and maintained. This explains the difficulty most people have in changing the amount of their body fat. There is frequently no clear difference between the amount of food eaten by obese people and by nonobese people. The belief that all obese people overeat is inaccurate. The defect seems to be in energy needs and expenditures, with some people being predisposed to obesity (Considine et al, 1996). Some people are blatantly hostile toward overweight people. It is no longer acceptable to stigmatize people on the basis of race or ethnic origin and therefore obesity remains one of the last socially acceptable forms of prejudice. Obese individuals may suffer from job discrimination because employers assume they are less healthy, less diligent, and less intelligent than their thinner peers. In stores, obese customers may be treated with less respect and less consideration. When obese people eat in public, they are often given disapproving looks and comments from thinner people. Frequent exposure to such treatment increases feelings of hurt and failure. Being bombarded with antifat values further increases the obese person's level of self-disgust. Health care professionals add to this discrimination by viewing obesity not only as a health hazard but also as an indication of emotional disturbance. In fact, it is the internalization of the culture's hatred and rejection, rather than body weight and size, that contributes to psychological problems (Stunkard and Sobal, 1995).

People who are 35% or more above ideal body weight are at high risk for developing a number of medical conditions. These include diabetes mellitus, hypertension, cardiovascular disease, hyperlipidemia, gallbladder disease, arthritis, and complications of pregnancy. The risk of mortality is higher for women than men and higher for the young than the old (Stunkard and Sobal, 1995).

A wide variety of treatment approaches have been tried. In all the approaches, there is a general tendency to regain lost weight. At this point, preventing obesity is more effective than treating it.

Knowledge Base: Anorexia and Bulimia

Behavioral Characteristics

Anorexia

Anorexic young women have a desperate need to please others. Their self-worth depends on responses from others, rather than on their own self-approval. Thus, their behavior is often overcompliant; they always try to meet the expectations of others in order to be accepted. They may overachieve in academic and extracurricular activities, but these accomplishments are usually an attempt to please parents rather than a source of self-satisfaction.

To control themselves and their environment, they develop rigid rules and moralistic guidelines about all aspects of life. Their decision-making ability is hampered by their need to make absolutely correct decisions. Such rigidity often develops into obsessive rituals, particularly concerning eating and exercise. Cutting all food into a predetermined size or number of pieces, chewing all food a certain number of times, allowing only certain combinations of food in a meal, accomplishing a fixed number of exercise routines, and having an inflexible pattern of exercises are rituals common to anorexic people. These rules and rituals help keep anxiety beyond conscious awareness. If the rituals are disrupted, the anxiety becomes intolerable. Paradoxically, all these efforts to stay in control lead to out-of-control behaviors (Beumont, 1995; Fichter and Pirke, 1995).

Many people with anorexia are hyperactive and discover that overexercise is a way to increase their weight loss. Solitary running tends to be the exercise of choice and there are often obsessional qualities to it. For example, they feel that before they can eat, they have to earn calories by exercising. Conversely, if they overeat, they feel they have to punish themselves with excessive exercise (Beumont, 1995).

Hopeless, helpless, and ineffective is how people with anorexia often feel. Because of being overcompliant with their parents, they believe they have always been controlled by others. Their refusal to eat may be an attempt to assert themselves and gain some control within the family.

Phobias in people with anorexia are common. Initially, the fear is of weight gain, but it develops into a secondary food phobia. The mechanism of phobic avoidance in anorexic people is different from that in others. In nonanorexic people, the phobia has an external stimulus, such as an animal or object, a place or situation. Avoidance prevents the escalation of anxiety, but the person receives no pleasure in the process. In people with anorexia, the phobia has an internal stimulus: the fear of being fat. Avoidance of food provides a feeling of control and a sense of pleasure when weight is lost.

> Inez is a high school junior who has lost 35 pounds (15.9 kg) in the past year and now weighs 90 pounds (40.9 kg). She typically goes 2–3 days without eating. She has a rigid, 2½-hour exercise routine, which she does before and after school. When her parents force her to eat, she focuses on her superstitious number of 7; that is, she will only eat 7 peas or 7 kernels of corn or drink 7 tiny sips of milk. She chews everything 7 times and must complete her meal in 7 minutes.

Bulimia

Unlike those with anorexia, people who begin their eating disorder with a bulimic pattern are often overweight before the onset of the disorder. Olivardia and colleagues (1995) found that young men who become bulimic often do so to make a specific wrestling weight or to improve other athletic performance. Typically, people with bulimia focus on changing specific body parts, and their usual motive is to remove flab

and increase muscle size. This behavior is common among dancers, actors, models, jockeys, and other athletes. They often learn this maladaptive pattern of weight control from peers who have used purging as a method of losing weight. This sort of bulimia may go undetected for years because often there is no significant weight loss. For both males and females, the behavior rapidly becomes compulsive, and the frequency and severity of the eating disorder tend to increase.

> Amy states that when she was 15 years old, she weighed 140 pounds (63.6 kg). One of her friends said to her, "I see you're working on a stomach there." She describes that incident as the beginning of her bulimic behavior.

There is a cyclic behavioral pattern in bulimia. It begins with skipping meals sporadically and overstrict dieting or fasting. In an effort to refrain from eating, the person may use amphetamines, which can lead to extreme hunger, fatigue, and low blood glucose levels. The next part of the cycle is a period of binge eating, in which the person ingests huge amounts of food (about 3500 kcal) within a short time (about 1 hour). Binges can last up to 8 hours, with consumption of 12,000 kcal. Binge eating usually occurs when the person is alone and at home, and is most frequent during the evening. The cycle may occur once or twice a month for some and as often as five or ten times a day for others. The binge part of the cycle may be triggered by the ingestion of certain foods, but this is not consistent for everyone. Although eating binges may involve any kind of food, they usually consist of junk foods, fast foods, and high-calorie foods.

The final part of the cycle is purging the body of the ingested food. After excessive eating, people with bulimia force themselves to vomit. They often abuse laxatives and diuretics in an attempt to purge their bodies of the food. Some use as many as 50–100 laxatives per day. In rare cases, they may resort to syrup of ipecac to induce vomiting. After the purging, the cycle begins all over again, with a return to strict dieting or fasting. Binge eating and purging begin as a way to eat and stay slim. Before long, the behavior becomes a response to stress and a way to cope with negative feelings such as anger, anxiety, and depression. For some it is poor impulse control, and for others it is an expression of rebellion against family members.

People with bulimia may engage in sporadic excessive exercise, but they usually do not develop compulsive exercise routines. They are more likely to abuse street drugs to decrease their appetite and alcohol to reduce their anxiety. Since their binges are often expensive, costing as much as $100 per day, they may resort to stealing food or money to buy the food (Beumont, 1995). The binge/purge cycle can become so consuming that activities and relationships are disrupted. To keep the secret, the person often resorts to excuses and lies.

> Akera, 23 years old, is a senior nursing student whose bulimia has been carefully hidden from family, friends, and teachers for the past 3 years. During a typical day after school, she stops at the local grocery store to buy 2 pounds of cookies, which she consumes on the way to the ice cream store. There she buys a gallon of ice cream. She eats that quickly and continues on to a fast-food restaurant, where she has three cheeseburgers, fries, and two milkshakes. Before she goes home, she stops at the drugstore, buys a pack of gum, and steals a box of laxatives so the clerks won't suspect she has an eating disorder. As soon as Akera arrives home, she forces herself to vomit and then takes the entire package of laxatives. This cycle repeats itself at home during the evening, when she eats any available food.

Affective Characteristics

Anorexia

People with anorexia are often beset by fears. Some fear becoming mature and assuming adult responsibilities. Because of their need to please others with high levels of achievement, some fear they are not doing well enough. Almost all have an extreme terror of weight gain and fat. A paradoxical response occurs when this fear actually increases as body weight decreases. If weight gain (real or imagined) occurs, anxiety surfaces to the conscious level and is perceived as a threat to the entire being. Anorexic people also fear a loss of control. Although this fear is usually related to losing control over eating, it may extend to other physiological processes such as sleeping, urination, and bowel functioning. The steady loss of weight becomes symbolic of mastery over self and environment. However, if anorexic people lose control and eat more than they believe to be appropriate, they experience severe guilt (Beumont, 1995).

Bulimia

Because of their need for acceptance and approval, people with bulimia repress feelings of frustration and anger toward others. Repressing feelings and avoiding conflict protect them from rejection. As the ability to identify feelings decreases, they often confuse negative emotions with sensations of being hungry. Food then becomes a source of comfort and a way to defend against anger and frustration (Garfinkel, 1995).

Like people with anorexia, bulimic people experience multiple fears. They fear a loss of control, not only over their eating but also over their emotions. They are extremely fearful of weight gain and, with real or perceived changes in their weight, they feel panic. Motivating much of their behavior is fear of rejection (Silva, 1995).

The binge/purge cycle can be understood from the affective perspective as well as the behavioral perspective. Anxiety increases to a high level, at which point the person engages in binge eating to decrease the anxiety. Afterward, the person experiences guilt and self-disgust because of the loss of control. Guilt and disgust increase the anxiety, and purging, through vomiting and other methods, is then used to decrease this anxiety. Because this behavior is an indirect and ineffective way to manage anxiety, the levels rebuild, and the cycle starts anew. Some are able to talk about their feelings of helplessness, hopelessness, and worthlessness, while others do not seem to have the language to talk about their feelings.

> Andrea, a 19-year-old college student, lives at home with her parents and younger brother. She has just been admitted to the eating disorders unit. She states that the only reason she has been admitted is because "my mother says I'm not eating right. She has been on me forever. She told me if I didn't eat I would have to get out of the home. I came in here so she would leave me alone." Andrea is angry at her mother for treating her like a baby on the one hand and threatening her with abandonment on the other.

Cognitive Characteristics

Anorexia

The desire to be thin and the behavioral control over eating are ego-syntonic in the anorexic client. **Ego-syntonic behavior** is behavior that agrees with one's thoughts, desires, and values. Anorexic people regard their obsessions with food and eating as conventional behavior. The major defense mechanisms for defining the behavior in an ego-syntonic manner are denial of sensations of hunger, denial of physical exhaustion, and denial of any disorder or illness.

People with anorexia experience distortions in the thinking process that are similar to those experienced by sufferers of mental disorders. These cognitive distortions are considered errors in thinking that continue even when there is obvious contradictory evidence (Silva, 1995). These cognitive distortions involve food, body image, loss of control, and achievement. One type of distortion is **selective abstraction,** or focusing on certain information while ignoring contradictory information. Another distortion is **overgeneralization,** in which the person takes information or an impression from one event and attaches it to a wide variety of situations. Using such words as "always," "never," "everybody," and "nobody" indicates that the client is overgeneralizing. Anorexic people also have a tendency toward **magnification,** attributing a high level of importance to unpleasant occurrences. Through **personalization,** or **ideas of reference,** they believe that what occurs in the environment is related to them, even when no obvious relationship exists. There is also a tendency for **superstitious thinking,** in which the person believes that some unrelated action will magically influence a course of events. A further distortion is **dichotomous thinking,** an all-or-none type of reasoning that interferes with people's realistic perceptions of themselves. Dichotomous thinking involves opposite and mutually exclusive categories such as eating or not eating, all good or all bad, and celibacy or promiscuity. Table 10.1 gives examples of cognitive distortions.

> Rachael, 18, has been diagnosed with anorexia. She does not believe that her 5 ft 9 in frame is underweight at 102 pounds (46.3 kg). Rachael believes she will look better when she reaches 85 pounds (38.6 kg). She says that when she goes to college, she wants to be active in student government and that fat people are never elected. Her superstitious thinking relates to white clothing, which she feels decreases her hunger.

People suffering from anorexia experience a severely distorted body image that often reaches delusional proportions. Incapable of seeing that their bodies are emaciated, they continue to perceive themselves as fat. Some perceive their total body as obese, whereas others focus on a particular part of the body

Table 10.1 **Examples of Cognitive Distortions**

Distortion	Example
Selective abstraction	"I'm still too fat—look at how big my hands and feet are."
Overgeneralization	"You don't see fat people on television. Therefore, you have to be thin to be successful at anything in life."
Magnification	"If I gain 2 pounds, I know everyone will notice it."
Personalization	"Jim and Bob were talking and laughing together today. I'm sure they were talking about how fat I am."
Superstitious thinking	"If I wear all white, I'll lose weight faster." "Sitting still will cause my weight to go up rapidly."
Dichotomous thinking	"If I gain even 1 pound, that means I am totally out of control and I might as well gain 50 pounds." "If I eat one thing, I will just keep eating until I weigh 300 pounds." "If I'm not thin, I'm fat."

as fat, such as their hips, stomach, thighs, or face. While others see these people as starving and disappearing, they view themselves as strong and in the process of creating a whole new person. Anorexic individuals believe they are in charge of their lives and in complete control. The disorder becomes an issue of autonomy because no one can make them eat or make them gain weight.

They think of food not as a necessity for survival but as something that threatens survival. Cognitively, fat represents need and loss of control; thinness represents strength and control. These people are frequently secretive about their behavior. The secrecy is not viewed as manipulative but rather protective. From their point of view, anorexia is the solution, not the problem.

Anorexic people have distorted perceptions of internal physical sensations, a distortion referred to as *alexithymia*. Hunger is not recognized as hunger. When they eat a small amount of food, they often complain of feeling too full. There is also a decreased internal perception of fatigue, so they often push their bodies to physical extremes. Even after long and strenuous exercise, they seem unaware of any sensations of fatigue.

Young people with anorexia are overly concerned with how others view them. Many are convinced that other people have more insight into who they are than they do themselves. This self-depreciation and fear of self-definition contribute to beliefs and fears of being controlled by others. Feeling they have no power in their interpersonal relationships, they attempt to please and placate significant others whom they perceive to be more powerful.

People with anorexia develop perfectionistic standards for their behavior. They are in such dread of losing control that they impose extremes of discipline on themselves. During the times they are able to maintain control, their perfectionistic behavior and dichotomous thinking lead them to believe they are better than other people. However, these standards of behavior become self-defeating when the anorexic person fails to achieve them consistently.

While it is unclear whether anorexia is a type of obsessive-compulsive disorder, anorexic people typically exhibit obsessive-compulsive symptoms. They spend a great deal of time obsessing about their weight and their bodies. They are preoccupied with thinking about food. Often they develop complex rituals around food preparation, even though they refuse to eat the final product. Even after long-term weight recovery, their obsessions and compulsions continue (Thiel et al, 1995).

Bulimia

In contrast to people with anorexia, bulimic individuals are troubled by their behavioral characteristics. They experience **ego-dystonic behavior,** behavior that does not conform to the person's thoughts, wishes, and values. Another facet of ego-dystonic symptoms is that one feels the symptoms are beyond personal control. The person feels compelled to binge, purge, and fast; helpless to stop the behavior; and full of self-disgust for continuing the pattern.

Although bulimic people are not pleased with their body shape and size, they usually do not experi-

ence the delusional distortions of anorexic people. There is a direct correlation between the frequency and severity of the disorder and the degree of perceived distortion of body size. Many were overweight before the disorder, so there is an obsessional concern about not regaining the lost weight. It is difficult for them to think of anything other than food. Since they eat in response to hunger, appetite, and thoughts of food, the obsessions also involve getting rid of the food ingested in an effort to counteract the caloric effects of binge eating.

People with bulimia also experience the cognitive distortions discussed for anorexic people. They tend to relate their problems to weight or overeating. Their fantasy is that if they could only be thin and not overeat, all other problems would be solved. Another example of this all-or-none thinking is the belief that one bite will automatically lead to binge eating. The person may say, "As long as I have eaten one cookie, I have failed, so I might as well eat the entire package."

Bulimic people are perfectionistic in their personal standards of behavior. Even with their typically high level of professional achievement, they are extremely self-critical and often feel incompetent and inadequate. They set unrealistic standards of weight control and feel like failures when unable to maintain these standards. The thought of failure is a contributing factor to the binge phase of the cycle. Following the purge phase, they promise themselves to be more steadfast and disciplined with their diet. Because these resolutions are unrealistic, they set themselves up for another failure (Thiel et al, 1995).

Characteristics of people with anorexia and bulimia are listed in Table 10.2.

Social Characteristics

Women's bodies, much more so than men's, have always been perceived as unfinished and in need of revamping to make them conform to the cultural standards of beauty. From Chinese women with bound feet in the 12th and 13th centuries, to corsets in the 19th century, to binding breasts in the early 20th century, to today's lean and physically fit body, women have tried to change their bodies to "look good."

In American society, female attractiveness is strongly equated with thinness. Models, actresses, and the media glamorize extreme thinness, which is then equated with success and happiness. This cultural obsession for an extremely thin female body has led

◼ *Table 10.2* Characteristics of Eating Disorders

Characteristic	People with Anorexia	People with Bulimia
Self-evaluation	Are dependent on response from others; are self-depreciating.	Are self-critical; view themselves as incompetent.
Decision making	Need to make perfect decisions.	Need to make perfect decisions.
Rituals	Are obsessive in eating and exercise.	Perpetuate the binge/purge/fast cycle.
Sense of control	Create a sense of control and achievement by refusing to eat.	Set unrealistic standards for own behavior; feel out of control.
Phobia	Initially fear weight gain; develop food phobia.	None specific.
Exercise	Have obsessive routines.	Exercise sporadically.
Fears	Fear not being perfect, weight gain, fat, loss of control.	Fear loss of control, weight gain, rejection.
Guilt	Experience guilt when they eat more than they believe appropriate.	Experience guilt when they binge and purge.
Defense mechanisms	Deny hunger, exhaustion, disease.	Do not deny hunger.
Insight into illness	Are ego-syntonic; do not believe they have a disorder; see anorexia as the solution, not the problem.	Are ego-dystonic; are disgusted with self but helpless to change.
Cognitive distortions	Practice selective abstraction, overgeneralization, magnification, personalization, dichotomous thinking.	Practice selective abstraction, overgeneralization, magnification, personalization, dichotomous thinking.
Body image	Experience delusional distortion.	See themselves as slightly larger.
Relationships	Attempt to please and placate others.	Experience conflicts between dependency and autonomy.
Social isolation	Tend to isolate themselves to protect against rejection; tend to be more introverted.	Need privacy for binge eating and purging; tend to be extroverted.
Weight loss	Experience 25–50% weight loss.	Maintain normal weight or experience slight weight loss.
Death	Results usually from starvation, when body proteins are depleted to half the normal levels.	Often results from hypokalemia, a deficiency of potassium (leading cause), and suicide (second most frequent cause).

to widespread prejudice against overweight people. This prejudice has a significant impact on overall self-esteem and self-acceptance. Self-worth is enhanced for those who are judged attractive and diminished for those deemed unattractive. Box 10.1 lists the cultural values that are extremely harmful to all women, whether overweight, normal weight, or underweight (Fontaine, 1991; Wilfley and Rodin, 1995).

Magazines marketed for adolescent women often present diet and weight control as the solutions for adolescent crises and contain 90% more articles and advertisements promoting dieting as compared to magazines read by young men. Thus, the body

becomes the central focus of existence, and self-esteem becomes dependent on the ability to control weight and food intake. This preoccupation with body image continues throughout women's lives. In fact, dieting and concerns about weight have become so pervasive that they are now the norm for American women (Andersen, 1995; Sobal, 1995).

Fear of fat is a constant companion. Young girls are often rewarded for their attempts at weight control. Peers, family members, gym teachers, dance teachers, and others may actively support the attainment or maintenance of low body weight. Those who go on to develop eating disorders may have internal-

Box 10.1

Cultural Values Harmful to All Women

Thinness equals power and control, and fat equals helplessness and lack of self-control. Those who are fat are viewed as helpless people who are weak-willed, nonachieving, and out of control. What often goes unrecognized, however, is the fact that it's the compulsion for thinness that is out of control.

Thinness equals beauty, and fat equals ugliness. Thinness is the most important aspect of physical attractiveness, and fat women are considered to be sexually unattractive.

Thinness equals happiness, and fat equals unhappiness. The main determining factor of joy in life becomes tied to body size and shape. A slim body is seen as the only way to achieve a happy life.

Thinness equals goodness, and fat equals immorality. The message is that those who diet and are thin are good, whereas those who eat normally are fat and bad. Because fat is considered a moral issue, discrimination is accepted as an appropriate response.

Thinness equals fitness, and fat equals laziness. The fitness movement has perpetuated the glorification of thinness as the cultural ideal. Those people who are overweight or even normal weight are considered lazy and have only themselves to blame for their body size.

ized an exaggerated version of the cultural ideal, the basis of which is that women define their value and worth in terms of being attractive to and obtaining love from men. No wonder eating disorders occur when women have grown up in a culture that is fat phobic, where they may have been ridiculed for being overweight or may have participated in ridiculing others. Discovering that thin girls frequently have more friends, go on more dates, and receive higher grades in school, they believe they can win approval, parental love, and social recognition by a frantic pursuit of thinness (Fontaine, 1991).

Young women with anorexia usually find that severe dieting does not produce the reward of being sought after by young men. In response to this real or perceived rejection, they feel even more unattractive

and undesirable. To protect themselves, they begin to lose interest in social activities and withdraw from their peers. Dating is minimal or nonexistent, and they purport to have no interest in sexual activities. High scholastic achievement may be an attempt to compensate for the lack of peer relationships (Sobal, 1995).

In one study of 135 men with eating disorders, 27% identified themselves as gay or bisexual compared to 1–6% of the general male population. This data supports other surveys that have shown that homosexual men are more dissatisfied with their body weight and shape than heterosexual men and that they consider their physical appearance to be more important to their sense of self (Carlat, Camargo, and Herzog, 1997).

People with bulimia experience shame and guilt about their behavior and may withdraw socially to hide it. They also need privacy for binge eating and purging, which contributes further to their isolation. The more isolated they become, the more the behavior tends to escalate, as food is used to fill the void and provide a source of comfort. Generally, they do not become as socially isolated as those with anorexia. Although they are sexually active, they have difficulty enjoying sex because of fears relating to loss of control. Feeling inadequate and incompetent, they may fear the intimacy of a long-term relationship.

Culture-Specific Characteristics

There is considerable evidence that eating disorders occur predominately in industrialized, developed countries and that they are uncommon outside the Western world. Thus, anorexia and bulimia could be considered to be culture-reactive syndromes.

A surprising influence in a girl's vulnerability may be her ethnic background. Recent studies have found, for instance, that African American women's perceptions of beauty are less media-driven than those of European American women. Dieting is less rampant, and African American teens may be more accepting of the way they look. This physical acceptance may stem from a strong identification with their culture. Eating disorders are probably more prevalent in Mexican American women than originally thought. Mexican American media are currently presenting thin ideal body sizes for women, similar to those presented in the Anglo media (Joiner and Kashubeck, 1996; Wilfley and Rodin, 1995).

Women in other cultures experience behaviors and symptoms that superficially appear to be similar but may not be identical in the causes or meanings of the disorder. Arab women in Quatar experience a culture-bound syndrome characterized by nausea, poor appetite, breathing difficulty, palpitations, faintness, and fatigue. The majority of these victims are either unmarried or have fertility problems. The disorder is rooted in the cultural belief that the value of women is based on their husbands and the children they have. As women become more educated and are exposed to Western media, they discover the different female/male relationships of more developed nations. Thus they find themselves caught between traditional cultural values and new values and role expectations. Women in Zar cults in North Africa and parts of Asia experience a culture-bound syndrome called "Zars," which is the possession by spirits. Symptoms include anorexia, nausea, depression, anxiety, headaches, and fertility problems (Silverstein and Perlick, 1995).

Physiological Characteristics

There are many physiological effects of starvation and purging of the body. Electrolyte imbalance may cause muscle weakness, seizures, arrhythmias, and even death, with hypokalemia being the most critical electrolyte abnormality. There are several ways hypokalemia develops. With vomiting, there is some loss of potassium itself. Perhaps more important is metabolic alkalosis, which results from the loss of stomach acid through vomiting. This, in turn, causes a shift of potassium from the extracellular space into the cells, thereby lowering the serum potassium level. In addition, laxative abuse causes loss of potassium through the lower GI system (Greenfeld et al, 1995).

Decreased blood volume results in lowered blood pressure and postural hypotension. Lessened sympathetic nervous system activity is reflected in symptoms such as hypotension, bradycardia, and hypothermia. Elevated blood urea nitrogen (BUN) indicates decreased blood flow to the kidneys, which predisposes these individuals to edema (Beumont, 1995).

Gastrointestinal complications such as constipation, cathartic colon, and laxative dependence may develop. When food is in short supply, gastric emptying slows to improve the efficiency of nutrient absorption. This also delays the expenditure of energy required for digestion, absorption, and storage (Robinson and McHugh, 1995). Frequent vomiting can lead to esophagitis, with scarring and stricture. If perforation or rupture of the esophagus occurs, there is a 20% mortality rate even with immediate treatment. Gastric rupture, fortunately a fairly rare occurrence, carries a mortality rate of 85%. Repeated vomiting decreases tooth enamel, causing dental caries and tooth loss. There may be a chronic sore throat, and salivary glands are usually swollen and tender. Some people with bulimia may demonstrate **Russell's sign,** a callus on the back of the hand, formed by repeated trauma from the teeth when forcing vomiting. Amenorrhea is an extremely common occurrence in females with anorexia, and irregular menses are frequently associated with bulimia. Although the exact mechanism is unclear, menstrual problems are thought to be related to the degree of stress the person is experiencing, the percentage of body fat lost, and altered hypothalamic function. There are also abnormalities in the secretion of luteinizing hormone and follicle-stimulating hormone, resulting in low estrogen and progesterone levels. With low estrogen levels, these young women are at higher risk for osteoporosis. In a similar fashion, testosterone levels drop in male sufferers. In an adaptive effort to limit energy expenditure and conserve protein, thyroid hormone levels drop (Fichter and Pirke, 1995).

People with anorexia usually experience a weight loss of 25%, but a loss as high as 50% is possible. People with bulimia do not reach such low levels of weight and may, in fact, remain at normal weight. Since a large food intake speeds up the gastric emptying rate, a significant number of calories are absorbed before the purging begins.

The physiological effects of malnutrition and vomiting are widespread throughout the body. In some cases, death occurs as a result of these disruptions.

Concomitant Disorders

The most frequently observed disorder is depression. In some cases this may be the result of abnormal eating and weight loss. In other cases, the depression is the primary disorder to which the eating disorder is a response. And for other people, the depression and eating disorder are both primary disorders (McGown and Whitbread, 1996).

Social phobias may occur in people with eating disorders, possibly in response to others' awareness of their abnormal eating behaviors. Obsessive-compulsive symptoms are common, especially among people with anorexia. Panic attacks are likely when anorexic people are prohibited from exercising their usual behavior patterns. It is unclear whether these are primary disorders or are secondary to the eating disorders. Eating-disordered people often abuse substances. In some, this may be an effort to self-medicate the symptoms of anxiety or depression. Others may abuse substances in an effort to decrease their appetite (Halmi, 1995; Schuckit et al, 1996).

Eating disorders share many features with problem drinking. Both begin with a decrease in anxiety in response to the behavior (drinking or not eating). Eventually both groups of people lose control over the behavior and continue on a path of self-destruction. There is a compulsive need to engage in the behavior with considerable distress if the behavior is disrupted. Denial is the central defense mechanism of both disorders, and both have a chronic course with frequent relapses (Halmi, 1995).

Causative Theories

The causes of eating disorders are multiple, in individuals and across a variety of people. Fatness and thinness are outcomes of biological, psychological, and social processes. Weight is determined by the balance between energy intake and expenditure and this balance is the product of many influences. Having a knowledge base about the major theories will help you understand individual clients from a composite perspective.

Neurobiological Theory

Recent studies indicate that neurotransmitter dysregulation may be involved in eating disorders, particularly serotonin (5-HT). Being full of food to the point of satisfaction is referred to as satiety. Normally, a low level of 5-HT decreases a person's satiety and thereby increases food intake. In contrast, a high level of 5-HT increases satiety and thereby decreases food intake. Carbohydrates (CHO) are involved in the synthesis of 5-HT by increasing tryptophan, the precursor of 5-HT. The neurotransmitter hypothesis of bulimia is that the recurrent binge episodes may result from a deficiency in 5-HT and low satiety levels. Since people with bulimia tend to binge on high-CHO foods, this may be a reflection of the body's adaptive attempt to increase 5-HT levels. The neurotransmitter hypothesis of anorexia is that decreased food intake is related to excess 5-HT and increased satiety (Hedaya, 1996). A comparison of the neurotransmitter hypothesis for anorexia and bulimia is shown in Figure 10.1.

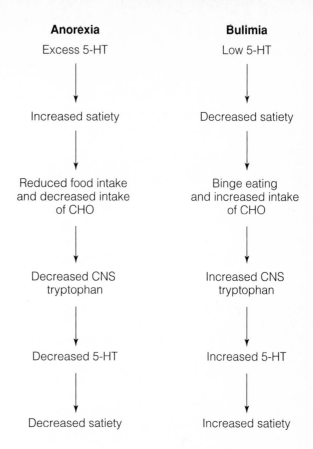

Figure 10.1 **The neurotransmitter hypothesis for eating disorders.**

Endogenous opioids, such as endorphins, are associated with food intake and mood. Opioids increase food intake and enhance positive mood states; therefore, insufficient levels cause decreased food intake and depressed mood. It has been found that underweight people have significantly lower levels of endorphins compared to healthy volunteers. When the person's weight is returned to normal levels, the endorphin level is also within normal limits (Kaye, 1995).

Family risk studies demonstrate that relatives of eating-disordered clients are four to five times more likely to develop an eating disorder. Twin studies show that the concordance rate for monozygotic twins is 47–56% and for dizygotic twins, 7–10%. These data suggest that there may be a genetic predisposition to eating disorders (Treasure and Holland, 1995).

Intrapersonal Theory

Intrapersonal theorists believe that girls at higher risk for eating disorders are those who have low self-esteem, experience significant adolescent turmoil, and are having difficulty with identity formation. Personality characteristics of people with anorexia are anxiety intolerance, a lack of personal effectiveness and self-direction, and difficulty achieving the maturational tasks of adolescence. People with bulimia are described in terms of affective instability and poor impulse control.

Motivation for losing weight is viewed in terms of how the person sees herself relating to others. For some, the motivation is an attempt to create closeness by gaining attention from parents, siblings, and friends. Others are motivated to create distance by avoiding identification with a disliked parent. The third possible motive is deliberate action against people, using eating behavior to express anger and control parental behavior. The intense concern over food says, "This is an area in which I am in control and can defy the demands of others," while at the same time saying, "I am only a little child who has to be looked after" (Dare and Crowther, 1995).

Cognitive Theory

Cognitive theorists believe that cognitive distortions and dysfunctional thoughts such as dichotomous thinking and catastrophizing (exaggerating failures in one's life) contribute to disordered eating patterns. The extreme belief is: "It is absolutely essential that I be thin." This belief leads to dieting, avoidant behavior, and increased isolation, which in turn cause a lack of responsiveness to alternative cognitive input. Given the cultural emphasis on thinness, there is a sense of gratification, self-control, mastery, and approval of or concern from others (DeSilva, 1995).

Behavioral Theory

Behavioral theorists are concerned with what the disordered behavior accomplishes rather than why the behavior occurs. Eating disorders are considered phobias. In this context, anxiety rises with eating and decreases with fasting or purging. Anxiety reduction is the reinforcer for both anorexia and bulimia (DeSilva, 1995).

Family Theory

Most family theorists believe family issues are not specific to eating disorders. The family is viewed more as an enabler of the disorder than as a primary causative factor. Some eating-disordered people are survivors of childhood or adolescent sexual abuse, which may or may not have occurred within the family or extended family system (Rorty, Yager, and Rossotto, 1994). (Sexual abuse is discussed further in Chapter 19.)

Some families of people with anorexia are enmeshed; that is, the boundaries between the members are weak, interactions are intense, dependency on one another is high, and autonomy is minimal. Everybody is involved in each member's concerns; within the family, there is a great deal of togetherness and minimal privacy. The enmeshed family system becomes overprotective of the children, possibly resulting in an intense focus on the children's bodily functions. In contrast, current research indicates that families of people with bulimia are less enmeshed than those of anorexic people. Family members tend to be isolated from one another, and eating behavior may be an attempt to decrease feelings of loneliness and boredom (Eisler, 1995). Many families of those with eating disorders have difficulty with conflict resolution. An ethical or religious value against disagreements within the family supports the avoidance of conflict. When problems are denied for the sake of family harmony, they cannot be resolved, and growth of the family system is inhibited. The anorexic child often protects and maintains the family unit. In some family systems, the parents avoid conflict with each other by uniting in a common concern for the child's welfare. In other family systems, the issues of marital conflict are converted into disagreements over how the anorexic child should be managed. In both systems, the marital problems are camouflaged in an effort to prevent the disruption of the family unit. See Chapter 2 for more details.

Many families of clients with eating disorders are achievement- and performance-oriented, with high ambitions for the success of all members. In these families, body shape is related to success, and priorities are established for physical appearance and fitness. The family's focus on professional achievement as well as on food, diet, exercise, and weight control may be obsessional (Eisler, 1995).

Feminist Theory

From the feminist perspective, eating disorders arise out of a conflict between female development and traditional developmental theories. Western culture has viewed male development as the norm, and autonomy as the opposite of dependency. For women, the opposite of dependency is isolation. Conflict arises when women believe they must become autonomous and minimize relationships in order to be recognized as mature adults. For some, this conflict is acted out in self-destructive eating behavior (Striegel-Moore, 1995).

Cultural stereotypes contribute to women's preoccupation with their bodies. Attractiveness is determined by how closely a woman's appearance matches the cultural ideal of thinness. Thus, identity and self-esteem are dependent on physical appearance. Being disgusted with one's flesh is the same as having an adversarial relationship with the body—a relationship that often results in eating disorders.

Psychopharmacological Interventions

A number of medications are being tested for clients with eating disorders. So far, they seem to be more effective in treating bulimia than anorexia. The tricyclic antidepressant Tofranil (imipramine) produces a 70% decrease in the frequency of binge eating and reduces the preoccupation with food, as well as anxiety and depressive symptoms. Another tricyclic antidepressant, Norpramine (desipramine), appears to decrease binge eating in those who do not have current symptoms of depression. Tricyclic antidepressants are started at very low doses (10–25 mg/day) and over a period of 3–4 weeks are increased to 3 mg/kg of body weight. Prozac (fluoxetine), an SSRI, is also effective for these clients, when given at the higher dose of 60 mg per day. Typically, the medication is continued until 6 months following the disappearance of symptoms. In some studies, lithium has been used alone or in conjunction with tricyclic antidepressants. Caution must be taken when prescribing lithium for a client who is purging, however. Vomiting will decrease intracellular potassium, and lithium may exacerbate this effect (McGown and Whitbread, 1996; Wolfe, 1995).

Multidisciplinary Interventions

Treatment of clients with eating disorders must have a multidisciplinary approach. Medical treatment may include a feeding schedule, appetite stimulants, potassium supplements, and bed rest. Tube feeding and parenteral nutrition are avoided unless absolutely necessary because they do not help clients assume responsibility for their own health. Psychological treatment may include individual therapy, group work, family therapy, cognitive therapy, and systematic desensitization. The majority of centers that treat clients with eating disorders use behavior modification to change the disordered eating pattern.

The Nursing Process

Assessment

A focused nursing assessment, which includes a physiological assessment, must be taken for clients with eating disorders. (See the Focused Nursing Assessment table.) You must be on the alert for medical emergencies such as acute cardiac failure, acute gastric dilatation, esophageal bleeding, and massive peripheral edema.

Clients with bulimia may welcome the opportunity to talk about their disorder with a caring, nonjudgmental nurse. Moreover, learning that they are not alone in having bulimia may relieve some of their anxiety and distress. Clients with anorexia, on the other hand, may not be as willing to talk about their disorder. Client denial of problems or illness may interfere with your ability to obtain an accurate nursing assessment. A supportive and caring approach is necessary to establish rapport with these clients.

In general, nursing assessment includes: a detailed analysis of eating patterns and weight fluctuations, methods of weight control, food avoided and the reasons they are avoided, and the occurrence of binge eating and purging. In addition, you explore the individual's and family's beliefs about nutrition and attitudes toward eating.

Diagnosis

After analyzing and synthesizing the client assessment data, you develop nursing diagnoses. The client's level of malnourishment must be identified because, in some cases, death could be imminent. The client's binge eating and/or purging patterns must be identified, as well as their fears, their cognitive distortions, and their relationships with family and friends. For nursing diagnoses for clients with eating disorders, see the Nursing Diagnoses box on page 220.

Text continues on page 220

Focused Nursing Assessment

CLIENTS WITH EATING DISORDERS

Behavior Assessment

What type of eating patterns do you have?

Do you have rules for eating, such as places to eat? Combination of foods? Number of pieces of food? Number of times to chew food?

What time of day do you usually binge? Where do you do this? How often? How long does it last? Foods that trigger a binge? Favorite foods to eat on a binge?

After binge eating, how do you rid your body of the food? Vomit? Laxatives? Diuretics?

How much time do you spend exercising each day?

How does the use of alcohol or drugs help you cope with your problems?

Affective Assessment

Describe any of the following fears: gaining weight, being fat, rejection by others, losing control over eating.

What kinds of situations make you feel guilty? Ashamed? Anxious? Frustrated? Helpless?

What are your feelings when you eat more than your diet allows?

Cognitive Assessment

Do you believe your eating pattern is in any way unusual?

Do you have any desire to alter your eating behavior?

Describe your body to me.

Describe what an attractive person looks like.

What would your life be like if you were as thin as you wished?

What will happen if you gain weight?

Social Assessment

How often do you socialize with friends? What activities do you do together?

How close are the members of your family?

What are the family rules about disagreements?

Describe your family's standards for physical fitness and appearance.

How do other members of the family control their weight?

Physiological Assessment

Weight

What is your present weight?

What is the most you have ever weighed?

What is the least you have ever weighed?

Endocrine

Are you having menstrual periods?

Describe your usual cycle to me.

Cardiovascular

Do you get dizzy when you stand up from a lying position?

Have you experienced any heart palpitations? Irregular heartbeat?

Are you having any problems with your ankles and feet swelling? Your fingers?

Gastrointestinal

Have you had an increase in the number of dental caries?

Have you lost any teeth?

Do you have frequent sore throats?

Do you experience heartburn?

Do you have problems with constipation?

Neurological

Have you experienced any seizures or convulsions?

Nursing Diagnoses

Clients with Eating Disorders

Alteration in nutrition: less than body requirements related to reduced intake; purging.

Anxiety related to fears of gaining weight and losing control.

Alteration in thought process related to dichotomous thinking, overgeneralization, personalization, obsessions, and superstitious thinking.

Body image disturbance related to delusional perception of body in anorexia.

Impaired social interaction related to withdrawal from peer group and fears of rejection.

Potential for injury related to excessive exercise.

Powerlessness related to having no control over bulimic pattern.

Outcome Identification

Once you have established diagnoses, you and the client mutually identify goals for change. Client outcomes are specific behavioral measures by which you, clients, and significant others determine progress toward goals. The following are examples of some of the outcomes appropriate to people with eating disorders:

- verbalizes decreased need to please others
- demonstrates more flexible daily routines
- exercises appropriately
- decreases frequency of binge eating and purging
- verbalizes fewer fears
- achieves target weight
- identifies secondary gains
- verbalizes fewer cognitive distortions
- family problem-solves together

See also the Critical Pathway for a Client with Anorexia Nervosa on pages 222–226.

Nursing Interventions

Most clients will be seen in an outpatient setting. Inpatient care is necessary when clients are in life-threatening circumstances related to starvation, are at risk for suicide, or are experiencing extreme social isolation. It is a challenge to develop a therapeutic alliance with eating-disordered clients. They often resist interventions and are angry about being in treatment. You should use a kind, firm, and consistent approach and work toward a collaborative relationship. It is sometimes difficult to maintain the balance between setting clear limits on behaviors and helping these clients grow in autonomy. The ultimate goal is to have them take responsibility for their own behavior. See the nursing interventions classification (NIC) box for clients with eating disorders.

Physiological: Basic: Nutritional Support

Eating Disorders Management

People with anorexia or bulimia have multiple anxieties, most of which get translated into fears of weight gain and loss of control. Help them identify underlying fears, such as a fear of rejection, that have been transformed into a fear of gaining weight. Those with bulimia typically confuse negative emotions as sensations of hunger and binge eat as a source of comfort. Help them label a variety of negative feelings and begin to distinguish these from hunger pangs. The fear of weight gain can be all-consuming. The term "weight restoration" may be more acceptable because the term "weight gain" often creates an instant phobic response. Provide repeated assurance that they will not be allowed to become fat.

It is important that a target weight be identified. This is usually set at 90% of the average weight for the person's age and height. Identifying a reasonable target weight reassures clients that they will not be forced to become overweight. It is best to choose a weight range of 4–6 pounds rather than a single target weight, since this helps clients learn to accept a certain amount of normal weight fluctuation. Clients should only be weighed once or twice a week to decrease the amount of time spent in obsessing about weight. Be alert to techniques of artificially increasing weight, such as concealing heavy objects in clothing or drinking large amounts of water.

$\mathcal{N}$*ursing* $\mathcal{I}$*nterventions* $\mathcal{C}$*lassification*

CLIENTS WITH EATING DISORDERS

DOMAIN: Physiological: Basic

Class: *Nutrition Support*

> **Interventions:** *Eating Disorders Management:* Prevention and treatment of severe diet restriction and overexercising or binge eating and purging of food and fluids

DOMAIN: Behavioral

Class: *Cognitive Therapy*

> **Interventions:** *Cognitive Restructuring:* Challenging a patient to alter distorted thought patterns and view self and the world more realistically

DOMAIN: Family

Class: *Life Span Care*

> **Interventions:** *Family Involvement:* Facilitating family participation in the emotional and physical care of the patient

Source: McCloskey and Bulechek, 1996.

Negotiate with clients a reasonable contract that states how much to eat for each meal and snack. The contract usually begins with a moderate amount, such as 1000–1500 kcal per day, which is gradually increased. Begin with a diet low in fats and milk products, since starvation has led to an insufficiency of the bowel enzymes necessary for digestion of these foods. The sensation of bloating may lessen if the calories are spread across six meals a day. A food diary is often helpful to both clients and staff. Clients are to keep the diary with them at all times and record all food eaten as well as any binge eating and purging. They are also to include notation of their thoughts and feelings associated with eating or not eating.

There are a number of ways you can assist people to decrease binge eating. Talk over the difference between emotions and sensations of hunger, since misinterpretation of emotions contributes to binge eating. Through the food diary, have them analyze which particular foods trigger binge eating. Review situations that precede binge eating, and explore alternative coping behaviors. Insight into high-risk situations will help clients gain control of binges. Encourage delay in responding to the urge to binge by trying alternative behaviors such as talking to a teacher or counselor, calling a friend, or using relaxation techniques. The delay interrupts the habitual cycle of behavior. Confer with clients on ways to avoid privacy at the usual time of binges, since most binge eating occurs in isolation. Being with other people decreases opportunities to binge eat. Other methods of inhibiting binge eating behavior include avoiding fast-food restaurants, formulating a list of "safe" foods, and shopping for food with a friend. Teach clients to eat three to six meals a day, since this interrupts the fasting part of the cycle. They should include a carbohydrate at each meal, since deprivation may trigger binge eating.

Another client goal is to discontinue purging activities. Discuss how purging is used to manage negative feelings. When they make the connection between purging and anxiety, guilt, and self-disgust, they may be able to identify healthier behaviors. Clients who typically purge after meals are not allowed to use the bathroom unsupervised for 2 hours after eating. Since anxiety often escalates in relation to eating and the prevention of purging, one-to-one support is often necessary before, during, and after meals. Clients are encouraged to talk to staff, parents, friends when they feel the urge to vomit and thus increase their control over impulsive behavior.

Text continues on page 226

Critical Pathway for a Client with Anorexia Nervosa

Expected length of stay 24–32 days	Date _____ Days 1–3	Date _____ Days 4–7	Date _____ Days 8–14
Daily outcomes	Client will: ■ Remain free of malnutrition, infection, electrolyte and cardiac abnormalities. ■ Identify initial goals for hospitalization. ■ Remain oriented to time, place, and person with prompting. ■ Participate in assessment. ■ Identify current dietary pattern and food preferences. ■ Identify current elimination pattern. ■ Identify current self-care patterns, including sleep, physical activity, and hygiene. ■ Remain free of dehydration. ■ Maintain oral intake of 1000 cc/day. ■ Ingest food provided as per contract. ■ Remain free of self-induced vomiting.	Client will: ■ Remain free of malnutrition, infection, electrolyte and cardiac abnormalities. ■ Participate in development of transdisciplinary treatment plan. ■ Participate in menu plan for balanced meal. ■ Remain free of dehydration evidenced by moist mucous membranes and urine output > 30 cc/hr. ■ Maintain oral intake of 1000 cc/day. ■ Ingest food provided as per contract. ■ Gain 1/2 lb each day. ■ Remain free of self-induced vomiting.	Client will: ■ Remain free of malnutrition, infection, electrolyte and cardiac abnormalities. ■ Identify two positive attributes of self. ■ Participate in transdisciplinary plan. ■ Remain oriented to time, place, and person. ■ Consume diet as per menu plan. ■ Remain free of dehydration evidenced by moist mucous membranes and urine output > 30 cc/hr. ■ Maintain oral intake of 1200 cc/day. ■ Ingest food provided as per contract. ■ Make dietary choices consistent with a well-balanced diet. ■ Gain 1/2 lb each day. ■ Remain free of self-induced vomiting.
Assessments, tests, and treatments	Complete psychosocial assessment to include mental status, mood, affect, behavior, and communication q shift and PRN. Contract for safety. Observe for safety per protocol. Complete nursing database assessment. Weight. CBC, urinalysis. Chemistry profile. Thyroid profile. EKG. Other laboratory studies as ordered. Vital signs BID.	Psychosocial assessment q shift and PRN. Observe for safety per protocol. Monitor dietary intake, sleep pattern, and bowel elimination pattern. Monitor effects of and compliance with medications. Routine vital signs.	Daily psychosocial assessment. Observe for safety per protocol. Monitor dietary intake, sleep pattern, and bowel elimination pattern. Monitor effects of and compliance with medications. Routine vital signs. Repeat laboratory studies if indicated.
Knowledge deficit	Orient client and family to clients, staff, and program. Review initial plan of care. Assess learning needs of client and family.	Review unit orientation with emphasis on program. Reinforce behavior-modification program.	Review plan of care. Include family in teaching. Continue behavior-modification program.

	Date _____ Days 1–3 *continued*	Date _____ Days 4–7 *continued*	Date _____ Days 8–14 *continued*
Knowledge deficit *continued*	Instruct client and family regarding behavior-modification program. Assess understanding of teaching.	Assess understanding of teaching.	Assess understanding of teaching.
Diet	Nutritional assessment. Dietary consultation. Monitor dietary intake. Diet as tolerated; encourage small, frequent feedings from all food groups. Provide preferred snacks and foods. Encourage fluids. Provide pleasant mealtime environment.	Monitor dietary intake. Diet per menu plan. Encourage fluids; encourage small, frequent feedings from all food groups. Provide preferred snacks and foods. Provide pleasant mealtime environment.	Monitor dietary intake. Diet per menu plan; encourage small, frequent feedings from all food groups. Provide preferred snacks and foods. Provide pleasant mealtime environment.
Activity	Assess safety needs and maintain appropriate precautions. Encourage brief periods of activity and interaction. Engage client in identifying reasonable activity/exercise plan.	Maintain safety precautions. Encourage activities during the day. Client will participate in exercise program of moderate intensity and duration.	Maintain safety precautions. Encourage involvement in 50–75% of activities. Client will participate in exercise program of moderate intensity and duration.
Psychosocial	Observe behavior. Assess level of anxiety. Encourage verbalization of feelings and thoughts. Listen attentively, giving adequate time to respond. Approach with nonjudgmental and accepting, calm, matter-of-fact attitude and positive expectation. Formulate initial plan of care with client and family. Identify current support system. Provide information regarding illness and treatment. Provide ongoing support and encouragement to client and family. Meet with client 4 times each shift for 5–10 min periods focused on establishing relationship.	Observe behavior Assess level of anxiety. Encourage verbalization of concerns and feelings. Approach with nonjudgmental and accepting, calm, matter-of-fact attitude and positive expectation. Provide information and ongoing support and encouragement to client and family. Provide simple structured activities. Identify potential support system and strategies to access additional supports. Prompt to attend group therapy. Acknowledge accomplishments. Meet with client 10–15 min twice a shift during waking hours and focus on working on initial goals. Avoid discussion of food and eating habits. Discuss problem-solving strategies.	Observe behavior. Assess level of anxiety. Encourage verbalization of concerns and feelings. Approach with nonjudgmental and accepting, calm, matter-of-fact attitude and positive expectation. Provide information and ongoing support and encouragement to client and family. Review strategies to access support system using problem-solving strategies. Attend group therapy independently with spontaneous involvement × 1. Acknowledge accomplishments. Meet with client 15 min every shift during waking hours to work on therapeutic goals. Explore effective coping strategies. Explore fears related to sexuality and weight gain. Practice problem-solving strategies.

continued ➤

Critical Pathway for a Client with Anorexia Nervosa *continued*

	Date _____ Days 1–3 *continued*	Date _____ Days 4–7 *continued*	Date _____ Days 8–14 *continued*
Medications	Routine meds as ordered.	Routine meds as ordered.	Routine meds as ordered.
Referrals and discharge plan	Family assessment. Establish discharge objectives with client and family.	Review discharge objectives with client and significant others. Initiate referrals for discharge care.	Review progress toward discharge objectives with client and significant others. Make appropriate referrals to support groups.

	Date _____ Days 15–21	Date _____ Days 22–26	Date _____ Days 27–Discharge Day
Daily outcomes	Client will: ▪ Remain free of malnutrition, infection, electrolyte and cardiac abnormalities. ▪ Communicate feelings spontaneously and appropriately in 1:1 and group activities. ▪ Identify method in which strengths can be used to improve coping skills. ▪ Participate in transdisciplinary plan. ▪ Begin to explore issues of body image and self-esteem. ▪ Maintain oral intake of 1,200 cc/day. ▪ Ingest food provided as per contract. ▪ Make dietary choices consistent with a well-balanced diet. ▪ Begin to verbalize accurate assessment of body size and nutritional needs.	Client will: ▪ Remain free of malnutrition, infection, electrolyte and cardiac abnormalities. ▪ Communicate feelings spontaneously and appropriately. ▪ Spontaneously and appropriately participate in 1:1 and group activities. ▪ Identify methods in which strengths can be used to improve coping skills. ▪ Verbalize plan to use strengths to enhance coping skills. ▪ Participate in transdisciplinary plan. ▪ Realistically discuss issues related to body image and self-esteem. ▪ Maintain oral intake of 1,200 cc/day. ▪ Ingest food provided as per contract. ▪ Make dietary choices consistent with a well-balanced diet. ▪ Continue to verbalize accurate assessment of body size and nutritional needs. ▪ Participate in discharge planning.	Client remains free of malnutrition, infection, electrolyte and cardiac abnormalities. Client expresses a positive self-perception and self-esteem. Client expresses less anxiety about weight gain. Client verbalizes accurate assessment of body size and nutritional needs. Client communicates feelings honestly and openly. Client participates in activities that promote physical health. Client develops sustaining relationships with friends and family members. Client verbalizes/demonstrates home care instructions including the importance of ongoing mental health care. Client demonstrates ability to adaptively cope with ongoing stressors. Client verbalizes positive attributes regarding self. Client accepts positive feedback.

	Date _____ Days 15–21 *continued*	Date _____ Days 22–26 *continued*	Date _____ Days 27–Discharge *continued*
Assessments, tests, and treatments	Daily psychosocial assessment. Observe for safety. Monitor dietary intake, sleep pattern, and bowel elimination pattern. Weigh. Monitor effects of and compliance with medications. Routine vital signs.	Daily psychosocial assessment. Observe for safety. Monitor dietary intake, sleep pattern, and bowel elimination pattern. Monitor effects of and compliance with medications.	Psychosocial assessment. Monitor dietary intake, sleep pattern, and bowel elimination pattern. Monitor effects of and compliance with medications.
Knowledge deficit	Review plan of care. Include family in teaching. Initiate teaching regarding coping strategies utilizing client strengths. Review current level of knowledge regarding medications, treatments, symptom management, and follow-up care. Assess understanding of teaching.	Review plan of care with client and family. Reinforce current level of knowledge regarding medications, treatments, symptom management, and follow-up care. Assess understanding of teaching.	Client and/or significant other verbalizes understanding of discharge teaching including activity level and exercise program, safety measures, diet, signs and symptoms to report, follow-up care, and MD appointment, medications: name, purpose, dose, frequency, route, dietary interactions, and side effects, and follow-up care arrangements. Assess understanding of teaching. Make referrals to community caregivers for any knowledge deficits regarding medications, treatments, symptoms management, and follow-up care.
Diet	Diet as tolerated; encourage small, frequent feedings from all food groups. Encourage fluids. Provide preferred snacks and foods. Provide adequate time for meals and snacks. Monitor dietary intake. Provide pleasant mealtime environment.	Diet as tolerated; encourage small, frequent feedings from all food groups. Encourage fluids. Provide preferred snacks and foods. Provide adequate time for meals and snacks. Monitor dietary intake. Provide pleasant mealtime environment.	Diet as tolerated; encourage small, frequent feedings from all food groups. Encourage fluids. Provide preferred snacks and foods. Provide adequate time for meals and snacks. Monitor dietary intake. Provide pleasant mealtime environment.
Activity	Maintain safety precautions. Encourage involvement in 75–100% of activities. Engage client and family in identifying reasonable activity plan following discharge. Client will participate in exercise program of moderate intensity and duration.	Maintain safety precautions. Encourage involvement in 100% of activities. Client will participate in exercise program of moderate intensity and duration.	Maintain safety precautions. Client is independently involved in 100% of activities. Client will participate in exercise program of moderate intensity and duration.

continued ➤

Critical Pathway for a Client with Anorexia Nervosa *continued*

	Date _____ Days 15–21 *continued*	Date _____ Days 22–26 *continued*	Date _____ Days 27–Discharge *continued*
Psychosocial	Assess level of anxiety. Support client in implementing stress-and anxiety-reducing strategies. Provide information and ongoing support and encouragement to client and family. Attend scheduled group therapy sessions independently. Reinforce skills learned in group therapy. Identify progress with cognitive restructuring and reinforce learning. Acknowledge accomplishments. Encourage verbalization of feelings and concerns. Meet with client 15 min every shift during waking hours to discuss progress in terms of therapeutic goals. Encourage client to discuss body image and self-esteem as well as role in family. Encourage client to acknowledge accomplishments. Provide ongoing support and encouragement to client and family.	Assess level of anxiety. Reinforce stress- and anxiety-reduction strategies. Encourage verbalization of concerns and feelings. Provide information and ongoing support and encouragement to client and family. Attend group therapy independently. Provide specific, realistic feedback. Encourage constructive expression of feelings. Provide ongoing support and encouragement to client and family. Meet with client 15 min every shift during waking hours to discuss progress in terms of therapeutic goals. Encourage client to discuss relationship to others in family. Encourage realistic discussion of body image. Encourage client to acknowledge accomplishments.	Assess level of anxiety. Reinforce stress- and anxiety-reduction strategies. Encourage verbalization of concerns and feelings. Provide information and ongoing support and encouragement to client and family. Client will attend group therapy independently. Meet with client 15 min every shift during waking hours to discuss progress in terms of therapeutic goals. Acknowledge accomplishments. Provide ongoing support and encouragement to client and family.
Medications	Routine meds as ordered.	Routine meds as ordered.	Routine meds as ordered.
Consults and discharge plan	Review discharge objectives with client and family.	Review discharge objectives with client and significant others. Complete referrals for discharge care.	Refer to support group and ongoing mental health care. Review need for any discharge referrals. Discharge with referrals.

Behavioral: Cognitive Therapy

Cognitive Restructuring

Suggest that clients write a list of the pros and cons of their eating disorder. Often they have been warned of the dangers of their disorder but have never identified the benefits. Treatment will not be successful if they do not compensate for the loss of these benefits. To this end, you should help clients identify secondary gains, that is, the ultimate purpose the disorder serves. There are many possible purposes, and accurate identification will lead to effective interventions. For some, the purpose is the attainment of the ideal body, with thoughts that this will protect them from all future pain. For others, eating disorders are a way of gaining a sense of control, as well as individuating and separating from parents. Eating disorders may develop in response to competition with siblings for parental attention. For some, it is a response to depressive feelings. Superimposed on the teenage crisis of identity, eating disorders may represent a regression to a younger and safer time in life. To plan nursing interventions that will help these clients meet their needs in constructive and healthy ways, it is vital that secondary gains of the disorder be identified.

If the secondary gain of the eating disorder is a sense of being in control of oneself, point out to clients that the binge/purge cycle that began as a method of control is now *out of control*. As clients develop insight into the paradox of the behavior, they can begin to explore alternative behaviors for maintaining control. As they learn to identify their own pleasurable activities, ways to spend their leisure time, and vocational interests, they increase their ability to define and control themselves, while decreasing their feelings of powerlessness. Increased self-acceptance decreases dependency on others.

To facilitate movement from a negative and distorted body image, clients keep a body image diary. In this they record situations that provoke concerns over their appearance, their body image beliefs, and the effect of these on their mood and behavior. As they recognize their maladaptive thoughts, they can begin to reframe those thoughts in positive affirmations or distract themselves by focusing on more pleasing aspects of their appearance.

It is important that clients consider sociocultural factors and body image issues. Topics include the pressures for women to be thin, the consequences of evaluating oneself largely in terms of weight, and how the female body is used in advertising and in the media. It is important that they see themselves as being in control rather than as passive sex objects valued mainly for appearance.

Several interventions are effective for clients who believe that achieving an ideal body will solve all problems in life. Point out the cognitive process of overgeneralization in developing the belief that all life's problems will be solved if enough weight is lost. You can help clients identify how losing weight is symbolic of other problems, and begin to separate interpersonal problems from physical problems. After you and the client generate a list of problems together, the problems can be prioritized and tackled one by one.

Medication Teaching

Clients with Eating Disorders

Antidepressants

The effect of the medication may not be felt for 2–3 weeks.

Use a sunscreen and wear protective clothing to prevent sunburn.

Rise slowly from a sitting or lying position to prevent a sudden drop in blood pressure.

This medication decreases the seizure threshold, making it more likely that a seizure will occur. Because alcohol and some drugs also lower the seizure threshold, do not use these substances while taking this medication.

Family: Life Span Care

Family Involvement

Education for the client and family about eating disorders is another primary concern for nurses. The general public has many misconceptions that interfere with effective treatment. Both families and clients need to be made aware of the seriousness of the disorders and the potential complications if left untreated. Accurate information will assist families in solving problems together, rather than blaming one another for the onset of the disorder. Be prepared to answer questions honestly and admit limitations of your own knowledge. Give clients and family members a list of self-help groups to support them throughout the long-term treatment process (see the Self-Help Groups section at the end of the chapter). Teach clients who are taking antidepressants all you can about their medication (see the Medication Teaching box).

The family needs to let the client take responsibility for her or his own eating behavior. Conflict about food is likely to be counterproductive. On the other hand, families must not ignore evidence that relapse is occurring. Psychoeducation may include discussions on family cohesion, the degree of emotional bonding that occurs within a family. At one end of the continuum of cohesion is the family system that is disengaged, that is, the family members are isolated and alienated from one another. At the other end of the continuum is the enmeshed family system in which the members are immersed in and absorbed by one another. Eating disorders often lead to an enmeshed family system as everyone becomes concerned and involved with the eating behavior of one family member. The family may also develop rigid rules and expectations for the identified client. Since the most adaptive family systems function between the two extremes of disengaged and enmeshed, families may need help in problem-solving ways to achieve a health balance. Increasing the autonomy of young people may decrease the use of food as a passive-aggressive adolescent rebellion and increase feelings of self-control.

Evaluation

In response to the unrelenting demand of the cultural ideal, fat has become a feminist issue. It is time for nursing to *challenge the cultural ideal* and respond appropriately to people suffering from eating disorders. Nurses must become leaders in fostering a humane approach to body size.

Because we, as nurses, are products of our culture, we have probably internalized the prejudice against fat. Before intervening with clients, we must rethink our values and rid ourselves of unrealistic ideals. When working with overweight clients, we must understand that they do not necessarily have more emotional problems than people of normal weight. Their emotional problems are most likely a result of prejudice and stigma and the cultural pressure to lose weight. Decreasing the stigma as well as the internalized disgust will greatly benefit overweight clients. We must be careful not to perpetuate the misconception that losing weight will solve all other problems in life. A thin body is neither a magical cure nor a guarantee for living happily ever after.

You can actively challenge idealized cultural values by eliminating all negative references to overweight people in verbal and written communications. You can support people of average weight and express concern for people who are severely underweight. You can speak up about the potential life-threatening aspect of dieting behavior. You can help expand the standard of feminine beauty. We can teach our daughters how to defend against cultural pressures for weight loss and how to love, respect, and celebrate their bodies. We can teach our sons that women are not ornaments or sex objects, teach them

to respect and appreciate women who have many qualities and many sizes and shapes. Finally, we must help all clients view themselves as competent people who have many talents and traits—creativity, humor, empathy, warmth, and wisdom. All of us must work together to eliminate the depreciation of women and instead celebrate womanhood (Fontaine, 1991).

Evaluation of the effectiveness of the nursing care plan is based on the expected outcomes. Because changes occur slowly, you and your clients must have a great deal of patience. If clients are not involved in the planning, implementation, and evaluation processes, success will be minimal.

Thus far, only short-term studies have been conducted to evaluate the effectiveness of treatment plans for people with bulimia. In the 1-year follow-up studies, approximately two-thirds were no longer suffering from bulimia. As the binge eating and purging decreased, clients experienced less depression and less anxiety (Hebebrand et al, 1997).

People with anorexia fare less well. About 50% relapse within 1 year of discharge. Long-term studies indicate that 50–60% of clients maintain normal weight, and 11–20% remain dangerously underweight. Even those who maintain normal weight do not necessarily develop healthy eating attitudes and behavior. Two-thirds are still intensely preoccupied and obsessed with weight and dieting (Keel and Mitchell, 1997).

At present, there are no long-term successful treatment programs for weight loss in the obese population. Those who are successful in losing weight often gain the weight back within 1 or 2 years. Research continues in a variety of diet and behavioral therapy programs to find some combination that will help people stabilize at a reduced weight.

Clinical Interactions

A Client with Anorexia

Lorna, 23 years old, entered the eating disorders unit at the urging of her husband and physician. Lorna and her husband would like to start a family, and she has been told that her eating disorder (anorexia) would be very dangerous to a fetus. She weighed 95 pounds (43 kg) when she was admitted, and now, 3 weeks later, weighs 102 pounds (46 kg). In the interaction, you will see evidence of:

- denial
- distorted body image
- obsessions
- fear of gaining weight

NURSE: You said that you still have difficulty believing you have a problem.

LORNA: Well, my doctor says I do, but it's just hard for me to see it.

NURSE: What do you see?

LORNA: I see a lot of fat.

NURSE: You see a lot of fat—on yourself? You mean, you look in the mirror and see yourself as fat?

LORNA: Yes. That's all I can see.

[Period of silence.]

LORNA: All I think about is food. My mind is like a computer—it just keeps going on thinking about food.

NURSE: Do you feel trapped?

LORNA: Very trapped. It's like a habit. I just can't stop it. And now, here on the unit, we spend so much time talking about food and weight and everything. I think you are all as obsessed as I am.

NURSE: Do you think the staff are as out-of-control as you feel you are? That might be a scary thought.

LORNA: No, not really. I'm just so frustrated. Getting on the scale every few days is frightening. Seeing the numbers going up—I just want to stop it. I want to lose weight—go back to where I was. Yet I want a future, too. I want to have a baby, and part of me knows that I have to get healthier before I can get pregnant. So it's an immense conflict every single day.

NURSE: As painful as the conflict sounds, I also see some progress in you. When you first came to the unit, you believed there was nothing dangerous with your lack of eating. Now it sounds like you understand that your eating disorder is a real problem, especially in terms of becoming a mother.

LORNA: Yeah, I know. My husband's being very supportive. I just wish I didn't have to gain this weight in order to become pregnant. ∎

Self-Help Groups

Clients with Eating Disorders

American Anorexia/Bulimia Association, Inc.
133 Cedar Lane
Teaneck, NJ 07666
(201) 836-1800

Anorexia and Bulimia Hotline
(800) 772-3390

Anorexia Nervosa and Related Eating Disorders, Inc.
P.O. Box 5102
Eugene, OR 97405
(503) 344-1144

Bulimic Anorexic Self-Help, Inc.
6125 Clayton Avenue, Suite 215
St. Louis, MO 63139
(800) 227-4785; (314) 567-4080

Center for the Study of Anorexia and Bulimia
1 West 91st Street
New York, NY 10024
(212) 595-3449

National Anorexic Aid Society, Inc.
P.O. Box 29461
Columbus, OH 43229
(614) 895-2009

National Association of Anorexia Nervosa and Associated Disorders, Inc.
P.O. Box 7
Highland Park, IL 60035
(312) 831-3438
e-mail: anad20@aol.com

Key Concepts

Introduction

- People with anorexia lose weight by dramatically decreasing their food intake and sharply increasing their amount of physical exercise.

- People with bulimia remain at near-normal weight and develop a cycle of minimal food intake, followed by binge eating and then purging.

- The two disorders have many features in common, and a person can revert from one disorder to the other.

Knowledge Base: Obesity

- Psychosocial factors contributing to the development of obesity include learned patterns of eating, overeating to manage negative feelings, and viewing food as a reward.

- Leptin, produced by a gene for obesity, travels to the brain, where it affects appetite and metabolic rate.

- Obese people are no more prone to emotional problems than are people of normal weight. It is the internalization of the culture's hatred and rejection that contributes to the psychological problems of obese people.

Knowledge Base: Anorexia and Bulimia

- Behaviors associated with anorexia and bulimia are compulsions and rituals about food and exercise, phobic responses to food, eating binges, purging, and the abuse of laxatives and diuretics.

- Affective characteristics include multiple fears, dependency, and a high need for acceptance and approval from others.

- Cognitive characteristics include selective abstraction, overgeneralization, magnification, personalization, superstitious thinking, dichotomous thinking, distorted body image, self-depreciation, and perfectionistic standards of behavior.

- In American society, thinness is equated with attractiveness, success, and happiness. This is a contributing factor to eating disorders.

- Eating disorders are considered to be culture-reactive syndromes in the Western world.

- Physiological characteristics include fluid and electrolyte imbalances, decreased blood volume, cardiac arrhythmias, elevated BUN, constipation, esophagitis, potential rupture of the esophagus or stomach, tooth loss, swollen salivary glands, Russell's sign, menstrual problems, and weight loss.

- Concomitant disorders include depression, social phobias, panic attacks, obsessive-compulsive symptoms, and substance abuse.

- Neurobiological factors in the development of eating disorders include 5-HT dysregulation, low levels of endorphins, and a genetic predisposition.

- Intrapersonal theorists consider low self-esteem, problems with identity formation, anxiety intolerance, and maturational problems to be factors in the development of eating disorders.

- Cognitive theorists believe that cognitive distortions and dysfunctional thoughts contribute to disordered eating patterns.

- The family system of a person with an eating disorder may be enmeshed. Family members may have difficulty with conflict resolution and have high ambitions for achievement and performance.

- Feminist theorists consider that women's preoccupation with their bodies results from the cultural ideal of thinness, and that their identity and self-esteem depend on physical appearance.

- Antidepressant medication is more helpful in treating bulimia than anorexia.

Nursing Process

- Eating disorders cause multiple physical complications. Accurate physical assessment may prevent death.

- The client's level of malnourishment must be identified, as well as binge eating and/or purging patterns, fear, cognitive distortions, and relationships with family and friends.

- Help clients discuss their fears related to weight gain and loss of control.

- Clients contract for the amount of food to be eaten in a day; a target weight is established, usually at 90% of average weight for the client's age and height.

- Contract for a reasonable intake, beginning with 1000–1500 kcal per day.

- Help clients identify situations that precede a binge and explore alternative coping behaviors. Discussion also focuses on how purging is used to cope with feelings.

- Clients may find it helpful to keep a food diary and a body image diary.

- Secondary gains must be identified in order to design interventions that will help clients meet these needs in constructive and healthy ways.

- The family needs to let the client take responsibility for her/his own eating behavior.

- Nurses must be leaders in actively challenging idealized cultural values in an effort to help women accept and value themselves as they are, and to prevent a continued increase in eating disorders.

- It appears that people with bulimia are more responsive to treatment than people with anorexia, who often remain intensely preoccupied with weight and dieting.

- At present, there are no long-term successful treatment programs for weight loss in the obese population.

Review Questions

1. Your client says to you, "If I'm not thin, I'm fat." You would document this as which type of cognitive distortion?

   a. selective abstraction

   b. superstitious thinking

   c. overgeneralization

   d. dichotomous thinking

2. Your client has been diagnosed with anorexia. You would expect to find which of the following exercise patterns?

   a. a fixed pattern of overexercise

   b. 1 hour of exercise a day

   c. a sporadic pattern

   d. a step aerobics class

3. Which one of the following lab values indicates the greatest need for immediate intervention?

   a. Na 125 mEq

   b. K 2.3 mEq

   c. Hgb 14.3 g/dL

   d. BUN 110 mg/100 mL

4. Which of the following medications will likely be ordered for Karen, who is suffering from bulimia?

   a. Thorazine, an antipsychotic agent

   b. Xanax, an antianxiety agent

   c. BuSpar, an antianxiety agent

   d. Prozac, an antidepressant

5. Karen believes that all her problems in life will be solved if she loses enough weight. The most appropriate intervention is to

   a. identify the secondary gains of her disorder.

   b. discuss how losing weight is symbolic of other problems.

   c. discuss how regression is a way to manage anxiety.

   d. tell her she has many more problems than her eating disorder.

References

Anderson, A. E. (1995). Eating disorders in males. In K. D. Brownell & C. G. Fairburn (Eds.), *Eating Disorders and Obesity* (pp. 177–182). New York: Guilford Press.

Beumont, P. J. V. (1995). The clinical presentation of anorexia and bulimia nervosa. In K. D. Brownell & C. G. Fairburn (Eds.), *Eating Disorders and Obesity* (pp. 151–158). New York: Guilford Press.

Carlat, D. J., Camargo, C. A., & Herzog, D. B. (1997). Eating disorders in males. *Am J Psychiatry, 154*(8), 1127–1132.

Considine, R. V., et al. (1996). Serum immuno-reactive-leptin concentrations in normal-weight and obese humans. *N Engl J Med, 334*(2), 292–295.

Dare, C., & Crowther, C. (1995). Psychodynamic models of eating disorders. In G. Szmukler, C. Dare, & J. Treasure (Eds.), *Handbook of Eating Disorders* (pp. 125–135). New York: Wiley.

DeSilva, P. (1995). Cognitive-behavioral models of eating disorders. In G. Szmukler, C. Dare, & J. Treasure (Eds.), *Handbook of Eating Disorders* (pp. 141–153). New York: Wiley.

Eisler, I. (1995). Family models of eating disorders. In G. Szmukler, C. Dare, & J. Treasure (Eds.), *Handbook of Eating Disorders* (pp. 155–176). New York: Wiley.

Fairburn, C. G., et al. (1996). Bias and bulimia nervosa. *Am J Psychiatry, 153*(3), 386–391.

Fichter, M. M. & Pirke, K. M. (1995). Starvation models and eating disorders. In K. D. Brownell & C. G. Fairburn (Eds.), *Eating Disorders and Obesity* (pp. 83–107). New York: Guilford Press.

Fontaine, K. L. (1991). The conspiracy of culture: Women's issues in body size. *Nurs Clin North Am, 26*(3), 669–676.

Garfinkel, P. E. (1995). Classification and diagnosis of eating disorders. In K. D. Brownell & C. G. Fairburn (Eds.), *Eating Disorders and Obesity* (pp. 125–134). New York: Guilford Press.

Greenfeld, D., et al. (1995). Hypokalemia in outpatients with eating disorders. *Am J Psychiatry, 1562*(1), 60-63.

Hedaya, R. J. (1996). *Understanding Biological Psychiatry*. New York: Norton.

Halmi, K. A. (1995). Current concepts and definitions. In G. Szmukler, C. Dare, & J. Treasure (Eds.), *Handbook of Eating Disorders* (pp. 39–42). New York: Wiley.

Hebebrand, J., et al. (1997). Prediction of low body weight at long-term follow-up in acute anorexia nervosa by low body weight at referral. *Am J Psychiatry, 154*(4), 566–569.

Joiner, G. W., & Kashubeck, S. (1996). Acculturation, body image, self-esteem, and eating-disorder symptomatology in adolescent Mexican American women. *Psych Women Quart, 20*, 419--35.

Kaye, W. H. (1995). Neurotransmitters and anorexia nervosa. In K. D. Brownell & C. G. Fairburn (Eds.), *Eating Disorders and Obesity* (pp. 255–260). New York: Guilford Press.

Keel, P. K., & Mitchell, J. E. (1997). Outcome in bulimia nervosa. *Am J Psychiatry, 154*(3), 313–321.

McCloskey, J., & Bulechek, G. M. (1996). *Nursing Interventions Classification (NIC)*, 2nd ed. St. Louis: Mosby.

McGown, A., & Whitbread, J. (1996). Out of control! The most effective way to help the binge-eating patient. *J Psychosoc Nurs, 34*(1), 30–36.

Olivardia, R., et al. (1995). Eating disorders in college men. *Am J Psychiatry, 152*(9), 1279–1284.

Owen, S. V., & Fullerton, M. L. (1995). A discussion group in a behaviorally oriented inpatient eating disorder program. *J Psychosoc Nurs, 33*(11), 35–40.

Robinson, P. H., & McHugh, P. R. (1995). A physiology of starvation that sustains eating disorders. In G. Szmukler, C. Dare, & J. Treasure (Eds.), *Handbook of Eating Disorders* (pp. 109–123). New York: Wiley.

Rorty, M., Yager, J., & Rossotto, E. (1994). Childhood sexual, physical, and psychological abuse in bulimia nervosa. *Am J Psychiatry, 151*(8), 1122–1127.

Schuckit, M. A., et al. (1996). Anorexia nervosa and bulimia nervosa in alcohol-dependent men and women and their relatives. *Am J Psychiatry, 153*(1), 74–82.

Silva, P. D. (1995). Cognitive-behavioral models of eating disorders. In G. Szmukler, C. Dare, & J. Treasure (Eds.), *Handbook of Eating Disorders* (pp. 141–153). New York: Wiley.

Silverstein, B., & Perlick, D. (1995). *The Cost of Competence*. Oxford, England: Oxford Univ. Press.

Sobal, J. (1995). Social influences on body weight. In K. D. Brownell & C. G. Fairburn (Eds.), *Eating Disorders and Obesity* (pp. 73–77). New York: Guilford Press.

Striegel-Moore, R. H. (1995). A feminist perspective on the etiology of eating disorders. In K. D. Brownell & C. G. Fairburn (Eds.), *Eating Disorders and Obesity* (pp. 224–229). New York: Guilford Press.

Stunkard, A. J., & Sobal, J. (1995). Psychosocial consequences of obesity. In K. D. Brownell & C. G. Fairburn (Eds.), *Eating Disorders and Obesity* (pp. 417–421). New York: Guilford Press.

Sullivan, P. F. (1995). Mortality in anorexia nervosa. *Am J Psychiatry, 152*(7), 1073–1074.

Thiel, A., et al. (1995). Obsessive-compulsive disorder among patients with anorexia nervosa and bulimia nervosa. *Am J Psychiatry, 152*(1), 72–75.

Treasure, J., & Holland, A. (1995). Genetic factors in eating disorders. In G. Szmukler, C. Dare, & J. Treasure (Eds.), *Handbook of Eating Disorders* (pp. 65–81). New York: Wiley.

Wilfley, D. E., & Rodin, J. (1995). Cultural influences on eating disorders. In K. D. Brownell & C. G. Fairburn (Eds.), *Eating Disorders and Obesity* (pp. 78–82). New York: Guilford Press.

Wolfe, B. E. (1995). Dimensions of response to antidepressant agents in bulimia nervosa. *Arch Psychiatr Nurs, 9*(3), 111–121.

CHAPTER 11

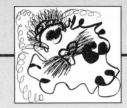

Mood Disorders

Karen Lee Fontaine

Objectives

After reading this chapter, you will be able to:

- Compare and contrast people who have unipolar disorder (major depression) with people who have bipolar disorder.
- Analyze the sociocultural factors that contribute to the incidence of depression.
- Discuss the impact of mood disorders on the family.
- Explain altered neurotransmission in people with mood disorders.
- Apply the nursing process to clients who have mood disorders.

Key Terms

affect
anhedonic
bipolar disorder
catastrophizing
circadian rhythms
cyclothymic disorder
dysthymic disorder
electroconvulsive therapy (ECT)
family therapy
major depression
manic-depressive disorder
mood
schizoaffective disorder
seasonal affective disorder (SAD)
somatization
unipolar disorder

*M*ood is defined as a sustained emotional state and how you subjectively feel. The way in which you communicate your mood to others is called **affect.** Affect is the immediate and observable emotional expression of mood which you communicate verbally and nonverbally. Verbal cues we may use to describe our emotional state are words such as elation, happiness, pleasure, frustration, anger, or hostility. Nonverbal cues to feelings include facial expressions such as smiling, frowning, and looking blank; motor activities such as making hands into fists and pacing; and physiological responses such as profuse sweating and increased respirations. We may choose not to communicate verbally to another person, but it is almost impossible to prevent nonverbal expression of our feelings.

A variety of descriptors of affect are used to facilitate communication among health care professionals. Table 11.1 defines the terminology and provides behavioral examples. Affect and mood can be pictured along a continuum ranging from depression through normal to mania. The normal range of mood is stable and appropriate to the situation. People diagnosed with mood disorders experience disrupting disturbances at varying points along the continuum.

The mood disorders are characterized by changes in feelings ranging from severe depression to inordinate elation. They are best understood as syndromes with a core cluster of symptoms. The two types of depressive disorders are major depression and dysthymic disorder. The medical diagnosis of **major depression** (also called **unipolar disorder**) is made when, along with a loss of interest in life, a person experiences a depressed mood that moves from mild to severe, with the severe phase lasting at least 2 weeks. Some people with major depression also experience delusions and hallucinations. When this occurs it is referred to as *Severe Depression with Psychotic Features,* although in the future it may be listed as a distinct syndrome. Those who have psychotic symptoms in one episode are much more likely to exhibit psychotic features in future episodes (Coryell et al, 1996). **Dysthymic disorder** is a chronic disorder in which periods of depressed mood are interspersed with normal mood. Symptoms in dysthymic disorder tend to be less severe than those in major depressive disorder, and there are fewer physiological symptoms (disturbed sleep, altered appetite, and weight loss or gain).

The bipolar disorders are a group of mood disorders that include main episodes, mixed episodes, depressed episodes, and cyclothymic disorder. The medical diagnosis of **bipolar disorder** (also called **manic-depressive disorder**) is given when a person's mood alternates between the extremes of depression and elation, with periods of normal mood in between the pathological phases. *Bipolar I Disorder* is characterized by the occurrence of one or more manic episodes and one or more depressive episodes. *Bipolar II Disorder* is on the less severe end of the continuum and is characterized by one or more hypomanic episodes and one or more depressive episodes. Bipolar disorder is further clarified as:

- Mixed: The person has rapidly alternating moods.

- Manic: The person is presently in the manic phase.

- Depressed: The person is in the depressed phase but has a history of manic episodes.

Cyclothymic disorder is characterized by a mood range from moderate depression to hypomania, which may or may not include periods of normal mood, lasting at least two years. Clients with cyclothymic disorder do not experience the severe symptoms that qualify for a diagnosis of manic disorder or major depressive disorder.

All of these disorders may be recurrent and are often chronic. Figure 11.1 shows the ranges of the mood disorders. **Schizoaffective disorder** is diagnosed when clients suffer from symptoms that appear to be a mixture of schizophrenia and the mood disorders. The person experiences one or more of the following symptoms: delusions, hallucinations, disorganized speech, disorganized behavior, or negative symptoms (see Chapter 12 for more detailed discussion of these symptoms). In addition, the person experiences symptoms of the mood disorders: major depressive symptoms, manic symptoms, or mixed symptoms. Clients often have difficulty maintaining job or school functioning, experience problems with self-care, are socially isolated, and often suffer from suicidal ideation.

Major depression is ten times more common than bipolar disorder. During any 6-month period approximately 10 million people in the United States are suffering from depression. It is thought that 8–12% of

Table 11.1 Descriptors of Affect

Affect	Definition	Behavioral Example
Appropriate	Mood is congruent with the immediate situation.	Juan cries when learning of the death of his father.
Inappropriate	Mood is not related to the immediate situation.	When Sue's husband tells her about his terrible pain, Sue begins to laugh out loud.
Stable	Mood is resistant to sudden changes when there is no provocation in the environment.	During a party, Dan smiles and laughs at the appropriate social interchanges.
Labile	Mood shifts suddenly in a way that cannot be understood in the context of the situation.	During a friendly game of checkers, Dorothy, who has been laughing, suddenly knocks the board off the table in anger. She then begins to laugh and wants to continue the game.
Elevated	Mood is one of euphoria not necessarily related to the immediate situation.	Sean bounces around the dayroom, laughing, singing, and telling other clients how wonderful everything is.
Depressed	Mood is one of despondency not necessarily related to the immediate situation.	Leo sits slumped in a chair with a sad facial expression, teary eyes, and minimal body movement.
Overreactive	Mood is appropriate to the situation but out of proportion to the immediate situation.	Karen screams and curses when her child spills a glass of milk on the kitchen floor.
Blunted	Mood is a dulled response to the immediate situation.	When Tom learns of his full-tuition scholarship, he responds with only a small smile.
Flat	There are no visible cues to the person's mood.	When Juanita is told about her best friend's death, she says "Oh" and does not give any indication of an emotional response.

men and 18–25% of women will suffer a major depression in their lifetime. Estimates are that only 25–50% of these individuals will seek and receive treatment. An untreated major depression may last 6 months to a year. The incidence of depression is increasing with each passing decade and the age of onset is lowering into adolescence and even childhood.

Of people admitted to the hospital for depression, 25% are suffering from psychotic symptoms. They may believe they are dying of incurable diseases or being punished for grave sins. They may hear voices telling them they are bad or to kill themselves (Hedaya, 1996; Zajecka, 1996).

Men and women are equally at risk for bipolar disorder, which affects 1.2% of the adult population, although women are more likely to develop the rapid-cycling form of the illness. The disorder most commonly begins during adolescence but has often been underrecognized and misdiagnosed in this age group. Untreated, the depressive phase may last 6–9 months

and the manic phase 2–6 weeks. It is difficult to predict the course of the disorder; some may have only one episode every 10 years, while others may have several episodes a year. Four or more episodes a year lead to the diagnosis of bipolar disorder, rapid cycling. People with bipolar II disorder have a higher frequency of episodes than those who have bipolar I disorder (Coryell et al, 1995; McElroy et al, 1997; Pollack, 1996).

Although 10–15% of pregnant women meet criteria for depression, they often remain undiagnosed because the symptoms of depression are similar to the somatic changes of pregnancy. Mood disorders in women after delivering a child are fairly common. Symptoms can be described along a continuum from postpartum blues to postpartum depression to the rare form, postpartum psychosis. *Postpartum blues* begin on the first to fourth day postpartum and last up to 10 days, with symptoms disappearing spontaneously. The mood may be unstable, accompanied by

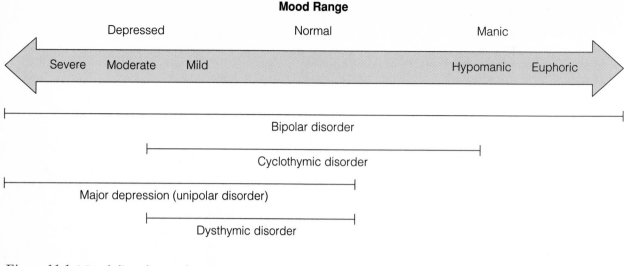

Figure 11.1 **Mood disorders and ranges.**

sadness, weepiness, irritability, anxiety, and fatigue. As many as 80% of new mothers may experience these symptoms, which are thought to be caused by hormonal fluctuations. Most of these women had not had previous emotional problems (Spinelli, 1997).

Postpartum depression is estimated to occur in 10–15% of new mothers beginning within 3 months of delivery. Women with this disorder experience mood swings, periods of crying, and feelings of despair, as they ruminate over perceived inadequacies as a parent. These symptoms are more intense and longer lasting than those in postpartum blues. Contributing factors are hormonal changes, feeling overwhelmed by parenting tasks, changes in family dynamics, and inadequate support (Blumenthal, 1996).

One woman in a thousand experiences a *postpartum psychosis*—a medical emergency where the woman may harm herself and/or her baby. The symptoms usually occur between the first 3 to 6 weeks after delivery and include insomnia, hallucinations, agitation, and bizarre feelings or behavior. An inordinate concern with the baby's health, guilt about lack of love, and delusions about the infant's being dead or defective also may be present. The mother may deny having given birth or hear voices that command her to hurt the baby. In extreme cases, the mother may even kill the child or herself (Thurtle, 1995; Ugarriza, 1995).

The high rate of mood disorders makes them a major concern for nurses. Mood-disordered clients are found in the community and in all types of clinical settings and are not restricted to psychiatric settings. It is vital that you be alert to cues because one of the tragic results in untreated depression is suicide.

Knowledge Base

People with mood disorders display a variety of characteristics involving changes in behavior, affect, cognition, and physiology. Depression occurs within a person's sociocultural context, and interactions with others are often disrupted.

Behavioral Characteristics

One of the changes in people with mood disorders is their level of desire to participate in activities. Initially, in depression, there is a decreased desire to engage in activities that do not bring immediate gratification. As the depression deepens, there is a further decrease in participation, and clients regard themselves as incompetent and inadequate. This further contributes to feelings of discouragement and, in severe depression, results in an inability to do anything, even the simplest ADLs. If you suggest that clients attempt

ADLs, they will often respond with something like "It's pointless to even try because I can't do it."

In the early stages of an elevated mood (hypomania), people with bipolar disorder increase their work productivity. This leads to positive feedback from employers and family members, which contributes to increased self-esteem around the issues of competency and power. When they reach the manic end of the continuum, however, their productivity decreases because of a short attention span. People in a manic phase are interested in every available activity and are supremely confident of being able to accomplish them all perfectly. Poor judgment can result in reckless driving, spending sprees, and foolish business investments.

> Jorge and Ava have been married for 12 years and are experiencing severe marital problems centering on financial issues. Jorge has had multiple episodes of bipolar disorder. Eighteen months ago they took a $10,000 home equity loan to pay off all the bills Jorge had run up during a manic phase. At that time they agreed that their credit cards would be used only for an emergency. Two weeks ago Ava needed to use the credit card to pay for some medication and found that the card was up to its limit of $5000. During a confrontation with Jorge, Ava found out that he had received two new credit cards and had taken a cash advance of $5000 on each card. He could not explain what he had done with the $15,000.

Interaction with others is altered in people with a mood disorder. In depression, the tendency is to withdraw from most social interactions because they are too demanding and require too much effort. Depressed people say they feel lonely but also say they feel incapable of halting the process of withdrawal and isolation. Family and friends, frustrated with the withdrawal, often respond with criticism and anger, further contributing to isolation.

During manic episodes, people are unusually talkative and gregarious. Unable to control the impulse to interact with everyone in the environment, they are oblivious to the social convention of not interrupting a private discussion. While interacting with others, they may share intimate details of their lives with anyone who will listen. When their mood returns to its normal range, they are often embarrassed about what they have said to others.

A change in affiliation needs also occurs in the mood disorders. During a depressive episode, normally self-sufficient people experience an increase in dependency. They may seek advice and assistance in work responsibilities and leisure activities. Affiliation needs are frequently expressed as demands or through whining complaints. Those experiencing a shift in mood toward elation show a decreased need for affiliation. Neither seeking nor heeding advice, they view themselves as completely autonomous.

Affective Characteristics

During depression, the mood begins with an intermittent sense of sadness. Statements are made such as "I feel down in the dumps." As depression deepens, people become more gloomy and dejected. You might hear such statements as "There is no joy in my life anymore" or "I feel really unhappy." In severe levels of depression, there is a sense of desolation. Depressed people despair over the past, present, and future; the misery is uninterrupted. A cue to the depth of the feeling might be something like "I'll always feel this awful; I'll never be any better."

On the manic end of the continuum, there is an unstable mood state. Beginning with cheerfulness, it escalates toward euphoria. People in this state are exuberant, energetic, and excitable. You will hear statements such as "Everything is just wonderful" or "I feel so high and great." The instability of mood is observed when, with minimal environmental stimulus, the person suddenly becomes irritable, argumentative, openly hostile, and even combative. As the stimulus is withdrawn, however, the person's mood returns to euphoric.

Guilt is another common affective experience on which depressed people focus. For some, the source of guilt is vague; for others, it is specific. Cues are such statements as "I have a loving wife and good children, a nice house, and no money problems. But I'm so unhappy. I shouldn't be feeling this way. It's terrible for me to be so miserable." Depressed people ruminate over incidents they feel guilty about, and it is difficult to change their focus of attention.

During a manic episode, people are unable to experience any sense of guilt. Confronted with behavior that has hurt another person, they respond with indifference, laughter, or anger. The ability to experience guilt returns when their affect returns to a normal level.

Crying spells may occur during a depressive state. In mild and moderate depressions, people have an increased tendency to cry in situations that would not normally provoke tears. In a severe depression, there is often a complete absence of crying. Some people do not even have the energy to cry. During the manic state, sudden and unpredictable crying spells may occur. These may last only 20–30 seconds before a rapid return to a euphoric mood.

People's feelings of gratification are altered in mood disorders. In depression, participation in normally pleasurable activities decreases, and people may become **anhedonic,** that is, incapable of experiencing pleasure. The change in mood is evidenced by such remarks as "I don't enjoy playing the piano anymore. It doesn't do anything for me. I just sit and watch TV all day" and "I can't seem to get interested in my stamp collection any more. I used to enjoy spending an hour a day working on it." Manic people, on the other hand, try to participate in every available pleasurable activity. Skillfulness is not a concern; they enjoy the activity regardless of the outcome. There is a constant need for fun, excitement, and stimulation.

Accompanying a depressive state is a loss of emotional attachment. People often become indifferent to family and friends and feel dissatisfied with these relationships. A cue may be: "I just don't care about anyone anymore." People in the manic state form intense emotional attachments very rapidly. They feel affectionate toward everyone in the environment and may "fall in love" in a matter of minutes and with a number of people. During a manic state, a person may think nothing of having simultaneous sexual relationships. Accompanying this is a preoccupation with sex, which others may find offensive.

> Juanita, a nurse, is doing a nursing history admission on Sid, a 73-year-old man with bipolar disorder, manic phase. He is sexually preoccupied throughout the interview. When asked what his major strengths are, he replies, "Making love." When asked how he handles stress at home, the response is, "Making it with as many girls as I can."

Alterations in the affective experience of people suffering from mood disorders are both broad and deep. In depression, there is an overall sense of hopelessness that the future will never bring any changes in mood or any pleasure or loving relationships. In a manic state, there is little recognition that they have not always felt this euphoric and wonderful.

> Carla describes her changes in this way: "I worry about what's going to happen to me. I mean, I didn't have this numbness a month ago. I could be lying here dying and not even know it. I just don't have any feeling anymore."

> Dales describes himself in this way: "I feel so good since I stopped taking my lithium. I'm not sick and I never needed it anyway. You know Susan, who just came into the group home yesterday? Well, we really hit it off and are thinking about getting married as soon as we can."

Perceptual Characteristics

Major depression can be accompanied by psychotic symptoms, often with depressive themes. Clients may hear voices telling them that they are bad or to kill themselves, or they may have delusions that they have a terminal illness or are responsible for some disaster. Hallucinations occur in 15–25% of people with mood disorders and may be the result of sleep deprivation. They may be reluctant to talk about their delusions and hallucinations if they realize that their thinking processes are not quite right (Zajecka, 1996).

> Sonja was brought in to the local mental health clinic by her husband. He said he was very concerned because he discovered she had recently purchased a gun, believeing the FBI was after her. She considers herself to be a bad person and that everything she does is bad. She believes she is dying soon and that there is no hope for the future. She states: "I don't know what I'm going to do. What do you think I should do? Nobody can help me. The FBI is after me. I know what I did wrong. I didn't do what I was supposed to do, I didn't keep my house clean. I can't afford to pay for therapy. So they'll take me to jail, won't they?"

Cognitive Characteristics

A person's thoughts about personal worth and value contribute to an overall sense of self-esteem. In the mood disorders, there is an alteration in the ability to self-evaluate objectively. When depressed, people focus much of their attention on past, present, and future failures. This magnification of failures is called **catastrophizing.** Such negative thoughts make them feel more depressed, which causes further self-depreciation.

Wendy is a severely depressed young woman. She verbalizes her negative expectations in this way: "Dr. Lee isn't doing anything. The antidepressants aren't working. I'm getting worse, and I won't get better this time. There is nothing anyone can do to help me and no one cares. I wish I could just die."

People on the manic end of the continuum have an exaggerated self-concept. They have *grandiose beliefs* about their physical and intellectual talents. In any undertaking, there is a supreme sense of self-confidence. During manic episodes, they do not regard their behavior as inappropriate, nor do they realize their need for professional assistance.

Steve is telling Keasha, his nurse, about firing his divorce lawyer right before coming into the hospital.

Steve: [Angry tone of voice.] I didn't like how he was handling the case. I know what I want to happen with the divorce. I want to make sure my daughters are taken care of.

Keasha: What was your lawyer doing that you felt like he wasn't handling things right?

Steve: I don't know; it was just the way he did things. I could do much better. I already filed five motions before I came here. The paperwork is not a problem. I've always had this instinct about things like the law. I've always liked to read. What got me so angry is that the judge was against me because I'm handling my own case. She just doesn't know what a great job I can do.

People's decision-making ability deteriorates in mood disorders. In depression, there is a decreased ability to concentrate on a subject long enough to formulate a decision. A person might stand in front of the closet for 20 minutes, trying to decide what clothes to wear. Planning meals, shopping, or concentrating on homework may be very difficult. In severe depression, people are incapable of making decisions. Because they cannot concentrate, they cannot recall information from the past to help them. Lack of concentration also interferes with their ability to compare alternatives and potential outcomes in the problem-solving process.

During manic episodes, people also have difficulty making decisions. Easily distracted by stimuli in the environment, they cannot concentrate long enough to go through the problem-solving process. Their short attention span causes them to respond impulsively to environmental stimuli. Because of their inability to think through the consequences of behavior before impulsively engaging in it, manic people often have poor judgment and self-control.

Flow of thought is disrupted in people with mood disorders. In depression, there may be slowed speech, an inability to think of specific words, or an inability to complete sentences. During manic episodes, *flight of ideas* is often present. The flow of thought is fragmented by any external stimuli. Thoughts come so quickly that there is not enough time to completely express one idea before another is stimulated. These thoughts may be connected by a theme or by alliteration or rhymes.

"I want to see my little niece. I haven't seen her yet. She's only 3 weeks old. Her name is Diamond. Do you like diamonds? I got my mother a necklace like that (pointing to the case manager's necklace) and earrings to match when I was 14 and I'm still paying on it. I insured it. I got life insurance. I'm completely insured. Even my fingernails are insured. I got in an accident. Someone hit me in the rear end. I got $10,000 for it because I was insured. It was my Dad's car. I'm going to call my Dad."

Thoughts about body image are also distorted in those with mood disorders. During a depressive episode, people believe they are unattractive and may actually erroneously perceive their body as being disfigured or deformed. People in a manic state have exaggerated self-esteem, which may contribute to believing they look like well-known people or famous beauties. If others challenge this perception, they often respond with a great deal of anger.

Meg states: "I want to go into the bathroom to put on some makeup. I used to be a model, you know. Don't you think I'm pretty? I was fine until I was diagnosed with this disease. I had a very high-profile job, I was making a lot of money, and I drove very fancy cars. I was very rich. I hung out only with important people."

Faulty perceptions of body image may escalate into delusions. Depressed people may experience somatic delusions, in which they believe themselves to be hopelessly ill or that part of the body has been infected or contaminated by outside agents. An example is the person who says, "I'm afraid I might have rabies because my friend spit in my throat. My sister has rabies because a wild rabid wolf pissed on her cocaine." Manic people may experience delusions of grandeur focusing on beliefs of being famous or having a personal relationship with prominent, well-known people. These delusions may include paranoid content. People with mood disorders may experience ambivalence about treatment which may be related to denial. They may minimize or deny the reality of a prior episode, their own behavior, and often the consequences of their behavior. People who deny that they have a serious disorder are not likely to seek treatment. Some clients may be reluctant to give up the experience of mania. The increased energy, euphoria, and heightened self-esteem may be very desirable and enjoyable.

> Aida, 40 years old, lives in a group home. She states, "I was hospitalized 23 years ago because I wasn't having fun in school and I was overweight." She states she is in the group home because "I am the way I am and because I couldn't figure out why I was gaining weight. I think my gallbladder operation 4 years ago has something to do with it."

Loss of faith is a common experience during depressive episodes. People lose faith in their ability to ever again feel love for family members, in the possibility of their negative thoughts ever going away, and in their religion. Unable to find meaning in their illness, they feel a sense of injustice in life. This loss of faith contributes to an overwhelming sense of spiritual distress.

Social Characteristics

The impact of mood disorders on the family must not be underestimated. Many families report that for several of their extended family and friends, mental illness is still associated with moral weakness or failure. This results in being treated differently or stigmatized. The family's frustration, confusion, and anger in response to the multiple changes in their loved ones are all understandable. Initially, family members may react with support and concern but in some families, when the depression does not improve, support changes to frustration and anger. A vicious cycle may be established. Increased conflict causes increased symptoms, further rejection, and deepening depression. Other families may become overly solicitous and assume total care of the depressed person. Total care

may contribute to increased symptoms because the person feels helpless and indebted to the family.

Nearly every family who has a loved one with bipolar disorder perceives the illness as a moderate to severe burden. About 33% of people with bipolar I disorder are unable to live independently. During manic episodes, a person's family may be subjected to bizarre, hostile, and even destructive behavior. Family members often call the police to protect themselves and their property. Untreated bipolar disorder can devastate individual and family life and often leads to a downward spiral in interpersonal, economic, and occupational functioning (Solomon, 1996).

There has been increasing awareness of the impact of parental mood disorders on children and adolescents. During an acute episode, youngsters must try to cope with parental behavior that is not easily understood. They may also experience repeated separations from the parent. Since both genetic and psychosocial influences are involved in the transmission of these disorders from parent to child, they are at higher risk for experiencing symptoms by the end of their adolescence (Mohit, 1996).

Mood disorders often disrupt a couple's sex life. Depressed people lose interest in sexual activity, both autoerotic and with their partner. The person and the partner must understand that this lack of sexual desire is a symptom of the depression, not necessarily a reflection of the relationship. During a manic state, there is an exaggerated sexual desire, and normal standards of sexual activity are not observed. Seductive behavior, frequency of activity, and number of partners may all increase. Families are often angry and hurt, and this may be the particular behavior that forces treatment or hospitalization. When mood levels return to normal, they often feel embarrassed and guilty about their behavior.

Culture-Specific Characteristics

Appropriate expressions of mood are largely culturally determined. For example, situations in which people are expected to experience sadness, anger, loneliness, frustration, joy, or happiness are defined by the culture. The culture also determines how people are to behave when experiencing a variety of feelings. For example, cultural expectations of grieving individuals may be self-control and a "stiff upper lip" or may be loud mourning and ripping of clothing. Extreme pleasure may be expressed with a nod and a smile or may be expressed with loud laughter and exuberant behavior.

The Western interpretation of feelings is that emotions are intrapersonal. In contrast, in Micronesia, emotions are considered to be not within a person but rather between people. In some Middle Eastern, African, Hispanic, and Chinese cultures, emotions are viewed and expressed in somatic (bodily) terms. The process by which psychological distress is experienced and communicated in the form of somatic symptoms is called **somatization.** Because these cultures are not subject to the mind/body dualism of Western thinking, psychological distress is viewed as arising from bodily imbalances (Hulme, 1996).

Throughout the world, women experience more depression than do men. Certainly there are cross-cultural similarities in the way women are socialized and in the inferior status that they experience in many societies. Psychosocial stressors, including multiple work and family responsibilities, poverty, sexual and physical abuse, gender discrimination, lack of social supports, and traumatic life experiences may contribute to women's increased vulnerability to depression (Blumenthal, 1996).

Emotions of dysphoria and depression have dramatically different meaning and forms of expression in different cultures. Many Americans view suffering as unexpected or unacceptable and perceive depression as something to overcome through personal striving. Latin American cultures associate suffering with a deep sense of tragedy. Shi'ite Muslims view suffering within a religious context of martyrdom, while Buddhist cultures view suffering as a positive feature of life. Throughout the entire world, most cases of depression are experienced and expressed in bodily terms such as fatigue, headaches, heart distress, dizziness, and so on. It is only in Western cultures that depression is considered to be a mental disorder. When assessing clients from cultures different from your own, it is important to understand that the expression of depression is culturally determined (Silverstein and Perlick, 1995).

Physiological Characteristics

People experience many physiological symptoms during episodes of the mood disorders. A change in appetite is not unusual. Many people lose their desire for food when depressed, and statements such as "Nothing tastes good to me" and "I can't eat, I feel like there is a big knot in my throat" are common. Others discover their appetites increase when they become depressed, and their eating patterns cause them to gain weight. Manic people may not obtain sufficient food and fluid because they cannot remain still long enough to eat a meal. The consequences of a change in appetite depend on the severity of the reduction or increase in food and fluid intake. The changes could become life-threatening.

Sleep patterns are disrupted in people with mood disorders. During mild or moderate depression, people may sleep more than usual or they may awaken earlier than usual. In severe depression, people usually have difficulty falling asleep and may sleep for only a few hours a night. During a manic state, people experience a dramatic decrease in their amount of sleep. Although they may sleep only 1 or 2 hours a night, they are full of energy throughout the day. They have great difficulty taking naps or relaxing during the day to compensate for their lack of sleep.

Another change characteristic of mood disorders is in activity level. Some experience extremely slowed motor activity, while others experience constant and nonpurposeful activity such as wringing the hands, picking at the skin, or agitated pacing. In the manic state, people experience hyperactivity without being aware of fatigue. They move constantly and have great difficulty remaining seated for more than a few minutes. Because they are unaware of fatigue, they are in danger of total physical exhaustion.

Bowel activity may be a problem in both unipolar and bipolar disorder. A marked decrease in food and fluid intake and decreased physical activity can result in constipation. During manic episodes, people may be unable to take the time to have a bowel movement.

Physical appearance is often indicative of an altered mood state. Depressed people may wear the same clothes for days without laundering them. Personal hygiene may be poor because they do not have the energy to brush their teeth, shower, or wash their hair. During a manic state, people may change clothes as often as every hour. Personal hygiene may become a problem if distractibility interferes with normal ADLs. Women who wear makeup and jewelry have extravagant tastes during an elevated mood state. Their cosmetics tend to be very bright and may be carelessly applied.

For a review of the behavioral, affective, cognitive, sociocultural, and physiological characteristics of people with mood disorders, see Table 11.2.

Table 11.2 Characteristics of Mood Disorders

Characteristic	Depressed State	Manic State
Behavioral		
Desire to participate in activities	Decreased to absent.	Interested in all activities.
Interaction with other people	Limited; client withdraws.	Talkative, gregarious.
Affiliation needs	Increased dependency.	Independent, self-sufficient.
Affective		
Mood	Despair, desolation.	Unstable: euphoric and irritable.
Guilt	High level.	Unable to experience guilt.
Crying spells	Frequent crying to inability to cry.	May have brief episodes.
Gratification	Loss of interest in pleasurable activities.	Constantly seeking fun and excitement.
Emotional attachments	Indifference to others.	Forms intense attachments rapidly.
Cognitive		
Self-evaluation	Focuses on failures; sees self as incompetent; catastrophizes and personalizes.	Grandiose beliefs about self.
Expectations	Believes present and future hopeless; overgeneralizes one experience or fact.	Inordinate positive expectations; unable to see potential negative outcomes.
Self-criticism	Harshly critical of self; is a perfectionist; anticipates disapproval from others.	Approves of own behavior; irate if criticized by others.
Decision-making ability	Decreased ability or inability to make decisions.	Difficulty due to distractibility and impulsiveness.
Flow of thought	Decrease in rate and number of thoughts.	Flight of ideas.
Body image	Believes self unattractive or ugly.	Believes self unusually beautiful.
Delusions	Somatic delusions.	Delusions of grandeur.
Hallucinations	Occur in 15–25% of cases.	Occur in 15–25% of cases.
Sociocultural		
Sexual desire	Loss of desire.	Increase in activity and partners.
Physiological		
Appetite	Increased or decreased in mild and moderate depression; decreased in severe depression.	Difficulty eating due to inability to sit still.
Amount of sleep	Increased or decreased in mild and moderate depression; decreased in severe depression.	Sleeps only 1 or 2 hours a night.
Activity level	Motor activity retarded.	Hyperactivity.
Bowel activity	Constipation.	Constipation.
Physical appearance	Unkempt; poor hygiene.	Bright clothing; frequently changes clothing.

Concomitant Disorders

Severe depression and anxiety disorders frequently occur at the same time. Studies indicate that as many as 40% of those suffering from agoraphobia, 35% of those experiencing panic attacks, and 17% of those with generalized anxiety disorder are also clinically depressed. Individuals with bipolar disorder are 26 times more likely to have concomitant panic disorder than the general population. People with both disorders have fewer personal and social resources and demonstrate poorer overall functioning (Brown et al, 1996; Chen and Dilsaver, 1995).

The rate of comorbidity between mood disorders and substance-related disorders is high. In some cases the primary diagnosis is a mood disorder, with substance abuse being an attempt to self-medicate. In other situations, the substance-related disorder is the primary diagnosis. An example is the person who becomes depressed on withdrawal from amphetamines or cocaine. A third possibility is that the person has both disorders as primary. In bipolar disorder, substance abuse may be a natural result of the impulsive, expansive lifestyle and poor judgment during a manic episode, which may worsen the course of bipolar disorder. Treatment for both disorders should be concurrent (Winokur, 1995).

Up to 25% of people with certain medical conditions—diabetes, myocardial infarction, stroke, Alzheimer's disease, Parkinson's disease, or cancer, for example—will develop major depression during the course of their medical illness. It is vital that you be alert to cues for depression in medical clients, since as many as 15% of people with mood disorders go on to commit suicide (Zajecka, 1996). Suicidal behavior and prevention is covered in Chapter 17.

Causative Theories

Multiple theories have been developed to explain the cause of mood disorders. It is thought that these disorders are largely a clinical syndrome with common features caused by a variety of factors. In understanding the individual from these theoretical perspectives, you must look at how these different factors interacted within the person's past and how they interact in present circumstances. A person may have a genetic predisposition to changes in neurotransmission. The actual changes may occur only if certain psychological mechanisms are present, and these mechanisms may operate only if particular social inter-actions occur. Many factors in both the individual and the environment increase or decrease the risk of mood disorders. By applying the neurobiological, intrapersonal, learning, cognitive, social, and feminist theories, you approach the client from a holistic perspective.

Neurobiological Theory

Some evidence suggests that people who experience mood disorders have a *genetic predisposition*. The risk to first-degree relatives of people diagnosed with either unipolar or bipolar disorder is 5–20 times higher than in the general population. Relatives of those with bipolar disorder may develop either bipolar or unipolar disorder, whereas relatives of those with unipolar disorder primarily develop unipolar disorder. Studies of the incidence in twins documented that in 75% of monozygotic twins, both twins developed a mood disorder, compared with only 20% of dizygotic twins. Additional evidence from adoption studies reveals that there is a three-times greater incidence of depression in biological relatives of depressed persons as compared to their adopted relatives. There is a 25% rate of depression in the first-degree relatives (parents, siblings) of people with depression. However, it is important to note that depression also occurs in individuals who have no family history.

Studies suggest that a complex mode of inheritance exists, rather than a single dominant gene. It is probably the individual mix of these multiple genes that determines differences such as age of onset, symptoms, severity, and course. At the present time, there is evidence to link mood disorders and abnormalities on chromosomes 4, 11, 18, and 21 (Blumenthal, 1996; Gershon, 1996; Reich, 1997; Sevy, 1995).

Recent studies have zeroed in on a tiny, thimble-size nodule of the brain located about 2½ inches behind the bridge of the nose (the subgenual prefrontal cortex) as being an important site in the control of emotions. It is thought that this area of the brain may act as a set of brakes for emotional responses, and when it does not function properly, widely abnormal swings in mood may occur (Gorman, 1997).

The neurotransmission hypothesis is specifically concerned with the levels of serotonin (5-HT), dopamine (DA), norepinephrine (NE), and acetylcholine (ACH) in the central nervous system. It is believed that there is a functional deficiency of these neurotransmitters during a depressive episode and a functional excess during a manic episode (Thase and Howland, 1995).

Most likely there are different combinations of problems with the neurotransmitter systems. Both DA and the balance between DA and ACH are responsible for difficulties with motivation. ACH is implicated in the sleep disturbances of both bipolar and unipolar disorders. NE is important in motor arousal and movement. The principal neurotransmitter for mood states is 5-HT, which is associated with anxiety and aggression, especially self-destructive behavior. In addition, endogenous opioids are necessary to moderate sad moods. The interactions between these different neurotransmitters explain how clinical features tend to vary from client to client (Mann et al, 1996).

One way this imbalance may occur is through the action of the enzyme monoamine oxidase (MAO), which is responsible for deactivating neurotransmitters after they have been released from the receptor sites. If there is an excess of MAO, neurotransmitter levels will be low, resulting in decreased impulse transmission. If levels are not sufficient to deactivate the neurotransmitters, they will accumulate at the synapse and increase the transmission of impulses.

This hypothesis may be one explanation for the higher incidence of depression in women and older people. Throughout life, women and older adults have consistently higher levels of MAO than do men and younger people. The result may be a functional decrease in the necessary neurotransmitters.

Another part of the hypothesis concerns the sensitivity of the receptors to the neurotransmitters. During depression, the receptors may be subsensitive, so that fewer impulses are transmitted. During the manic state, receptors may be supersensitive, resulting in an increase in the transmission of impulses. The sensitivity of the receptors is influenced by the thyroid hormone triiodothyronine (T_3). Thus, people with hypothyroidism are at higher risk for a depressive episode, and those with hyperthyroidism are at higher risk for a manic episode (Zajecka, 1996).

Continuing research into the relationship between stress and mood disorders indicates that the limbic system of the brain is the major site of stress adaptation. With stress, neurotransmitter production in the limbic system increases. When the stress becomes chronic or recurrent, the body can no longer adapt as efficiently, and a shortage of neurotransmitters results. During manic episodes, there appears to be a defective feedback mechanism in the limbic system. Even after the stressful event has been resolved, the limbic system continues to produce excessive neurotransmitters; the increased transmission of impulses continues. Different areas of the limbic system play a major role in the regulation of emotions such as fear, rage, excitement, and euphoria. The signs and symptoms of limbic dysfunction correlate to the characteristics seen in the mood disorders (Hammen and Gitlin, 1997; Zajecka, 1996).

Another hypothesis involves biological rhythms. **Circadian rhythms** are regular fluctuations of a variety of physiological factors over 24 hours. The rhythms, which are often altered during mood disorders, include adrenal, thyroid, and growth hormone–secreting patterns, as well as temperature, sleep, arousal, energy, appetite, and motor activity patterns. The biological "clock," or internal pacemaker located in the hypothalamus, may be desynchronized by external or internal factors. An example of external desynchronization is jet lag, in which rapid time zone changes result in decreased energy level and ability to concentrate, as well as mood variations. In some individuals, internal desynchronization may result in depression. The tendency toward internal desynchronization is probably inherited, but it is also influenced by stresses, lifestyle, and normal aging. However, it is unclear whether changes in circadian rhythms cause mood disturbances or whether changes in mood alter circadian rhythms (Hedaya, 1996; Mann et al, 1996).

Some forms of mood disorders are related to the time of year and the amount of available sunlight. In **seasonal affective disorder (SAD)**, depression occurs annually during fall and winter, and normal mood or hypomania occurs in spring and summer. The depressive state appears to be directly related to the amount of light because symptoms disappear if the person is exposed to more sunlight. Light has an inhibiting effect on the production of melatonin, a hormone that affects mood, sensations of fatigue, and sleepiness. Seasonal light changes are not the only trigger. A change of living quarters, such as a move into a darker basement apartment or into a windowless office, can cause the disorder in some people. The majority of SAD sufferers are women with a family history of mood disorders. Unlike major depression, in which symptoms for children and adults differ, children and adults with SAD exhibit similar symptoms: fatigue, decreased activity, irritability, sadness, crying, worrying, and decreased concentration. A symptom seen more frequently in SAD, compared to the other mood disorders, is increased appetite, carbohydrate craving, and weight gain (Hedaya, 1996). A secondary cause of depression may be related to a variety of medications and medical conditions. Medications implicated in secondary depression include antianxiety agents, antihypertensives, corticosteroids, estrogen/progesterone, and chemotherapeutic agents. Metabolic disorders that may cause depression include hyperthyroidism, hypothyroidism, Addison's disease, and vitamin B_{12} deficiency. Neurological disruptions include brain tumors or acute traumatic brain injury (especially in the frontal or basal ganglia areas), CVA, Huntington's disease, multiple sclerosis, Parkinson's disease, and Alzheimer's disease (Zajecka, 1996).

Intrapersonal Theory

Intrapersonal theory focuses on the theme of loss, either real or symbolic. The loss may be of another person, a relationship, an object, self-esteem, or security. When grief concerning the loss is unrecognized or unresolved, depression may result. A normal feeling accompanying all losses is anger. People who have been taught it is inappropriate to experience and express anger learn to repress it. The result is that anger is turned inward and against the self. Some theorists believe the repressed anger and aggression against the self are the cause of depressive episodes. Other theorists believe the cause of depression is an inability to achieve desired goals, the loss of these goals, and a feeling of lack of control in life.

Learning Theory

Learning theory states that people learn to be depressed in response to an external locus of control, as they perceive themselves lacking control over their life experiences. Throughout life, depressed people experience little success in achieving gratification, and little positive reinforcement for their attempts to cope with negative incidents. These repeated failures teach them that what they do has no effect on the final outcome. The more that stressful life events occur, the more their sense of helplessness is reinforced. When people reach the point of believing they have no control, they no longer have the will or energy to cope with life, and a depressive state results.

Cognitive Theory

The cognitive schemas influence the way people with mood disorders experience themselves and others. Those who are depressed focus on negative messages in the environment and ignore positive experiences. These negative schemas contribute to a view of the self as incompetent, unworthy, and unlikable. All present experiences are viewed as negative, and there is no hope for the future. In the manic phase, people focus on positive messages in the environment and ignore negative experiences. These positive schemas contribute to a grandiose view of themselves. Everything that occurs is seen as positive, and the future holds no limits. When people get caught up in this process, a number of cognitive distortions may occur (see Table 1.5 in Chapter 1).

Social Theory

A variety of sociocultural conditions may contribute to a person's depressive feelings of powerlessness, hopelessness, and low self-esteem. Racism, classism, sexism, ageism, and homophobia are predominant sociocultural characteristics in the United States. Whatever way minorities are defined, they experience discrimination psychologically, educationally, vocationally, and economically. When one is the subject of cultural stereotypes in comments or jokes, it is difficult not to feel inadequate and shameful. When education has been substandard, one cannot expect to be successful without remedial work. When promotions are based on race, gender, age, or sexual orientation, it is difficult to feel hopeful about advancing in one's career. It is also difficult to combat the helplessness felt when one's financial compensation is clearly inadequate for the job being done.

There is a much higher rate of depression among women than among men. One of the contributing factors in Western society may be the stress of being a single parent. With the high divorce rate, there are increasing numbers of single parents, 85% of them women. These women must deal with financial hardships, parenting problems, loneliness, and lack of a supportive adult relationship. A major predisposing factor for depression in women is having three or more children under the age of 14 living at home. When the children grow up and leave, the rate of depression decreases. This is contrary to the theory that depression results from the empty-nest syndrome. It appears that being responsible for children is a source of stress that contributes to depression (Gotlib and Hammen, 1992).

Another sociocultural factor that may contribute to depression is the occurrence of stressful life events. Some events cause expansion of the family system: marriage, births, adoptions, other people moving into the home. Other events cause a reduction of the family system: children leaving, marital separations, divorce, death. Some life events involve a threat, as in job problems, difficulties with the police, and illness. Others can be emotionally exhausting, such as holidays, changing residences, and arguing with family and friends. Many people who experience major stressful events do not become depressed. However, for those who are vulnerable to depression, stressors may play a significant role in the exacerbation and course of the disorder (Cui and Vaillant, 1996; Kendler et al, 1995).

A number of factors influence the degree of stress that accompanies significant life events (Figure 11.2). The presence of a social support network can decrease the impact an event may have on a person. People who have developed adaptive coping patterns such as problem solving, direct communication, and use of resources are more likely to maintain their normal mood. Those who feel out of control, are unable to problem-solve, and ignore available resources are more apt to feel depressed. Thus, an individual's perception and interpretation of significant events may contribute to depression.

Feminist Theory

In the definition of mental health there has, in the past, been a double standard for women and men. A healthy woman has been described as acquiescent, subdued, dependent, and emotionally expressive. A healthy man, on the other hand, has been described as logical, rational, independent, aggressive, and unemotional. These stereotypes have had unfortunate consequences for both women and men. However, there is movement toward an androgynous definition of mental health. This perspective stresses positive human qualities such as assertiveness, self-reliance, sensitivity to others, intimacy, and open communication—qualities that legitimately belong in the repertoire of both women and men.

Gender socialization differences may be a factor in the higher rate of depression in women. It starts early, when many girls are encouraged to play with dolls and help take care of other children in the family. Girls are taught to be "nice," nonargumenative, and docile. They become more concerned than boys about fitting in and backing down in the face of conflict. Gradually they begin to question the worth of their abilities and opinions, which decreases self-esteem. Boys are socialized to be individualistic, to speak up, to raise their hands more in class. Gradually they begin to see themselves as autonomous individuals with good self-esteem.

Rigid expectations about gender roles continue to linger and contribute to higher rates of depression among women. Women who are full-time homemakers may develop no identity other than that of wife and mother. The tremendous duties of managing a household are often invisible to others and lack prestige. Positive feedback or positive reinforcement such as compliments, a paycheck, and retirement benefits are uncommon. And the position is continuous, 24 hours a day. Since one lives in the workplace, there is no stimulation from a change in the environment. Indeed, being a full-time homemaker is one of the most isolating professions in society today.

Women who are employed outside the home, in both professional and blue-collar positions, are less depressed than those who remain at home. This is true even for women who must assume the responsibility for two full-time jobs with minimal or no support from other family members (Faludi, 1991). Employed women must often accept lower pay, inferior jobs, and fewer opportunities for career advancement. The legal system has been slow to redress employment discrimination, which increases women's frustration, anger, and distress. Thoughts of the future focus on the helplessness of their situations and contribute to depression.

Feminist theory can also be applied to the situation in which some older adults find themselves. In a society that places a premium on youth, older people feel useless, unimportant, incapable, and at times even repulsive. Role changes and losses may threaten their self-esteem. With aging, physiological changes may lead to a self-perception of being unfit, which then extends to further thoughts of being ineffectual and inferior. All these changes may contribute to despair about one's entire life and a sense of hopelessness about the limited future. Considering these effects, it is not surprising to find a higher rate of depression among older people.

Table 11.3 summarizes the causative theories of mood disorders, with specific relevance to women and older adults.

Psychopharmacological Interventions

The initial phase of medical intervention for clients with mood disorders begins with an in-depth assessment. The physician or nurse practitioner must determine whether any drugs are contributing to or causing the depression. Most commonly, these drugs are alco-

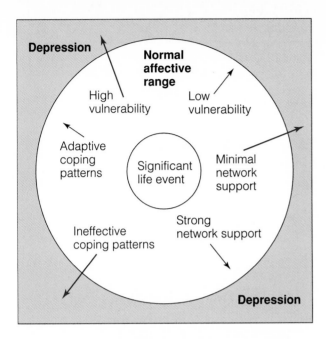

Figure 11.2 **The relationship between life events and depression.**

hol, barbiturates, tranquilizers, and certain antihypertensive agents. The primary care provider also treats any medical conditions, because poor physical health may increase the severity of a clinical depression.

Antidepressant and mood-stabilizing medications are often prescribed for clients with mood disorders (Table 11.4). Because depressions are heterogeneous in terms of which neurotransmitters are depleted, different people respond differently to various antidepressants. (See Chapter 8 for a detailed discussion of these medications.) At times, a period of trial and error is necessary to determine which medication is the most effective. Maintenance continues until clients are free of symptoms for 4 months to 1 year; then the drugs are slowly discontinued. One of the difficulties with taking these medications may be the presence of undesirable side effects. For example, men may experience ejaculatory problems and women may become nonorgasmic. Given these dysfunctions, some people personally elect to stop taking their medication.

Antidepressants do not cause dependence, tolerance, addiction, or withdrawal. Therapeutic response is better determined by blood plasma levels than by dosages (Table 11.5 on page 250). It takes an average of 10–14 days for the beginning effect of most antidepressants, and the full effect may not be apparent for 4–6 weeks. Approximately 30% of clients do not respond after a trial of 4–6 weeks. At that point, the physician may try a different antidepressant or augment with other medications. A significant number of clients improve when 600 mg of lithium is added to the antidepressant treatment. Other clients improve when triiodothyronine (T_3) is administered daily. For clients who are delusional or severely agitated, antipsychotic medication may be indicated. Use of these medications is often necessary because it may take 7 to 10 days or longer before lithium and/or antidepressants are clinically effective (Marangell et al, 1997; Mulsant et al, 1997).

When prescribing antidepressants for older clients, particular care must be taken for several reasons. The older person may metabolize medications at a slower rate because of a decrease in hepatic enzyme activity. Also, as people age, they develop more body fat in comparison to their total body mass. This results in a longer duration of action of these medications because they are stored in body fat. In addition, the CNS of an older person is more sensitive to psychoactive medications because of changes in the blood-brain barrier.

The primary care provider must determine whether the benefits of antidepressant therapy outweigh the risks for the older client. The anticholinergic properties of these medications may lead to short-term memory problems, disorientation, and impaired cognition. These side effects may be mistaken for organic brain disease (pseudodementia). The physician can determine if the client's confusion is due to the antidepressant therapy by administering physostigmine, 1–2 mg IM. This medication increases acetylcholine at the sites of cholinergic transmission, and the symptoms are temporarily reversed if they are related to the side effects of the medication.

There are additional problems with the anticholinergic properties of these medications. If the client has dentures, an extremely dry mouth can lead to gingival erosion. If the older male client has prostatic enlargement, the anticholinergic effect of urinary retention can cause very serious problems. Anticholinergic properties can also intensify unsuspected glaucoma, resulting in increased intraocular pressure. Antidepressant medications may also cause orthostatic hypotension, resulting in a higher risk of dizzy spells and falls.

Table 11.3 Causative Theories of Mood Disorders

Theory	Main Points	Relevance to Women and Older Adults
Genetic	Increased sensitivity to chemical changes related to stress.	
Neurotransmitter	Impaired neurotransmission; limbic dysfunction.	Higher levels of MAO in CNS in women and older people.
Biologic rhythms	Internal desynchronization of circadian rhythms.	
Sunlight	Decreased exposure to sunlight increases production of melatonin.	Older people do not go outside as much during the winter months.
Intrapersonal	Loss of person, object, self-esteem; hostility turned against the self; goals unachieved.	Women are more dependent on others for self-esteem; older people suffer multiple losses.
Learning	Lack of control over experiences; learned helplessness; failure to adapt.	Expectation of women's dependency reinforces helplessness; older people have increased stress with decreased resources, which contributes to loss of control.
Cognitive	Negative view of self, the present, and the future; focus on negative messages; cognitive errors.	
Feminist	Internalization of cultural norms of behavior; rigid gender-role and age expectations.	Women's identity may be limited to home-maker role; employment positions less prestigious; may hold two full-time jobs. Older people suffer from the cultural value on youth; many role changes and losses.

Compared to younger adult clients, older clients are started on antidepressants at lower levels, which are gradually increased to lower maximum levels. Tofranil (imipramine) and Elavil or Endep (amitriptyline) have a maximum level of 100 mg/day for the older client. Pertofrane or Norpramin (desipramine) have a maximum daily dosage level of 150–200 mg. The drugs of choice for older clients are Wellbutrin (bupropion), Prozac (fluoxetine), Zoloft (sertraline), Norpramin (desipramine), Pamelor (nortriptyline), and Vivactil (protriptyline) because they are the least sedating and have the fewest anticholinergic effects (Thase and Kupfer, 1996). Monoamine oxidase inhibitors (MAOIs) do not cause dependence, tolerance, addiction, or withdrawal. In clients experiencing atypical symptoms of depression, MAOIs may be more effective than heterocyclic medications. Adding lithium may speed up the effects of MAOIs (Glod, 1996).

Because the production of MAO increases with age, MAOIs may be more effective for older clients.

Another benefit to older people is the absence of anticholinergic side effects. However, there is a higher risk of hypotension, which may be a contributing factor in falls. The disadvantage of this group of antidepressant medications is the strict dietary limitations. The nutritional options of many older clients are limited because of their finances; they may find it difficult to follow the severely restricted diet. (For dietary restrictions with MAOIs, see Chapter 8.)

It is thought that for a person in a manic state, sodium has replaced potassium in the CNS intercellular spaces. Treatment is directed toward replacing sodium with lithium in these locations. This process is believed to affect the action of NE and 5-HT. It takes anywhere from 7 to 21 days for the therapeutic effect to be clinically visible. If clients have a high salt intake with foods such as pizza, popcorn, or pretzels, the lithium blood level will be lowered. When clients have a very low-salt diet, have a fever, or engage in strenuous exercise with much sweating, they run the risk of a high lithium blood level (Hedaya, 1996).

Table 11.4 Antidepressant Medications

Class	Generic Name	Trade Name	Adult Dosage
Aminoketone	bupropion	Wellburtin	100–450 mg/day
Selective Serotonin Reuptake Inhibitor (SSRI)	fluoxetine	Prozac	20–80 mg/day
	fluvoxamine	Luvox	50–300 mg/day
	paroxetine	Paxil	50–200 mg/ day
	sertraline	Zoloft	50–200 mg/day
Serotonin-Norepinephrine Inhibitor (SNRI)	venlafaxine	Effexor	75–375 mg/day
	nefazodone	Serzone	200–600 mg/day
Tricyclic	amitriptyline	Elavil, Endep	50–300 mg/day
	amoxapine	Asendin	50–400 mg/day
	clomipramine	Anafranil	75–250 mg/day
	desipramine	Norpramin, Petrofrane	50–300 mg/day
	doxepin	Adapin, Sinequan	50–300 mg/day
	imipramine	Tofranil	50–300 mg/day
	nortriptyline	Aventyl, Pamelor	30–125 mg/day
	protriptyline	Vivactil	10–60 mg/day
	trimipramine	Surmontil	50–300 mg/day
Tetracyclic	maprotiline	Ludiomil	50–225 mg/day
	mirtazapine	Remeron	15–45 mg/day
Phenylpiperazine	trazodone	Desyrel	50–600 mg/day
MAOI	isocarboxazid	Marplan	10–30 mg/day
	phenelzine	Nardil	45–90 mg/day
	tranylcypromine	Parnate	30–60 mg/day

When lithium therapy is initiated, blood levels are monitored three times a week until a therapeutic level is achieved, and then monthly during maintenance therapy. For accuracy, lithium levels should be measured 12 hours after the last lithium dose. The early side effects are identical to signs of toxicity, and blood levels are the only indicator of toxicity. Since the side effects disappear after 4 weeks, clients are cautioned to report the following toxic signs to their doctor: nausea and vomiting, diarrhea, ataxia, blurred vision, tremors, confusion, and seizures. Toxicity can cause myocardial infarction and cardiovascular collapse.

Clients who experience fewer episodes of bipolar disorder are more responsive to lithium than those who are rapid-cyclers. In studying the frequency of relapse in a time period of 2 years, it has been found that 20–40% of clients on lithium will relapse, compared to 65–90% of those who are not on lithium (Fenn et al, 1996).

Lithium toxicity may occur with conditions that cause fluid loss, such as vomiting or diarrhea, or with decreased glomerular filtration rate, which is most often seen in older or pregnant clients. In the normal aging process, there may be a decreased glomerular filtration rate in the kidneys. When an older client is on lithium therapy for bipolar disorder, there is delayed excretion of the lithium and therefore an increased risk of lithium toxicity. If the older client is concurrently on a sodium-depleting diuretic, the risk of toxicity increases rapidly. The therapeutic range of blood lithium levels for the younger adult is 1.0–1.5 mEq/L in the acute phase and 0.6–1.2 mEq/L in the maintenance phase. In the older adult, the therapeutic range lowers to 0.5–1.0 mEq/L (Fenn et al, 1996).

Table 11.5 Therapeutic Blood Level Responses to Mood Disorder Medications

Generic Name	Trade Name	Blood Level
bupropion	Wellburtin	10–29 ng/mL
amitriptyline	Elavil, Endep	50–250 ng/mL
amoxapine	Asendin	200–600 ng/mL
desipramine	Norpramin, Petrofrane	70–260 ng/mL
doxepin	Adapin, Sinequan	150–250 ng/mL
imipramine	Trofranil	150–250 ng/mL
nortriptyline	Aventyl, Pamelor	70–260 ng/mL
protriptyline	Vivactil	70–260 ng/mL
trimipramine	Surmontil	100–200 ng/mL
maprotiline	Ludiomil	200–600 ng/mL
trazodone	Desyrel	800–1,600 ng/mL
lithium	Eskalith, Lithane, Lithobid, Cibalith-S	1.0–1.5 mEq/L, acute
		0.6–1.2 mEq/L, maintenance
carbamazepine	Tegretol	8–12 µg/mL
valproate	Depakene, Depakote	50–100 mg/mL

Sources: Goodnick, 1992; Maxmen, 1991; Rakel, 1993.

About 30% of clients in a manic state either fail to respond to lithium or cannot tolerate the side effects. Recent research has found that two anticonvulsant drugs, Tegretol (carbamazepine) and Depakene (valproate), are possible alternatives to lithium. Tegretol is related to the tricyclic antidepressants and has a similar CNS effect. Depakene potentiates GABA, which in turn regulates an abnormal circadian cycle (Bowden, 1996). Clients taking these medications must be carefully assessed for suicide because they may choose to overdose. The older antidepressant medications have very high overdose potential, and as little as 30–40 mg/kg of body weight may be fatal for adults. A 10-day supply of MAOIs can be lethal if taken at one time. Lithium is fatal at a dose of 10–60 g, which is indicated by a blood level of 4–5 mEq/L.

Multidisciplinary Interventions

Electroconvulsive therapy (ECT) may be useful for a variety of clients. ECT is a safer alternative for highly suicidal clients, those who suffer from psychotic depression, and those who are medically deteriorated. During pregnancy, ECT is a safer choice than medications because uterine muscle does not automatically contract as part of a generalized tonic-clonic seizure. Clients who do not respond to medications, or who cannot tolerate the side effects, often respond positively to ECT. In addition, ECT may be safer for older clients at high risk from the anticholinergic side effects of medications (Finnerty and Levin, 1996; Zajecka, 1996). See Chapter 7 for further information on ECT.

Another medical treatment for depression is sleep deprivation. This may be total, for 36 hours, or partial, with the person being awakened after 1:30 AM and kept awake until the next evening. During this time, clients may be alone, in a group, or participating in activities. Some improve steadily after only one night of sleep deprivation. Others respond better if the deprivation is conducted once a week for several weeks. Merely advancing the sleep period to begin at 5:00 PM and end at 12:00 midnight for two to three weeks leads to an improvement of depression in 75% of clients (Berger et al, 1997).

Phototherapy is often the treatment of choice for SAD. Clients are exposed to very bright full-spectrum fluorescent lamps for 2–6 hours a day. Clinical improvement is typically seen within 3–5 days. Phototherapy may be used prophylactically with clients susceptible to SAD. It is thought that the bright light suppresses the production of melatonin and normalizes the disturbance in circadian rhythms (Terman et al, 1996).

When one family member suffers from a mood disorder, there is frequently a detrimental effect on all family members. Families need information and support during this time, and **family therapy** is often very beneficial. Roles and relationships must be redefined during acute episodes and clients and families may need help with this process. If family interactions are dysfunctional, therapists may be able to assist in the development of healthier and more adaptive coping behaviors. Most family members want to be involved in treatment and believe that it is difficult to support the person with a mood disorder if they are excluded from the therapeutic process (Badger, 1996).

The Nursing Process

Assessment

Assessing clients with mood disorders is often done in segments of 15–20 minutes each. Those who are depressed do not have the energy to talk for longer periods, and those who are in a manic phase are unable to concentrate and sit still for longer periods. You must exercise a great deal of patience when assessing these clients. Clients who are depressed may take a long time to answer your questions, and you may need to repeat them. If family members are present, discourage them from answering questions for the client who is responding slowly. Clients in a manic phase with flight of ideas must frequently be refocused on the topic at hand. Their elevated mood may interfere with their ability to give accurate information. See the Focused Nursing Assessment table on the following pages. You may wish to use the Beck Depression Inventory (Table 11.6 on page 254). This is a self-rating scale that measures levels of depression.

At times your assessment will be focused toward differentiating between depression and grief. See Table 11.7 on page 256 for the differences and refer to Chapter 16 for further information on grief and loss.

Diagnosis

Assessment provides the data you use to develop the nursing diagnoses. To guide this process, ask the following questions:

- Is any of the client's behavior a danger to self or others (eg, suicide, impulsive behavior)?
- Are there any physiological signs and symptoms that are of priority concern (eg, inadequate intake, exhaustion)?
- In what areas does the client have the most difficulty functioning (ADLs, problem solving, interpersonal relationships)?

The Nursing Diagnoses box on page 257 contains those diagnoses most commonly identified for clients with mood disorders.

Outcome Identification

Once you have established diagnoses, you and the client mutually identify goals for change. Client outcomes are specific behavioral measures by which you, the client, and significant others determine progress toward these goals. The following are examples of outcomes that may be pertinent to the client with a mood disorder:

- remains safe
- verbalizes decreasing suicidal ideation
- establishes a routine schedule that balances exercise and quiet time
- accomplishes ADLs
- utilizes the problem-solving process
- makes appropriate decisions
- verbalizes logical thought processes
- socializes appropriately with others
- becomes a self-advocate
- reports purpose and joy in life and a sense of connectedness to others

See the Critical Pathway for a Client with Depression Without Psychotic Features or Agitation on pages 258–263 and the Critical Pathway for a Client with Bipolar Disorder, Manic Phase on pages 264–269.

Nursing Interventions

Goals and outcome criteria help focus your nursing care. The overall goal is to help clients improve the response to mood disorders and develop effective coping behaviors. See the box on page 270 for an overview of the nursing interventions classification (NIC) for people with mood disorders.

Safety: Crisis Management

Suicide Prevention
The first priority of care is client safety. Since as many as 15% of clients with mood disorders commit suicide, it is extremely important that you assess for suicide potential. Chapter 16 gives detailed information on assessment and interventions for clients who are suicidal.

Behavioral Assessment	Affective Assessment	Cognitive Assessment
How are you managing your work/household/school responsibilities?	How would you describe your overall mood?	What qualities do you like about yourself?
What are your leisure activities?	Do you have mood swings?	Give me an example of past success in your life.
Do you feel isolated from others?	How much time each day do you spend thinking about failure or guilt?	Overall, how would you evaluate your life in the past?
	How often do you cry?	Are you having difficulty concentrating?
	What activities have given you pleasure in the past ? In the present?	Does it seem as though your thoughts come slowly or quickly?
		Do you make decisions easily?

Family members need to be taught the following: people who talk about suicide are at high risk; suicide attempts may follow the loss of an important person, position, or possession; social isolation and substance abuse increase the risk of a suicide attempt; suicide attempts may increase as the depression is beginning to improve, since thought patterns are still negative but the person now has enough energy to make the attempt; and getting one's "life in order" is a high-risk signal.

Safety: Risk Management

Hallucination Management

Hallucinations are frightening experiences and most individuals welcome opportunities to discuss them. It is critical that you monitor the hallucinations for content that is self-harmful, suicidal, or violent toward others. Encourage clients to express these feelings appropriately rather than act on the violent messages.

Encourage clients to validate their perceptions with people whom they trust, such as yourself or family members. If a client asks you to verify a hallucination, point out that you are not experiencing the same stimuli. Arguments about the validity of the hallucination should be avoided. If hallucinations are interfering with a conversation, try to refocus the client to the topic. If that is unsuccessful, focus the discussion on the underlying feelings, rather than the content of the hallucination. You may say something like: "That sounds like a very frightening experience." Some people find that participation in reality-based activities such as a game or cooking may distract from the hallucination. Other find that music may "drown out" the voices (McCloskey and Bulechek, 1996). Further information on hallucinations is found in Chapter 6.

Behavioral: Behavioral Therapy

Behavior Management/Overactivity

Clients experiencing a manic episode may become exhausted when excessive levels of activity are combined with decreased awareness of fatigue. When intervening you must first get clients' attention by calling their name or lightly touching the arm. If the environment (a person or a situation) is overstimulating, you may need to redirect or remove the client to a quieter area to facilitate self-control. Clients experiencing hypomanic or manic episodes should avoid stimulating places such as bars or busy shopping malls. Limiting intake of caffeinated food and fluids may also facilitate self-control. Clients should establish a routine schedule that includes a balance of structured time (activities such as work, writing, painting, or crafts) and quiet time and post this in a visible place.

Social Assessment	Cultural Assessment	Physiological Assessment
Who lives in your household?	What is your ethnic identity?	How is your appetite?
With whom do you communicate most easily?	What do you believe is the source of your problems?	Are you having difficulty sleeping?
What roles and responsibilities do you assume in your family?	What home remedies have you tried to make yourself better?	Do you tire easily or have a high level of energy?
What kinds of losses have you sustained during the past year?		Has your partner commented on a change in your level of sexual desire?

If you are helping clients who are hyperactive to follow a procedure, give instructions or explanations in simple, concrete language and ask them to repeat what they heard before beginning the task. Allow clients to carry out one instruction before being given another and provide positive feedback for the completion of each step.

Manic episodes cause some people to become interested in every person and every activity in the environment. Thus, they may be very intrusive in other people's conversations and create socially awkward situations. You, or family members, need to set limits on intrusive or interruptive behaviors. Appropriate social roles and the appropriate expression of feelings need to be taught and reinforced (McCloskey and Bulechek, 1996).

Behavior Management: Sexual

Adult clients who are depressed often experience a diminished interest in sex. You should introduce the topic of sexuality with the client and partner, to enable them to share concerns. Teaching includes explaining that sexual desire usually returns as the depression recedes. Understanding that lack of desire is a symptom of depression will decrease feelings of hurt, inadequacy, and guilt. Stress the importance of nonsexual expressions of affection, such as hugging and holding each other, as reassuring forms of communication. If the lack of desire continues after the depression has lifted, suggest that the couple consider sex therapy.

Clients in a manic episode often exhibit an impulsive increase in their sexual activity. Family members must understand that such behavior is a symptom of the manic state and is not within the client's control. As much as possible, the client should be protected from sexual acting-out until he or she is able to assume control over this behavior.

Behavioral: Cognitive Therapy

Cognitive Restructuring

Assess clients for altered thought processes such as overgeneralization, dichotomous thinking, catastrophizing, or personalization. Help them identify negative self-statements by asking questions such as: "What do you say about yourself? Is that true? Have these thoughts increased with your depression?" This helps clients understand that negative thinking is part of the disorder and not necessarily fact. Point out examples of dysfunctional thinking as it occurs. Remind clients and families that depression is neither related to personal failure nor a sign of inferiority.

Text continues on page 256

Table 11.6 Beck Depression Inventory

The Beck Depression Inventory is a self-rating scale that measures depression. The patient can complete the questionnaire in about 10 minutes. The total score provides an estimate of the degree of severity of the depressed mood. Add the raw scores. The mean scores can be interpreted as follows

Total Score	Levels of Depression
1–10	Normal ups and downs
11–16	Mild mood disturbance
17–20	Borderline clinical depression
12–30	Moderate depression
30–40	Severe depression
Over 40	Extreme depression

(A persistent score of 17 or above indicates professional treatment might be necessary)

1.
   - 0   I do not feel sad.
   - 1   I feel sad.
   - 2   I am sad all the time and I can't snap out of it.
   - 3   I am so sad or unhappy that I can't stand it.

2.
   - 0   I am not particularly discouraged about the future.
   - 1   I feel discouraged about the future.
   - 2   I feel I have nothing to look forward to.
   - 3   I feel that the future is hopeless and that things cannot improve.

3.
   - 0   I do not feel like a failure.
   - 1   I feel I have failed more than the average person.
   - 2   As I look back on my life, all I can see is a lot of failures.
   - 3   I feel I am a complete failure as a person.

4.
   - 0   I get as much satisfaction out of things as I used to.
   - 1   I don't enjoy things the way I used to.
   - 2   I don't get real satisfaction out of anything anymore.
   - 3   I am dissatisfied or bored with everything.

5.
   - 0   I don't feel particularly guilty.
   - 1   I feel guilty a good part of the time.
   - 2   I feel quite guilty most of the time.
   - 3   I feel guilty all of the time.

6.
   - 0   I don't feel I am being punished.
   - 1   I feel I may be punished.
   - 2   I expect to be punished.
   - 3   I feel I am being punished.

7.
   - 0   I don't feel disappointed in myself.
   - 1   I am disappointed in myself.
   - 2   I am disgusted with myself.
   - 3   I hate myself.

8.
   - 0   I don't feel I am worse than anybody else.
   - 1   I am critical of myself for any weaknesses or mistakes.
   - 2   I blame myself all the time for my faults.
   - 3   I blame myself for everything bad that happens.

9.
   - 0   I don't have any thoughts of killing myself.
   - 1   I have thoughts of killing myself, but I would not carry them out.
   - 2   I would like to kill myself.
   - 3   I would kill myself if I had the chance.

Table 11.6 continued

10. 0 I don't cry any more than usual.
    1 I cry more now than usual.
    2 I cry all the time now.
    3 I used to able to cry, but now I can't even though I want to.

11. 0 I am no more irritated by things than I ever am.
    1 I am slightly more irritated now than usual.
    2 I am quite annoyed or irritated a good deal of the time.
    3 I feel irritated all the time now.

12. 0 I have not lost interest in other people.
    1 I am less interested in other people than I used to be.
    2 I have lost most of any interest in other people.
    3 I have lost all of my interest in other people.

13. 0 I make decisions about as well as I ever could.
    1 I put off making decisions more than I used to.
    2 I have greater difficulty in making decisions than before.
    3 I can't make decisions at all anymore.

14. 0 I don't feel that I look any worse than I used to.
    1 I am worried that I am looking old or unattractive.
    2 I feel that there permanent changes in my appearance that make me look unattractive.
    3 I believe that I look ugly.

15. 0 I can work about as well as before.
    1 I takes an extra effort to get started doing something.
    2 I have to push myself very hard to do anything.

---

  3 I can't do any work at all.

16. 0 I can sleep as well as usual.
    1 I don't sleep as well as I used to.
    2 I wake up 1–2 hours earlier than I used to and cannot get back to sleep.
    3 I wake up several hours earlier than I used to and cannot get back to sleep.

17. 0 I don't get more tired than usual.
    1 I get tired more easily than I used to.
    2 I get tired from doing almost anything.
    3 I am too tired to do anything.

18. 0 My appetite is no worse than usual.
    1 My appetite is not as good as it used to be.
    2 My appetite is much worse now.
    3 I have no appetite at all anymore.

19. 0 I haven't lost much weight, if any, lately.
    1 I have lost more than 5 pounds.
    2 I have lost more than 10 pounds.
    3 I have lost more than 15 pounds.

20. 0 I am no more worried about my health than usual.
    1 I am worried about physical problems such as aches and pains, or upset stomach, or constipation.
    2 I am very worried about physical problems and it's hard to think of much else.
    3 I am so worried about my physical problems that I cannot think about anything else.

21. 0 I have not noticed any recent change in my interest in sex.
    1 I am less interested in sex than I used to be.
    2 I am much less interested in sex now.
    3 I have lost interest in sex completely.

Beck et al, 1961.

Table 11.7 Differences Between Depression and Grief

Trait	Depression	Grief
Trigger	Specific trigger not necessary	Trigger usually loss or multiple losses
Active/passive	Passive behavior tends to keep them "stuck" in sadness	Actively feel their emotional pain and emptiness
Emotions	Generalized feeling of helplessness, hopelessness	Experience a range of emotions that are usually intense
Ability to laugh	Likely to be humorless and incapable of being happy or even temporarily cheered up; likely to resist support	Sometimes will be able to laugh and enjoy humor; more likely to accept support
Activities	Lack of interest in previously enjoyed activities	Can be persuaded to participate in activities, especially as they begin to heal
Self-esteem	Low self-esteem, low self-confidence; feels like a failure	Self-esteem usually remains intact; does not feel like a failure unless it relates directly to the loss
Feeling of failure	May dwell on past failures, catastrophize	Any self-blame or guilt relates directly to the loss; feelings resolve as they progress toward healing

Sources: Klebanoff and Smith, 1997; Silverstein and Perlick, 1995.

It is not unusual for people with bipolar disorder to deny the disorder and the need for treatment. Frequently this occurs at the onset but may recur throughout the course of the disorder. When treatment is initiated and they start to feel better, they may again deny the illness and the need for medication.

Clients working toward self-management typically go through several cognitive phases. The first phase is the realization of a need. In other words, individuals must accept that they have a disorder in order to be motivated to seek information. Phase two is the process of seeking information. You may need to alert clients and families to reliable resources so they can obtain the information they desire. The third phase has been identified as being a critical juncture in treatment. The information they receive must be perceived as being applicable to themselves. If clients are to move on to self-management, they must also have the energy and the will to succeed in self-care. Phase four is the process of self-management. In this advanced phase clients select useful self-management strategies, including problem-solving skills, and learn how to deal with and overcome barriers to self-management (Pollack, 1995).

Behavioral: Communication Enhancement

Active Listening

People with mood disorders experience either slowed or racing thought processes, both of which result in problems with communication. You can assist these clients through active listening. To do this you must clear your mind of preoccupying personal concerns, eliminate environmental distractions, and focus completely on the interaction. Listen for clients' unexpressed messages and feelings as well as the overt content of the conversation. You must clarify the message through use of questions and feedback and finally verify your understanding of what was communicated.

People in the manic phase of bipolar disorder often experience flight of ideas. Since flight of ideas is partially in response to multiple stimuli in the environment, you should decrease environmental stimuli by suggesting that the two of you go to a quieter area. If you cannot follow what is being said, say you are having difficulty such as, "Your thoughts are coming too quickly for me to follow what you are trying to say." Ask the person to try to slow

Nursing Diagnoses

Clients with Mood Disorders

High risk for violence, self-directed, related to suicidal ideation or suicide plan.

High risk for violence, directed at others, related to impulsive behavior and labile affect.

Impaired verbal communication related to retardation in flow of thought; flight of ideas.

Decisional conflict related to inability to concentrate; need to make perfect decisions.

Altered role performance related to high affiliation needs.

Hopelessness related to negative expectations of self and future.

Deficit in diversional activity related to decrease in gratification; short attention span and high energy level.

Fatigue related to lack of energy and tiring easily; hyperactivity and decreased awareness of physical exhaustion.

Bathing/hygiene self-care deficit related to low energy level; distractibility in completing ADLs.

Altered thought process related to overgeneralization, dichotomous thinking, catastrophizing, or personalization.

Self-esteem disturbance related to guilt, criticism, and negative self-evaluation; delusions and grandiosity.

Spiritual distress related to no purpose or joy in life; lack of connectedness to others; misperceived guilt.

down the communication in an effort to help organize their thinking. You might say, "Let's talk about one thought at a time" or "Let's stay with this idea for a minute." Try to identify the theme of the client's flight of ideas to increase your comprehension of what the client is attempting to communicate. In order to promote successful communication, you should provide clients the opportunity to validate or correct your perception. You might say, "You seem to be mentioning your mother often. Are you having some concerns about her?"

Socialization Enhancement

People who are depressed often experience a decreased desire to interact with others, which results in social isolation. However, the more alone and isolated people are, the more depressed they feel. When people connect to and interact with others, they feel less lonely and their mood often begins to lift. In severe depression it may be necessary for either you or one family member to participate with the person in solitary activities in the beginning. As the mood lifts, more people and more activities may be planned into the day. Encourage clients and families to identify the benefits of social interaction, as this reinforces the positive change in behavior.

Peer counseling may be another activity to enhance clients' socialization. Peer counseling is a free, safe, and effective self-help tool that encourages expression of feelings. It puts clients in control of their own healing process. In a peer counseling session, two people agree to spend a certain amount of time together, dividing the time equally, paying attention to each others' issues, needs, and distresses. Judging, criticizing, and giving advice are not allowed.

Behavioral: Coping Assistance

Coping Enhancement

Nurses can enhance coping by teaching clients to utilize the problem-solving process. This process is presented in more detail in Chapter 5. Initially, you must evaluate clients' abilities to problem-solve while discouraging decision making under situations of severe stress or during the acute phase of a mood disorder. Together, you, clients, and families can explore previous methods of dealing with life problems and the success or failure of those past attempts. Next, help them identify appropriate short- and long-term goals while ensuring that these are broken down into small, manageable steps (outcomes). Clients and families next choose which strategies they wish to implement to solve the problem. Following the actual implementation, they evaluate the process on the basis of how well their outcomes were achieved and how close they have come to meeting their goals.

Other activities to encourage coping include exploring clients' previous achievements of success, encouraging clients to identify their own strengths and abilities, and facilitating the evaluation of their own behavior. You can help them problem-solve situations

Text continues on page 272

Critical Pathway for a Client with Depression without Psychotic Features or Agitation

Expected length of stay: 8 days	Date _____ Day 1	Date _____ Days 2–3	Date _____ Day 4
Daily outcomes	Client will: ■ Remain free of self-inflicted injury. ■ Communicate suicidal ideation. ■ Contract for safety. ■ Identify initial goals for hospitalization. ■ Verbalize need for medications. ■ Remain oriented to time, place, and person with prompting. ■ Participate in assessment. ■ Identify current dietary pattern and food preferences. ■ Identify current elimination pattern. ■ Identify recreation and leisure interest and capabilities. ■ Identify current self-care patterns including sleep, physical activity, and hygiene.	Client will: ■ Remain free of self-inflicted injury. ■ Communicate feelings related to depressed mood. ■ Maintain contract for safety. ■ Participate in development of transdisciplinary treatment plan. ■ Identify name, dose, and major side effects of medications. ■ Demonstrate orientation to time, place, and person. ■ Participate in menu plan for balanced meal. ■ Identify need for laxative if no BM in 3 days. ■ Attend 25% of leisure activities as scheduled with prompting and support.	Client will: ■ Remain free of self-inflicted injury. ■ Identify at least one reason for living. ■ Identify 3 positive attributes of self. ■ Identify one false perception of misbelief. ■ Communicate feelings related to managing loss and stress. ■ Participate in transdisciplinary plan: Identify changes in symptoms as a result of medications; remain oriented to time, place, and person; consume diet as per menu plan; attend 50% of scheduled activities independently; identify need for laxative; perform self-care activities independently 50% of time.
Assessments, tests, and treatments	Complete psychosocial assessment to include mental status, mood, affect, behavior, and communication q shift and PRN. Assess suicidal ideation, gestures, threats, plans, and means. Contract for safety. Observe for safety per protocol. Complete nursing database assessment. Weight. Initiate suicide precautions as indicated. CBC, urinalysis. Chemistry profile Thyroid profile. RPR. Other laboratory as ordered. Vital signs BID.	Psychosocial assessment q shift and PRN. Observe for safety per protocol. Monitor dietary intake, sleep pattern, and bowel elimination pattern. Continue suicide assessment. Reinforce safety contract. Suicide precautions as indicated. Monitor effects of and compliance with medications. Routine vital signs.	Daily psychosocial assessment. Observe for safety per protocol. Monitor dietary intake, sleep pattern, and bowel elimination pattern. Continue suicide assessment. Reinforce safety contract. Suicide precautions as indicated. Monitor effects of and compliance with medications. Routine vital signs.

	Date _____ Day 1 *continued*	Date _____ Days 2–3 *continued*	Date _____ Day 4 *continued*
Knowledge deficit	Orient client and family to patients, staff, and program. Review initial plan of care. Assess learning needs of client and family. Initiate medication teaching. Assess understanding of teaching.	Review unit orientation with emphasis on program. Continue medication teaching. Assess understanding of teaching.	Review plan of care. Include family in teaching. Initiate teaching regarding anxiety, depression, treatment modalities, and preventive techniques. Assess medication teaching response and need for additional teaching. Assess understanding of teaching.
Diet	Monitor dietary intake. Diet as tolerated; encourage small, frequent feedings from all food groups. Provide preferred snacks and foods. Provide adequate time for meals and snacks. Encourage fluids. Low tyramine diet if on MAOIs.	Monitor dietary intake. Diet per menu plan; encourage fluids; encourage small, frequent feedings from all food groups. Provide preferred snacks and foods. Provide adequate time for meals and snacks. Encourage fluids. Low tyramine diet if on MAOIs.	Monitor dietary intake. Diet per menu plan; encourage fluids; encourage small, frequent feedings from all food groups. Provide preferred snacks and foods. Provide adequate time for meals and snacks. Encourage fluids. Low tyramine diet if on MAOIs.
Activity	Assess safety needs and maintain appropriate precautions. Encourage client to be in milieu 10 hr/day. Encourage brief periods of activity and interaction. Provide sleep-enhancing atmosphere for 45 min prior to sleep.	Maintain safety precautions. Encourage activities during the day; prompt client to attend 25% of activities. Prompt and assist with hygiene as necessary. Encourage to participate in simple exercise. Prompt to engage in simple structured activities. Provide sleep-enhancing atmosphere for 45 min prior to sleep.	Maintain safety precautions. Encourage involvement in 50–75% of activities. Prompt with hygiene as necessary. Prompt to participate in exercise.
Psychosocial	Observe behavior. Assess level of anxiety. Encourage verbalization of feelings and thoughts. Listen attentively, giving adequate time to respond. Approach with nonjudgmental and accepting manner. Formulate initial plan of care with client and family.	Observe behavior. Assess level of anxiety. Encourage verbalization of concerns and feelings. Provide information and ongoing support and encouragement to client and family. Provide simple structured activities.	Observe behavior. Assess level of anxiety. Encourage verbalization of concerns and feelings. Provide information and ongoing support and encouragement to client and family.

continued ➤

Critical Pathway for a Client with Depression without Psychotic Features or Agitation continued

	Date _____ Day 1 continued	Date _____ Days 2–3 continued	Date _____ Day 4 continued
Psychosocial *continued*	Offer realistic hope to client and family. Identify current support system. Encourage structured activities. Provide information regarding illness and treatment. Provide ongoing support and encouragement to client and family. Meet with client 4 times each shift for 5-min periods focused on establishing relationship.	Identify potential support system and strategies to access additional supports. Prompt to attend group therapy. Acknowledge accomplishments. Meet with client 10–15-min twice a shift during waking hours and focus on working on initial goals.	Provide increasingly complex structured activities. Initiate cognitive restructuring. Review strategies to access support system using problem-solving strategies. Encourage group therapy independent attendance with spontaneous involvement × 1. Acknowledge accomplishments. Meet with client 15 min every shift during waking hours to work on therapeutic goals.
Medications	Identify target symptoms. Antidepressants as ordered. Routine meds as ordered.	Identify target symptoms. Antidepressants as ordered. Routine meds as ordered Colace/Metamucil if indicated. PRN laxative if no BM in 3 days.	Assess target symptoms. Antidepressants as ordered. Routine meds as ordered. Colace/Metamucil if indicated. PRN laxative if no BM in 3 days.
Consults and discharge plan	Family assessment. Establish discharge objectives with client and family. Occupational and recreational therapist.	Review discharge objectives with client and significant others. Initate referrals for discharge care.	Review progress toward discharge objectives with client and significant others. Make appropriate referrals to support groups.

	Date _____ Day 5	Date _____ Day 6	Date _____ Days 7–8 to Discharge
Daily outcomes	Client will: ■ Remain free of self-inflicted injury. ■ Verbalize at least one reason for living. ■ Communicate feelings spontaneously and appropriately in 1:1 and group activities. ■ Identify method in which strengths can be used to improve coping skills. ■ Describe how distorted perceptions affect coping.	Client will: ■ Remain free of self-inflicted injury. ■ Verbalize at least one reason for living. ■ Communicate feelings spontaneously and appropriately. ■ Spontaneously and appropriately participate in 1:1 and group activities. ■ Identify method in which strengths can be used to improve coping skills.	Client is free of self-inflicted injury and verbalizes reasons for living. Client express a positive self-perception and self-esteem. Client communicates feelings honestly and openly. Client participates in activities that promote physical health. Client identifies cues to increasing depression.

	Date _____ Day 5 *continued*	Date _____ Day 6 *continued*	Date _____ Days 7–8 to Discharge *cont.*
Daily outcomes *continued*	■ Begin to reframe false beliefs. ■ Participate in transdisciplinary plan: consume diet as per menu plan; perform self-care independently 75% of time; attend 75% of scheduled activities independently; identify need for laxative; identify changes in symptoms as a result of medications; verbalize awareness of long-term medication needs for depression; identify discharge activity pattern; remain oriented to time, place, and person.	■ Describe how distorted perceptions affect coping ■ Reframe distorted beliefs. ■ Verbalize plan to use strengths to enhance coping skills. ■ Participate in transdisciplinary plan: consume diet as per menu plan; perform self-care independently 100% of time; attend 100% of scheduled activities independently; identify need for laxative; identify changes in symptoms as a result of medications; demonstrate self-administration of medication safely and correctly; verbalize awareness of and commitment to long-term medication needs for depression; remain oriented to time, place, and person.	Client develops sustaining relationships with friends and family members. Client utilizes strengths and skills in managing current and ongoing stressors. Client is alert and oriented. Client verbalizes/demonstrates home care instructions including the importance of ongoing mental health care. Client attains maximum independence in self-care. Client demonstrates ability to adaptively cope with ongoing stressors.
Assessments, tests, and treatments	Daily psychosocial assessment. Observe for safety. Monitor dietary intake, sleep pattern, and bowel elimination pattern. Weight. Continue suicide assessment. Reinforce safety contract. Suicide precautions as indicated. Monitor effects of and compliance with medications. Routine vital signs.	Daily psychosocial assessment. Observe for safety. Monitor dietary intake, sleep pattern, and bowel elimination pattern. Continue suicide assessment. Reinforce safety contract. Suicide precautions as indicated. Monitor effects of and compliance with medications.	Psychosocial assessment. Monitor dietary intake, sleep pattern, and bowel elimination pattern. Suicide assessment. Suicide precautions as indicated. Monitor effects of and compliance with medications.
Knowledge deficit	Review plan of care. Include family in teaching. Review teaching regarding anxiety. Initiate teaching regarding coping strategies utilizing client strengths.	Review plan of care with client and family. Reinforce current level of knowledge regarding medications, treatments, symptom management, and follow-up care.	Client and/or significant other verbalizes understanding of discharge teaching including activity level and exercise program, safety measures, diet, signs and symptoms to report, follow-up care and MD appointment, medications (name, purpose, dose, frequency, route, dietary interactions, and side effects), and follow-up care arrangements.

continued ➤

Critical Pathway for a Client with Depression without Psychotic Features or Agitation continued

	Date _____ Day 5 *continued*	Date _____ Day 6 *continued*	Date _____ Days 7–8 to Discharge *cont.*
Knowledge deficit *continued*	Review current level of knowledge regarding medications, treatments, symptom management, and follow-up care. Assess understanding of teaching.	Assess understanding of teaching.	Assess understanding of teaching. Make referrals to community caregivers for any knowledge deficits regarding medications, treatments, symptoms management, and follow-up care.
Diet	Diet as tolerated; encourage small, frequent feedings from all food groups. Encourage fluids. Provide preferred snacks and foods. Provide adequate time for meals and snacks. Monitor dietary intake. Low tyramine diet if on MAOIs.	Diet as tolerated; encourage small, frequent feedings from all food groups. Encourage fluids. Provide preferred snacks and foods. Provide adequate time for meals and snacks. Monitor dietary intake. Low tyramine diet if on MAOIs.	Diet as tolerated; encourage small, frequent feedings from all food groups. Encourage fluids. Provide preferred snacks and foods. Provide adequate time for meals and snacks. Monitor dietary intake. Low tyramine diet if on MAOIs.
Activity	Maintain safety precautions. Encourage involvement in 75–100% of activities. Prompt with self-care. Provide sleep-enhancing atmosphere for 45-min period before sleep. Engage client and family in activity plan following discharge.	Maintain safety precautions. Encourage involvement in 100% of activities. Encourage independance in self-care. Provide sleep-enhancing atmosphere for 45-min period before sleep. Identify plan to create sleep-enhancing environment in after-discharge setting.	Maintain safety precautions. Independently involved in 100% of activities. Independent in self-care. Provide sleep-enhancing atmosphere for 45-min period before sleep.
Psychosocial	Assess level of anxiety. Support client in implementing stress- and anxiety-reduction strategies. Provide information and ongoing support and encouragement to client and family. Reinforce and utilize role playing strategies as approach to developing support system. Client attends scheduled group therapy session independently. Reinforce skills learned in group therapy.	Assess level of anxiety. Reinforce stress- and anxiety-reduction strategies. Encourage verbalization of concerns and feelings. Provide information and ongoing support and encouragement to client and family. Client attends scheduled group therapy session independently. Provide specific, realistic feedback. Encourage constructive expression of feelings.	Assess level of anxiety. Reinforce stress- and anxiety-reduction strategies. Encourage verbalization of concerns and feelings. Provide information and ongoing support and encouragement to client and family. Client attends scheduled group therapy session independently. Meet with client 15 min every shift during waking hours to work on therapeutic goals.

	Date _____ Day 5 *continued*	Date _____ Day 6 *continued*	Date _____ Day 7–8 *continued*
Psychosocial *continued*	Identify progress with cognitive restructuring and reinforce learning. Acknowledge accomplishments. Encourage verbalization of feelings and concerns. Meet with client 15 min every shift during waking hours to work on therapeutic goals. Encourage client to acknowledge accomplishments. Provide ongoing support and encouragement to client and family.	Meet with client 15 min every shift during waking hours to work on therapeutic goals. Reinforce strategies for cognitive restructuring and reinforce learning. Encourage client to acknowledge accomplishments. Provide ongoing support and encouragement to client and family.	Acknowledge accomplishments. Reinforce progress with and strategies for cognitive restructuring and reinforce learning. Provide ongoing support and encouragement to client and family.
Medications	Assess target symptoms. Antidepressants as ordered. Routine meds as ordered. Colace/Metamucil if indicated. PRN laxative if no BM in 3 days.	Assess target symptoms. Antidepressants as ordered. Routine meds as ordered. Colace/Metamucil if indicated. PRN laxative if no BM in 3 days.	Assess target symptoms. Antidepressants as ordered. Routine meds as ordered. Colace/Metamucil if indicated. PRN laxative if no BM in 3 days.
Transfer/ discharge plan	Review discharge objectives with client and family.	Review discharge objectives with client and significant others. Complete referrals for discharge care.	Review progress toward discharge objectives. Review need for any discharge referrals. Discharge with referrals.

Critical Pathway for a Client with Bipolar Disorder, Manic Phase

Expected length of stay: 14 days	Date _____ Day 1	Date _____ Days 2–4	Date _____ Days 5–7
Daily outcomes	Client will: ■ Remain free of injury to self or others. ■ Identify initial goals for hospitalization. ■ Contract for management of intrusive behaviors. ■ Participate in transdisciplinary treatment plan: participate in assessment; identify most recent medication regime; drink 2000 cc of fluids each day; identify current dietary pattern and food preferences. ■ Remain oriented to time, place, and person.	Client will: ■ Remain free of injury to self or others. ■ Identify initial goals for hospitalization. ■ Maintain contract for management of intrusive behaviors. ■ Participate in transdisciplinary treatment plan: participate in assessment; begin to verbalize need for medication; participate in menu planning; drink 2000 cc of fluids each day; participate in physical activity groups as scheduled; respond to redirection while participating in physical activity groups; establish rest/sleep-promoting environment. ■ If sleep period less than 4 hr, client will increase sleep period by 5%. ■ Remain oriented to time, place, and person.	Client will: ■ Remain free of injury to self or others. ■ Identify initial goals for hospitalization. ■ Maintain contract for management of intrusive behaviors. ■ Participate in transdisciplinary treatment plan: verbalize reasons for medications; consume diet per menu plan; drink 2000 cc of fluids each day; listen and respond to topic for a few minutes; increase sleep period by 5%; participate in physical activity groups as scheduled; respond to redirection while participating in physical activity groups; perform self-care activities independently 50% of time; establish rest/sleep-promoting environment; stay focused on simple task for a few minutes. ■ Remain oriented to time, place, and person.
Assessments, tests, and treatments	Psychosocial assessment to include mental status, mood, affect, behavior, and communication q shift and PRN. Complete nursing database assessment. Observe behavior and activity level. Weight. Monitor fluid intake. CBC, urinalysis. Thyroid profile. Chemistry profile. Drug screen. RPR. Electrolytes. Lithium level. Other laboratory as ordered. Vital signs BID and PRN.	Psychosocial assessment q shift and PRN Observe for safety per protocol. Monitor behavior and activity level. Monitor effects and compliance with medication. Monitor fluid intake. Assess sleep pattern. Lithium level day 3. Routine vital signs.	Psychosocial assessment q shift and PRN. Observe for safety per protocol. Monitor behavior and activity pattern. Monitor effects and compliance with medication. Monitor fluid intake. Assess sleep pattern. Lithium level day 7. Routine vital signs.

	Date _____ Day 1 *continued*	Date _____ Days 2–4 *continued*	Date _____ Days 5–7 *continued*
Knowledge deficit	Orient client/family to unit and program. Assess learning needs of client and family. Review initial plan of care Initiate medication teaching. Assess understanding of teaching.	Review unit orientation with emphasis on program. Continue medication teaching. Assess understanding of teaching.	Review plan of care. Include family in teaching. Initiate teaching regarding treatment modalities and preventive techniques. Assess medication teaching response and need for additional teaching. Assess understanding of teaching.
Diet	Monitor dietary intake. Diet as tolerated; encourage small frequent feedings from all food groups. Provide preferred snacks and foods. Encourage fluids and finger foods, making them accessible throughout the day.	Monitor dietary intake. Diet as tolerated; encourage small frequent feedings from all food groups. Provide preferred snacks and foods. Encourage fluids and finger foods, making them accessible throughout the day.	Monitor dietary intake. Diet as tolerated; encourage small frequent feedings from all food groups. Provide preferred snacks and foods. Encourage fluids and finger foods, making them accessible throughout the day.
Activity	Assess safety needs and maintain appropriate precautions. Observe activity level. Develop schedule for stimulus titration (quiet time and periods in the milieu). Manage agitation with periods of physical activity. Provide sleep-enhancing atmosphere for 45 min prior to sleep.	Maintain safety precautions. Observe activity level. Maintain schedule for stimulus titration. Manage agitation with periods of physical activity. Prompt to attend physical activity groups. Prompt and assist with hygiene as necessary. Provide sleep-enhancing atmosphere for 45 min prior to sleep.	Maintain safety precautions. Observe activity level. Maintain schedule for stimulus titration. Manage agitation with periods of physical activity. Prompt to attend physical activity groups. Encourage to attend small group activities. Prompt with hygiene as necessary. Provide sleep-enhancing atmosphere for 45 min prior to sleep.
Psychosocial	Approach with nonjudgmental and accepting manner. Observe and monitor behavior. Provide structure activities and contracts. Direct to structured activities as per contract. Minimize environmental stimuli and provide a safe environment. Redirect intrusive behaviors: sexual, aggressive, and/or manipulative.	Approach with nonjudgmental and accepting manner. Observe and monitor behavior. Provide structure activities and contracts. Direct to structured activities as per contract. Minimize environmental stimuli and provide a safe environment. Redirect intrusive behaviors: sexual, aggressive, and/or manipulative.	Approach with nonjudgmental and accepting manner. Observe and monitor behavior. Provide structure activities and contracts. Direct to structured activities as per contract. Minimize environmental stimuli and provide a safe environment. Redirect intrusive behaviors: sexual, aggressive, and/or manipulative.

continued ➤

Critical Pathway for a Client with Bipolar Disorder, Manic Phase *continued*

	Date _____ Day 1 *continued*	Date _____ Days 2–4 *continued*	Date _____ Days 5–7 *continued*
Psychosocial *continued*	Provide information regarding illness and treatment to client and family. Avoid power struggles by maintaining kind but consistent approach. Redirect frequent requests and attempt to meet needs in effective manner. Maintain scheduled contacts.	Provide information regarding illness and treatment to client and family. Avoid power struggles by maintaining kind but consistent approach. Redirect frequent requests and attempt to meet needs in effective manner. Maintain scheduled contacts.	Provide information regarding illness and treatment to client and family. Avoid power struggles by maintaining kind but consistent approach. Redirect frequent requests and attempt to meet needs in effective manner. Maintain scheduled contacts.
Medications	Identify target symptoms. Lithium as ordered. Carbamazepine or valproic acid as ordered. Antipsychotics as ordered. Routine meds as ordered.	Assess target symptoms. Lithium as ordered. Carbamazepine or valproic acid as ordered. Antipsychotics as ordered. Routine meds as ordered.	Assess target symptoms. Lithium as ordered. Carbamazepine or valproic acid as ordered. Antipsychotics as ordered. Routine meds as ordered.
Consults and discharge plan	Family assessment. Consult with internist if ordered. Occupational and recreational therapist. Establish discharge objectives with client and family.	Review with client and significant others discharge objectives. Complete discharge planning.	Review with client and significant others progress toward discharge objectives. Make appropriate referrals to support groups.

	Date _____ Days 8–9	Date _____ Days 10–12	Date _____ Days 13–14 to Discharge
Daily outcomes	Client will: ■ Remain free of injury to self or others. ■ Discuss goals for hospitalization. ■ Contract for management of intrusive behaviors. ■ Participate in transdisciplinary treatment plan. ■ Verbalize reasons for medications and understanding of side effects of medication. ■ Consume diet per menu plan. ■ Participate in physical activity groups as scheduled.	Client will: ■ Remain free of injury to self or others. ■ Discuss goals for hospitalization. ■ Contract for management of intrusive behaviors. ■ Participate in transdisciplinary treatment plan. ■ Verbalize reasons for medications and need for long-term therapy. ■ Consume diet per menu plan. ■ Participate in physical activity groups as scheduled.	Client is free of injury to self or others. Client is alert and oriented. Client communicates feelings of self-worth. Client's weight is stable. Client achieves maximum independence in self-care. Client adaptively uses listening skills. Client enjoys 6 hr. of uninterrupted sleep. Client identifies plan if symptoms recur.

	Date _____ Days 8–9 *continued*	Date _____ Days 10–12 *continued*	Date _____ Days 13–14 to Discharge *cont.*
Daily outcomes *continued*	▪ Listen and respond to topic. ▪ Increase sleep period by 5%. ▪ Begin to identify consequences of manic behavior. ▪ Respond to redirection when participating in physical activity groups. ▪ Perform self-care activities independently 75% of time. ▪ Establish sleep/rest-promoting environment. ▪ Stay focused on simple task for 10-min period. ▪ Maintain usual elimination patterns. ▪ Remain oriented to time, place, and person.	▪ Adaptively use listening skills. ▪ Respond to redirection when participating in physical activity groups. ▪ Perform self-care activities independently 100% of time. ▪ Establish sleep/rest-promoting environment. ▪ Stay focused on simple task for 15-min period. ▪ Maintain usual elimination patterns. ▪ Remain oriented to time, place, and person.	Client eats a well-balanced diet inclusive of all food groups. Client drinks 2000 cc of fluids each day. Client has resumed readmission urine and bowel elimination pattern. Client verbalizes/demonstrates home care instructions including the importance of ongoing mental health care. Client participates in regular exercise program. Client demonstrates ability to adaptively cope with ongoing stressors.
Assessments, tests, and treatments	Psychosocial assessment BID and PRN. Observe for safety per protocol. Monitor behavior and activity pattern. Monitor effects and compliance with medication. Monitor fluid intake. Assess sleep pattern.	Psychosocial assessment QD PRN. Observe for safety per protocol. Monitor behavior and activity pattern. Monitor effects and compliance with medication. Monitor fluid intake. Assess sleep pattern. Lithium level day 12.	Psychosocial assessment. Observe for safety per protocol. Monitor behavior and activity pattern. Monitor effects and compliance with medication. Monitor fluid intake. Assess sleep pattern.
Knowledge deficit	Review plan of care. Include family in teaching. Review current level of knowledge regarding medications, treatments, symptom management, and follow-up care. Assess understanding of teaching.	Review plan of care with client and family. Reinforce current level of knowledge regarding medications, treatments, symptom management, and follow-up care. Assess understanding of teaching.	Client and/or significant other verbalizes understanding of discharge teaching including activity level and exercise program, safety measures, diet, signs and symptoms to report, follow-up care and MD appointment, medications (name, purpose, dose, frequency, route, dietary interactions, and side effects), and follow-up care arrangements. Assess understanding of teaching. Make referrals to community caregivers for any knowledge deficits regarding medications, treatments, symptoms management, and follow-up care.

continued ➤

Critical Pathway for a Client with Bipolar Disorder, Manic Phase continued

	Date _____ Days 8–9 *continued*	Date _____ Days 10–12 *continued*	Date _____ Days 13–14 to Discharge *cont.*
Diet	Monitor dietary intake. Diet as tolerated; encourage small frequent feedings from all food groups. Provide preferred snacks and foods. Encourage fluids and finger foods, making them accessible throughout the day.	Monitor dietary intake. Diet as tolerated; encourage small frequent feedings from all food groups. Provide preferred snacks and foods. Encourage fluids and finger foods, making them accessible throughout the day.	Monitor dietary intake. Diet as tolerated; encourage small frequent feedings from all food groups. Provide preferred snacks and foods. Encourage fluids and finger foods, making them accessible throughout the day.
Activity	Maintain safety precautions. Observe activity level. Maintain schedule for stimulus titration. Works at activities until completion. Manage agitation with periods of physical activity. Encourage to eat meals in dining room. Prompt with hygiene as necessary. Provide sleep-enhancing atmosphere for 45 min prior to sleep.	Maintain safety precautions. Observe activity level. Maintain schedule for stimulus titration. Manage agitation with periods of physical activity. Encourage independent attendance at physical activity groups. Encourage independence in self-care. Provide sleep-enhancing atmosphere for 45 min prior to sleep.	Maintain safety precautions. Observe activity level. Maintain schedule for stimulus titration. Manage agitation with periods of physical activity. Prompt to attend physical activity groups. Client is independent in self-care. Provide sleep-enhancing atmosphere for 45 min prior to sleep.
Psychosocial	Approach with nonjudgmental and accepting manner. Observe and monitor behavior. Provide structure activities and contracts. Direct to structured activities as per contract. Minimize environmental stimuli and provide a safe environment.	Approach with nonjudgmental and accepting manner. Observe and monitor behavior. Provide structure activities and contracts. Direct to structured activities as per contract. Minimize environmental stimuli and provide a safe environment.	Approach with nonjudgmental and accepting manner. Observe and monitor behavior. Provide structured activities and contracts. Direct to structured activities as per contract. Minimize environmental stimuli and provide a safe environment.

	Date _____ Days 8–9 *continued*	Date _____ Days 10–12 *continued*	Date _____ Days 13–14 to Discharge *cont.*
Psychosocial *continued*	Redirect impulsive behaviors: sexual, aggressive, and/or manipulative. Provide information regarding illness and treatment to client and family. Avoid power struggles by maintaining kind but consistent approach. Redirect frequent requests and attempt to meet needs in effective manner. Prompt to attend physical activity groups. Client independently attends short small-group activities. Prompt to start attending group therapy as tolerated. Meet with client 2 times each shift for 5-min periods focused on activities of daily living and behavior. Maintain scheduled contacts.	Redirect intrusive behaviors: sexual, aggressive, and/or manipulative. Provide information regarding illness and treatment to client and family. Avoid power struggles by maintaining kind but consistent approach. Redirect frequent requests and attempt to meet needs in effective manner. Client eats meals in dining room without prompting. Client independently attends group therapy for increasingly longer period. Client independently attends short small-group activities. Client attends discharge planning group. Meet with client 2 times each shift for 5-min periods to work on discharge goals. Maintain scheduled contacts.	Redirect intrusive behaviors: sexual, aggressive, and/or manipulative. Provide information regarding illness and treatment to client and family. Avoid power struggles by maintaining kind but consistent approach. Redirect frequent requests and attempt to meet needs in effective manner. Meet with client 2 times each shift for 5-min periods to discuss after-discharge care and management. Maintain scheduled contacts.
Medications	Monitor target symptoms. Lithium as ordered. Carbamazepine or valproic acid as ordered. Antipsychotics as ordered. Routine meds as ordered.	Monitor target symptoms. Lithium as ordered. Carbamazepine or valproic acid as ordered. Antipsychotics as ordered. Routine meds as ordered.	Monitor target symptoms. Lithium as ordered. Carbamazepine or valproic acid as ordered. Antipsychotics as ordered. Routine meds as ordered.
Transfer/ discharge plan	Review discharge objectives with client and significant others.	Review progress toward discharge objectives with client and significant others. Complete referrals for discharge care.	Discharge with referrals.

Nursing Interventions Classification

CLIENTS WITH MOOD DISORDERS

DOMAIN: Safety

Class: *Crisis Management*

    Interventions: *Suicide Prevention:* Reducing risk of self-inflicted harm for a patient in crisis or severe depression

Class: *Risk Management*

    Interventions: *Hallucination Management:* Promoting the safety, comfort, and reality orientation of a patient experiencing hallucinations

DOMAIN: Behavioral

Class: *Behavioral Therapy*

    Interventions: *Behavior Management/Overactivity:* Provision of a therapeutic milieu which safely accommodates the patient's overactivity while promoting optimal function

    Behavior Management: Sexual: Delineation and prevention of socially unacceptable sexual behaviors

    Limit Setting: Establishing the parameters of desirable and acceptable patient behavior

Class: *Cognitive Therapy*

    Interventions: *Cognitive Restructuring:* Challenging a patient to alter distorted thought patterns and view self and the world more realistically

Class: *Communication Enhancement*

    Interventions: *Active listening:* Attending closely to and attaching significance to a patient's verbal and nonverbal messages

    Socialization Enhancement: Facilitation of another person's ability to interact with others

Class: *Coping Assistance*

    Interventions: *Coping Enhancement:* Assisting a patient to adapt to perceived stressors, changes, or threats which interfere with meeting life demands and roles

    Guilt Work Facilitation: Helping another to cope with painful feelings of responsibility, actual or perceived

    Mood Management: Providing for safety and stabilization of a patient who is experiencing dysfunctional mood

    Self-Esteem Enhancement: Assisting a patient to increase his/her personal judgment of self-worth

    Spiritual Support: Assisting the patient to feel balance and connection with a greater power

Class: *Patient Education*

    Interventions: *Teaching: Disease Process:* Assisting the patient to understand information related to a specific disease process

Class: *Psychological Comfort Promotion*

    Interventions: *Simple Guided Imagery:* Purposeful use of imagination to achieve relaxation and/or direct attention away from undesirable sensations

    Simple Relaxation Therapy: Use of techniques to encourage and elicit relaxation for the purpose of decreasing undesirable signs and symptoms such as pain, muscle tension, or anxiety

DOMAIN: Family

Class: *Life Span Care*

    Interventions: *Caregiver Support:* Provision of the necessary information, advocacy, and support to facilitate primary patient care by someone other than a health care professional

    Family Involvement: Facilitating family participation in the emotional and physical care of the patient

    Family Mobilization: Utilization of family strengths to influence patient's health in a positive direction

    Family Therapy: Assisting family members to move their family toward a more productive way of living

DOMAIN: Physiological: Basic

Class: *Activity and Exercise Management*

    Interventions: *Exercise Promotion:* Facilitation of regular physical exercise to maintain or advance to a higher level of fitness and health

Class: *Elimination Management*

    Interventions: *Constipation Management:* Prevention and alleviation of constipation

Class: *Nutritional Support*

    Interventions: *Nutritional Management:* Assisting with or providing a balanced dietary intake of food and fluids

Class: *Self-Care Facilitation*

    Interventions: *Self-Care Assistance:* Assisting another to perform activities of daily living

    Sleep Enhancement: Facilitation of regular sleep/wake cycles

Source: McCloskey and Bulechek, 1996.

in which they can become more autonomous, especially through vocational, social, and community activities.

Many people with mood disorders feel they have lost control over their own lives, rights, and responsibilities, and have lost the ability and right to effectively advocate for themselves. Nursing activities designed to help clients advocate for themselves give them hope and self-esteem. The following steps are a guide to assisting clients in this process:

- Encourage them to believe in themselves.
- Inform them of their rights.
- Help them clarify what they need and want by setting clear goals.
- Provide them with accurate information, preferably in writing.
- Help them strategize by using the problem-solving process.
- Facilitate their identification of resources such as friends, family, self-help groups, and advocacy organizations.
- Encourage them to identify the best person(s) to assist them with this problem.
- Foster effective communication so they can get their message across by suggestions such as: be brief, stick to the point, don't get diverted, and state your concern and how you want things changed.
- Promote firmness and persistence so they can get what they need for themselves.

Another activity to enhance clients' coping abilities is through the development of advance directives. While not legally binding in all states, these plans assist family and caregivers who must make decisions for clients when they are unable to make them for themselves. Advance directives are initiated by the client, formulated between acute episodes, and include:

- Symptoms that indicate the person is not able to make decisions at this time.
- The names and phone numbers of at least three people, including health care professionals, and family members who should make decisions in their behalf.
- A listing of medications, other treatments, and treatment facilities—ranked as preferred, acceptable, and unacceptable—including reasons.

Clients are encouraged to develop their own mental health file containing information about their diagnoses, medications, self-help strategies, and resources. The advance directives should be kept in this file and a copy should be given to each specific supporter or health care professional.

Guilt Work Facilitation

In the midst of a severe depression, many people experience feelings of guilt, often more perceived than real. You can help clients identify and express their painful feelings of guilt and explore the situations in which these feelings are experienced. Encourage them to identify how they behaved in those situations. Following these discussions, you can use reality testing to help clients identify possible irrational beliefs. Global statements about guilt and inadequacy contribute to low self-esteem. More realistic evaluation will help correct cognitive distortions.

Impulse Control Training

Cognitive disruptions for clients in the manic phase of bipolar disorder often result in impulsive behavior which may or may not be dangerous to themselves or others. There are a number of actions you can take to assist clients in impulse control training. You want to help clients identify situations that require thoughtful action and then teach them to cue themselves to "stop and think" before acting impulsively. In addition, they should identify other courses of action and the potential benefits of each course of action. An example might be impulse buying. Clients may decide that every time they take out their wallet, they must "stop and think" if they really need the item they are about to purchase. They might choose to leave their credit cards and checkbooks at home as well. If absolutely necessary, they may elect to have another person control access to credit cards, checkbooks, ATMs, and cash disbursements. The benefits from these decisions are financial stability and self-management.

Mood Management

It is easier to help clients manage mood instability before the episode has cycled into a severe depression or a manic phase. The development and maintenance of an early warning signs chart facilitates this process by helping clients and families identify symptoms that indicate the beginning of a relapse. For example, many people report that fatigue, isolating behaviors, and indecision are early warning signs of depression.

Insomnia, racing thoughts, and rapid speech may be signs of mania. Each evening before bedtime, clients can review the chart to see if any of these warning signs have appeared during the day. If they have, or if they recur for several days, they may need to take a preplanned action to alleviate the symptoms.

Recreation Therapy

People who are depressed often say they have no energy or motivation to participate in social activities and they often forget to do the things they enjoy that make them feel better. In contrast, people experiencing a manic episode are interested in every activity whether appropriate or not. Nursing activities include assisting clients to choose recreational activities that are consistent with their physical, emotional, and social capabilities. For clients in the acute phase of a mood disorder, it is most helpful to keep activities simple and short, thus ensuring success and boosting self-esteem. You will want to avoid activities requiring intense concentration since their attention span is insufficient for success. Clients with manic behavior will manage better with nonstimulating activities, thereby avoiding the escalation of their mood by competition or sensory stimulation.

In the nonacute phase of mood disorders, clients find it helpful to make a list of things they enjoy doing, which becomes an easy reference when they are having a harder time. The list might include going for a walk, listening to music, working in the garden, watching funny videos, or visiting with friends. Part of self-management is making the time to include one or more of these activities in a regular schedule.

Self-Esteem Enhancement

People suffering from depression often experience self-esteem disturbances related to criticism and negative self-evaluation. One nursing activity that may be helpful is setting limits on the amount of time clients spend discussing past failures, since rumination intensifies guilt and low self-esteem. Help clients identify the significance of culture, religion, race, gender, and age on self-esteem. Based on this, assist them in setting realistic goals to achieve higher self-esteem. From there you can move on to encouraging review of past achievements and present successes. Determine clients' locus of control and encourage behaviors that foster an internal locus of control. Help them develop confidence in their own judgment by conveying your confidence in their ability to handle various situations and by helping them acknowledge positive responses from others.

Spiritual Support

In the midst of depression, many people experience spiritual distress related to a lack of purpose or joy in life and feeling disconnected with others. Be open to their expressions of loneliness and powerlessness. Review their past joys and successes in life and help them identify "small" purposes of current life such as contributions to their family, value to friends, and goals for next month. Help them identify possible new functions or purposes in life to counteract the depressed feelings. Review with them the availability of supportive people, as those people will increase their sense of connectedness to others. For clients who are religious, use spiritual resources to decrease distress. Facilitate their use of meditations, prayer, and other religious traditions and rituals. For many people religious beliefs improve self-esteem, life satisfaction, and the ability to cope.

Behavioral: Patient Education

Teaching: Disease Process

People who are self-managers say that it is absolutely essential to learn everything they can about their particular diagnosis and possible treatment strategies. Education is part of taking responsibility for wellness and facilitates appropriate decision making. This educational process must be continuous to keep clients and families up-to-date with the latest findings about their disorder. More detailed information on client and family teaching is found in Chapter 5.

Some individuals may reject the information you provide. One reason may be that they believe that they know all about their disorder and have no need to learn anything else. Others may reject information because they are in total denial of having a disorder (Pollack, 1996). Barriers to learning must be identified and managed if your teaching is to be effective.

Family: Life Span Care

Caregiver Support

Mood disorders affect not only the client but also family and friends. During acute episodes, clients may be very dependent and needy or may need firm direction and limit setting. You must consider all

Medication Teaching

Clients with Mood Disorders

Antidepressants

It may take as long as 4 weeks before you feel the effects of this medication.

Do not abruptly stop taking this medication. If you do, you might get symptoms such as headache, dizziness, insomnia, and depression.

Call your doctor immediately if you experience any of the following symptoms: sore throat, fever, tiredness, bruising easily, severe headache, fast heart rate, difficulty urinating, rash, or hives.

If you experience drowsiness or dizziness, do not drive or operate dangerous machinery. Sedation usually improves with time on this medication. If you continue to feel tired during the day, discuss with your doctor the possibility of taking the medication at bedtime.

If you get dizzy when arising from bed, sit at the side of your bed for several minutes before moving to a standing position.

Use a sunscreen and wear protective clothing because your skin may be more susceptible to sunburn.

If you experience a dry mouth, take frequent sips of water, chew citrus-flavored sugarless gum, or suck on ice chips or hard candy. Frequent brushing of your teeth is also helpful.

If you experience constipation, increase your fluid intake if it is low, increase your consumption of vegetables and fiber, and increase your exercise.

You may experience some weight gain while taking this medication. Weigh yourself weekly, develop good eating habits, and increase your exercise. (Prozac and Zoloft may cause weight loss.)

Some people develop sexual dysfunctions from this medication, such as decreased desire for sex, erectile problems, impaired ejaculation, and orgasm problems. If any of these occurs, discuss the problem with your doctor. A different antidepressant medication may or may not be helpful.

Sources: Fenn, 1996; Glod, 1996; Thase and Kupfer, 1996.

If you are taking your medication several times a day and you forget to take a dose, do the following: If within 1–2 hours of the missed time, take the medication; if more than 2 hours after the missed dose, skip the dose and take the next dose at the regularly scheduled time.

Mood Stabilizers

Take with meals to decrease the chance of GI upset.

Daily fluid intake should range from 2500–3000 mL/day.

Avoid heavy intake of caffeine, which increases urine output.

Maintain normal dietary sodium levels.

Report any sudden weight gain and/or edema to your doctor.

Report any event or condition that results in sweating, diarrhea, or increased urine output to your doctor.

Immediately report any sign of toxicity: persistent nausea and vomiting, severe diarrhea, ataxia (lack of muscle coordination), blurred vision, or ringing in the ears.

Follow your doctor's directions on the frequency of monitoring blood lithium levels. Blood should be drawn 12 hours after the last lithium dose.

Use the following medications very cautiously and only under a doctor's direction:

- Aminophylline, sodium bicarbonate: wash lithium out of body.
- Muscle relaxants: lithium increases their effect.
- Nonsteroid anti-inflammatory drugs: increase the risk of toxicity.
- Thiazide diuretics: increase the risk of toxicity.

If you forget to take a dose, do the following: If within 2 hours of the next dose, do not take the missed dose. If you are taking sustained-release capsules, do not take the missed dose if it is within 6 hours of the next dose.

significant others to be recipients of your care. Help these caregivers acknowledge the client's dependency issues and assume appropriate responsibility. Be alert for family interaction problems related to the care of the client. Provide information about the client's condition in accordance with client preferences, remembering the issue of confidentiality. Inform caregivers of community resources and encourage them to participate in support groups. See the Self-Help Groups section at the end of this chapter.

Family Mobilization

Family mobilization includes education, communication skills training, and problem-solving skills training. In mobilizing the family, you apply the same principles that you use with clients. Assess how the family's behavior affects the client and how the client's behavior affects the family. Discuss how family strengths and resources can be used to enhance the health status of the client and the family's ability to cope. Collaborate with families and clients in planning and implementing lifestyle changes.

Teach families and clients how to identify early signs and symptoms of manic or depressive episodes. Such identification can help ensure that treatment is begun as early as possible in the course of a relapse. Relapse prevention and early recognition are important concepts in self-management.

Family Therapy

When caring for families, observe interactional behaviors and verbal communications to assess for functional or dysfunctional patterns of behavior. For example, you might look for messages to children that they are bad or deficient, or that the world is a hostile place. Repeated messages such as "You're not good," "I wish you had never been born," and "This is an unfair world—I hate it" contribute to a negative and distorted way of viewing oneself and the world. Help the family determine areas of dissatisfaction and/or conflict and see whether they want to resolve these issues. The goal is to help family members identify and change behaviors that maintain depression and dependency within the family system. Because family therapy is a specialized area of nursing practice and requires additional education, you should collaborate closely with colleagues who possess advanced practice skills.

Physiological: Basic: Activity and Exercise Management

Exercise Promotion

Exercise is the least expensive and most available antidepressant. It is nature's way of increasing neurotransmitters and endorphins, thus decreasing feelings of sadness and tension. A daily walk or some other kind of enjoyable exercise makes most people feel better.

Teach clients to begin slowly and increase the intensity and length of the exercise gradually. Have them keep a record of their physical activities as a way to monitor their own behavior. Clients who are depressed may tell you that they will exercise when they feel better. Teach them that, in contrast, they will feel better when they exercise. Finding an "exercise buddy" may facilitate this aspect of self-management.

Physiological: Basic: Elimination Management

Constipation Management

You may need to institute measures to relieve constipation which may result from decreased activity, reduced intake, side effects of antidepressant medications, or ignoring bodily signals. Baseline data are established by reviewing clients' normal patterns of bowel activity and having them keep a record of current patterns. In addition to exercise, nutritional measures such as increased fiber in the diet and adequate fluid intake are helpful.

Physiological: Basic: Nutritional Support

Nutritional Management

Dietary modifications are being explored as an adjunct to more traditional interventions. The neurotransmitters that are implicated in the neurobiology of mood disorders are synthesized from dietary proteins. Specific protein intake might be increased, depending on which neurotransmitter is depleted. Tryptophan is the precursor of 5-HT and niacin. If the body has more than enough niacin, tryptophan will be forced to choose the 5-HT pathway. Vitamin B_6 might be depleted by the use of antidepressants, birth control pills, and antihypertensive agents. By increasing tryptophan in the diet as well as adding niacin and vitamin B_6, the 5-HT levels are increased. If the mood disorder involves decreased levels of NE or DA, the diet is increased in tyrosine. Choline is increased in the diet when higher levels of ACH are desired. This evolving field of dietary pharmacology will become more important as neurobiology continues to be explored. St. John's Wort, a wild flowering plant available in health food stores, contains a chemical component called hypericin, which has been found to produce an antidepressant effect. It is most effective in relieving cases of mild to moderate depression. As herbology becomes more recognized as an alternative healing method, it is anticipated that more herbs will be recognized and approved by the FDA (NAMI, 1997).

Physiological: Basic: Self-Care Facilitation

Sleep Enhancement

Another nursing intervention is helping clients re-establish normal sleep patterns. People who are depressed or in a manic episode experience insomnia and frequent awakening. Ask clients what measures to improve sleeping have been successful in the past and help them find ways to adjust the environment of their bedroom to promote sleep. Implementing natural sedative measures may improve sleeping patterns. These methods include increased physical activity during the day but not right before bedtime, decreased amount of daytime napping, relaxation techniques, avoidance of caffeine, and a warm bath or a warm drink just before bed. When clients are unable to sleep, encourage them to get out of bed to read or watch television. Since nighttime often increases feelings of hopelessness, clients tend to spend sleepless periods ruminating over problems. Redirection to other activities minimizes concentrating on negative thoughts.

Evaluation

Evaluation is accomplished by determining the client's progress toward achieving the outcome criteria. If progress is not being made, determine whether the interventions or diagnoses need to be modified. It is through evaluation that the nursing process is validated. You may use the following questions to guide evaluation of clients' progress:

- Is the client participating in appropriate available activities?
- Are interactions with others socially appropriate?
- Is the client able to balance dependency on others with independent actions?
- Is the client's mood stable and appropriate to the situation?
- Is the client able to experience pleasure without constantly seeking excitement?
- How does the client describe personal strengths and limitations?
- How does the client describe expectations of the future?
- Is the client able to make appropriate decisions?
- Are you able to follow the client's flow of thought?
- Is the client able to concentrate?
- Does the client and family utilize self-help groups?
- Has the client and family established a self-management program?

Clinical Interactions

A Client with Bipolar Disorder

Ken, age 36, has been in a partial hospitalization program for the past 2 months. Both of his parents are deceased, and his two siblings are uninvolved with him. His mood ranges from euphoria to irritability. He believes he is very handsome, intelligent, and superior to other people. He is often preoccupied with sexual topics. The nurse is meeting Ken for the first time. In the interaction, you will see evidence of:

- Ken's grandiose beliefs about himself
- his flight of ideas
- his labile moods

KEN: You would like to talk and help me?
NURSE: I would like to get to know you first.
KEN: You will find me really interesting. I am rich.

NURSE: I would like to know a little bit about who you are, Ken.

KEN: I was a chosen child.

NURSE: Can you help me understand what that means, to be a chosen child?

KEN: I was my parents' favorite child and they treated me special.

NURSE: What does "special" mean to you?

KEN: Love would come from my mother to me. Jesus is the love child. Did you know that?

NURSE: Ken, let's concentrate on you and your family. You were telling me that your mother loved you very much.

KEN: Yes, she showed me how to love, but she died and left me. She went away. My father died later when I was 26.

NURSE: How did your parents' deaths affect you?

KEN: I like women. There is no room for homosexuals. I'm a heterosexual.

NURSE: Ken, let's concentrate on the topic of you and your parents. How did you feel when your parents died?

KEN: My father was a big man.

NURSE: Your father was a strong figure to you?

KEN: Big man. He would slap my mother. [Acts out how his father would slap his mother; seems to be getting angry and aggressive.]

NURSE: Ken, did that anger you when your father hit your mother? Can you tell me about those times?

KEN: My father would slap my mother and hit me here. [Jumps up and points to his backside and legs.]

NURSE: That must have been painful. How did you feel when that happened?

KEN: He had to show me the way. Like God the Father.

NURSE: Ken, let's continue on with your childhood father.

KEN: I signed up for the army and went to Vietnam. I killed the evil people. [Angry tone and then starts laughing.]

NURSE: You sound angry about having killed but yet you laugh.

KEN: I had to kill those liars. My brother and sister were jealous.

NURSE: Ken, I don't understand. Slow down. Let's talk about the jealousy.

KEN: I was chosen. My mother loved me [loudly]. I came home with shell shock. I have a tattoo on my nose and a fracture on my skull. I'm tired of talking. I'll see you later. ■

Self-Help Groups

Clients with Mood Disorders

Depression After Delivery
P.O. Box 1282
Morrisville, PA 19067
(800) 944-4773

National Alliance for the Mentally Ill (NAMI)
2101 Wilson Boulevard, Suite 302
Arlington, VA 22201
(800) 950-NAMI
www.nami.org

National Depressive and
Manic Depressive Association
730 North Franklin, Suite 501
Chicago, IL 60610
(312) 642-0049
www.ndmda.org

National Foundation for Depressive Illness
P.O. Box 2257
New York, NY 10116
(212) 370-7190
www.depression.org

National Organization for Seasonal Affective
Disorder (NOSAD)
P.O. Box 40133
Washington, DC 20016

Key Concepts

Introduction

- The mood disorders are major depression (unipolar disorder), dysthymic disorder, bipolar disorder, cyclothymic disorder, and schizoaffective disorder.

- Affect is the verbal and nonverbal expression of one's internal feelings or mood. Descriptors are appropriate versus inappropriate, stable versus labile, elevated versus depressed, and overreactive versus blunted or flat.

- Postpartum mood changes range along a continuum from postpartum blues to major depression.

Knowledge Base

- People who are depressed withdraw from activities and other people; experience feelings of despair, guilt, loss of gratification, and loss of emotional attachments; and suffer from self-depreciation, negative expectations, cognitive distortions, and self-criticism. They also have difficulty making decisions and experience a retarded flow of thought.

- People who are in a manic phase engage in any available activity, are effusive in interactions with others, and form intense emotional attachments quickly. They experience feelings of euphoria but may become suddenly irritable. Thoughts focus on grandiose expectations for themselves, exaggerated accomplishments, and a positively distorted body image. Distractibility and flight of ideas interfere with decision making.

- Families may be oversolicitous or may become frustrated when a family member is unable to change affect, behavior, or cognition. If the person is hostile and destructive, police may be called upon to intervene.

- The sex life of couples is often disrupted by mood disorders. People who are depressed have little interest in sex, and people who are manic are obsessed with sex.

- Appropriate expressions of mood are largely culturally determined.

- Throughout the world, most cases of depression are experienced and expressed in somatic terms.

- Physiologically, people who are depressed experience loss of appetite, insomnia, decreased mobility, and constipation, while people in the manic phase experience hyperinsomnia and hyperactivity.

- Concomitant disorders include agoraphobia, panic attacks, GAD, and substance-related disorders.

- There appears to be a genetic predisposition to mood disorders, most likely a mixture of multiple genes.

- In the mood disorders, there is a change in the amount of neurotransmitters or a change in the sensitivity of the receptors, thus altering the transmission of electrical impulses.

- The mood disorders may involve a desynchronization of circadian rhythm in some people.

- Seasonal affective disorder (SAD) is cyclic and related to the amount of available sunlight.

- Depression may be secondary to prescribed medications, metabolic disorders, and neurological disruptions.

- Repressed hostility, losses, unachieved goals, learned helplessness, and cognitive distortions contribute to mood disorders.

- Racism, classism, sexism, ageism, and homophobia contribute to depression by increasing feelings of powerlessness, hopelessness, and low self-esteem.

- People experiencing multiple significant life events along with minimal support networks and maladaptive coping patterns are at higher risk for developing a depressive disorder.

- Rigid expectations about gender roles and being isolated within the home may contribute to higher rates of depression among women. Role changes and losses may contribute to higher rates of depression among older adults.

- Antidepressants, MAOIs, mood stabilizers, ETC, sleep deprivation, and phototherapy may be used in the treatment of mood disorders. Blood plasma levels are important in determining the dosage of many medications.

Nursing Assessment

- Nursing assessment must often be conducted in segments of 15–20 minutes for clients who have little energy or for those who are hyperactive.

Nursing Diagnosis

- Some clients are a danger to themselves or others; therefore, *High risk for violence* is a priority nursing diagnosis. Other diagnoses include *Impaired verbal communication, Decisional conflict, Altered role performance, Hopelessness, Deficiency in diversional activity, Fatigue, Bathing/hygiene self-care deficit,*

Altered thought processes, Self-esteem disturbance, and *Spiritual distress.*

Nursing Interventions

- The first priority of care is client safety. Safety concerns include monitoring for suicide potential and management of hallucinations.

- Behavioral interventions include prevention of physical exhaustion, limit setting with intrusive behavior, and protection from impulsive sexual behavior.

- Cognitive interventions include identifying distorted cognitive processes and gently confronting these.

- Clients working toward self-management go through several cognitive phases: realization of a need, seeking information, critical juncture, and self-management.

- Identifying themes and focusing on one topic at a time are helpful for clients who are experiencing flight of ideas.

- Peer counseling may enhance clients' socialization levels.

- Interventions to enhance coping include problem solving, self-advocacy, advance directives, management of mood swings, impulse control training, self-esteem enhancement, and spiritual support.

- Families will benefit from education, communication skills training, and caregiver support. Dysfunctional families will benefit from family therapy.

- Exercise and dietary modifications are natural ways to increase beneficial neurotransmitters.

- Implementing natural sedative measures may improve sleeping patterns.

Evaluation

- Evaluation is accomplished by determining the client's progress toward achieving the outcome criteria. Modification of the plan of care is based on evaluation data.

Review Questions

1. Sue gave birth to a baby 3 weeks ago. Ten days ago she began to experience mood swings, feelings of despair, and thoughts of being an inadequate mother. She is suffering from

    a. normal postpartum feelings.

    b. postpartum blues.

    c. postpartum depression.

    d. postpartum psychosis.

2. Tom is unable to experience pleasure as a result of his depression. You would document this as

    a. anhedonia.

    b. catastrophizing.

    c. somatization.

    d. secondary gain.

3. Lithium toxicity may occur in which of the following situations?

    a. a tennis match in hot weather

    b. swimming 20 laps in a pool

    c. gardening

    d. walking 1 mile

4. In working with Jorge, you do the following activities: inform him of his rights, facilitate the identification of resources, and problem-solve. Your interventions are part of helping him

    a. manage his moods.

    b. increase his self-esteem.

    c. develop a treatment preference plan.

    d. advocate for himself.

5. Exercise works as an antidepressant by

    a. getting people out in fresh air.

    b. improving one's body image.

    c. increasing neurotransmitters.

    d. providing diversional activity.

References

Badger, T. A. (1996). Living with depression. *J Psychosoc Nurs, 34*(1), 21–9.

Beck, A. T., et al. (1961). Inventory for measuring depression. *Arch Gen Psychiatry, 4,* 561–571.

Berger, M., et al. (1997). Sleep deprivation combined with consecutive sleep phase advance as a fast-acting therapy in depression. *Am J Psychiatry, 154*(6), 870–872.

Blumenthal, S. J. (1996). Women and depression, *Decade of the Brain, 7*(3), 1–4.

Bowden, C. L. (1996). Relation of serum valproate concentration to response in mania. *Am J Psychiatry, 153*(6), 765–771.

Brown, C., et al. (1996). Treatment outcomes for primary care patients with major depression and lifetime anxiety disorders. *Am J Psychiatry, 153*(10), 1293–1300.

Chen, Y. W., & Dilsaver, S. C. (1995). Comorbidity of panic disorder in bipolar illness. *Am J Psychiatry, 152*(2), 280–282.

Coryell, W., et al. (1995). Long-term stability of polarity distinctions in the affective disorder. *Am J Psychiatry, 152*(3), 385–390.

Coryell, W., et al. (1996). Importance of psychotic features to long-term course in major depressive disorder. *Am J Psychiatry, 153*(4), 483–489.

Cui, X., & Vaillant, G. E. (1996). Antecedents and consequences of negative life events in adulthood. *Am J Psychiatry, 153*(1), 21–26.

Faludi, S. (1991). *Backlash: The Undeclared War Against American Women.* New York: Anchor Books.

Fenn, H. H., et al. (1996). Trends in pharmacotherapy of schizoaffective and bipolar affective disorders. *Am J Psychiatry, 153*(5), 711–713.

Finnerty, M., & Levin, Z. (1996). Acute manic episodes in pregnancy. *Am J Psychiatry, 153*(2), 261–263.

Gershon, E. S. (1996). Genetic discoveries in depression and mania. *Decade of the Brain, 7*(2), 3–4.

Glod, C. A. (1996). Recent advances in the pharmacotherapy of major depression. *Arch Psychiatr Nurs, 10*(6), 355–364.

Gorman, C. (1997, May 5). Anatomy of melancholy. *Time, 149*(18), 78.

Gotlib, J. H., & Hsammen, C. L. (1992). *Psychological Aspects of Depression.* New York: Wiley.

Hammen, C., & Gitlin, M. (1997). Stress reactivity in bipolar patients and its relation to prior history of disorder. *Am J Psychiatry, 154*(6), 856–857.

Hedaya, R. J. (1996). *Understanding Biological Psychiatry.* New York: Norton.

Hulme, P. A. (1996). Somatization in hispanics. *J Psychosoc Nurs, 34*(3), 33–37.

Kendler, K. S., et al. (1995). Stressful life events, genetic liability, and the onset of an episode of major depression in women. *Am J Psychiatry, 152*(6), 833–842.

Klebanoff, N. A., & Smith, N. M. (1997). *Behavioral Management in Home Care.* Philadelphia: Lippincott.

Mann, J. J., et al. (1996). Demonstration in vivo of reduced serotonin responsivity in the brain of untreated depressed patients. *Am J Psychiatry, 153*(2), 174–182.

Marangell, L. B., et al. (1997). Inverse relationship of peripheral thyrotropin-stimulating hormone levels to brain activity in mood disorders. *Am J Psychiatry, 154*(2), 224–230.

McCloskey, J., & Bulechek, G. M. (1996). *Nursing Interventions Classification (NIC),* 2nd ed. St. Louis: Mosby.

McElroy, S. L., et al. (1997). Phenomenology of adolescent and adult mania in hospitalized patients with bipolar disorder. *Am J Psychiatry, 154*(1), 44–49.

Mohit, D. L. (1996). Management and care of mentally ill mothers of young children. *Arch Psychiatr Nurs, 10*(1), 49–54.

Mulsant, B. H., et al. (1997). Low use of neuroleptic drugs in the treatment of psychotic major depression. *Am J Psychiatry, 154*(4), 559–562.

NAMI. (1997). St. John's Wort for depression? *NAMI Advocate, 18*(5), 14.

Pollack, L. E. (1996). Information seeking among people with manic-depressive illness. *IMAGE, 28*(3), 259–265.

Reich, R. (1997). Genetic studies in bipolar disorder. *Decade of the Brain, 7*(4), 5–6.

Sevy, S. (1995). Genetic research in bipolar illness. In E. E. Beckham & W. R. Leber (Eds.), *Handbook of Depression* (2nd ed.) (pp. 203–212). New York: Guilford Press.

Silverstein, B., & Perlick, D. (1995). *The Cost of Competence.* Oxford, England: Oxford Univ. Press.

Solomon, D. A. (1996). Serum lithium levels and psychosocial function in patients with bipolar I disorder. *Am J Psychiatry, 153*(10), 1301–1308.

Spinelli, M. G. (1997). Interpersonal psychotherapy for depressed antepartum women. *Am J Psychiatry, 154*(7), 1028–1030.

Thase, M. E., & Howland, R. H. (1995). Biological processes in depression. In E. E. Beckham & W. R. Leber (Eds.), *Handbook of Depression* (2nd ed.) (pp. 213–279). New York: Guilford Press.

Thase, M. E., & Kupfer, D. J. (1996). Pharmachotherapy for the treatment of depression. *Decade of the Brain, 7*(2), 5–6.

Thurtle, V. (1995). Post-natal depression: The relevance of sociological approaches. *J Adv Nurs, 22*(3), 416–424.

Terman, M., et al. (1996). Predictors of response and nonresponse to light treatment for winter depression. *Am J Psychiatry, 153*(11), 1423–1429.

Ugarriza, D. N. (1995). A descriptive study of postpartum depression. *Perspect Psychiatr Care, 31*(3), 25–29.

Winokur, G. (1995). Alcoholism in manic-depressive (bipolar) illness. *Am J Psychiatry, 152*(3), 365–372.

Zajecka, J. (1996). Update on major depression. *Decade of the Brain, 7*(2), 1–3.

VISIT OUR WEBSITE!
www.awnursing.com

CHAPTER 12

Schizophrenic Disorders

Karen Lee Fontaine

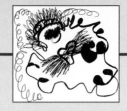

Objectives

After reading this chapter, you will be able to:

- Define the positive and negative characteristics of schizophrenic disorders.
- Describe the multiple etiologies of the schizophrenic syndrome.
- Discuss the psychopharmacological interventions for persons with schizophrenia.
- Identify the principles of psychiatric rehabilitation.
- Apply the nursing process to clients who have schizophrenic disorders.

Key Terms

delusions
hallucination
extrapyramidal side effects (EPS)
loose association
negative characteristics
positive characteristics
schizophrenia
schizoaffective disorder

Schizophrenia is a disorder of the brain like epilepsy or multiple sclerosis. It is diagnosed in about 1% of the U.S. population and affects not only the individual but also family, friends, and the community as a whole. Although it is referred to as a single disease, it is more accurately a syndrome, characterized by a broad range of symptoms, physiological malfunctions, etiologies, and prognoses. **Schizophrenia** is a combination of disordered thinking, perceptual disturbances, behavioral abnormalities, affective disruptions, and impaired social competency. This means the person has difficulty thinking clearly, knowing what is real, managing feelings, making decisions, and relating to others. Typically the person is fairly normal early in life, experiences subtle changes after puberty, and undergoes severe symptoms in the late teens to early adulthood. The early age of onset often shatters the lives of its victims and robs them of the opportunity for a productive adult life.

The onset and progression of schizophrenia is quite variable. It is believed that people with an abrupt onset of the illness suffer from a different form of schizophrenia than those whose onset is more insidious. The vast majority develop the disorder in adolescence or young adulthood, with only 10% of cases first diagnosed in people over the age of 45. In some cases, the disorder progresses through exacerbations and remissions; in other cases, it takes a chronic, stable course; while in still others, a chronic, progressively deteriorating course evolves. Much too often the illness results in lifelong problems in coping with everyday living that reflect irreversible neurobiological deficits. Early diagnosis and treatment may reduce the chronicity and improve the prognosis of people suffering from schizophrenia. Women tend to have a later onset of illness, shorter and less frequent exacerbations, and an overall higher quality of life than do their male counterparts (Grossberg, 1997; Lewine et al, 1996; Wyatt and Henter, 1997).

In **schizoaffective disorder,** clients suffer from symptoms that appear to be a mixture of schizophrenia and the mood disorders. The person experiences one or more of the following symptoms: delusions, hallucinations, disorganized speech, disorganized behavior, or negative characteristics (see Table 12.1). In addition, the person experiences symptoms of the mood disorders, which may be major depressive symptoms, manic symptoms, or mixed symptoms. Clients

Table 12.1 **Characteristics of Schizophrenia**

Positive Characteristics	Negative Characteristics
Behavioral	
Hyperactivity	Decreased activity level
Bizarre behavior	Limited speech; conversation difficult
	Minimal self-care
Affective	
Inappropriate affect	Blunted or flat affect
Overreactive affect	Anhedonia
Hostility	
Perceptual	
Hallucinations	Inability to understand
Sensory overload	sensory information
Cognitive	
Delusions	Concrete thinking
Disorganized thinking	Attention impairment
Loose associations	Memory deficits
Suspiciousness	Impaired problem solving
	Lack of motivation
Social	
Aloof and stilted interactions	Social withdrawal, isolation
	Poor rapport with others
	Inadequate social and occupational skills

often have difficulty maintaining job or school functioning, experience problems with self-care, are socially isolated, and often suffer from suicidal ideation. Schizoaffective disorder, like schizophrenia, usually begins in adolescence or early adulthood.

Knowledge Base

The classic subtypes described in the *DSM-IV* (undifferentiated, catatonic, paranoid, and disorganized) have given way to new systems of classification. The most widely used system is one of positive characteristics, negative characteristics, and thought disorganization. This arrangement represents symptom types that are probably semi-independent of each other. To make sense of these groups, you must understand that positive does not mean good, and negative does not mean bad. Rather, **positive characteristics** are added behaviors that are not normally seen in mentally healthy adults. For example, healthy adults do not experience delusions; therefore, delusions are a positive characteristic. Positive characteristics are most likely the result of physiological changes, including increased dopamine (DA) function in the subcortical areas of the brain and decreased glucose utilization in the brain. Medication is often successful in diminishing positive characteristics.

Negative characteristics are the absence of behaviors that are normally seen in mentally healthy adults. For example, healthy adults are able to complete their ADLs; therefore, an inability to care for oneself is a negative characteristic of schizophrenia. Negative characteristics are most likely related to anatomic changes as well as decreased DA function in the prefrontal cortex. These characteristics have been more treatment-resistant (Kahn, Davidson, and Davis, 1996; Kapur and Remington, 1996; Keltner, 1996).

Thought disorganization or cognitive difficulties can also be described as positive or negative characteristics (refer back to Table 12.1).

Behavioral Characteristics

Positive behavioral characteristics include hyperactivity and bizarre behavior. *Hyperactive behavior* most typically occurs during a period of exacerbation. The excitement may become so great that it threatens the person's safety or that of others. Schizophrenia can cause people to engage in bizarre behavior such as repeating rhythmic gestures, doing ritualistic postures, or demonstrating freakish facial or body movements. Some people will imitate other people's movements or words or may senselessly repeat the same word or phrase for hours or days.

Negative behavioral characteristics are decreased activity level, limited speech, and minimal self-care. The *decreased activity level* includes a reduction of energy, initiative, and spontaneity. There is a loss of natural gracefulness in body movements that results in poor coordination; activities may be carried out in a robot-like fashion. People with schizophrenia often have *limited speech*, which makes it difficult for them to carry on a continuous conversation or say anything new.

Another difficulty for individuals and their significant others is a deterioration in appearance and manners. *Self-care* may become *minimal;* they may need to be reminded to bathe, shave, brush their teeth, and change their clothes. Because of confusion and distraction, they may not conform to social norms of dress and behavior.

Affective Characteristics

Positive affective characteristics include inappropriate affect, overreactive affect, and hostility. *Inappropriate affect* occurs when the person's emotional tone is not related to the immediate circumstances. An *overreactive affect* is appropriate to the situation but out of proportion to it. With little warning, some people with schizophrenia become *hostile* as anger turns into aggression with the intent to do harm.

Negative affective characteristics include blunted or flat affect and anhedonia. A *blunted affect* describes a dulled emotional response to a situation, and a *flat affect* describes the absence of visible cues to the person's feelings. Schizophrenia can make it difficult for people to clearly express their emotions. They show less emotion, laugh less, and cry less. *Anhedonia,* the inability to experience pleasure, causes many people with schizophrenia to feel emotionally barren. They may not take much interest in the things around them, even things they used to find enjoyable. If the world feels "flat as cardboard," they may not feel that it is worth the effort to get out and do things. See Table 12.2 for examples of affective characteristics of schizophrenia.

Perceptual Characteristics

Positive perceptual characteristics include hallucinations and sensory overload. A **hallucination** is the occurrence of a sound, sight, touch, smell, or taste without an external stimulus to the corresponding sensory organ. Hallucinations are very real to the person and may be triggered by anxiety and by functional

Table 12.2 Affective Characteristics of Schizophrenia

Affect	Example
Inappropriate	When told it's time to turn off the TV and go to bed, Joe begins to laugh uproariously.
Overreactive	When Kathy wins at cards, she jumps up and down and does a cheer for herself.
Blunted	Tom has been looking forward to his wife's visit. When she arrives on the unit, he is only able to give her a small smile.
Flat	When Juanita's mother tells her that her favorite dog has died, Juanita simply says, "Oh," and does not give any indication of an emotional response.

changes in the CNS. The most common type is *auditory hallucination,* or the hearing of voices. The voice is often that of God, the devil, a neighbor, or a relative; the voice may say either bad or good things; and the voice seems to be coming from an external source. The next most common type is *visual hallucination,* which is usually nearby, clearly defined, and moving. Visual hallucinations are often accompanied by auditory hallucinations. *Tactile, olfactory,* and *gustatory hallucinations* are uncommon and are more likely to occur in people who are undergoing substance withdrawal or abuse.

Hallucinations may considerably control the person's behavior. It is not unusual for people having auditory hallucinations to carry on a conversation with one of the voices. After a period of time, many people realize that if they admit they hear voices, they will be labeled "sick" or "crazy." To avoid being labeled, they may be very evasive about their hallucinations.

Kari, a nurse, is on a home visit with Lisa, a 44-year-old client who lives in supervised housing. Lisa is filling out a piece of paper that Kari gave her yesterday.

KARI: "How are you doing with the self-image exercise?"

LISA: "He tells me what to say." (laughing softly)

KARI: "Who tells you what to say?"

LISA: "He does. I never tell anyone about him. I've only told a couple of people." (makes brief eye contact)

KARI: "Is he here right now?"

LISA: "Yes, he just walked around the corner." (looks across the room)

KARI: "How do you feel when this voice talks to you?"

LISA: "I'm used to it. I've known him since I was little. Let's see. What do I value the most? Myself. No, he said I can't put that. He says I have to put my loved ones." (looking down at piece of paper)

KARI: "You value yourself the most, but the voice won't let you write that down?"

LISA: "Yes."

Our sensory systems receive information from the environment and from our bodies through stimuli transmitted to the brain. However, we do not consciously perceive much of this sensory information. Sensory information is processed in a series of relay stations within the brain where irrelevant stimuli are inhibited. This allows us to filter out unnecessary and distracting information—a process called *selective perception*—and focus on what is important at the given moment. Schizophrenia often disrupts the filtering process, causing sensory overload. When there are too many messages arriving at the cortex at the same time, thinking becomes disorganized and fragmented. See Figure 12.1 for a representation of impaired sensory filtering.

The negative perceptual characteristic in schizophrenia is the inability to understand sensory information. People with schizophrenia sometimes have a hard time making sense of everyday sights, sounds, and feelings. Their perception of what is going on around them may be distorted so that ordinary things appear distracting or frightening. They may be extra sensitive to background noises and colors and shapes.

Cognitive Characteristics

Positive cognitive characteristics of schizophrenia are delusions, disorganized thinking, and loose associations.

Delusions are false beliefs that cannot be changed by logical reasoning or evidence. When there is an

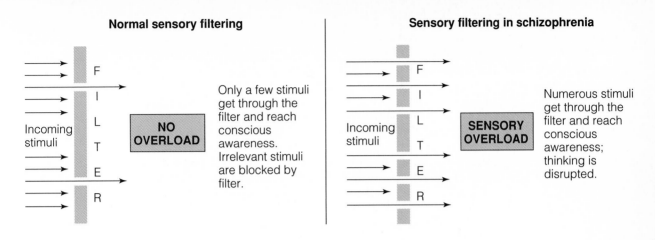

Figure 12.1 **Impaired sensory filtering in schizophrenia.**

extensively developed central delusional theme from which conclusions are deducted, the delusions are termed *systematized*. There are a number of delusional types: grandiosity (delusions of grandeur), persecution, control, somatic, religious, erotomanic, ideas of reference, thought broadcasting, thought withdrawal, and thought insertion. It is thought that delusions represent dysfunctions in the information-processing circuits within and between the hemisphere. The severity of delusions can be a valuable indicator in monitoring the course of the illness (Moller, Rice, and Murphy, 1996).

Grandiosity, also known as *delusions of grandeur*, is an exaggerated sense of importance or self-worth. It is often accompanied by beliefs of magical thinking.

> Shane lives in a group home and is introducing himself to the nursing student who will be there every Wednesday for the next 6 weeks. "I am Jeramiah the prophet, and this is just the body I reside in. My doctor is the descendent from hell. He has trouble relating to me because I am the Angel of Death. I am having a delusion right now that you are my girlfriend, but I can't marry you because I am marrying Elaine this afternoon."

People with schizophrenia may experience *delusions of persecution*. They may believe someone is trying to harm them and, therefore, any personal failures in life are the fault of these harmful others.

> Vanessa believes she is a victim of a plot. She states that people live in her attic and that they

followed her on a recent trip to Florida. She believes these people are spraying her with a toxic chemical that creates somatic symptoms. "They have somehow chosen me to be a victim in an attempt to disrupt the water waves."

Delusions of control occur when the person believes that feelings, impulses, thoughts, or actions are not one's own but are being imposed by some external force.

> Samuel believes that a group of doctors are doing long-distance laser surgery on his back. He says his back twitches when they do the surgery, and he can hear the voices of the doctors talking. "I have computer chips in my brain, and the computer sends out electrical impulses and tells me what to do. I really shouldn't be telling you this because now the security people are going to follow you."

Religious delusions involve false beliefs with religious or spiritual themes.

> The case manager has been called by Miguel's family to make a home visit. He has been sitting in front of a homemade altar and prays with a rosary to God all day long. He has been fasting intermittently for 7 weeks and has lost 30 pounds. He tells the case manager that he is being controlled by the devil, needs to be freed by God, and is fasting to atone for his sins. He states, "I don't eat because God is nourishing me."

Table 12.3 Types of Delusions

Delusion	Example
Grandiosity (delusions of grandeur)	"I've been a member of the President's Cabinet since the Kennedy years. No president can do without me. If it weren't for me, we would probably be in World War IV by now."
Persecution	"The CIA and the FBI are both out to get me. I am constantly being followed. One of the other patients in here is really a CIA agent and is here to spy on me."
Control	"I have this wire in my head, and my family controls me with it. They make me wake up and make me go to sleep. They control everything I say. I can't do anything on my own."
Religious	"As long as I wear these ten religious medals and keep all these pictures of Jesus pinned to my clothes, nothing bad can happen to me. No one can hurt me as long as I do this."
Erotomanic	"Julia Roberts is really my wife. We got married last week. She adores me and will be here soon to visit."
Sin and guilt	"I know I often hurt my parents' feelings when I was growing up. That's why I can't ever keep a job. When I get a job and start doing good, I have to quit it to make up for my bad behavior."
Somatic	"My esophagus is being torn apart. I have this rat in my stomach, and sometimes he comes all the way up to my throat. He's eating away at my esophagus. Look in my throat now—you can probably see the rat."
Ideas of reference	"People on TV last night told me I was in charge of saving the environment. That's why I'm telling everyone to stop using their cars. It's my job because that's what they told me last night."
Thought broadcasting	"I'm afraid to think anything. I know you can read my mind and know exactly what I'm thinking."
Thought withdrawal	"I can't tell you what I'm thinking. Somebody just stole my thoughts."
Thought insertion	"You think what I'm telling you is what I'm thinking, but it isn't. My father keeps putting all these thoughts in my head. They are not my thoughts."

Erotomanic delusions are beliefs that a person, usually someone famous and of higher status, is in love with her or him. Preoccupation with the "fantasy" lover may lead to stalking. Occasionally the stalker turns violent, not because of hatred of the person, but because the person cannot fulfill the romantic delusions.

Somatic delusions occur when people believe something abnormal and dangerous is happening to their bodies.

> Rachel, looking at an orange she is holding, says: "I had a bowel movement yesterday. It looked like this. It was one of my ovaries or it might have been a tumor."

Ideas of reference are remarks or actions by someone else that in no way refer to the person but are interpreted as related to her or him. *Thought broadcasting* occurs when people believe that their thoughts can be heard by others. *Thought withdrawal* is the belief that others are able to remove thoughts from one's mind. *Thought insertion* is the belief that others are able to put thoughts into one's mind.

Table 12.3 provides examples of the different types of delusions. Further information about delusions is found in Chapter 5.

Disorganized thinking is another effect of schizophrenia. Adaptation to the environment and effective coping depend not only on learned responses but also on the flexibility of the brain in organizing this incoming information. The accuracy of perceptions and organization of information influence the brain's ability to organize effective behavioral responses (Moller, Rice, and Murphy, 1996).

Because speech is a reflection of cognitive functioning, **loose association** is an indication of disorganized thinking. The person is described as having loose association when verbal ideas shift from one topic to another, there is no apparent relationship between thoughts, and the person is unaware that the topics are unconnected. At times the person may change topic and direction so frequently that she or he is incoherent or impossible to understand.

> Ming Lee states: "The thing is the ozone level is going away and people aren't told about it. Do you know why my bed is so soft? It doesn't matter. Everybody's got to die and the babies are going away. God bless America."

The negative characteristics of schizophrenia are concrete thinking, attention impairment, memory deficits, impaired problem solving, and lack of motivation. These symptoms are most likely related to dysfunctions in the cerebral cortex.

Concrete thinking is characterized by a focus on facts and details, and an inability to generalize or think abstractly. *Attention impairment* interferes with the processing of information and the response to such information. The person has poor concentration and is easily distracted. Disturbances include responding to irrelevant external stimuli and difficulty completing tasks. *Memory deficits* occur when the person is unable to retain learning. You will recall from Chapter 3 that there are two types of long-term memory: declarative and procedural. Declarative memory is memory for people and facts, is consciously accessible, and can be verbally expressed. Procedural memory does not require conscious awareness and involves the memory of motor skills and procedures. Memory problems in schizophrenia include forgetfulness, disinterest, and lack of compliance.

Impaired problem solving may occur for a number of reasons. The person may be unaware that a problem exists, have impaired judgment, be unable to think logically, be unable to make a decision, or be unable to plan or follow through on a decision. Since one of the problems with this disorder is faulty information processing, a person with schizophrenia needs more time to think and problem-solve. *Lack of motivation* is the inability to persist in goal-directed activities. People may have trouble starting projects or following though with things once begun. At the extreme, they may have to be reminded to do simple things like taking a bath or changing clothes.

Social Characteristics

The primary positive social characteristic of schizophrenia is one of *aloof and stilted interactions* with others. People with schizophrenia may use outdated or very formal language.

The negative social characteristics of schizophrenia are social withdrawal/isolation, a poor rapport with others, and inadequate social and occupational skills.

Social withdrawal/isolation may result from paranoid delusions, from severe difficulty participating in conversations, or an inability to experience feelings of friendship or intimacy. *Inadequate social skills* can interfere with the ability to develop *rapport* with others. These ineffective skills may drive away friends and family members who do not understand the behavior, further increasing the sense of isolation. People with schizophrenia may be socially incompetent in part because they are unable to perceive the subtle cues that are critical to interpersonal interactions. In order to understand body cues during an interaction, one must be able to think abstractly. People with schizophrenia understand concrete cues much better than abstract cues. For example, while they can identify and recall what someone said and did, they are less able to identify the emotional tone behind the words or comprehend the motivation for the interaction (Corrigan and Green, 1993). *Occupational skills* may be inadequate because of cognitive disruptions, behavioral abnormalities, inability to manage feelings, or inadequate social skills.

Most people with schizophrenia experience cycles of exacerbation and remission. Families who have a loved one suffering from a chronic medical illness, such as debilitating heart disease, usually receive social support and sympathy. But members of families with a loved one suffering from schizophrenia are often avoided. Many families are drained financially from the expense of long-term therapy, medications, and intermittent hospital stays. Mental health services are poorly covered in most medical insurance policies.

People suffering from schizophrenia are not indifferent to their emotional and social environments. The emotional climate of the family has been shown to play a role in the relapse of the disorder. In one study, clients who lived at home in families who were highly critical, hostile, and overinvolved had a 51% relapse rate within 9 months, compared to 13% of clients living in a supportive and caring family system (Potkin, Albers, and Richmond, 1993).

Approximately one-third of the *homeless* population suffers from psychiatric disability, many of these with schizophrenia. The figures rise to 66% when chemical dependence is included in the estimate. In addition, all people, if left homeless for a sufficient period, will develop less effective coping skills and demonstrate some type of mental disorder or disability

(Murray, 1996; Wolff, 1997). Perhaps nothing is more upsetting than the sight of an individual who is homeless and clearly experiencing severe psychiatric problems. The image of a disheveled man angrily responding to voices only he can hear is an example of society's failure to address the problem of both homelessness and psychiatric disability. Homeless mentally ill women represent one of the most vulnerable segments of our society. They frequently face a choice between the dangers of life on the street and the hazards of overcrowded, unsafe, and poorly supervised shelters. Rape and physical battery are a daily risk for these women.

Homeless psychiatrically disabled people are often fearful and distrustful of the mental health system. In community health nursing, you must be prepared to work with homeless people in nonclinical settings, including streets, shelters, subways, bus terminals, and other public areas. You will need a combination of patience, persistence, and understanding. Depending on the needs and wants of a particular person, providing food, clothing, or simply company can be essential in developing a therapeutic relationship.

Culture-Specific Characteristics

Schizophrenia is recognized worldwide and affects about 1% of the population in different cultures, although there are small areas of population with increased incidence. The symptoms tend to be universal, with minimal influence by the specific culture.

Physiological Characteristics

Some individuals with schizophrenia experience a decreased sensitivity to physical pain associated with illness and injury. Studies have demonstrated an absence of pain in 21% of clients with acute peptic ulcers, 37% of those with acute appendicitis, and 82% of those with myocardial infarction. This reduced sensitivity to pain also shows up in other medical conditions such as fractures, burns, arthritis, and post-operative experience. Because pain is a symptom of many problems, insensitivity may leave these individuals vulnerable to injury or severe medical problems (Schizophrenia Bulletin, 1996).

Concomitant Disorders

Many who suffer from schizophrenia use alcohol or drugs in an effort to self-medicate and feel better. More than 50% of people with schizophrenia have problems with alcohol or drugs at some point during their illness. Prompt recognition and treatment of this *dual diagnosis* problem is essential for effective treatment.

Suicide accounts for the majority of premature deaths among people with schizophrenia. It is estimated that as many as half of this population experience suicidal ideation, make suicide attempts, or both. Ten to 13 percent are successful suicides. Risk factors include more severe illness, frequent relapses, and significant depressive symptoms, especially hopelessness (Fenton et al, 1997).

Twenty-five percent of people with schizophrenia also experience obsessions and compulsions and of this group, 8% can be diagnosed with obsessive-compulsive disorder. Most typically, people are preoccupied with the content of their delusions and may ruminate for hours over their upsetting thoughts (Eisen et al, 1997).

Causative Factors

Schizophrenia is not a single disorder but rather a syndrome with multiple variations and multiple etiologies, both of which are complex and inadequately understood. In some, a genetic defect may contribute to abnormal development of the brain or a neurochemical malfunction, while in other cases factors such as nutrition, toxins, or trauma might interact in a genetically vulnerable person, resulting in schizophrenia. In other cases the cause may be completely environmental, such as viral infections or birth complications.

Neurobiological Factors

That there is a *genetic component* in schizophrenia is well recognized. However, the exact genetic vulnerability is not known, as no single gene has been identified as a risk factor for schizophrenia. Research is focusing on chromosomes 6, 18, and 22. It is likely that more than one gene is involved and that different families may have different genes involved. A person has an 8% risk of schizophrenia if a sibling has the disorder, a 12% risk if one parent is affected, a 14% risk of sharing the disorder with a dizygotic twin, a 39% risk if both parents are affected, and a 50% risk if a monozygotic twin has schizophrenia (Kennedy, 1996; Straub, 1997).

In monozygotic twins, prenatal factors do not always affect each twin to the same extent. Because the hands are formed at the same time cells are migrating to the cerebral cortex during the second trimester of pregnancy, they have been a site for indirectly studying brain development. In studying sets of twins in which one has schizophrenia and the other does not, it was found that affected twins had a number of small deformities in their hands and greater differences in their fingerprints compared to their siblings. There was also a significant prenatal size difference between the twins during the second trimester. Conditions that could result in brain injury at this stage of development include anemia, anoxia, ischemia, maternal alcohol or drug abuse, toxin exposure, or viral infection (Davis and Bracha, 1996).

Neurodevelopmental studies demonstrate evidence of abnormal brain development. The basic flaw seems to be that certain nerve cells migrate to the wrong areas when the brain is first taking shape, leaving small regions of the brain permanently out of place or miswired. In some cases, the neurons of the cortex may be deficient. From a developmental perspective we do not know whether these cells form normally and then fail to thrive or whether they are malformed from the beginning.

You may be wondering why, if schizophrenia begins in utero, does it not manifest for 20 years. Recent studies show that some people with schizophrenia may have early signs that are overlooked or misunderstood. For example, a child might sit up a month later than other children, or speak three months later. These signs may indicate a slight maturational lag in brain function that is later associated with schizophrenia. Later in childhood there may be evidence of lagging development and cognitive perceptual abnormalities. One factor related to the delay in the appearance of significant symptoms may be the myelin sheath, which does not form on the outside of many brain cells until late adolescence. Between the ages of 16 and 22, there are also progressive changes in cortical interactions, especially between the left prefrontal and temporal regions. This failure of the cortex to reorganize during adolescence may be the final neurodevelopmental failure of schizophrenia (Hedaya, 1996).

Neurodegeneration, the loss of neurons and brain tissue through destruction or deterioration, is a separate process that seems to occur with the onset of the illness. At this time, the mechanism responsible for the neurodegeneration is unknown. Early diagnosis and effective treatment at the onset of the illness may prevent the damage from occurring and thus improve the clinical course of schizophrenia (Lieberman, 1997).

Neurochemical factors likely involve dopamine (DA), serotonin (5-HT), norepinepherine (NE), glutamate, and GABA neurotransmission. At times neurotransmitters work together (synergistically) to trigger the same biochemical reaction, while at other times they act as antagonists, with one inhibiting the action of another. Abnormalities in the DA systems may be the result of a decrease in GABA and/or glutamate activity. Excessively high levels of NE are associated with positive symptoms, while paranoid symptoms have been related to increased DA activity. No single neurotransmitter is clearly responsible for schizophrenia. The important concept may be homeostasis: the absolute level of any neurotransmitter being much less important than its relative level with respect to all other transmitters. There may also be an undiscovered neurochemical factor yet to be found. It will be a long time before this is understood clearly (Busatto et al, 1997; Meltzer et al, 1997).

On a larger scale, new *brain imaging* studies have revealed abnormalities of brain structure in schizophrenia. Although no single brain region has been found to be involved in the pathology of schizophrenia, the areas most noted for abnormalities include the prefrontal cortex, the temporal lobes, the hippocampus, the limbic system, the thalamus, and the ventricles. The reason people with schizophrenia may not "look the same" clinically may be a function of individual deviations in brain structure. In some cases there is decreased tissue volume in specific areas, in others there is disrupted cerebral blood flow, in some cases there is decreased utilization of glucose and oxygen, and in others there is increased ventricular size. See Box 12.1 for a list of brain abnormalities. An example of one deviation is that decreased blood flow to the thalamus may affect the ability of the brain to filter sensory signals, causing the person to be flooded with sensory information (refer back to Figure 12.1). Changes in cerebral blood flow suggest abnormalities in the density, size, or configuration of blood vessels in the person with schizophrenia (Buchsbaum et al, 1996; Keltner, 1996; Lim et al, 1996; Yugelun-Todd et al, 1996). Structural abnormalities are really only the end result of some abnormal process and do not tell us much about what that process may be.

For some people with schizophrenia there is a deficiency of nicotinic receptors in the hippocampus, an area of the brain important in attention to new sensory stimuli and memory formation. Clients who smoke may be self-medicating with nicotine, which

Box 12.1

Structural Abnormalities in Schizophrenia

Decreased Volume
- Temporal lobes
- Hippocampus
- Cortical gray matter
- Limbic system

Decreased Cerebral Blood Flow
- Temporal lobes
- Basal ganglia
- Thalamus

Decreased Blood Glucose and Oxygen Utilization
- Frontal lobes
- Basal ganglia

Increased Ventricular Size

improves their attentiveness and ability to lay down memories. Since cigarette smoking is unhealthy behavior, perhaps use of nicotine skin patches may be useful in decreasing some of the cognitive symptoms of schizophrenia (Levin, 1997).

In summarizing the neurobiological factors in schizophrenia, it is believed that biological vulnerabilities (very likely genetically transmitted) interact with developmental, environmental, and social processes to produce the schizophrenic syndrome. Current research suggests that this begins during fetal development and continues through late adolescence and early adulthood (Hedaya, 1996).

Sociocultural Factors

It appears that people in lower socioeconomic levels have a slightly greater chance of developing schizophrenia than those in higher socioeconomic levels. Poor prenatal care, increased obstetric complications, and inadequate early childhood medical care may be contributing factors. Children born into poverty are exposed to excessive environmental stressors such as

poor nutrition, inadequate clothing, crime, and street violence. Schizophrenia may be a consequence of the deprivation and distress associated with poverty. Recently a significant association has been found between the age at onset of schizophrenia and a history of obstetric complications. Those who develop schizophrenia before the age of 22 are more likely to have experienced complications such as breech or abnormal presentation or a complicated cesarean delivery. Both of these complications can cause anoxia, which may cause perinatal brain damage, possibly a factor leading to the early onset of schizophrenia (Hedaya, 1996; Verdoux et al, 1997).

There is growing evidence that social support may be an important factor in impacting the course of schizophrenia. Studies indicate that people who are in positive, reciprocal relationships often function at a higher level. Social support may protect the person with schizophrenia against stress, increase self-esteem, boost the sense of well-being, and contribute to the perception of the world as a safe place. Components of social support may influence the different outcomes in levels of functioning (Buchanan, 1995).

Psychopharmacological Interventions

Conventional Antipsychotic Medications

Conventional antipsychotic medications are generally more successful at relieving the positive characteristics of schizophrenia than the negative ones. It may take 2–4 weeks to see clinical improvement from these medications. Although no evidence suggests the superiority of any one conventional antipsychotic agent, some people respond better to one drug than another. Approximately 15–30% of clients are resistant to conventional antipsychotic medications. Half of the people will get one or more side effect and, in response, many will discontinue their medication (Tollefson et al, 1997). See Table 12.4 for a summary of medications used for schizophrenia. You are encouraged to reread Chapter 7 for more detail on the medications used in treating schizophrenia.

The most common side effects of conventional antipsychotic medications include anticholinergic effects, photosensitivity, and extrapyramidal side effects (see Table 12.5). Smooth body movements depend on a critical ratio of DA to acetylcholine (ACH) in the brain. When medications block DA receptors, they lower this ratio, and **extrapyramidal side effects (EPS)** occur. *Dystonia* has an abrupt onset, with frightening

Critical Thinking

Ricardo is a 24-year-old client who is being treated for schizoaffective disorder. He is depressed, withdrawn, and disheveled. He often looks upward and listens intently. He does not offer conversation and reacts in a hostile manner when spoken to, while retreating to the corner of his room.

Mohammed is a 19-year-old client on the same psychiatric unit who is being treated for schizophrenia. Mohammed has a flat affect, paces his room for hours, stomps on spiders that are not present, seldom socializes, and often accuses others of trying to steal his clothing.

1. In what ways does Ricardo's illness differ from Mohammed's?

Suggested answers can be found in Appendix D.

2. What are the positive and the negative characteristics of schizophrenia?

3. What data support the positive characteristics of schizophrenia for Ricardo? For Mohammed?

4. What data support the negative characteristics of schizophrenia for Ricardo?

5. Both Ricardo and Mohammed are being treated with antipsychotic drugs that can produce tardive dyskinesia. How will you know if either of these clients is developing this drug side effect?

6. If you were Ricardo or Mohammed's nurse, how would you intervene during their chronic hallucinatory episodes?

Table 12.4 Antipsychotic Medications

Class	Generic Name	Trade Name	Adult Dosages (mg/day)
Atypical antipsychotics	clozapine	Clozaril	300–900
	olanzapine	Zyprexa	5–20
	quetiapine	Seroquel	150–750
	risperidone	Resperdal	4–16
	sertindole	Serlect	12–24
	ziprasidone	Zeldox	80–160
Phenothiazines	acetophenazine	Tindal	40–120
	chlorpromazine	Thorazine	30–800
	fluphenazine	Prolixin, Permitil	1–40
	mesoridazine	Serentil	75–300
	perphenazine	Trilafon	8–64
	thioridazine	Mellaril	150–800
	trifluoperazine	Stelazine, Suptazine	15–20
	triflupromazine	Vesprin	60–150
Thioxanthenes	chlorprothixene	Taractan	75–600
	thiothixene	Navane	6–120
Butyrophenones	haloperidol	Haldol	1–50
Dibenzoxazepine	loxapine	Loxitane	10–160
Dihydroindolone	molindone	Moban	15–225
Diphenylbatylperidine	pimozide	Orap	1–10

Table 12.5 Side Effects of Conventional Antipsychotics and Counteracting Measures

Side Effect	What this means . . .	Measures
Akathisia	<ul><li>Feeling restless or jittery</li><li>Needing to fidget, pace around</li></ul>	Beta-blocker, such as Inderal (propranolol)
Dystonia	<ul><li>Sudden muscle spasm</li><li>Oculogyric crisis</li><li>Laryngospasm</li></ul>	Benadryl (diphenhyramine) Cogentin (benztropine)
Parkinsonism	<ul><li>Tremor, stiffness, stooped posture, shuffling gait</li><li>Akinesia—feeling slowed down</li></ul>	Cogentin (benztropine) Symmetrel (amantadine) Akineton (biperiden) Kemadrin (procyclidine) Benadryl (diphenhyramine)
Neuroleptic malignant syndrome	<ul><li>Muscle rigidity</li><li>Hyperpyrexia</li><li>Hypertension</li><li>Confusion, delirium</li></ul>	Supportive measures Discontinue antipsychotic medication May give muscle relaxants
Tardive dyskinesia	<ul><li>Involuntary movements of face and body</li><li>Swallowing problems</li></ul>	Goal is prevention Reduce dose of antipsychotic medication
Anticholinergic physical effects	<ul><li>Dry mouth</li><li>Blurry vision</li><li>Trouble urinating</li><li>Constipation</li></ul>	Medications as below Rinse mouth with water; chew sugar-free gum Drink 6–8 glasses of fluid each day Eat bulky foods
Anticholinergic mental effects	<ul><li>Memory difficulties</li><li>Confusion</li></ul>	Akineton (biperiden) Cogentin (benztropine) Artane (trihexyphenidyl) Kemadrin (procyclidine) Symmetrel (amantadine)
Weight gain	<ul><li>Up to 40% of clients gain weight</li></ul>	Decrease caloric intake Exercise daily
Sexual difficulties	<ul><li>Loss of sexual desire</li><li>Loss of erection or ejaculation</li><li>Anorgasmia</li></ul>	Try different antipsychotic medications Discuss problem with client and partner

muscle spasms in the head and neck. Oculogyric crisis and laryngospasm are terms used to describe dystonic reaction in specific body regions. These reactions usually occur within the first 5 days of therapy or when dosage is significantly increased. Males and younger people are at higher risk for dystonia.

Parkinsonism is evidenced in clients' stooped posture and shuffling gait. Their faces resemble masks, and they may drool. They experience tremors and pill-rolling motions of the thumb and fingers at rest. This reaction is likely to begin within the first 30 days of treatment and occurs throughout the use

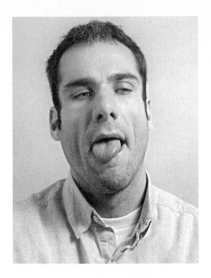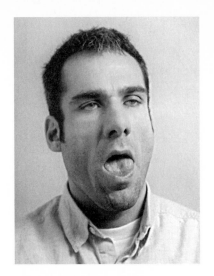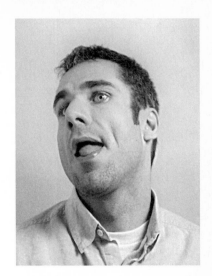

Figure 12.2 **Tardive dyskinesia: abnormal movements of the mouth, tongue and jaw.**

of the medication. *Akathisia* is the inability to sit or stand still, along with a feeling of anxiety. This side effect usually begins within the first 60 days of treatment and persists as long as the client is on medication. This side effect is extremely distressing to people and is a frequent cause of medication noncompliance. It is less responsive to treatment than are parkinsonism and dystonia. A number of medications may be used to lessen the EPS effects of the conventional antipsychotics. These medications reduce ACH, thereby restoring the DA-ACH ratio (Kapur and Remington, 1996).

Neuroleptic malignant syndrome (NMS) is a potentially fatal extrapyramidal symptom. It affects 1–2% of clients who take conventional antipsychotic medication. The risk is higher when clients are on two or more of these medications. Symptoms of NMS develop suddenly and include muscle rigidity and respiratory problems. Hyperpyrexia ranges from 101F to 107F (38C–41.6C). During the next 2–3 days, clients develop tachycardia, hypertension, respiratory problems, confusion, and delirium. The mortality rate with NMS is 14–30%; it is estimated that 1000–4000 people die every year. There is no specific treatment for NMS other than supportive measures and discontinuation of the medication. Parlodel (bromacriptine) may be of some help in halting the DA blockage. Muscle relaxants may lessen the rigidity (American Psychiatric Association, 1997).

Tardive dyskinesia occurs in 20–25% of clients who take conventional antipsychotic medications for over 2 years. Females and older people are at higher risk for tardive dyskinesia. Many of the cases are mild, but the disorder can be socially disfiguring. Symptoms include frowning, blinking, grimacing, puckering, blowing, smacking, licking, chewing, tongue protrusion, and spastic facial distortions (Figure 12.2). Abnormal movements of the arms and legs include rapid, purposeless, irregular movements; tremors; and foot tapping. Body symptoms include dramatic movements of the neck and shoulders and rocking, twisting pelvic gyrations and thrusts. Because tardive dyskinesia is often irreversible, the goal is prevention. If symptoms begin to appear, the medication is reduced or the person is switched to a newer antipsychotic medication (American Psychiatric Association, 1997).

Because of the side effects, many people do not like the way their bodies feel when taking conventional antipsychotic medication. Interference with sexual functioning is fairly common. Almost half report weight gain. Anticholinergic side effects are unpleasant and can occur in 15–50% of people treated with these drugs. Identifying and managing side effects may help people stay on the medication and maintain a higher level of functioning, thus avoiding acute hospitalization. Some people will stop taking their medication and relapse, while others relapse first and, as a result of their symptoms, stop taking their medication.

New or Atypical Antipsychotic Medications

Negative symptoms impose great suffering on people by interfering with their psychosocial functioning. *Atypical antipsychotic medications* are characterized by:

- effectiveness in eliminating the negative as well as the positive characteristics of schizophrenia
- effectiveness for many people who are not responsive to conventional antipsychotic agents
- effectiveness for people who also experience depressive symptoms
- a significantly lower incidence of EPS effects, which increases compliance

Research suggests that people on *Clozaril (clozapine)* have fewer relapse episodes and significantly fewer hospitalizations. Clozaril affects DA receptors primarily in the limbic system. About 1% of those taking Clozaril develop agranulocytosis, which carries a 40% fatality rate; therefore, weekly blood tests are essential for the first 6 months. Thereafter, WBCs are measured every other week. It is desirable that the white blood count stay above 3500/mm. Side effects occur most typically during the first few weeks of therapy and include sedation, weight gain, and hypersalivation. Because of the sedating and hypotensive effects, this drug may be problematic for older clients (Grossberg, 1997).

Risperdal (risperidone) is different from both Clozaril and conventional antipsychotic medications. It antagonizes both DA and 5-HT receptors. It lacks most of the serious side effects of Clozaril and has fewer motor side effects than do conventional antipsychotic medications. Other advantages are low anticholinergic side effects, low sedation, and more effectiveness for affective symptoms (Grossberg, 1997).

New medications receiving FDA approval in 1997 include *Zyprex (olanzapine)*, *Serlect (sertindole)*, and *Seroquel (quetiapine)*. These drugs affect all of the DA receptors, many of the 5-HT receptors, and the histamine receptors. Studies have shown these drugs to be effective and safe in long-term treatment of schizophrenia. Common side effects are sedation, weight gain, and hypotension. They appear to be relatively free of EPS effects. A similar medication, Zeldox (ziprasidone), is under FDA investigation at the current time (American Psychiatric Association, 1997).

Ancillary Medications

When added to antipsychotic medications, mood-stabilizing agents such as *lithium carbonate*, *Tegretol (carbamazepine)*, and *Depakote (valproate)* enhance the effectiveness of the response and improve negative symptoms specifically. They are also effective for people experiencing affective symptoms.

Benzodiazepines may also be used as adjuncts to antipsychotic medications. Studies have demonstrated reductions in anxiety, agitation, and psychotic symptoms with the use of these agents. See Chapter 7 for a more detailed explanation of these ancillary medications.

Multidisciplinary Interventions

Psychiatric Rehabilitation

The field of psychiatric or psychosocial rehabilitation grew out of a need to create opportunities for people suffering from psychiatric disabilities. The rehabilitation approach emphasizes the development of skills and supports necessary for successful living, learning, and working in the community. This approach creates collaborative partnerships with all interested people—consumers, families, friends, and mental health providers. It is assumed that the consumer will be "in charge" with regard to setting goals for where and how to live, work, learn, socialize, and recreate (see Box 12.2). Rehabilitation is a process, not a quick fix. It is also different than the traditional approach to long-term clients, which assumed that people with schizophrenia could not make decisions and would continue to deteriorate in spite of interventions. We now know that a substantial number of people with schizophrenia make good adjustments and lead satisfactory lives.

People with mental illness differ little from the general population. They want work that is meaningful and self-enhancing and the opportunity to socialize with others. Psychiatric rehabilitation is anchored in the values of hope and optimism that people can grow, learn, and make changes in their lives. Other values include the promotion of choices, self-determination, and individual responsibility. The essential element of self-help is power. People who are psychiatrically disabled need power and control in their relationships with professionals, in their own lives, and in the way resources are allocated. This allows them to take personal responsibility for where they are in their lives and where they are going. As a

Box 12.2

Beliefs and Values in Psychiatric Rehabilitation

Beliefs

- The most severely disabled psyciatric client has a potential for productivity
- The opportunity to be gainfully employed is a generative force in human beings
- Work can enhance self-esteem and reduce symptoms of mental illness
- People require opportunities to be together socially

Values

- Hope, optimism
- Wellness
- Choices
- Self-determination
- Individual responsibility
- Compassion

---

nurse who functions as a resource for clients, you must not only be competent but also compassionate and caring. This includes searching for talents and skills until you find them, even when they are obscured by multiple relapses and low self-esteem. Your role is to teach skills, to coach skills as needed in a variety of social and work situations, and to identify supports in the community of choice. In this way you will promote independent living and successful coping for people with psychiatric disabilities (Carling, 1995; Farrell and Deeds, 1997; Palmer-Erbs, 1996).

Group Therapy

Group therapy is an effective psychosocial treatment modality for persons with schizophrenia. It helps prevent the withdrawal and social isolation that may occur for people who are psychiatrically disabled. For people who live alone, the group may be their primary opportunity to relate to others. The group setting also provides an opportunity to discuss and help each other solve problems in everyday living, employment difficulties, or interpersonal conflicts. There are several types of group therapy. Some groups are

highly structured, while others may be more spontaneous. Some may have a very narrow topic range such as assertiveness training, while others may have a broader range such as general problems in living in the community. Groups focus on peer support, with an emphasis on development skills and changing behavior. Groups are also used for teaching and social support. See Chapter 6 for more information on group therapy.

Case Management

Case management is intended to increase consumers' access to care and to ensure that they receive coordinated, continuous, and comprehensive services. There are a number of activities for which case managers are responsible. Case managers *identify clients*. They determine whose needs are congruent with the available services and resources. They may be involved in increasing access to services in the form of outreach to the homeless population. Once case managers identify clients, they must *assess individual needs and strengths*. Case managers work with other providers to determine the best way to meet those needs and support skills and strengths. This planning determines the next step in treatment, which is *linkage*. The case manager links clients to available services by helping them meet the qualifying criteria. They also serve as *advocates* when they negotiate with agencies and policy makers in an effort to gain resources for consumers. Almost all case managers also provide *direct care* in the form of a therapeutic relationship, supportive psychotherapy, and crisis response. If appropriate, they may help clients shop, cook, obtain medical cards, and learn activities of daily living (American Psychiatric Association, 1997).

Treatment Settings

People with schizophrenia may receive their care in a variety of settings. These settings vary with regard to the types of services offered, the amount of support, structure, and restrictiveness, and the hours of operation.

Supportive housing is a program used for consumers who do not live with their families and who would benefit from some degree of assistance in self-care and self-management. These programs can increase social and vocational functioning and quality of life and decrease homelessness and rehospitalization. See Box 12.3 for descriptions of the types of residential facilities.

Box 12.3

Types of Residential Facilities

Transitional Halfway Houses

- Provide room and board until suitable housing is available

Long-Term Group Residences

- On-site staff
- Appropriate for psychiatrically disabled persons
- Length of stay is indefinite

Cooperative Apartments

- No on-site staff
- Staff make regular visits to assist residents

Intensive-Care or Crisis Community Residences

- Used to help prevent hospitalization or shorten length of hospitalization
- On-site nursing staff and counseling staff

Foster or Family Care

- In private homes
- Close supervision of foster family to assure a therapeutic environment

Nursing Homes

- Appropriate for some geriatric or medically disabled consumers
- Activity programs and psychiatric supervision

Psychosocial clubhouses are therapeutic communities where staff function as administrators whose role is to encourage the decision making and socialization of the "members" of the club. Club activities focus on recreational, vocational, and residential functions. The approach is transitional, with individuals gradually assuming more responsibilities and privileges.

Day treatment programs are open only during the day and are used to provide ongoing supportive care. They are usually not time-limited (that is, they are not limited in duration to a specific number of months or years). They provide structure and programs to help prevent relapse and to improve social and vocational functioning. Day treatment programs have low staff-to-client ratios and minimal or no nursing staff.

Day hospitalization can be used as an alternative to inpatient care or following a brief hospitalization. The advantage over inpatient care is less disruption of the person's life and treatment in a less restrictive environment. The person should not be at risk of harming self or others and should be able to cooperate minimally in treatment. The day hospital is staffed similarly to the staffing of the day shift on an acute inpatient unit.

Treatment in *hospitals* has the advantage of providing a safe, structured, and supervised environment, which reduces stress on both consumers and family members. It allows the health care team to closely monitor the level of symptoms and reactions to treatments. Hospitalization is indicated for those people who are considered at risk of harm to themselves or others or who are so severely disorganized or under the influence of delusions or hallucinations that they are unable to care for themselves.

There remains a small group of clients who require *long-term hospitalization* for their own safety as well as for the protection of family and community. These individuals profit most from treatment programs that emphasize highly structured behavioral interventions such as a token economy, point systems, and skills training that can improve their level of functioning.

The Nursing Process

Assessment

The assessment of clients' responses to their illness and their functional status includes assessment of clients' reports, family or caregiver reports, and direct observation of performance. Clients who are not acutely ill are usually able to provide accurate information about their past history with mental illness and their current experiences. Identification of functional disabilities leads to the formulation of nursing diagnoses.

If clients are acutely ill, it may be difficult to obtain information directly from them. This is especially true for those who are experiencing delusions and hallucinations. Family members, roommates, friends, group home supervisors, or case managers may be the initial data source when there is an admission to the acute care setting. The Focused Nursing Assessment table provides questions that can be used in the home, the residential or group home setting, or in the acute care setting.

Diagnosis

There are many potential nursing diagnoses for clients suffering from schizophrenia. In synthesizing the assessment data, consider how well clients are functioning in daily life, what their skills and talents are, how stable their affect is, how well they are able to communicate, how well they are getting along with others, and how well they function at work. See the Nursing Diagnoses box at the right for some of the more common nursing diagnoses you may be applying to your clients.

Outcome Identification

Once you have established diagnoses, you and the client mutually identify goals for change. Client outcomes are specific behavioral measures by which you, clients, and significant others determine progress toward goals. The following are examples of some of the outcomes appropriate to people with schizophrenia:

- communicates clearly
- completes ADLs appropriately
- exhibits increased attention span
- makes appropriate decisions
- affect is appropriate to the situation
- denies hallucinations
- verbalizes logical thought processes
- interacts well with others
- develops occupational skills

See also the Critical Pathway for a Client with Schizophrenia on pages 299–304.

Nursing Diagnoses

Clients with Schizophrenia

Altered thought process related to delusions, loose association, autistic thinking, concrete thinking, symbolic thinking.

Sensory-perceptual alterations related to hallucinations (auditory, visual).

High risk for violence, self-directed, related to command hallucinations.

High risk for violence, directed at others, related to suspiciousness, fear, command hallucinations.

Self-care deficit related to an inability to remember steps in self-care; preoccupation with the symptoms of the disorder.

Social isolation related to withdrawal, preoccupation with symptoms, lack of a supportive network, negative reaction by others to client's social behavior.

Impaired verbal communication related to poverty of speech, autistic thinking, neologisms, anxiety.

Self-esteem disturbance related to feeling different from others, chronic nature of the disorder.

Ineffective family coping related to not understanding the disorder and the treatment process; inability to adapt to client's illness.

Nursing Interventions

Nurses have many opportunities to assist people with schizophrenia in a variety of settings as previously described. These contacts may be long-term relationships or may be during crisis periods of time. Families, significant others, or caregivers should be actively involved in the plan of care and be taught to implement many of these interventions. See the box on page 305 for an overview of the nursing interventions classification (NIC) for people with schizophrenia.

Behavioral: Communication Enhancement

Complex Relationship Building

The nature of the nurse-client relationship is one of the most effective nursing interventions. With rapport, communication, and trust, we are able to help our clients meet the outcome criteria they have identified. Review the material on communicating with clients in

Text continues on page 304

Focused Nursing Assessment

CLIENTS WITH SCHIZOPHRENIA

Behavior Assessment	Affective Assessment	Cognitive Assessment	Sociocultural Assessment
Describe your usual pattern of activities throughout the day.	What kinds of activities/situations give you pleasure? Anxiety? Anger? Guilt?	Have you ever heard voices? Are you hearing voices now? What do the voices say to you? What feelings are associated with the voices?	Who are the people most significant to you?
What are your responsibilities at home? At work? At school?		Have you ever seen things other people don't see? What things do you see? What feelings are associated with seeing things?	When do you prefer to be alone?
What do you do for leisure activities?		Do you believe that you are someone very important?	When do you prefer to be with others?
		Do you feel anyone is trying to harm you?	How do you relate to others?
		Do you feel anyone is controlling you?	How do you resolve conflict with others?
		Do you think about religion a lot?	
		Do you believe that you are very guilty for something you have done?	
		Do you think anything abnormal is happening to your body?	
		Do you think people are talking about you often?	
		Do you believe others can hear your thoughts?	
		Do you believe others can take away your thoughts?	
		Do you believe others can put thoughts into your head?	
		Do you have thoughts of harming yourself? Harming others?	
		Have you ever thought you have special powers that other people do not have?	

Critical Pathway for a Client with Schizophrenia*

Expected length of stay: 10–14 days	Date _____ Day 1	Date _____ Days 2–4	Date _____ Days 5–7
Daily outcomes	Client will: ▪ Remain free of injury to self or others. ▪ Identify initial goals for hospitalization. ▪ Participate in transdisciplinary treatment plan. ▪ Participate in assessment. ▪ Identify most recent medication regime. ▪ Drink 2000 cc of fluids each day. ▪ Identify current dietary pattern and food preferences.	Client will: ▪ Remain free of injury to self or others. ▪ Identify initial goals for hospitalization. ▪ Maintain contract for management of impulsive acts. ▪ Participate in transdisciplinary treatment plan. ▪ Participate in assessment. ▪ Begin to verbalize need for medications. ▪ Participate in menu planning. ▪ Drink 2000 cc of fluids each day. ▪ Respond to redirection PRN. ▪ Establish rest/sleep-promoting environment. ▪ Remain oriented to time, place, and person. ▪ Verbalize feelings appropriately. ▪ Seek help appropriately when experiencing increasing anxiety. ▪ Cooperate in self-care activities. ▪ Use physical activity to manage tension.	Client will: ▪ Remain free of injury to self or others. ▪ Identify initial goals for hospitalization. ▪ Maintain contract for management of impulsive acts. ▪ Participate in transdisciplinary treatment plan. ▪ Verbalize reasons for medications. ▪ Consume diet per menu plan. ▪ Drink 2000 cc of fluids each day. ▪ Listen and respond to topic for a few minutes. ▪ Participate in physical activity groups as scheduled. ▪ Participate in group activities as scheduled. ▪ Respond to redirection PRN. ▪ Perform self-care activities independently 50% of time. ▪ Establish rest/sleep-promoting environment. ▪ Stay focused on simple task for a few minutes. ▪ Remain oriented to time, place, and person. ▪ Seek help appropriately when anxiety level is increasing. ▪ Performs self-care activities with prompting. ▪ Use physical activity to manage tension.
Assessments, tests, and treatments	Psychosocial assessment to include mental status, mood, affect, behavior, and communication every shift and PRN. Complete nursing database assessment. Observe behavior and activity level. Weight. Monitor fluid intake. CBC, urinalysis.	Psychosocial assessment every shift and PRN. Observe for safety per protocol. Monitor behavior and activity level. Monitor effects and compliance with medication. Monitor fluid intake. Assess sleep pattern. Routine vital signs.	Psychosocial assessment every shift and PRN. Observe for safety per protocol. Monitor behavior and activity level. Monitor effects and compliance with medication. Monitor fluid intake. Assess sleep pattern. Routine vital signs.

*This critical pathway provides a sample guideline for nursing care. Variations of this pathway may be seen in your clinical setting or based on the client's condition.

continued ▶

Critical Pathway for a Client with Schizophrenia continued

	Date _____ Day 1 *continued*	Date _____ Days 2–4 *continued*	Date _____ Days 5–7 *continued*
Assessments, tests, and treatments *continued*	Chemistry profile. Drug screen. RPR. Electrolytes. Other laboratory as ordered. Vital signs BID and PRN.		
Knowledge deficit	Orient client/family to unit and program. Assess learning needs of client and family. Review initial plan of care. Initiate medication teaching. Assess understanding of teaching.	Review unit orientation with emphasis on program. Continue medication teaching. Assess understanding of teaching.	Review plan of care. Include family in teaching. Initiate teaching regarding treatment modalities and preventive techniques. Assess medication teaching response and need for additional teaching. Evaluate understanding of teaching.
Diet	Monitor dietary intake. Diet as tolerated—encourage small, frequent feedings from all food groups. Provide preferred snacks and foods.	Monitor dietary intake. Diet as tolerated—encourage small, frequent feedings from all food groups. Provide preferred snacks and foods.	Monitor dietary intake. Diet as tolerated—encourage small, frequent feedings from all food groups. Provide preferred snacks and foods.
Activity	Assess safety needs and maintain appropriate precautions. Observe activity level. Develop schedule for stimulus titration (i.e., quiet time and periods in the milieu). Provide sleep-enhancing atmosphere for 45 min prior to sleep.	Maintain safety precautions. Observe activity level. Maintain schedule for stimulus titration. Prompt and assist with hygiene as necessary. Provide sleep-enhancing atmosphere for 45 min prior to sleep.	Maintain safety precautions. Observe activity level. Maintain schedule for stimulus titration. Encourage to attend small group activities. Prompt with hygiene as necessary. Provide sleep-enhancing atmosphere for 45 min prior to sleep.
Psychosocial	Approach with nonjudgmental and accepting manner. Observe and monitor behavior. Provide structured activities and contracts. Direct to structured activities as per contract. Minimize environmental stimuli and provide a safe environment. Redirect impulsive acts.	Approach with nonjudgmental and accepting manner. Observe and monitor behavior. Provide structured activities and contracts. Direct to structured activities as per contract. Minimize environmental stimuli and provide a safe environment. Redirect impulsive acts.	Approach with nonjudgmental and accepting manner. Observe and monitor behavior. Provide structured activities and contracts. Direct to structured activities as per contract. Minimize environmental stimuli and provide a safe environment. Redirect impulsive acts.

	Date _____ Day 1 *continued*	Date _____ Days 2–4 *continued*	Date _____ Days 5–7 *continued*
Psychosocial *continued*	Provide information regarding illness and treatment to client and family. Use calm, consistent approach. Communicate in clear, direct terms. Provide positive feedback for reality-based focus and socially appropriate behavior. Maintain scheduled contacts.	Provide information regarding illness and treatment to client and family. Use calm, consistent approach. Communicate in clear, direct terms. Provide positive feedback for reality-based focus and socially appropriate behavior. Maintain scheduled contacts.	Provide information regarding illness and treatment to client and family. Use calm, consistent approach. Communicate in clear, direct terms. Provide positive feedback for reality-based focus and socially appropriate behavior. Maintain scheduled contacts.
Medications	Identify target symptoms. Antipsychotics as ordered. Monitor for extrapyramidal side effects. Administer antiparkinsonian medications as indicated. Routine meds as ordered.	Assess target symptoms. Antipsychotics as ordered. Monitor for extrapyramidal side effects. Administer antiparkinsonian medications as indicated. Routine meds as ordered.	Assess target symptoms. Antipsychotics as ordered. Monitor for extrapyramidal side effects. Administer antiparkinsonian medications as indicated. Routine meds as ordered.
Referrals and discharge plan	Family assessment. Consult with internist if ordered. Occupational and recreational therapist. Establish discharge objectives with client and family.	Review with client and significant others discharge objectives. Complete discharge planning.	Review with client and significant others progress toward discharge objectives. Make appropriate referrals to support groups.

	Date _____ Days 8–9	Date _____ Days 10–12	Date _____ Days 13–14
Daily outcomes	Client will: ■ Remain free of injury to self or others. ■ Discuss goals for hospitalization. ■ Contract for management of impulsive behaviors. ■ Participate in transdisciplinary treatment plan. ■ Verbalize reasons for medications and understanding of side effects of medication. ■ Consume diet per menu plan. ■ Participate in physical activity groups as scheduled. ■ Listen and respond to topic in group sessions. ■ Begin to identify consequences of impulsive behavior.	Client will: ■ Remain free of injury to self or others. ■ Discuss goals for hospitalization. ■ Contract for management of impulsive acts. ■ Participate in transdisciplinary treatment plan. ■ Verbalize reasons for medications and need for long-term therapy. ■ Consume diet per menu plan. ■ Participate in physical activity groups as scheduled. ■ Adaptively use listening skills. ■ Respond to redirection when participating in physical activity groups.	Client is free of injury to self or others. Client is alert and oriented. Client communicates ability to cope with current and ongoing stressors. Client identifies plan to access resources for increasing anxiety or stress levels. Client's weight is stable. Client achieves maximum independence in self-care. Client adaptively uses listening skills. Client enjoys 6 h of uninterrupted sleep. Client identifies plan if symptoms recur. Client eats a well-balanced diet inclusive of all food groups.

continued ➤

Critical Pathway for a Client with Schizophrenia continued

	Date _____ Days 8–9 *continued*	Date _____ Days 10–12 *continued*	Date _____ Days 13–14 *continued*
Daily outcomes *continued*	▪ Respond to redirection when participating in physical activity groups. ▪ Perform self-care activities independently 75% of time. ▪ Establish sleep/rest-promoting environment. ▪ Stay focused on simple task for 10 min period. ▪ Verbalize feelings appropriately. ▪ Seek help appropriately when anxiety level is increasing. ▪ Maintain usual elimination patterns. ▪ Remain oriented to time, place, and person.	▪ Perform self-care activities independently 100% of time. ▪ Establish rest/sleep-promoting environment. ▪ Stay focused on simple task for 15 min period. ▪ Seek help appropriately when anxiety level is increasing. ▪ Maintain usual elimination patterns. ▪ Remain oriented to time, place, and person.	Client drinks 2000 cc of fluids each day. Client has resumed readmission urine and bowel elimination pattern. Client verbalizes/demonstrates home care instructions including the importance of ongoing mental health care. Client participates in regular exercise program. Client demonstrates ability to adaptively cope with ongoing stressors.
Assessments, tests, and treatments	Psychosocial assessment BID and PRN. Observe for safety per protocol. Monitor behavior and activity pattern. Monitor effects and compliance with medication. Monitor fluid intake. Assess sleep pattern.	Psychosocial assessment QD PRN. Observe for safety per protocol. Monitor behavior and activity pattern. Monitor effects and compliance with medication. Monitor fluid intake. Assess sleep pattern.	Psychosocial assessment. Observe for safety per protocol. Monitor behavior and activity pattern. Monitor effects and compliance with medication. Monitor fluid intake. Assess sleep pattern.
Knowledge deficit	Review plan of care. Include family in teaching. Review current level of knowledge regarding medications, treatments, symptom management, and follow-up care. Assess understanding of teaching.	Review plan of care with client and family. Reinforce current level of knowledge regarding medications, treatments, symptom management, and follow-up care. Evaluate understanding of teaching.	Client and/or significant other verbalizes understanding of discharge teaching including activity level and exercise program, safety measures, diet, signs and symptoms to report, follow-up care and MD appointment, medications (name, purpose, dose, frequency, route, dietary interactions, and side effects), and follow-up care arrangements. Evaluate understanding of teaching. Make referrals to community caregivers for any knowledge deficits regarding medications, treatments, symptoms management, and follow-up care.

	Date _____ Days 8–9 *continued*	Date _____ Days 10–12 *continued*	Date _____ Days 13–14 *continued*
Diet	Monitor dietary intake. Diet as tolerated—encourage small, frequent feedings from all food groups. Provide preferred snacks and foods.	Monitor dietary intake. Diet as tolerated—encourage small, frequent feedings from all food groups. Provide preferred snacks and foods.	Monitor dietary intake. Diet as tolerated—encourage small, frequent feedings from all food groups. Provide preferred snacks and foods.
Activity	Maintain safety precautions. Observe activity level. Maintain schedule for stimulus titration. Work at activities until completion. Manage agitation with periods of physical activity. Encourage to eat meals in dining room. Prompt with hygiene as necessary. Provide sleep-enhancing atmosphere for 45 min prior to sleep.	Maintain safety precautions. Observe activity level. Maintain schedule for stimulus titration. Manage agitation with periods of physical activity. Independently attends physical activity groups Independent in self-care. Provide sleep-enhancing atmosphere for 45 min prior to sleep.	Maintain safety precautions. Observe activity level. Maintain schedule for stimulus titration. Manage agitation with periods of physical activity. Prompt to attend physical activity groups. Independent in self-care. Provide sleep-enhancing atmosphere for 45 min prior to sleep.
Psychosocial	Approach with nonjudgmental and accepting manner. Observe and monitor behavior. Provide structured activities and contracts. Direct to structured activities as per contract. Minimize environmental stimuli and provide a safe environment. Redirect impulsive behaviors. Provide information regarding illness and treatment to client and family. Use calm, consistent approach. Communicate in clear, direct terms. Provide positive feedback for reality-based focus and socially appropriate behavior. Prompt to attend physical activity groups. Independently attends short, small group activities. Prompt to start attending group therapy as tolerated. Meet with client 2 times each shift for 5 min periods focused on activities of daily living and behavior.	Approach with nonjudgmental and accepting manner. Observe and monitor behavior. Provide structured activities and contracts. Direct to structured activities as per contract. Minimize environmental stimuli and provide a safe environment. Redirect impulsive behaviors. Provide information regarding illness and treatment to client and family. Use calm, consistent approach. Communicate in clear, direct terms. Provide positive feedback for reality-based focus and socially appropriate behavior. Eats meals in dining room without prompting. Independently attends group therapy for increasingly longer period. Independently attends short, small group activities. Attends discharge planning group.	Approach with nonjudgmental and accepting manner. Observe and monitor behavior. Provide structured activities and contracts. Direct to structured activities as per contract. Minimize environmental stimuli and provide a safe environment. Redirect impulsive behaviors. Provide information regarding illness and treatment to client and family. Use calm, consistent approach. Communicate in clear, direct terms. Provide positive feedback for reality-based focus and socially appropriate behavior. Meet with client 2 times each shift for 5 min periods to discuss after discharge care and management. Maintain scheduled contacts.

continued ➤

Critical Pathway for a Client with Schizophrenia continued

	Date _____ Days 8–9 *continued*	Date _____ Days 10–12 *continued*	Date _____ Days 13–14 *continued*
Psychosocial *continued*	Maintain scheduled contacts.	Meet with client 2 times each shift for 5 min periods to work on discharge goals. Maintain scheduled contacts.	
Medications	Monitor target symptoms. Antipsychotics as ordered. Monitor for extrapyramidal side effects. Administer antiparkinsonian medications as indicated. Routine meds as ordered.	Monitor target symptoms. Antipsychotics as ordered. Monitor for extrapyramidal side effects. Administer antiparkinsonian medications as indicated. Routine meds as ordered.	Monitor target symptoms. Antipsychotics as ordered. Monitor for extrapyramidal side effects. Administer antiparkinsonian medications as indicated. Routine meds as ordered.
Referrals and discharge plan	Review discharge objectives with client and significant others.	Review progress toward discharge objectives with client and significant others. Complete referrals for discharge care.	Discharge with referrals.

Chapter 5. When we listen to clients, accept them for who they are, and understand their perspective, we are more likely to help empower them and thereby help them achieve their highest level of functioning.

Active Listening

Sometimes clients are not able to hold thoughts together enough for you to comprehend what is being said. They may not remember how they started a sentence or where their thoughts were taking them (loose association). They are often more able to understand others than to make themselves understood. When this occurs, *interrupt politely* but firmly and ask a question that will help them communicate in a more direct manner. Say something like, "I'm not understanding what you are saying. Could we try that again?" *Listening for themes* in the conversation may help you understand the current concerns of the person. When you try to understand the world the client is experiencing, the person is more likely to feel you are being helpful (Moller, Rice, and Murphy, 1998).

Sensory overload or the inability to screen out unimportant stimuli is frustrating and disorienting to clients and interferes with their abilities to listen and communicate. You can teach clients to decrease environmental stimuli by avoiding noise and confusion, including large crowds or large family gatherings.

Socialization Enhancement

Social difficulties frequently accompany schizophrenia, and *social skills training* is an appropriate nursing intervention. Because of the stigma attached to mental disorders and especially schizophrenia, consumers have had fewer opportunities to develop and practice social skills. This inexperience contributes to inappropriate responses when interacting with others. After specific skill deficits are identified, training strategies are designed to reduce these deficits and improve the level of functioning. Social skills training is a series of highly structured and organized sessions of practice in basic skills usually conducted in a group format. Group leaders model the appropriate skills. Through role-play and social reinforcement, members learn the same behaviors, step by step. Social skills training includes such areas as how to initiate a conversation, how to express ideas and feelings appropriately, how to avoid topics that are not appropriate for a casual conversation, how to ask about job openings, and how to interview for a job. Repeat practice can result in improvements in important areas of social adjustment, leading to less withdrawal and isolation.

Nursing Interventions Classification

CLIENTS WITH SCHIZOPHRENIA

DOMAIN: Behavioral

Class: *Communication Enhancement*

Interventions: *Complex Relationship Building:* Establishing a therapeutic relationship with a patient who has difficulty interacting with others.

Active Listening: Attending closely to and attaching significance to a patient's verbal and nonverbal messages.

Socialization Enhancement: Facilitation of another person's ability to interact with others.

Class: *Coping Assistance*

Interventions: *Self-Esteem Enhancement:* Assisting a patient to increase his/her personal judgment of self-worth.

Class: *Psychological Comfort Promotion*

Interventions: *Anxiety Reduction:* Minimizing apprehension, dread, foreboding, or uneasiness related to an unidentified source of anticipated danger.

Class: *Patient Education*

Interventions: *Teaching: Disease Process:* Assisting the patient to understand information related to a specific disease process.

Teaching: Prescribed Medications: Preparing a patient to safely take prescribed medications and monitor for their effects.

DOMAIN: Physiological: Basic

Class: *Activity and Exercise Management*

Interventions: *Energy Management:* Regulating energy use to treat or prevent fatigue and optimize function.

Class: *Self-Care Facilitation*

Interventions: *Self-Care Assistance:* Assisting another to perform activities of daily living.

DOMAIN: Safety

Class: *Crisis Management*

Interventions: *Suicide Prevention:* Reducing risk of self-inflicted harm for a patient in crisis or severe depression.

Class: *Risk Management*

Interventions: *Hallucination Management:* Promoting the safety, comfort, and reality orientation of a patient experiencing hallucinations.

Delusion Management: Promoting the comfort, safety, and reality orientation of a patient experiencing false, fixed beliefs that have little or no basis in reality.

Environmental Management: Violence Prevention: Monitoring and manipulation of the physical environment to decrease the potential for violent behavior directed toward self, others, or environment.

DOMAIN: Family

Class: *Life Span Care*

Interventions: *Family Integrity Promotion:* Promotion of family cohesion and unity.

Family Involvement: Facilitating family participation in the emotional and physical care of the patient.

Source: McCloskey and Bulechek, 1996.

Behavioral: Coping Assistance

Self-Esteem Enhancement

Many people with schizophrenia desperately desire to be "normal" and thus suffer from low self-esteem. *Self-esteem exercises* can be implemented one-to-one and in group settings. In a one-to-one exercise, you might ask clients to write out or verbalize their positive qualities. Keeping a self-esteem journal is appropriate for some clients. Look for opportunities to give positive reinforcement. In a group setting, clients may be asked to share their own positive qualities as well as to recognize those of their peers. Group experience is an opportunity to learn how to give and receive positive feedback.

A number of group exercises promote self-esteem. One is having clients make a collage. Materials include magazines, scissors, glue, and blank paper. Have clients look for pictures that tell something about themselves and their interests, cut them out, and glue them on the paper. Have each person take a turn in describing the significance of the collage to the other group members. You can emphasize the positive qualities each collage reveals.

Another self-esteem exercise focuses on the image we present to others and who we really are. Give group members two sheets of paper and crayons or markers. On one sheet of paper, have them draw the "real me," and on the other sheet, the "me others see." Each group member then presents the "me others see" and receives feedback from their peers as to the accuracy of this perception. Then the "real me" is presented and feedback is once again given. This exercise is most successful with clients who have some ability to think abstractly.

Behavioral: Psychological Comfort Promotion

Anxiety Reduction

Some persons with schizophrenia experience periodic symptoms of anxiety. Since anxiety can be contagious, remain calm and reassuring as you interact with clients. Your presence may help the anxious person feel more secure. Using relaxation techniques or meditation, reducing or eliminating caffeine intake, and moderating environmental stimuli often lower levels of anxiety. You may encourage clients to go for a walk, work at a simple concrete task, or play a noncompetitive game such as catch. Further interventions are found in Chapter 9.

Behavioral: Patient Education

Teaching: Disease Process

A *psychoeducation program* is an extremely important nursing intervention. The goal is to teach consumers about their illness and to cover the important behavioral, affective, cognitive, perceptual, and social problems they commonly experience. Another facet of psychoeducation is teaching clients to identify early signs of relapse. What exactly those early warning signs are vary from person to person but are repetitive for any one individual. Since early intervention may prevent a relapse, this self-surveillance strategy allows people to influence the course of the disease.

Teaching: Prescribed Medication

Some consumers will be unhappy or frustrated with their medication. Discontinuation of medication is a significant factor in relapse. *Helping clients understand the need for medication* is an important nursing intervention. The most common reasons for stopping medications include denial of the disorder and the desire to be "normal," an unwillingness to take the amount prescribed since they feel much better, self-medicating with drugs or alcohol, and the distress associated with side effects. A recent study indicates that clients' attitudes toward medication may be more positive than health care professionals have previously thought. The majority of consumers recognize that medications are important for their mental health and are necessary for functioning within the community (Van Dongen, 1997). For more information, see the Medication Teaching box.

Physiological: Basic: Activity and Exercise Management

Energy Management

Some clients pace much of the day and are in danger of exhaustion and must be monitored for evidence of excess physical fatigue. Set limits on hyperactivity by providing firm direction in taking short, frequent rest breaks. They often will manage this better if you stay with them for the designated rest time. Limit environmental stimuli to facilitate relaxation. Design diversional activities that are calming and restful. Clients should monitor their nutritional intake to ensure they have adequate energy resources (McCloskey and Bulechek, 1996).

Medication Teaching

Clients with Schizophrenia

When lying down, rise slowly to a sitting position, and dangle your feet while sitting. Then slowly stand up. This will prevent the dizziness that occurs when you get up too quickly.

If you experience a dry mouth, try sugar-free gum and candy, cool drinks, ice chips, and frequent brushing of your teeth.

If you are constipated, increase fiber in your diet, increase water intake, and exercise.

Call your doctor immediately if you experience a sore throat, high fever, or mouth or skin sores or rashes.

When outdoors, always use a sunscreen and limit your exposure to the sun.

If you forget to take a dose, you can take it up to 2 hours late. If more than 2 hours late, wait for the next scheduled dose. Do not double the dose.

Physiological: Basic: Self-Care Facilitation

Self-Care Assistance

Some clients will need assistance with *self-care* because of a change in activity level, confusion, or a perceptual impairment. They may need reminding or assistance with bathing, grooming, personal hygiene, and dressing. This assistance may be in the form of a list of step-by-step directions in the bathroom or bedroom, or gentle reminders such as "It's time for you to brush your teeth," "I think the dress you have chosen is not appropriate for work," or "Did you shower this morning?" Other self-care activities might involve household tasks such as cleaning, cooking, shopping, or money management. As clients progress toward their goals, they are rewarded with greater responsibility and more privileges. Although some clients may never live independently, they often can improve the quality of their lives through increased autonomy.

Safety: Crisis Management

Suicide Prevention

An important priority of care is client *safety*. Command hallucinations may order clients to harm, mutilate, or kill themselves or others. Others have suffered from delusions so intensely for so long that suicide seems like the only way to escape the pain of being persecuted or controlled by others. You must carefully assess for evidence of self-harm and direct care toward protecting clients until they can protect themselves. See Chapter 17 for care of a client who is suicidal.

Safety: Risk Management

Hallucination Management

The experience of hallucinations can be especially troublesome for the person who does not have anyone to talk to about them. *Discussion of hallucinations* is important to the development of reality-testing skills. Look and listen for clues that the person may be hallucinating, such as grinning or laughing inappropriately, talking to someone whom you cannot see, or slowed verbal responses. Ask the person to describe what is happening. If the person asks you, point out simply that you are not experiencing the same stimuli. The goal is to guide the person through the experience and let them know what is actually happening in the environment. Help the individual describe needs that may be reflected in the content of the hallucination. These needs may include having power and control of decisions that affect daily life, the ability to express anger, and self-esteem. For chronic hallucinations, the person might *keep a calendar* of when hallucinations occur and how long they last in an effort to identify the trigger (Moller and Murphy, 1996).

The person experiencing acute hallucinations has no voluntary control over the brain malfunction that is causing this symptom and needs immediate nursing interventions. Do not leave the client alone since the inability to sort out reality may overwhelm her or his ability to cope. You may need to *talk slightly louder* than usual, but use very short, simple phrases using the person's first name. The person may not be able to hear you but will see that your mouth is moving and know that you are trying to communicate. *Touching* the client, with her or his permission, or extending your hand and asking her or him to grab hold may be helpful in orientation to reality (Moller, Rice, and Murphy, 1998).

Delusion Management

Persons experiencing delusions have difficulty processing language; therefore, *nonverbal communication* is critically important. Approach the person with calmness and empathy. It is very normal to feel confused by a delusion. You must carefully *assess the content* of the delusion without appearing to probe or patronize the client. Do not attempt to logically explain the delusion nor underestimate the power of a delusion and the person's inability to distinguish the delusion from reality. Assess the duration, frequency, and intensity of the delusion. Since delusions are often triggered by stress, correlate the onset of the delusion with the onset of stress.

Fleeting delusions often will disappear in a short time frame. Fixed delusions may have to be *temporarily avoided*. Respond to the underlying feelings rather than the illogical nature of the delusion. This will encourage discussion of fears, anxieties, or anger without judging the person. Quietly listen and then give guidance for the immediate task at hand. The client may find it helpful to engage in distracting activities as a way to stop focusing on the delusion.

Environmental Management: Violence Prevention

Some clients may be at high risk for violence directed at others when they misperceive communication from others or when they perceive that they themselves are being threatened. Encouraging clients to talk out rather than act out feelings will assist in maintaining control over behavior. Clients often can identify triggering factors such as a noisy environment, unfamiliar people, or other anxiety-provoking situations. If clients begin to escalate and become more agitated, it helps to remain calm, use a low tone of voice, give them personal space, and avoid physical contact with them. Set limits on aggressive behavior. Depending on the clinical setting, seclusion may become necessary. See Chapter 6 for further interventions with clients who are at high risk for violence.

The suspicious client is always on the lookout for danger and functions at a steady level of hyperalertness. Avoid frightening these individuals, who may strike out to protect themselves from perceived danger. Always give them plenty of *personal space* and never touch them without specific permission. Because they are hyperalert to everything in the environment, be careful not to behave in ways that could be misinterpreted. Two people talking together in a soft tone of voice could be misperceived by a suspicious client as "They're talking about me." A group of nurses sharing a laugh could be misperceived as "They're all laughing at me."

Family: Life Span Care

Family Integrity

Schizophrenia often strikes adolescents or young adults, leaving their parents confused and frightened. Whether the child was living at home or away, employed or unemployed, all of the parents in one study reported feeling a never-ending sense of responsibility for their child, which was at times overwhelming. Parents are likely to experience sorrow and grief as they begin to deal with the impact of their child's illness. Knowing that this is likely to occur, nurses can offer anticipatory guidance and interventions. Parents desire information and some level of involvement in their child's treatment plan. They often seek advice on how to cope with the day-to-day challenges they face, what they might expect in the future, and sources of community support. The question that health care professionals have to answer is how to include the family within the context of client confidentiality (Eakes, 1995).

Family Involvement

Because so many people are afraid of and uninformed about schizophrenia, many families try to hide it from friends and deal with it on their own. We must reach out to these families and offer them support and education. *Family education* often is conducted in a group setting, which enables families to begin to build a support network. You must help them understand that they are not responsible for causing their loved one to develop schizophrenia and have no reason to feel guilty. They need to learn about the nature of schizophrenia and the variety of available treatment programs. They need practical solutions on how to manage on a day-to-day basis. You can assist families in achieving a balance between being protective and encouraging independence. For example, families should try to do things *with* them rather than *for* them, so that clients are able to regain their sense of self-confidence.

Families can encourage their loved ones to stick with the treatment program, take their medications, and avoid alcohol and drugs. It is important to recognize early signs of relapse to prevent acute episodes and rehospitalizations. Family members can ask the person with schizophrenia to agree that, if they notice warning signs of a relapse, it is okay for them to contact the physician so that the medication can be adjusted in an effort to stabilize the condition. All

Family Education

- Information about the disorder
- Managing symptoms
- Expectations during recovery
- Role of medications
- Handling crises
- Warning signs of suicide
- Early signs of relapse
- Housing and social resources
- Self-help groups

threats of suicide should be taken very seriously. Families should have an identified contact person they can call for help. If the situation becomes desperate, the family should call 911.

The family may need help in setting expectations and limits on inappropriate behavior. The positive characteristics of schizophrenia can cause a great deal of family stress. That is also true of the negative characteristics, which are often misinterpreted as laziness or uncooperativeness.

It is totally within the rights of a family to decide that a member who has an illness must get treatment for it. The family should also establish appropriate rules that must be followed. If the client is unwilling to comply, the family may choose to look for alternative living arrangements. For more information see the Family Education box and the Self-Help Groups section at the end of this chapter.

Consumers who are discharged from an acute hospitalization with medication as the primary intervention have a 50% rehospitalization rate within 6 to 9 months. In contrast, consumers discharged with medication and continuing *family therapy* only have a 2–10% rehospitalization rate. Family therapy moves beyond family education and helps people cope with the disorder of schizophrenia. Families learn how to manage conflict, avoid criticizing one another, decrease overprotective behaviors, and develop appropriate expectations of one another. Often this is best accomplished with the help of a family therapist.

Evaluation

For clients to be successful, they must set small, achievable, short-term goals. Positive outcomes include client safety, improved communication skills, improved social skills, improved self-esteem, compliance with prescribed medication, effective family functioning, and adaptation to living in the least restrictive setting. As research continues to help us understand neurobiology, the multiple causes of schizophrenia, and more effective treatment approaches, consumers will achieve higher levels of functioning and fewer disabilities in the future.

Clinical Interactions

A Client with Schizophrenia

Sara is 41 years old and has suffered with schizophrenia for the past 15 years. She has a history of childhood sexual abuse. She has been able to live at home with her husband except for a few brief periods of hospitalization. Lately, her thinking has become more disorganized, and her therapist has recommended that she come to the day treatment program. The themes of the interaction below include raping and hurting little children and a desire to return to infancy, a period of time when she felt safe and cared for. In the interaction, you will see evidence of:

- labile affect
- loose associations
- symbolism (attached at waist)
- somatic delusions
- grandiosity with magical powers

SARA: I killed a man when I was 6 years old and he was raping and killing little babies. I killed him. Then my friends told me to run, so I ran. I got away with my underpants on. My twin brother died—he committed suicide (crying).

NURSE: Would you like to talk about this?

SARA: Not right now. I loved my brother (sobbing). I really miss him. You know I build houses.

NURSE: You do?

SARA: Yes, I start out 14 feet tall and when I'm done I've shrinked to 14 inches (smiles and laughs).

NURSE: You shrink?

SARA: Yes. The aliens come and get me at night and tell me they'll make me safe and they make me into a baby and take care of me.

NURSE: Do you feel safe as a baby?

SARA: Yes; no one can hurt me then. They protect me (smiling).

NURSE: (Silence)

SARA: My husband exhibits me, you know (laughs).

NURSE: Can you explain "exhibits"? I don't understand.

SARA: He took movies of us having sex and set me down and showed them to me. He told me I had grown into a beautiful woman. He still loves me, you know, and I still love him even though I slapped him 3,600 times in the head.

NURSE: How did you feel about his exhibiting you?

SARA: It was okay because I really do love him. I was attached to my husband at the waist in the bedroom (laughs). (Puts finger to ear and pauses)

NURSE: Are you hearing voices?

SARA: No. I have synthetic eardrums and I hear a buzz sometimes. Do you know I saved little boys from Alcatraz? I saved them to keep them safe (laughs).

NURSE: I didn't know that. What did you save them from?

SARA: I saved them from the men raping them. They were raping and killing all those little boys. The President gave me permission to save as many as I could.

NURSE: Is it a good feeling when you are able to help others?

SARA: I build spaceships at night and escape to bars for smokes and men buy me whiskey.

NURSE: Could we talk about one thing at a time? You are skipping to other subjects too quickly for me.

SARA: Okay. ■

Self-Help Groups

American Schizophrenic Association Hotline
(800) 847-3802

ENOSH
PO Box 1593
Ramat Hasharon, 47-113
Israel

National Alliance for the Mentally Ill (NAMI)
200 N. Glebe Road, Suite 1015
Arlington, VA 22203
(800) 950-NAMI
www.nami.org

Schizophrenia Association of Ireland
4 Fitzwilliam Place
Dublin 2
Ireland

Schizophrenia Australia Foundation
223 McKean Street
North Fitzroy
3068 Victoria
Australia

Schizophrenia Fellowship
PO Box 593
Christchurch
New Zealand

Schizophrenia Society of Canada
75 The Donway West, Suite 814
Don Mills, Ontario M3C 3E9
Canada
1-800-809-HOPE
www.schizophrenia.ca

Key Concepts

Introduction

- Schizophrenia is a syndrome characterized by disordered thinking, perceptual disturbances, behavioral abnormalities, affective disruptions, and impaired social competency.

- Schizoaffective disorder is characterized by symptoms common to both schizophrenia and the mood disorders.

Knowledge Base

- The positive characteristics of schizophrenia are added behaviors not normally seen, such as delusions, hallucinations, loose associations, and overreactive affect.

- The negative characteristics of schizophrenia are the absence of normal behaviors, for example, flat affect, minimal self-care, social withdrawal, and concrete thinking.

- People with schizophrenia may exhibit purposeless or ritualistic behavior, or even pace for hours on end. Some have bizarre facial or body movements.

- The most common type of hallucination is auditory followed by visual. Tactile, olfactory, and gustatory hallucinations occur in people undergoing withdrawal from or abuse of alcohol and drugs.

- Delusions are false beliefs that cannot be changed by logical reasoning or evidence. It is thought that they represent dysfunctions in the information-processing circuits between the hemispheres.

- Having no apparent relationship between thoughts is referred to as loose association.

- Concrete thinking is a focus on facts and details and an inability to generalize or think abstractly.

- People with schizophrenia frequently have ineffective social skills, which increases their sense of isolation.

- Concomitant disorders include substance abuse, obsessions and compulsions, and suicide.

- Neurobiological factors of schizophrenia include genetic defects, abnormal brain development, neurodegeneration, disordered neurotransmission, and abnormal brain structures.

- It is believed that biological vulnerabilities interact with developmental, environmental, and social processes to produce the schizophrenic syndrome.

- Conventional antipsychotic medications are more effective in decreasing the positive characteristics than they are the negative characteristics.

- Extrapyramidal side effects (EPS) include dystonia, parkinsonism, akathisia, neuroleptic malignant syndrome, and tardive dyskinesia.

- The new or atypical antipsychotic medications are effective in eliminating both the positive and negative characteristics.

- Psychiatric rehabilitation emphasizes the development of skills and supports, considers the consumer to be in control, and promotes choices, self-determination, and individual responsibility.

- Group therapy helps prevent the withdrawal and social isolation that may occur for people who are psychiatrically disabled.

- Case management is intended to increase consumers' access to care and to ensure that they receive comprehensive services.

- People who are psychiatrically disabled may receive their care in a variety of settings, such as supportive housing, psychosocial clubhouses, day treatment programs, day hospitalization, hospital acute care, and long-term hospitalization.

Nursing Assessment

- Nursing assessment is based on interviews with clients, family members, friends, group home supervisors, or case managers.

Nursing Diagnosis

- Nursing diagnoses are based on assessment data focusing on how well clients are functioning in daily life, how stable their affect is, how effective their communication is, and how well they are getting along with others.

Outcome Identification

- Successful outcomes include client safety, improved communication skills, improved social skills, improved self-esteem, compliance with prescribed medication, effective family functioning, and adaptation to living in the least restrictive setting.

Planning and Nursing Interventions

- Opportunities to assist people with schizophrenia occur in a variety of settings, in long-term relationships, or in crisis periods.

- A priority of care is client safety, which includes measures to prevent self-harm, suicide, physical exhaustion, and striking out to protect themselves from perceived danger.

- Consumers may need assistance with self-care, ranging from gentle reminders to more step-by-step directions.

- Helping clients understand the need for medication is an important nursing intervention.

- Reduction of anxiety may be accomplished with relaxation techniques, eliminating caffeine, moderating environmental stimuli, walking, or talking out feelings with another person.

- Look and listen for clues that the person might be hallucinating; identify the needs that may be reflected in the hallucination, stay with the person, and speak in short, simple phrases. If asked, simply point out that you are not experiencing the same stimuli.

- Interventions for people who are experiencing delusions include assessing the content, duration, and frequency of the delusion; correlating it with stressful situations; responding to underlying feelings; and providing distracting activities.

- It is necessary to clarify communication when clients' thinking is disorganized. You should listen for themes in clients' conversations.

- Exercises to promote self-esteem include listing positive qualities, keeping a self-esteem journal, making a collage, and focusing on the image we present to others and who we really are.

- The goal of psychoeducation is to teach consumers about their illness, the problems they commonly experience, early signs of relapse, and the need for medication.

- Social skills training is a series of highly structured and organized sessions of practice in basic skills, which can result in improvements in important areas of social adjustment.

- Parents of young adult children stricken with schizophrenia often feel a sense of responsibility that, at times, can be overwhelming.

- Family education includes knowledge about the disease, available treatment programs, how to manage on a day-to-day basis, early signs of relapse, and suicide precautions.

- The family may need help in setting expectations and limits, coping with conflict, and developing appropriate expectations of one another.

Evaluation

- For clients to be successful, they must set small, achievable, short-term goals.

Review Questions

1. You have assessed that May is experiencing negative characteristics of schizophrenia. Which of the following would you document?

   a. minimal self-care

   b. delusions

   c. hallucinations

   d. hyperactive behavior

2. Jorge states that he has a rat in his stomach that can come all the way up to his throat. You would document this as which type of delusion?

   a. grandiosity

   b. control

   c. somatic

   d. ideas of reference

3. John hears voices telling him that he is a terrible person who would be better off dead. Which of the following would be the priority nursing diagnosis?

   a. *Impaired verbal communication*

   b. *High risk for violence, self-directed*

   c. *Sensory-perceptual alteration*

   d. *Impaired social interaction*

4. Ilse is taking conventional antipsychotic medication. Her mother notices one evening that she is experiencing muscle rigidity and respiratory problems. When she takes her temperature it is 104F. Which of the following problems is Ilse experiencing?

   a. neuroleptic malignant syndrome

   b. dystonia

   c. akathisia

   d. tardive dyskinesia

5. You are working in a psychiatric rehabilitation program. Which of the following interventions would be most appropriate?

   a. teaching and coaching social and work skills

   b. administering antipsychotic medications

   c. planning social activities for clients

   d. establishing suicide precautions

References

American Psychiatric Association. (1997). Practice guidelines for the treatment of patients with schizophrenia. *Am J Psychiatry, 154*(Suppl. 4), 1–63.

Buchanan, J. (1995). Social support and schizophrenia. *Arch Psychiatr Nurs, 9*(2), 68–76.

Buchsbaum, M. S., et al. (1996). PET and MRI of the thalamus in never-medicated patients with schizophrenia. *Am J Psychiatry, 153*(2), 191–199.

Busatto, G. F., et al. (1997). Correlation between reduced in vivo benzodiazepine receptor binding and severity of psychotic symptoms in schizophrenia. *Am J Psychiatry, 154*(1), 56–63.

Carling, P. J. (1995). *Return to Community*. New York: Guilford Press.

Corrigan, P. W., & Green, M. F. (1993). Schizophrenic patients' sensitivity to social cues: The role of abstraction. *Am J Psychiatry, 150*(4), 589–594.

Davis, J. O., & Bracha, H. S. (1996). Prenatal growth markers in schizophrenia. *Am J Psychiatry, 153*(9), 1166–1172.

Eakes, G. G. (1995). Chronic sorrow: The lived experience of parents of chronically mentally ill individuals. *Arch Psychiatr Nurs, 9*(2), 77–84.

Eisen, J. L., et al. (1997). Obsessive-compulsive disorder in patients with schizophrenia or schizoaffective disorder. *Am J Psychiatry, 154*(2), 271–273.

Farrell, S. P., & Deeds, E. S. (1997). The clubhouse model as exemplar. *J Psychosoc Nurs, 35*(1), 27–34.

Fenton, W. S., et al. (1997). Symptoms, subtype, and suicidality in patients with schizophrenia spectrum disorders. *Am J Psychiatry, 154*(2),199–204.

Grossberg, G. T. (1997). The older schizophrenic. *Treatment Today, 9*(2), 19–23.

Hedaya, R. J. (1996). *Understanding Biological Psychiatry*. New York: Norton.

Kahn, R. S., Davidson, M., & Davis, K. L. (1996). Dopamine and schizophrenia revisted. In S. J. Watson (Ed.), *Biology of Schizophrenia and Affective Disease* (pp. 369–391). Washington, D.C.: American Psychiatric Press.

Kapur, S., & Remington, G. (1996). Serotonin-dopamine interaction and its relevance to schizophrenia. *Am J Psychiatry, 153*(4), 466–476.

Keltner, N. L. (1996). Pathoanatomy of schizophrenia. *Perspect Psychiatr Care, 32*(2), 32–35.

Kennedy, J .L. (1996). Schizophrenia genetics. *Am J Psychiatry, 153*(12), 1513–1514.

Levin, E. D. (1997). Nicotine and schizophrenia. *NARSAD Reseach Letter, 13*(2), 3–9.

Lewine, R. R. J., et al. (1996). Sex differences in neuropsychological functioning among schizophrenic patients. *Am J Psychiatry, 153*(9), 1178–1184.

Lieberman, J. A. (1997). Untreated psychosis and the pathophysiology of schizophrenia. *Decade of the Brain, 8*(1), 4–6.

Lim, K. O., et al. (1996). Cortical gray matter volume deficit in patients with first-episode schizophrenia. *Am J Psychiatry, 153*(12), 1548–1553.

McCloskey, J. C., and Bulechek, G. M. (1996). *Nursing Interventions Classifications (NIC)*, 2nd. ed. St. Louis: Mosby.

Meltzer, H. Y., et al. (1997). Age at onset and gender of schizophrenic patients in relation to neuroleptic resistance. *Am J Psychiatry, 154*(4), 475–482.

Moller, M. D., Rice, M. J., & Murphy, M. F. (1998). *Psychiatric Protocols for Family Nurse Practitioners*. Philadelphia: Saunders.

Murray, R. B. (1996). Stressors and coping strategies of homeless men. *J Psychosoc Nurs, 34*(8), 16–22.

Palmer-Erbs, V. (1996). A breath of fresh air in a turbulent health-care environment. *J Psychosoc Nurs, 34*(9),16–21.

Potkin, S. G., Albers, L. J., Richmond, G. (1993). Schizophrenia. In D. L. Dunner (Ed.), *Current Psychiatric Therapy*. Philadelphia: Saunders.

Schizophrenia Bulletin. (1996). Pain sensitivity and schizophrenia. *NAMI Adovcate, 18*(1), 15.

Straub, R. E. (1997). Searching for schizophrenia genes. *NAMI, Decade of the Brain, 7*(4), 3–4.

Tollefson, G. D., et al. (1997). Olanzapine versus haloperidol in the treatment of schizophrenia and schizoaffective and schizophreniform disorders. *Am J Psychiatry, 154*(4), 457–465.

Van Dongen, C. J. (1997). Attitudes toward medications among persons with severe mental illness. *J Psychosoc Nurs, 35*(3), 21–25.

Verdoux, H., et al. (1997). Obstetric complications and age at onset in schizophrenia. *Am J Psychiatry, 154*(9), 1220–1227.

Wolff, N., et al. (1997). Cost-effectiveness evaluation of three approaches to case management for homeless mentally ill clients. *Am J Psychiatry, 154*(3), 341–348.

Wyatt, R. J., & Henter, I. D. (1997). Early intervention in schizophrenia. *Decade of the Brain, 8*(1), 1–2.

Yurgelun-Todd, D. A., et al. (1996). Functional magnetic resonance imaging of schizophrenic patients and comparison subjects during word production. *Am J Psychiatry, 153*(2), 200–205.

CHAPTER 13

Substance-Related Disorders

Karen Lee Fontaine

Objectives

After reading this chapter, you will be able to:

- List the commonly abused substances, the actions of these substances, and the signs and symptoms of chemical dependence.
- Explain the effects of substance abuse on the fetus and the newborn.
- Identify the effects of substance abuse on the family.
- Compare and contrast causative theories of substance abuse.
- Use the substance abuse history and focused nursing assessment when interviewing clients who abuse substances.
- Intervene with clients who are chemically dependent.

Key Terms

codependency
confabulation
dual diagnosis
enabling behavior
substance abuse
substance dependence
withdrawal

*I*n our society, many people use substances recreationally to modify mood or behavior. However, there are wide sociocultural variations in the acceptability of chemical use. Alcohol, caffeine, and tobacco are legal drugs, but the social acceptability of using them varies. Narcotics, sedatives, stimulants, and hallucinogens are illegal drugs, and the general population considers using them to be socially unacceptable.

The *DSM-IV* classifies the pathological use of chemicals as psychoactive substance–related disorders. **Substance abuse** is defined as the purposeful use, for at least 1 month, of a drug that results in adverse effects to oneself or others. This diagnosis can only be used for someone who has never been diagnosed as dependent. **Substance dependence** occurs when the use of the drug is no longer under control and continues despite adverse effects (American Psychiatric Association, 1994). This chapter focuses on substance dependence, which is the more severe form of the substance-related disorders. The words "substance" and "chemical" are used interchangeably.

Chemical dependence is a chronic, progressive disease that can be fatal if left untreated. While it is true that a disease is *not* defined as a deficiency of willpower, this disease is comprised of several biochemical processes that are subject to voluntary control. In addition, there are psychological, sociological, and spiritual aspects to chemical dependence.

A number of types of psychoactive substances are associated with chemical dependence. The days of the so-called "pure" drug addict or alcoholic are gone. Most people who are chemically dependent are polydrug abusers. They may use amphetamines or cocaine to get high, and alcohol, Valium, or marijuana to come down off the high. Some use sedatives to sleep and amphetamines to wake up. Whatever the pattern, clients must be treated for all secondary as well as primary addictions (Washton, 1995).

Substance use disorders in the United States cost over $300 billion a year, including the costs of treatment, related health problems, absenteeism, lost productivity, drug-related crime and incarceration, and efforts in education and prevention. Alcoholism (alcohol dependence) is a major health problem, one that is responsible for 100,000 deaths annually in the United States. More than 20 million people experience alcohol-related problems, but less than 10% seek any kind of treatment. Approximately 35% of

the population does not drink, and 55% consumes only 20% of the alcohol. The remaining 10% consumes 80% of the alcohol (Am J Psychiatry, 1995; Kinney, 1996). See Figure 13.1.

Studies indicate that alcohol is a factor in 50% of motor vehicle fatalities, 50% of domestic violence cases, 53% of all deaths from accidental falls, 64% of all fatal fires, and 80% of suicides. Alcoholism is the most expensive addiction for business and industry; 40% of industrial deaths and 47% of industrial injuries are caused by the use of alcohol (Am J Psychiatry, 1995; Coleman, 1993; Kinney, 1996). See Figure 13.2.

In general, women drink less heavily than men. However, the level of drinking for women age 35–64 has increased. Drinking typically begins during adolescence, with 92% of high school students and 90% of college students reporting the use of alcohol; 30% report drinking regularly. This rate has remained fairly stable for the past 20 years (Kinney, 1996). Statistics on the number of drug abusers are difficult to provide. The illicit nature of drug use makes it nearly impossible to retrieve accurate information. In the 1960s, hallucinogens and amphetamines were the illegal drugs most commonly used. In the 1970s, heroin, marijuana, and sedatives were the most popular drugs. The 1980s was the decade of cocaine. Judging by the increase in cocaine-related visits to hospital emergency departments, we continue to have hardcore cocaine abuse problems in the United States.

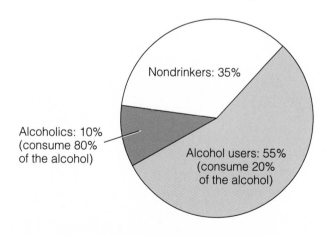

Figure 13.1 **Alcohol use in the United States.**

Source: Kinney, 1996.

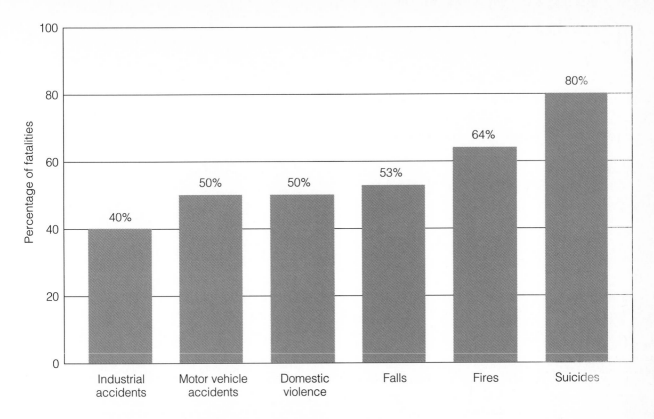

Figure 13.2 **Fatal accidents in which alcohol is a factor.**

Sources: Am J Psychiatry, 1995: Coleman, 1993; Kinney 1996.

Eight million Americans use cocaine regularly, with 2.2 million considered to be dependent. As many as 33% of all Americans age 12 and older have used an illegal drug during their lives.

Adolescents are quicker than adults to initiate and extend poly-drug abuse. Most adolescents abuse a wide number of substances, whereas adults tend to focus on one or two "drugs of choice." (For a list of the risk factors in teenagers, see Box 13.1 on page 320.) Men are more likely to abuse cocaine, marijuana, and opioids; women are more likely to abuse sedatives, antianxiety agents, and amphetamines (Am J Psychiatry, 1995; Kinney, 1996). Recent attention has been given to the severity of chemical dependence among health professionals, including nurses and physicians. When they have an addiction, the shame and guilt is magnified. After all, nurses are healers and nurturers. They are not expected to have their own problems, certainly not an addiction that could lead them to take drugs from clients or be less than 100 percent in

control when they are at work. Many state nurses' associations, supported by the national nursing organizations, have established peer support systems to help nurses who abuse substances recover.

Knowledge Base

This section begins with an overview of the commonly abused substances. Table 13.1 provides specific information for each of the categories. We then move on to discuss the general characteristics of substance-abusing individuals and their families.

Substances with Dependence Potential

Alcohol

Alcoholism is a heterogeneous disorder, thought to have two types. Type II alcoholism has an onset of heavy drinking before the age of 25 as well as at least

Text continues on page 320

Table 13.1 Substance Dependence Summarized

Substance	Types	Street Names	Mode of Administration	Behavioral Characteristics	Affective Characteristics
Alcohol	Beer, wine, liquor	Booze, sauce, oil	Oral	Lack of control of drinking, sneaking drinks, gulping drinks, shifting from one alcoholic drink to another, hiding bottles at home or work, telephonitis	Hostility, argumentativeness, tearfulness, crying, shame, depression, despair, jealousy
Amphetamine	Amphetamine, benzedrine, methedrine, dexedrine, methamphetamine	Crystal, meth, speed, uppers, pep pills, bennies, cartwheels, ice, dexies, Christmas trees	Oral, injection, IV, smoking	Hypervigilance, increased energy, rapid speech, decreased appetite	Euphoria, agitation, anxiety, irritability
Cannabis	Marijuana, hashish	Pot, mary jane, joint, reefer, grass, hash, weed, Acapulco gold, Colombian, roach	Smoking, oral	Passivity, sexual arousal	Pleasure that may progress to euphoria, apathy, anxiety that may progress to panic, detachment
Cocaine	Cocaine	Coke, crack, blow, snow, C, powder, dust	Smoking, inhalation, injection, IV	Hypervigilance, talkativeness, increased energy, heightened sexuality, violence	Feeling of well-being, euphoria followed by depression, agitation, anxiety
Hallucinogen	Phencyclidine hydrochloride (PCP), LSD, mescaline, MDMA	Acid, trip, tab, cactus, angel dust, superjoint, peace pill, ecstasy	Oral, IV, smoking, inhalation	Inability to perform simple tasks; facial grimacing, muscle rigidity, violent or bizarre behavior	Euphoria, anxiety, emotional lability, impulsiveness, hostility, depression

Cognitive Characteristics	Physiological Characteristics	Withdrawal	Complications	Cause of Death
Low self-esteem, grandiosity, denial, projection, minimization, rationalization, confusion, blackouts	Lack of coordination, slurred speech, flushed face	6–8 hours after last drink: irritability, anxiety, insomnia, tremors, tachycardia, hypertension; 6–96 hours after last drink: seizures, hallucinations; 3–14 days after last drink: DTs	Pancreatitis; hypoglycemia; ketoacidosis; myopathy; GI bleeding, especially from varices; hepatitis, cirrhosis; infections; Wernicke's encephalopathy; Korsakoff's psychosis; attempted suicide	Acute intoxication; respiratory arrest; chronic intoxication; DTs, ruptured GI varices
Extreme self-confidence, grandiosity, confusion	Tachycardia, arrhythmias, hypertension, vasoconstriction, altered respiration, headache, visual disturbances, insomnia	Excessive need to sleep, fatigue, anhedonia, depression	Malnutrition, seizures	Cerebrovascular accident, cardiovascular collapse, suicide
Slowed sense of time, altered perceptions	Dry mouth, tachycardia, dilated pupils, increased appetite, fatigue, impaired sperm count and motility	Craving, anxiety, physical withdrawal symptoms not demonstrated	Acute panic reactions, paranoia, hallucinations, bizarre behavior, hostility, vomiting, fever	Does not usually occur
Grandiosity, extreme self-confidence, impaired judgment, ideas of reference, paranoia hallucinations	Insomnia, anorexia, dilated pupils, tachycardia, hypertension, nausea or vomiting, weight loss, stuffy or runny nose, irritated nasal membrane	Severe craving for cocaine, fatigue irritability	Malnutrition, perforated nasal septum, seizures	Respiratory failure, cardiac arrest, cerebral hemorrhage
Grandiosity, hallucinations, paranoia, impaired judgment, body image changes	Intensified perceptions, sensation of slowed time, tachycardia, hypertension, tremors, lack of coordination, salivation	Generally believed not to occur	Rare	Suicide, accident

continued ➤

■ *Table 13.1* Substance Dependence Summarized *continued*

Substance	Types	Street Names	Mode of Administration	Behavioral Characteristics	Affective Characteristics
Opioid	Morphine, heroin, codeine, Dilaudid, Demerol, methodone	H, horse, smack, junk, shit, Miss Emma, lords, D, dollies	Oral, injection, IV, subcutaneous ("skin popping")	Sedated appearance, motor retardation, slurred speech	Euphoria, agitation, decreased emotional pain, apathy
Sedative/ hypnotic/ anxiolytic	Amytal, Nembutal, Seconal, Methaqualone, Valium, Librium, Ativan, Xanax, Rohypnol, GHB	Downers, ludes, red devils, blue angels, yellow jackets	Oral, IV	Sedated appearance, lack of coordination, talkativeness	Euphoria, emotional lability, irritability, anxiety

■ *Box 13.1*

Substance Dependence Risk Factors in Teenagers

Peer pressure, group norms: pro–substance use.

A greater here-and-now orientation than adults; drugs provide immediate gratification.

Rebellion against authority.

Alienation from traditional social and religious values; drugs viewed as a way to individuate and disconnect.

Stressful situations, such as a dysfunctional family.

Insecurity and low self-esteem: powerful triggers for compensatory substance abuse.

two social complications due to excessive use of alcohol. Those people not meeting the type II criteria are considered to be type I (George et al, 1997).

The pattern of *dependence* on alcohol varies from person to person. Some have a regular daily intake of large amounts of alcohol. Others restrict their use to drinking heavily on the weekends or days off from work. Some may abstain for long periods of time and then go on a drinking binge. The behavior may be inconsistent at the beginning of dependence. At times, people with alcohol dependence can drink with control, and at other times, they cannot control the drinking behavior. As the course of alcoholism continues, there may be behaviors such as starting the day off with a drink, sneaking drinks through the day, gulping alcoholic drinks, shifting from one alcoholic beverage to another, and hiding bottles at work and at home. They may give up hobbies and other interests in order to have more time to drink. It is not unusual for alcoholics to engage in what is known as telephonitis, making telephone calls to family and friends at inappropriate times, such as the middle of the night.

Cognitive Characteristics	Physiological Characteristics	Withdrawal	Complications	Cause of Death
Impaired attention/memory, decreased awareness, reduction of drives	Pinpoint pupils (may be dilated with severe hypoxia), drowsiness, nausea/vomiting	May occur within a few hours to a few days and may last for 1–2 weeks; craving, chill, sweats, goose-flesh, abdominal pain, muscle cramps, fearfulness, runny nose, diarrhea, irritability	Increased likelihood of exposure to HIV and hepatitis; malnutrition	Respiratory depression, potentiated by other CNS depressants
Impaired attention/memory, amnesia	Drowsiness, extended sleep, flushed face, brady-cardia, hypotension	Symptoms similar to alcohol withdrawal, seizures, altered perceptions/hallucinations, tachycardia, anxiety, tremors, depression	Dependence	CNS depression, respiratory depression, suicide

Blackouts, a fairly early sign of alcoholism, are a form of amnesia for events that occurred during the drinking period. The alcoholic may carry out conversations and elaborate activities with no loss of consciousness, but have total amnesia for those activities the next day. This may be explained by the toxic effects of alcohol on glutamate transmission necessary for memory storage. A more advanced CNS problem is *Wernicke's disease,* which is characterized by ataxia (lack of coordination), abnormal eye movements, and confusion. These symptoms result from chronic thiamine deficiency. About 80% of people with Wernicke's disease also develop *Korsakoff's syndrome,* characterised by intact intellecual functioning but an inability to retrieve long-term memory events or retain new information. **Confabulation,** making up information to fill memory blanks, develops in the person's attempt to protect self-esteem when confronted with memory loss. *Alcoholic dementia* is characterized by impaired abstract thinking and judgment, personality changes, and impaired memory. This is often seen in chronically heavy drinkers (Cummings and Trimble, 1995; Tsai et al, 1995).

Alcohol withdrawal syndrome typically begins about 6–8 hours after the last drink. Early symptoms include irritability, anxiety, insomnia, tremors, and a mild tachycardia. Withdrawal seizures typically occur 6–96 hours after the last drink, with 90% of the seizures occurring between 7 and 48 hours. Seizures are usually grand mal and may last for a few minutes or less. During withdrawal, hallucinations may occur at 6–96 hours, peaking at 48–72 hours and typically lasting 3 days. Hallucinations range from bad dreams to visual, auditory, olfactory, gustatory, and tactile hallucinations.

Delirium tremens (DTs) usually occur on days 4 and 5 but may appear as late as 14 days after the last drink. During DTs, the person experiences confusion, disorientation, hallucinations, tachycardia, hypertension or hypotension, extreme tremors, agitation, diaphoresis, and fever. DTs usually last about 5 days. With improved diagnosis and medical treatment, the mortality rate has dropped from 20% to 1% (Am J Psychiatry, 1995).

Cocaine

Cocaine acts as a local anesthetic similar to novocaine by blocking the conduction of sensory impulses within the nerve cells. This effect occurs when cocaine is snorted and the nasal and throat passages become temporarily numb.

The primary reason people use cocaine is to stimulate the CNS. Cocaine alters dopamine (DA) transmission and also affects the endorphins, GABA, and acetylcholine (ACH). DA, the neurotransmitter involved in movement, is used by the brain to "reward itself," to reinforce positive experiences. In normal neurotransmission, DA is released into the synapse, crosses over to the receptor site, is picked up by transporters, and is returned to the presynaptic neurons for future use. It is believed that cocaine binds to the DA transporters, preventing them from picking up DA, resulting in an accumulation of DA and an out-of-control reward system. The cumulative effect is an intense feeling of euphoria (Cummings and Trimble, 1995; Schlaepfer et al, 1997). Because of its action on the CNS, cocaine is a uniquely addicting drug. With its powerful rewarding properties, cocaine is even capable of making obsessive users of well-adjusted and mature individuals. *Positive reinforcement* occurs through the mood-altering effects of generalized euphoria, increased energy and mental alertness, a feeling of self-confidence, and increased sexual arousal. Tension, fatigue, and shyness disappear, and the person becomes more talkative and playful. Following cocaine use, the intense pleasure is replaced by equally unpleasant feelings. This is referred to as a rebound dysphoria, or "crash." *Negative reinforcement* occurs when the person experiences the crash and takes more cocaine to overcome the dysphoria. Both positive and negative reinforcement sustain the use of cocaine. With increased use, there is a progressive tolerance of the positive effects while the negative effects steadily intensify. In other words, the highs are not as high and the lows are much lower. Cocaine is addicting even when there is no physical discomfort during withdrawal. However, a person experiencing withdrawal has intense cravings for the drug (Am J Psychiatry, 1995).

Cocaine can be used in several ways. *Snorting* powdered cocaine into the nose, where it is absorbed through the mucous membrane, is a common method. There remains a persistent but erroneous belief that snorting cocaine is not addictive. It *is* addictive; it just takes longer. Snorting on a regular basis causes ulcerations of the nasal mucous membrane and may lead to perforation of the septum. The high is achieved about 2–3 minutes after use and may last as long as 20–30 minutes.

Smoking purified chips of cocaine, known as crack, has a higher potential for addiction and leads to more compulsive use than snorting. It is the most efficient way to deliver cocaine, taking only 6–7 seconds for the drug to reach the brain. The high lasts only 2–5 minutes, and the crash is more severe than with snorting. Crack cocaine can lead to marathon binge use, known as a "run," lasting many hours or even days. A run can cost hundreds or thousands of dollars and leave the person in a state of total dysfunction. Death can occur in as little as 2–3 minutes or up to 30 minutes after smoking crack. Tachycardia and cardiac arrhythmias occur from overstimulation of the adrenergic nervous system. Hypertension can lead to intracranial hemorrhage. Seizures are more likely because of the concentrated doses that reach the brain (Kinney, 1996). Another method is called *speedballing,* in which cocaine is mixed with heroin and injected intravenously. The high is reached in about 30–60 seconds. The appeal of a speedball is that the heroin decreases the unpleasant jitteriness and crash from cocaine. Speedballs are extremely dangerous. Heroin decreases the respiratory rate, as does cocaine in high enough doses. Heroin decreases the threshold for seizures, and cocaine is capable of inducing seizures. Mistakenly believing that the effects cancel each other out, some users overdose (Kinney, 1996).

Space-basing is smoking crack cocaine that has been sprinkled with PCP. This method may lead to intense panic and terror. People who have space-based sometimes become violent, and their behavior is uncontrollable.

Amphetamines

In small amounts, *amphetamines* create a sense of mental alertness, euphoria, and self-confidence. As use increases, people become hypervigilant, grandiose, agitated, and irritable. Some individuals alternate between using amphetamines to "get going" and sedatives to "calm down." It is believed that amphetamines inhibit the reuptake of DA, serotonin (5-HT), and norepinephrine (NE), resulting in CNS stimulation (Baberg et al, 1996).

Ice, the smokable form of methamphetamine, is sometimes used as a substitute for cocaine because it is more easily available and less expensive. The effects of ice are similar to those of crack cocaine except that the euphoric state may last as long as 12–30 hours. People who use ice are more likely to become violent and unpredictable in their behavior. Other forms of amphetamines are taken orally or intravenously (Baberg et al, 1996).

Cannabis

The drug classification of *cannabis* includes *marijuana* and *hashish*. These drugs are usually smoked and occasionally taken orally when mixed with food. Delta-9-tetrahydrocannabinol (THC) is the psychoactive ingredient in cannabis. The content of THC ranges from 1–5% in marijuana, while hashish can contain up to 15% THC. Cannabis is the most widely used illegal drug in the United States. Sixty million people have tried cannabis, and some 20 million use it regularly (Kinney, 1996).

Hallucinogens

Hallucinogens are natural and synthetic substances that cause hallucinations, primarily visual. The most common drugs are LSD (lysergic acid diethylamide), PCP (phencyclidine), and mescaline. These substances affect DA, 5-HT, and opioid receptors in the brain. The effects on the CNS are somewhat unpredictable and may be influenced by the environment, the experience, and the expectations of the user. One of the dangers is a "bad trip," during which the person is in a psychotic state and terrified by perceptual changes. Flashbacks occur when the person is drug-free but relives the experience of being on the drug. Hallucinogens can lead to violent and out-of-control behavior.

Designer or synthetic drugs are becoming increasingly available. Ecstasy, also known as XTC, love drug, Adam, and essence, is derived from methamphetamine and amphetamine. It acts as both a stimulant and a hallucinogen. Herbal ecstasy, also known as Cloud 9, X, and Ultimate Xphoria, is a legal (in many states) combination of herbs and other ingredients available cheaply at health food and drug stores as pills or tea. The main active ingredients are caffeine and ephedrine. Both of these drugs give a sense of euphoria and energy that lasts several hours. High doses can cause increased heart rate and blood pressure, heat stroke, stroke, and death (Kinney, 1996).

Opioids

This classification of drugs includes heroin, morphine, codeine, and synthetic drugs that act like morphine, such as methadone. *Opioids* can be taken orally, intravenously, by injection, or subcutaneously. Some people obtain the drugs from illegal sources, while others obtain them by prescription from a variety of physicians. Some people experience a high from the opioids, but most experience a sense of calm. Since most users "shoot up" and share needles, they are at high risk for hepatitis, HIV infection, and AIDS. Withdrawal symptoms usually begin within a few hours to a few days after the last dose and may last as long as 1–2 weeks.

Sedatives/Hypnotics/Anxiolytics

Sedatives, hypnotics, and *anxiolytics* are sleeping pills and medications for treating anxiety. The usual route of administration is oral, although some may be used intravenously. Prescribed to reduce anxiety, induce sleep, relieve muscle spasms, and reduce pain, they provide a sense of well-being and relaxation. They act by enhancing the action of GABA in the brain. Individuals who abuse amphetamines may use these drugs to "come down" after being high. If they are combined with alcohol, death may occur from CNS depression because the two substances potentiate each other.

Two new designer drugs, Rohypnol (roofies, forget pills, R2) and GHB (G-riffic, Grievous Bodily Harm, Liquid G), have been called "date rape" drugs since they have been used to render rape victims unconscious. They also cause short-term memory loss, leading to horrifying stories of women whose only memory is of waking up naked with a stranger. Initially they give a feeling of euphoria but combined with alcohol can lead to unconsciousness, coma, or, in some cases, death.

Inhalants

Substances inhaled include hydrocarbons such as solvents, paints, glues, and aerosols, and nitrites such as amyl nitrite, butyl nitrite, and nitrous oxide. Hydrocarbons produce euphoria, uninhibited behavior, sensation of floating, and perceptual changes including hallucinations. Problems associated with hydrocarbons include cardiac depression leading to "sudden sniffing death," respiratory depression, renal complications, and car accidents while intoxicated. Nitrites are used to postpone or enhance intercourse, may cause euphoria, and may alter perceptions. Problems associated with nitrites include panic reactions, nausea, dizziness, and hypotension. Nitrous oxide can cause a paranoid psychosis with confusion (Kinney, 1996).

Behavioral Characteristics

Lack of control in using chemicals is the central behavioral characteristic. Because alcohol and drugs decrease inhibitions, many substance abusers become hostile, argumentative, loud, boisterous, and even violent when they are under the influence of the chemical. Compulsive and long-term substance abusers are at higher risk for violence than are recreational or intermittent users. Other users become withdrawn, tearful, and socially isolated when they are under the influence (Volavka, 1995).

Behavioral characteristics are exhibited in the workplace as frequent absences. If workers are abusing substances at noon, their productivity decreases in the afternoon. They often have interpersonal problems at work that are related to their chemically dependent behavior. They may fail to get promoted or may lose a job, and frequent job changes are common (Kinney, 1996).

Users who obtain their drugs through prescriptions may be able to live normally without arousing suspicion, but those who use illegal drugs may have to alter their lifestyle. The latter group often becomes involved in a drug subculture in which self-protection, prostitution, theft, and burglary prevail. As a result of this kind of lifestyle, they often find themselves in legal difficulties.

Affective Characteristics

Psychoactive substances are used by some people as stimulants to overcome feelings of boredom and depression. Others use these substances to manage their anxiety and stress. The overall intention is to decrease negative feelings and increase positive feelings. People who abuse substances are often emotionally labile. They may be grandiose or irritable at one moment and morose and guilty the next. When they try to control their use of drugs and fail in this attempt, they experience feelings of guilt and shame. When the problem becomes public knowledge, they are likely to feel embarrassed and humiliated.

Cognitive Characteristics

Some people have low self-esteem prior to their chemical dependence. They may have turned to drugs as a way to feel better about themselves. Others develop low self-esteem as a result of their problems with substance abuse. Grandiose thoughts may be an attempt for both groups to compensate for low self-esteem.

Denial is the major defense mechanism that helps maintain a chemical dependence. *Denial,* which is self-deception and an unconscious attempt to maintain self-esteem in the face of out-of-control behavior, enables a person to underestimate the amount of drugs used and to avoid recognizing the impact of abusing behavior on others. Denial results from cultural standards of what is or is not appropriate behavior. Supporting the denial is the use of projection, minimization, and rationalization. *Projection,* seeing others as being responsible for one's substance abuse, is heard in: "My three teenagers are driving me crazy. It's their fault I drink." *Minimization,* not acknowledging the significance of one's behavior, is heard in: "Don't believe everything my wife tells you. I wasn't so high that I couldn't drive." *Rationalization,* giving reasons for the behavior, is heard in: "I only use Valium because I'm so unhappy in my marriage." These defense mechanisms are considered consequences, not causes, of chemical dependence. They serve to protect self-esteem by giving an explanation that helps the person conform to cultural standards (Wing, 1996).

Alcoholic denial has many aspects, including denial of facts, denial of implications, denial of change, and denial of feelings. Denial of facts is the outermost layer of protection and the most frequently used form of denial. It functions to avoid negative consequences. It is heard in: "I have not been drinking," and "I only had one or two beers." Denial of implications is used when some threatening fact gets established and that fact is made public, as in a DUI (driving under the influence). It functions to avoid the image of failure and is heard in: "Okay, I had a few, but I wasn't drunk," "I only smoke pot," and "Your sister drinks more than I do." Denial of change helps people resist making any real change. It functions to protect them from assuming responsibility for their own behavior. It is heard in: "So, I'm an alcoholic, so what?", "I'll try to stop," and "I wanted to stay sober, but I couldn't." Denial of feelings is aimed at shutting off feelings and protects people from being overwhelmed by strong emotions. It is heard in: "It doesn't bother me," and "I'm not angry!" (Kearney, 1996). Denial can be a major obstacle to treatment, for no treatment will be effective until the individual acknowledges that the substance abuse is out of control.

Social Characteristics

Social values contribute to the problem of substance abuse in the United States. The mass media promote the desire for immediate gratification and self-indulgence. Complex family problems are solved in 30 minutes on television. All forms of media push OTC medications for minor ailments, contributing to the expectation of a pain-free existence. Values such as these indirectly support the use and abuse of chemical substances.

Effects on the Family

Substance abuse is a family problem, and the most devastating impact occurs when the abuser is a parent. Power struggles between abusing and nonabusing partners destroy couples. Family relationships begin to deteriorate, and family members become trapped in a cycle of shame, anger, confusion, and guilt. In some families, substance abuse is a contributing factor to emotional neglect and physical or sexual abuse. Often family members and old friends will be abandoned for new relationships within the drug subculture. In other cases, chemically dependent people simply become more isolated as alcohol or drugs become the main focus of their lives. Some are successful in keeping their substance abuse hidden from their colleagues and most of their significant relationships.

Financial problems may arise from underemployment or unemployment as the compulsion to use chemicals takes precedence over work. However, many substance abusers continue to be employed. For those using illegal substances, the cost can be incredibly expensive. Illegal substance abusers may be criminally involved with the legal system. Some use prostitution or drug dealing as a way to pay for their drugs. Some become involved in minor crimes such as pickpocketing or shoplifting to obtain money for the drugs. Yet others turn to robberies and burglaries to support the high cost of their habit.

> Kendal, age 36, has a 20-year history of poly-drug abuse. At 16, he smoked pot every day, drank beer and wine, and used downers, Valium, and phenobarbital. He dropped out of school in the middle of his sophomore year. His sporadic employment history includes being a laborer and a short-order cook. The longest Kendal has ever been employed is 8 months. His wife has filed for divorce because of his financial problems, drinking, and verbal abuse. He has been living with his mother, but she recently told him to leave because he continues to abuse alcohol and other drugs. He has been charged with public intoxication five times and has been picked up on assault charges for disturbing the peace and resisting arrest while being intoxicated. Kendal appears to be dependent on others to take care of him or make decisions for him.

The inability to discuss substance abuse contributes to family denial. To avoid embarrassment, family members make excuses to outsiders for the addict's behavior. A nonabusing partner may remain in a relationship because of emotional dependency, money, family cohesion, religious compliance, or outward respectability. Other nonabusing partners may threaten to or actually leave the abuser. At this point, the abuser promises never to drink or use again, the family is reunited, the promise is usually broken, and the family becomes locked into a dysfunctional pattern.

Codependency

Codependency is a relationship in which a non-substance-abusing partner remains with a substance-abusing partner. The relationship is dysfunctional—the nonabusing partner being overresponsible and the abusing partner being underresponsible. Codependents operate out of fear, resentment, helplessness, hopelessness, and desire to control the user's behavior. Codependents try obsessively to solve the problems created by the user. When this is not effective, codependents become exhausted and depressed but are unable to stop the "helping" behaviors. They often suffer from low self-esteem and fear of abandonment. Codependents are caretakers, and this caretaking activity may be a compensation for feelings of inadequacy. Women may be more vulnerable to codependent behavior because they have been socialized to be responsible for the family and often feel they are expected to be loyal to their partner at all costs (Kinney, 1996).

Codependents often engage in **enabling behavior,** which is any action by a person that consciously or unconsciously facilitates substance dependence. Enabling behaviors, such as making excuses for the partner with the employer and lying to others about the abuse, protect the substance abuser from the natural consequences of the problem. Enabling is a response to addiction, *not* a cause of addiction. The purpose of enabling is the family's instinctual desire to stay together. It is a process of compensating for the dysfunction in one family member and avoiding the issues that threaten the breakup of the family.

Children of Alcoholics

It is estimated that one out of every eight Americans is a child of an alcoholic parent. Children who grow up in homes where one or both parents are alcoholics often suffer the effects their entire lives. Dysfunctional family roles develop around the impact of alcoholism. Despite mysterious events, nonsense language, and threats of impending doom, everyone in the family acts as if the situation were perfectly normal. It is extremely frightening to have a parent who switches from being a joking, pleasant person to a raging tyrant in the blink of an eye. It is terrifying to live with a drunken father who not only screams that he is going to kill the child but then attempts to do just that. At the same time, the parent convinces the child that if it weren't for what the child did, the parent would not be acting that way.

Very early in life, children of alcoholics learn to keep the secret and not talk about the alcohol problem, even within the family. They are taught not to talk about their own feelings, needs, and wants; they learn not to feel at all. Eventually, they repress all feelings and become numb to both pain and joy. The children become objects whose reason for existence is to please the alcoholic parent and serve his or her needs. Children of alcoholics are expected always to be in control of their behavior and their feelings. They are expected to be perfect and never make mistakes. However, within the family system, no child can ever be perfect "enough." Consistency is necessary for building trust, and alcoholic parents are very unpredictable. Children learn not to expect reliability in relationships. They learn very early that if you don't trust another person, you won't be disappointed (Evans and Sullivan, 1995).

Children of alcoholics tend to develop one of four patterns of behavior. The *hero*, often the oldest child, becomes the competent caretaker and works on making the family function. The *scapegoat* acts out at home, in school, and in the community. This child takes the focus off the alcoholic parent by getting into trouble and becoming the focus of conflict in the family. The behavior may also be a way to draw attention to the family in an unconscious attempt to seek help. The *lost child* tries to avoid conflict and pain by withdrawing physically and emotionally. The *mascot*, often the youngest child, tries to ease family tension with comic relief used to mask his or her own sadness (Williams, 1996).

In dysfunctional families, designated roles keep the family balanced. Each role is a way to handle the distress and shame of having an alcoholic parent. Every family member has a sense of some control, even though the roles do not change the family system's dysfunction.

> Leticia, a 14-year-old high school student, had been an excellent student when suddenly her grades dropped dramatically. She tearfully confessed to her school counselor that personal problems were affecting her grades. Leticia explained that her father had a "drinking problem" but had been going to AA for several years. Three months ago, Leticia's father lost his job and was unable to get another. A month ago, he started a pattern of binge drinking. Leticia was reluctant to talk because she knew her mother would be furious if she knew Leticia had revealed the family secret. Leticia's mother was working overtime to keep the family going. When Leticia's mother was home, she fought constantly with her husband about his drinking. Her father tried to get Leticia to buy alcohol for him after her mother poured his supply down the drain. When Leticia tried to explain that she was too young to purchase alcohol, her father screamed at her, "Get out of my sight! You're useless!" When her father was sober, he tried to be Leticia's best friend. Leticia stopped bringing friends home because she didn't know what to expect. She was too nervous to do homework, always worrying about what her father might do. Leticia told the counselor, "I don't want him to be my friend. I don't even want him for a father anymore!"

Adult children of alcoholics grow up denying the stresses of their dysfunctional families. Denial becomes a frequent defense mechanism that only makes things worse as they proceed through life. The sense of total obligation to the alcoholic parent makes it extremely difficult for adult children to criticize the addicted parent.

Adult children of alcoholics have grown up without mature adult role models and without experiencing healthy family dynamics. They expect all relationships to be based on power, violence, deceit, and misinformation. They often have difficulty expressing emotion and receiving expressions of feelings. Some grow up to repeat the family pattern by either becoming addicted themselves or marrying an addicted person.

Adult children of alcoholics often feel a need to change others or to control the environment for the good of others. They typically deny powerlessness and try to solve all problems alone. They blame themselves for not being able to achieve what no one can achieve. Obsessions are common forms of defense, such as constant worrying, preoccupations with work or other activities that bring about good feelings, and compulsive achievement. The obsessive pattern covers the feelings of helplessness and blocks the feelings of anxiety, inadequacy, and fear of abandonment (Evans and Sullivan, 1995).

Social Morality

Most Americans have a moralistic attitude about substance dependence. It is viewed as a sin or as the result of a weak will. Addicts are seen as totally responsible for their situation and are expected to use willpower to control themselves and become respectable members of society once again. Women are especially stigmatized by this perspective. Women are expected to be "ladylike" at all times, and when they drink too much or get high, they are quickly labeled "loose women," "sleaze-bags," or "drunks." Nurses who have moralistic views may have difficulty accepting the disorder in a clergyperson yet have no reservations acknowledging alcoholism among gang members or the homeless population (Wing, 1996).

Even more stigmatized by American society are lesbian alcoholics. They suffer as women in a male-dominated culture and also carry the double stigma of being lesbian and being alcoholic. Lesbian women have a higher rate of alcohol consumption than heterosexual women. They also attempt suicide seven times more often and have higher rates of completed suicide than do heterosexual, nonalcoholic women. In a homophobic culture, coming to terms with one's homosexuality and accepting a gay identity are very painful. It is thought that depression, alcohol use, and suicide among lesbians may be related to the effects of stigmatization (Skinner, 1994).

Women who have been abused physically and sexually are at greater risk for becoming alcoholics than nonabused women. It is believed that using alcohol may be an attempt to self-medicate while coping with the physical and emotional consequences of abuse (Evans and Sullivan, 1995). (Domestic violence is covered fully in Chapter 18, and sexual abuse is covered in Chapter 19.)

Culture-Specific Characteristics

Alcohol-related diseases affect 5–10% of the world's population each year. The social consequences of abuse of other substances is increasing in more and more countries. The money involved in the sale of illicit drugs rivals the income of oil industries (Desjarlais et al, 1995).

There are many different ethnic groups in the United States, each having its own unique values regarding the definition of substance abuse and how it should be regarded and treated. The use of naturally produced drugs is deeply rooted in many cultures. In some contexts, such as in communion in Christian chruches or in ceremonies of the Native American church, substances are considered sacred. The use of mind-altering drugs for treatment of medical conditions is legally permitted but controlled. In other circumstances, the use of these same drugs is considered criminal. Alcohol is frequently used to celebrate social interactions (Foulks and Pena, 1995).

European Americans have the highest overall rates of alcohol consumption. European American men are much more likely to be heavy drinkers, while only 8% of the women are classified as heavy drinkers. One-third of the women abstain completely (Kinney, 1996).

African Americans abstain more and drink less than European Americans. Only 4% of the women are classified as heavy drinkers. However, the leading cause of death among African American males between the ages of 15 and 34 is homicide, and alcohol and/or drugs are implicated in at least 70% of these incidents (Kinney, 1996).

Hispanic Americans are the second-largest minority population, next to African Americans, in the United States. They are predicted to be the largest minority group by the year 2000. Hispanic American men typically increase their drinking from their 20s to their 30s, then decrease it after age 40. Of the men, 36% drink moderately heavily, 42% drink moderately, and 22% abstain. The ability to consume large amounts of alcohol without appearing intoxicated is associated with "machismo." Hispanic American women are similar to African American women in that nearly half abstain from any use of alcohol (Kinney, 1996; Wing, 1996).

Asian Americans have the lowest consumption levels and rates of alcohol-related problems of all the major racial and cultural groups. A genetic predisposition to the flushing response, due to an inherited isoenzyme of aldehyde dehydrogenase in 50% of the

Asian American population, may be a protective factor. Chinese culture, for example, discourages solitary drinking and emphasizes social drinking associated with eating. Sharing a meal with others includes ritualistic toasting, which increases social interactions and increases the bonds of friendship (Desjarlais et al, 1995; Higuchi et al, 1995).

Alcohol was introduced to the Native American population by the Europeans. Because Native Americans are not a homogeneous group, there is considerable tribal variation in drinking patterns. In general, the magnitude of alcohol problems is greater among Native Americans than among other groups in the United States. The percentage of Native Americans who abstain is about the same as in the general population. However, among those who do drink, there are significantly fewer light or moderate drinkers and over twice as many heavy drinkers. As with other cultural groups, the men drink more than the women. Alcohol is associated with social situations, and there is little solitary drinking. Men tend to drink in groups and pass the bottle. It is considered rude or insulting to refuse the offer of a drink. Adolescents have a higher rate of substance abuse and are more likely to be poly-drug abusers than older people (Kinney, 1996). Hawk Littlejohn, the medicine man of the Cherokee Nation, Eastern Band, attributes this problem to the fact that Native Americans have lost the opportunity to make choices. They can no longer choose how they live or how they practice their religion. He believes that once people return to a sense of identification, they will begin to rid themselves of alcoholism (Spector, 1996).

Physiological Characteristics

Alcohol is a chemical irritant and has a direct toxic effect on many organ systems, as listed in Table 13.2. The rate of premature death from the abuse of alcohol is 11 times higher than that from the abuse of other substances (Hedaya, 1996).

Hospital emergency personnel have seen a sharp increase in the number of cocaine abusers who come for treatment. Cocaine-induced delirium is dramatic and may be fatal if not treated appropriately. *Delirium* usually begins with an acute onset of paranoia, followed by extremely violent behavior that necessitates the use of restraints. Other signs of delirium include decreased levels of alertness and awareness, altered perceptions, disorientation, cognitive impair-

Table 13.2 **Physiological Complications from Alcohol Dependence**

Body System, Organ, Function, or Condition	Toxic Effects
Gastrointestinal	Esophageal reflux, recurrent diarrhea, acute or chronic pancreatitis (75% of cases related to alcohol abuse)
Liver	Fatty liver, alcoholic hepatitis, cirrhosis
Cardiac	Hypertension, cardiomyopathy, arrhythmias
Respiratory	Pneumonia, bronchitis, tuberculosis
Neurologic	Seizures, peripheral neuropathy, Wernicke's disease, Korsakoff's syndrome, alcoholic dementia
Endocrine	Hyperglycemia, decreased thyroid function
Reproductive	Erectile problems, decreased testosterone, menstrual irregularities
Nutritional status	Thiamine deficiency, folic acid deficiency, vitamin A deficiency, magnesium deficiency, zinc deficiency

Sources: Hedaya, 1996; Washton, 1995.

ment, dilated pupils, and hyperthermia of 107F (41.6C) or more.

Toxic levels of cocaine can cause neurological complications. Seizures can be life-threatening, requiring immediate intervention. Death secondary to respiratory collapse or cardiac arrest may occur suddenly and without warning. Strokes often result in quadriplegia and aphasia. Sudden hemorrhage into the subarachnoid space may be a complication of cocaine abuse. When cocaine is used with alcohol, there is a twentyfold greater risk of cardiac arrest (Washton, 1995).

Individuals who have used hallucinogens may have dilated pupils, tachycardia, hyperglycemia, leukocytosis, and at times a marked rise in temperature. Their deep reflexes are hyperactive. People who have used PCP often are confused, delirious, and psychotic. They experience hypertension, muscle rigidity, seizures, and lowered body temperature. They may become comatose (Kinney, 1996).

People who abuse heroin experience respiratory depression and may have sudden irreversible pulmonary edema. They may have multiple abscesses on their extremities, edema of the hands, and the presence of "tracks"—darkened, hardened, and scarred veins (Kinney, 1996).

A rapid increase in sexually transmitted infections (STIs) has been associated with substance abuse, especially crack cocaine. Users of illegal substances may trade sex for the drug. Cocaine abusers often get involved in multiple-partner sex and are unable to consider safer sex practices when high. Since alcohol decreases inhibitions and judgment, there has been a rise in STIs among adolescents and young adults. Contaminated needles are a leading cause of the spread of hepatitis, HIV infection, and AIDS. As this problem grows, the premature death rate from drug abuse may approach that of alcohol abuse (Hedaya, 1996).

Substance-related disorders have a number of sexual consequences. Chronic alcohol abuse leads to erection problems for 40% of men as well as ejaculation difficulties in 10–25% of men. Among women entering treatment for alcoholism, 70–80 % have difficulty achieving orgasm, 30–40 % have problems with sexual arousal, and 30% have lost their desire for sex. People who use marijuana report enhanced sexual enjoyment with an intensification of touch and perception. They have increased attentiveness to their partner although sexual behavior remains the same. The initial use of amphetamines increases sex drive and sensations; long-term use leads to problems with arousal, function, and the sense of pleasure. Use of hallucinogens can create both extremely positive and negative sexual effects. The heightened sensory-perceptual stimuli may enhance or intensify sex or create a terrifying experience. Sexual performance may be impossible because of intoxication. People using opioids find their desire for sex has been replaced with their desire for the drug. They also experience decreased sexual arousal and difficulties with orgasm/ejaculation. Cocaine is associated with hypersexuality. Seventy percent of males and 30% of females report a strong link between cocaine use and a variety of sexual acting-out behaviors. Cocaine is a CNS stimulant which relaxes inhibitions, increases sexual fantasies, and increases sexual desire. High doses of cocaine can produce compulsive masturbation, multi-partner marathons, group sex, and even sexual abuse

of children. It is not uncommon for cocaine abusers to go on marathon binges of cocaine and sex (Crenshaw and Goldberg, 1996; Washton, 1995).

Professionals are concerned not just with the direct effects of alcohol and drugs on the brain but also with residual effects that cause recovering individuals to return to compulsive substance abuse. It is believed that each time a drug is used, specific brain structures are activated, leaving a memory trace that remains long after the drug has disappeared from the body. Each incidence of drug use is paired with environmental cues of persons, places, and things which then have the ability to trigger the same brain circuits even in the absence of the drug. Brain imaging techniques have been able to measure changes in specific brain areas in response to environmental triggers (O'Brien, 1997).

Intrauterine Substance Exposure

It is known that many of these chemicals cross the placental barrier and have harmful effects on unborn children. Alcohol is the most abused substance by pregnant women and causes abnormalities ranging from the subtle cognitive-behavioral impairments of *fetal alcohol effects (FAE)* to the symptoms of *fetal alcohol syndrome (FAS)*. FAS is the third-leading cause of birth defects in the United States. Defects include heart defects, malformed facial features, and mental retardation. Other effects are a slow growth rate, hyperactivity, and learning disabilities (Streissguth and O'Malley, 1997; Tiedje and Starn, 1996). Cocaine use is associated with an increased rate of prematurity, intrauterine growth retardation, microcephaly, and cerebral infarction. Cocaine is especially dangerous to the fetus if it is used during the first trimester of pregnancy when the brain is developing. Cocaine is such a potent vasoconstrictor that reduced blood supply to the fetus causes neurological abnormalities that may result in lifelong learning and behavioral problems. After birth, these infants tend to experience abnormal sleep patterns, tremors, poor feeding, irritability, and sometimes seizures. There is a tenfold greater risk of sudden infant death syndrome (SIDS) (Kinney, 1996).

At this time, we do not know whether early, intensive help can reverse a significant amount of the damage caused by exposure to cocaine in utero. In the best environment, these children may do fine. In a chaotic, abusive household, these children may be overwhelmed and have delayed development. Many have difficulty paying attention and controlling impulses.

Although they may be intelligent, they may have problems in school because they are distracted (Am J Psychiatry, 1995).

Children who have been exposed to opioids prior to birth have an increased rate of prematurity and a 5–10 times higher risk of SIDS. Newborns are very sensitive to noise; they are irritable and tremulous; they sweat and have nasal congestion. They may have uncoordinated sucking and swallowing reflexes, which cause feeding problems (Am J Psychiatry, 1995).

Concomitant Disorders/Dual Diagnosis

Clients must be assessed for **dual diagnosis,** the presence of substance abuse with a concurrent psychiatric disorder. A dual diagnosis indicates one of three things: two independent disorders occur together, substance abuse caused the other mental disorder, or the person with the mental disorder uses substances in an effort to self-medicate and feel better. Whatever the original cause of substance abuse, it usually complicates all other problems so much that it must be dealt with immediately. Substance abuse can precipitate prolonged psychotic relapses and contribute to medication noncompliance, as well as unstable relationships, financial mismanagement, disruptive behavior, and unstable housing.

Individuals with a psychiatric disorder are at higher risk for having a substance abuse disorder. Of the general population, 7–10% abuse substances. The risk is twice as high for those suffering from depression, bipolar disorder, or an anxiety disorder. For those who are young and psychiatrically disabled, the substance abuse rate is around 50%. About 70% of those diagnosed with antisocial personality disorder are chemically dependent (Brown et al, 1995; Miller, 1997).

The frequency of both suicide attempts and completed suicides is significantly higher among people with substance use disorders than it is in the general population. Substance use disorders are also associated with greater than average risk for other forms of violence, including homicide (Schuckit et al, 1997).

Causative Theories

Extensive research on the causes of substance dependence has yielded theories that combine biological, psychological, and sociocultural components. There are probably several subtypes of alcoholism, each having different combinations of predisposing factors. The abuse of other substances may be related to a variety of combinations. At present, it is thought that heredity determines 30–50% of one's susceptibility to alcoholism, with cultural and environmental factors accounting for the rest. Although the theories are presented separately, remember that they interact in ways that are not yet clearly understood.

Neurobiological Theory

Substance-related disorders are heterogeneous. Many studies have focused on families in an attempt to determine whether a predisposition to alcoholism or substance abuse is inherited. Twins and adoptees have been studied to determine the role of genetics, and it has been found that alcoholism clearly runs in families. It is thought that alcoholism itself is not inherited; rather, there is an underlying predisposition to develop the disease, which is most likely the result of the interaction of many genes. Genetic defects lead to deficiencies and imbalances in neurotransmitters, neuropeptides, and receptors. These chemical changes may give rise to a wide range of behavioral disturbances and a variety of compulsive disorders (Diamond and Gordon, 1995).

Cravings for alcohol, drugs, and food share an abnormal mechanism involving the reward system in the brain. Dopamine (DA) is not just the neurotransmitter that transmits pleasure signals, but it may, in fact, be the master molecule of craving and addiction. Organic defects affect DA neurotransmission by

- interfering with the normal release of DA at critical receptor sites in the reward centers of the brain.
- changing the structure of DA receptors, resulting in decreased DA binding.
- decreasing the number of DA receptors, leading to decreased DA binding.

Psychoactive drugs such as alcohol, cocaine, and morphine temporarily offset or overcome these defects by artificially inducing the release of abnormal amounts of DA. DA is directly responsible for the exhilarating rush that reinforces the desire to take drugs. Glucose probably has the same effect, thus causing a compulsive craving for food in some eating disorders. There is evidence that alcoholics have low levels of MAO. It is unclear whether the deficit occurs prior to the disease or if the brain's chronic exposure to alcohol decreases MAO production. Some studies indicate that alcoholics also have low levels of 5-HT (Little et al, 1996; Pace, 1995; Ruden, 1997). All genetic and neurobiological theories leave room for the substantial impact of environmental, social, and individual factors.

Intrapersonal Theory

For many years, intrapersonal theories were the only causative explanations for substance dependence, and they contributed to the moral perspective that still exists in the general population today. These theories describe substance dependence as being determined by personality traits and developmental failures. More recent research has made these theories much less popular.

One hypothesis is that the person's basic nature is to search for altered states of consciousness. The result of this unconscious search is chemical dependence. Another hypothesis is related to the person's desire to seek out and discover new experiences. Rebellion has also been proposed as an explanation for initiating the use of substances. Unlawful or undesirable behavior is one of the most effective means of expressing contempt or defiance of authority (Pace, 1995).

Behavioral Theory

Behavioral theory looks at the antecedents of substance use behavior, prior experiences with use, and the beliefs and expectations surrounding the behavior. This perspective considers which reinforcement principles operate in substance dependence. Consequences for continuing to use or deciding not to use, such as increasing pleasure or decreasing discomfort, are studied. Behavioral theorists also look at the activities associated with substance dependence, social pressures, rewards, and punishments.

Learning Theory

Learning theory states that chemically dependent people have learned maladaptive ways of coping. It is thought that substance dependence is a learned, maladaptive means of decreasing anxiety. Abusive behavior is viewed on a continuum from no use to moderate use, through excessive to dependent use. All these behaviors are learned responses. Learning theorists look at childhood exposure to role models, customs surrounding the use of chemicals, and the symbolic meaning of the drug (Kinney, 1996).

Sociocultural Theory

Sociocultural theory considers how cultural values and attitudes influence substance abuse behavior. Cultures whose religious or moral values prohibit or extremely limit the use of alcohol or drugs have lower rates of chemical dependence.

Sociocultural theory is based on the idea that values, perceptions, norms, and beliefs are passed on from one generation to another. Alcohol is part of everyday life in some families, while in other families, there is infrequent use or abstinence. The United States is a drug-oriented society. Advertisements offer medicinal cures not only for minor aches and pains but also for major health problems. Adolescents and young adults see their parents use various substances such as alcohol, caffeine, nicotine, antianxiety agents, and sedatives. With sanction from television advertising and parental examples, these young people see nothing wrong with trying various drugs.

Peer group pressure can cause drug use. Being in a peer group is important for adolescents and young adults. If some members are experimenting with drugs, other members are likely to follow suit.

One of the primary causes of substance abuse and dependence among African Americans and Hispanic Americans is sociocultural. Substance abuse is symptomatic of larger social problems. Racism creates a disparity in the socioeconomic systems of minority groups, who must manage the oppression that accompanies this inequality. Racism results in unemployment, and it is very painful to live in poverty in a culture with a materialistic ethic. Racism also results in dense clustering in substandard housing, environmental pollution, inadequate health care, and lack of power. When all this is combined with the relatively excessive availability of alcohol and other drugs, it is not surprising that there is a high rate of substance dependence among young people from minority populations (Kinney, 1996).

One example of sociocultural theory is seen in substance-related disorders among Native Americans who have suffered the loss of their historical traditions. The federal government made them relocate to reservations, forcing subservience on them. The stress of acculturation has been very high. Economically, most residents of the reservations are chronically depressed. Native Americans suffer from extreme poverty, poor health, inadequate health care, housing problems, and transportation problems. Short-term relief through drinking or using drugs may appear to outweigh the long-term damage that results from substance dependence (Kinney, 1996).

Feminist Theory

Feminist theory looks at the high cost of conforming to gender roles. Rigid gender socialization may keep people from experiencing life to the fullest. Women are denied access to their powerful selves, and men are denied access to their nurturant and expressive selves. Feminist theory believes that addiction may be a response to suppressed identity and self-concept. Women frequently have histories of physical, sexual, or emotional abuse and often state that addiction occurred as a response to severe stressors. When women's relationships fail or are dysfunctional, the use of substances often increases (Pace, 1995; Tiedje and Starn, 1996).

Psychopharmacological Interventions

Alcohol **withdrawal** is a serious medical problem, and the primary treatment goal is the prevention of DTs. Benzodiazepines are the medications of choice, with dosage determined by withdrawal symptoms. One of the following medications will be used: Librium (chlordiazepoxide), 25–50 mg, orally or IV, every 4–6 hours; Valium (diazepam), 5–10 mg, orally or IV, every 4–6 hours; Tranzene (clorazepate), 15 mg, orally, every 4–6 hours; or Ativan (lorazepam), 2 mg, PRN. These medications are titrated downward over a period of 5 days. High doses of thiamine are given during alcohol withdrawal to decrease the rebound effect of the nervous system as it adapts to the absence of alcohol. For clients with delirium, delusions, or hallucinations, antipsychotic medications may be used (Am J Psychiatry, 1995).

Some people suffering from alcoholism take *Antabuse* (disulfiram) as part of their rehabilitation treatment program. Antabuse inhibits aldehyde dehydrogenase and leads to an accumulation of acetaldehyde if alcohol is ingested. The reaction occurs within 5–10 minutes and may last from 30 minutes to several hours. Symptoms include flushing, nausea and copious vomiting, thirst, diaphoresis, dyspnea, hyperventilation, throbbing headache, palpitations, hypotension, weakness, and confusion. In severe reactions, coma, seizures, cardiovascular collapse, respiratory depression, and death can occur. Antabuse should be used only under careful medical and nursing supervision, and clients must understand the consequences of the therapy. See the Medication Teaching box.

Medication Teaching

Clients with Alcoholism
Antabuse

Avoid all exposure to alcohol and substances containing alcohol, including food, liquids, and substances applied to the skin.

Read all product labels to ensure that they do not contain alcohol.

Common products that contain alcohol include mouthwash, cough syrups, shaving lotion, and cologne.

If you are exposed to alcohol while taking Antabuse, you will experience a reaction within 5–10 minutes, and it may last from 30 minutes to several hours.

Symptoms of an Antabuse reaction include flushing, nausea and severe vomiting, thirst, sweating, shortness of breath, hyperventilation, throbbing headache, heart palpitations, low blood pressure, weakness, and confusion. In a severe reaction, you may experience seizures, coma, and cardiac or respiratory arrest.

Antabuse takes 14 days to be removed from your body following discontinuation of the medication. Do not drink or become exposed to alcohol during this time.

The opiate antagonist naltrexone (ReVia) has been shown to significantly decrease craving for alcohol and lower the relapse rate. This medication interferes with alcohol's intoxicating effects in the brain by blocking the opiate receptors. People who take naltrexone and drink report that they feel less "high," less uncoordinated, and less intoxicated than usual. Side effects can include difficulty sleeping, nervousness, and gastrointestinal distress. Since this drug can interfere with the use of narcotic analgesics in emergencies, the person must carry a medical alert card at all times. Some AA groups disagree with the use of naltrexone since the person is not "drug-free," while other AA groups support the use of this medication (Freed and Nattkemper, 1997; O'Malley et al, 1996).

Opioid overdose is a medical emergency that places the client in danger of respiratory arrest. The client is given 0.4–0.8 mg of Narcan (naloxone) intravenously. Since the medication is very short-lived, the client must be observed closely and most likely will need repeat doses (Am J Psychiatry, 1995). Methadone maintenance programs are used for some people who are addicted to heroin. The dose is titrated upward over a period of 2 weeks, with a daily maintenance dose of 60–80 mg. LAAM is a longer-acting preparation that can be administered less frequently, as little as three times a week. The opiate antagonist naltrexone is an alternative medication. The purpose of methadone or naltrexone is to reduce the craving for and block the effects of illegal opioids. The typical course of this narcotic substitution therapy program is 2–4 years (Am J Psychiatry, 1995).

Multidisciplinary Interventions

Treatment options include brief therapy, intensive outpatient or inpatient treatment, and residential treatment. Brief therapy is usually provided by trained professionals at a community drug treatment center. Clients learn specific behavioral methods for stopping or reducing their substance use, such as goal setting, self-monitoring, and identifying high-risk situations. Outpatient intensive programs allow clients to remain in their work and home settings while participating in treatment for 4 or 5 hours every day. It is appropriate for those who require intensive care but have a reasonable chance for abstinence outside a restricted setting. Inpatient treatment occurs in the emergency department and on acute care inpatient units. Hospitalization is appropriate for those at risk for severe withdrawal syndromes, those who are psychiatrically disabled, those who are a danger to themselves or others, and those who have not responded to less intensive treatment efforts. Residential treatment usually lasts 14–21 days and offers a safe and structured environment for those who lack social and vocational skills and drug-free social supports to be abstinent in a less restricted setting. Inpatient programs are downsizing and closing as third-party reimbursment is rapidly decreasing.

Drug rehabilitation is the recovery of optimal health through medical, psychological, social, and peer group support for chemically dependent people and their significant others. *Abstinence* is merely stopping the intake of the drug; it does not imply that any other behaviors have changed. People who abstain are often referred to as "dry drunks" because they continue all their other unhealthy behaviors. In contrast, *sobriety* implies that not only have these individuals stopped using the drug, but they have also achieved a centered or balanced state. Emotional growth is achieved through the development of positive values, attitudes, beliefs, and behaviors. Sobriety is the overall goal of drug rehabilitation (Kinney, 1996). The *recovery model* is a vital part of rehabilitation that views chemical dependence as a chronic, progressive, and often fatal disease. The responsibility for recovery is on the client, and any attempt to shift responsibility to others, such as family or friends, is confronted directly. Recovery is considered a lifelong, day-to-day process and is accomplished with the support from peers with the same addiction. Recovery programs typically are 12-step programs, first introduced by Alcoholics Anonymous (AA), in which honesty is a very high value. These programs are deeply spiritual, and recovery is thought to depend, in part, on faith in a higher power. Clients are referred to AA, Cocaine Anonymous, or Narcotics Anonymous. Partners are encouraged to join Al-Anon, children to join Alateen or Alatots, and adult children to join Adult Children of Alcoholics (ACOA) (Evans and Sullivan, 1995). Box 13.2 shows the 12 steps of AA. Treatment programs have traditionally been designed for men and many people believe that women require different, gender-specific approaches. Believing that causes of substance abuse are poor self-esteem, relationship problems, and histories of abuse and depression, treatment focuses on competence, strengths, and confidence. Women for Sobriety (WFS) is the first self-help support group founded specifically for women who are alcoholics. It is an emotional and spiritual growth program in which members use positive affirmation and share experiences to aid in the recovery process (Tiedje and Starn, 1996). Box 13.3 shows the 13 affirmations of WFS.

Family therapy helps family members identify situations in which they acted as enablers. They then suggest alternative actions or statements they could have used in those situations. These new behaviors are practiced in a variety of settings. The family then moves on to making a contract with the client to use new, nonenabling strategies in the future (Kinney, 1996).

Preventive education is another multidisciplinary intervention. Adolescents and preteens who have not used either alcohol or other drugs need some anticipatory guidance to help them cope with the inevitable choices they will have to make. Many community alcohol and drug projects have programs for parents and offer support groups and literature. This outreach to parents helps them develop guidelines relating to alcohol and drug use (Kinney, 1996).

Box 13.2

The 12 Steps of Alcoholics Anonymous

We

1. Admitted we were powerless over alcohol, that our lives had become unmanageable.

2. Came to believe that a Power greater than ourselves could restore us to sanity.

3. Made a decision to turn our will and our lives over to the care of God as we understood Him.

4. Made a searching and fearless moral inventory of ourselves.

5. Admitted to God, to ourselves, and to another human being the exact nature of our wrongs.

6. Were entirely ready to have God remove all these defects of character.

7. Humbly asked Him to remove our shortcomings.

8. Made a list of all persons we had harmed and became willing to make amends to them all.

9. Made direct amends to such people wherever possible, except when to do so would injure them or others.

10. Continued to take personal inventory and when we were wrong promptly admitted it.

11. Sought through prayer and meditation to improve our conscious contact with God as we understood Him, praying only for knowledge of His will for us and the power to carry that out.

12. Having had a spiritual awakening as the result of these steps, we tried to carry this message to alcoholics and to practice these principles in all our affairs.

Source: Alcoholics Anonymous World Services, 1952. Reprinted with permission.

Box 13.3

Levels of the New Life Program and Thirteen Affirmations: Women for Sobriety

Level I: Accepting alcoholism as a physical disease.

I have a drinking (life-threatening) problem that once had me.

Level II: Discarding negative thoughts, putting guilt behind, and practicing new ways of viewing and solving problems.

Negative thoughts destroy only myself.

Problems bother me only to the degree I permit them to.

The past is gone forever.

Level III: Creating and practicing a new self-image.

I am what I think.

I am a competent woman and have much to give life.

Level IV: Using new attitudes to enforce new behavior patterns.

Happiness is a habit I will develop.

Life can be ordinary or it can be great.

Enthusiasm is my daily exercise.

Level V: Improving relationships as a result of our new feelings about self.

Love can change the course of my world.

All love given returns.

Level VI: Recognizing life's priorities: emotional and spiritual growth, self-responsibility.

The fundamental object of life is emotional and spiritual growth.

I am responsible for myself and my actions.

The Nursing Process

Assessment

People who abuse substances rarely seek treatment because they believe they are drinking too much alcohol or using too many drugs. Typically, what brings them into the health care system are problems with their jobs, relationships, money, and/or the legal system. All who enter treatment are ambivalent about giving up the chemicals they have become dependent upon. If clients are coerced into treatment, expect them to feel angry, controlled, humiliated, fearful, defensive, and mistrustful.

The nursing assessment should be conducted in a nonjudgmental and matter-of-fact way. Give positive recognition that it was a personal choice to come into treatment. State that your goal is not to force them into doing anything but rather help achieve an assessment and understanding of the nature of their use of substances. Following the assessment you will be able to provide them with realistic feedback about their substance use behavior. Begin with less intrusive questions, such as "How many cigarettes do you smoke a day?" before asking questions about other substances. Follow with questions related to the use of prescription drugs. Then proceed to ask questions about the past and present use of alcohol and illegal drugs. Box 13.4 is an overview of a substance abuse assessment.

Mayfield, McCleod, and Hall (1974) developed the CAGE Questionnaire, which is simple and can be incorporated into any nursing assessment. One positive answer raises concern, and more than one positive answer is a strong indication of alcohol problems.

C   Have you ever felt that you should *cut down* on your drinking?

A   Have people *annoyed* you by criticizing your drinking?

G   Have you ever felt bad or *guilty* about your drinking?

E   Have you ever taken a drink in the morning, as an *"eye-opener"*?

The Focused Nursing Assessment table provides questions for assessing clients who are substance-dependent. The assessment has a twofold purpose: to identify problems and to increase clients' awareness of the toll that substance use may be taking on their lives.

Diagnosis

After completing the assessment and appraising the knowledge base, you are ready to analyze and synthesize the information. Answer the following questions:

1. How does the client view substance abuse?
2. How does the client view alcoholics or addicts?
3. What is the client's concept of disease?
4. What does the client claim to want out of treatment?
5. Is the client being forced to seek treatment by family, employer, or the legal system?

See the Nursing Diagnoses box for clients with substance-related disorders. Nursing diagnoses relating to acute overdose and chronic physical complica-

Box 13.4

Substance Abuse History

Assess for each substance:

Age begun:

Method of use: (oral, smoking, inhaling, injecting)

Amount and frequency of use:

Most recent use:

Withdrawal symptoms in the past:

Setting and circumstances of use: (people, places, things, moods, and emotional states associated with use. How and where drugs are procured.)

Benefits of use:

Proportion of income or savings spent on drugs:

Financial consequences of drug use: (overdue bills, credit card debts, does person sell drugs to offset cost)

Relationship, vocational, social problems associated with use:

tions of substance dependence are beyond the scope of this text. Refer to your medical-surgical text to review these diagnoses and the appropriate nursing responses.

Outcome Identification

Once you have established diagnoses, you and the client mutually identify goals for change. Client outcomes are specific behavioral measures by which you, clients, and significant others determine progress toward goals. The following are examples of some of the outcomes appropriate to people who have substance-related disorders:

- remains safe during the withdrawal process
- acknowledges the reality of the disorder
- acknowledges the negative consequences of substance-abusing behavior
- identifies triggers to relapse
- utilizes spiritual support resources
- demonstrates improved problem-solving skills
- improves levels of physical health and fitness
- participates in self-help groups

Focused Nursing Assessment

CLIENTS WITH SUBSTANCE-RELATED DISORDERS

Behavior Assessment	Affective Assessment	Cognitive Assessment	Social Assessment
When did you begin to have problems with substances?	In what way does your drug use decrease your anxiety? Boredom? Depression?	What kinds of things do you have difficulty remembering?	Who do you consider to be the most significant people in your life?
Have you ever missed work/school because of drug use?	What kinds of comments have others made to you about rapid mood swings?	Have you ever had blackouts?	Can you confide in these people?
What kinds of employment/school problems have you experienced?	What drug-abusing behavior has led you to feel guilty? Embarrassed? Ashamed? Humiliated?	Have you invented information or stories to make up for forgetting?	Which of these individuals abuse substances with you?
Have you missed family/social events because of drug use?		What reasons do you give others for your use of drugs?	Who knows about your substance abuse?
How hostile and argumentative do you become when using substances?		Have you experienced hallucinations?	Describe family arguments relating to your substance abuse.
Have you ever attempted to harm yourself or others while under the influence of these drugs?		Do you believe you have a chemical dependence that is out of your control?	Who protects you from the consequences of your abuse?
Have you had periods in your life when you were drug-free? How long did these last?			How has your sexual behavior changed with your substance use?
Have you ever received treatment for using drugs? If so, what kind?			

Nursing Diagnoses

Clients with Substance-Related Disorders

Altered thought process related to long-term chronic brain damage.

Ineffective individual coping related to using chemicals as a way to cope with life.

Social isolation related to a lifestyle of substance abuse.

Ineffective family coping related to codependent and enabling behavior; neglect or abuse of family members.

Powerlessness related to an inability to control the use of drugs.

Self-esteem disturbance, altered role performance related to lifestyle disrupted by substance abuse.

Ineffective denial related to believing that there is no problem with use of substances.

High risk for violence, self-directed, related to psychotic symptoms; hyperactivity; panic anxiety; hopelessness; suicidal ideation.

High risk for violence, directed at others, related to history of violence when using drugs; complications from withdrawal such as agitation, suspicion, paranoia; drug-induced impulsivity and angry outbursts.

Spiritual distress related to alienation from others; loss of faith in a higher being.

See also the Critical Pathway for a Client Experiencing Alcohol Withdrawal on pages 338–342.

Nursing Interventions

Substance dependence is not hard to see, but it is hard to treat. Clients must become invested in treatment and require intensive support from others. See the box on page 343 for an overview of the nursing interventions classification (NIC) for substance abuse.

Behavioral: Behavior Therapy

Substance Use Treatment: Alcohol Withdrawal

Emergency management of acute alcohol intoxication is necessary to save lives. Clients must be quickly assessed for life-threatening situations requiring imme-

Table 13.3 Blood Alcohol Levels and Symptoms

Blood Alcohol Level (Percentage of Alcohol in Blood)	Behavior
0.05	Changes in mood and normal behavior; loosening of judgment and restraint; person feels carefree
0.08–0.10	Voluntary motor action clumsy; legal level of intoxication
0.20	Brain motor area depression causes staggering; easily angered; shouting; weeping
0.30	Confusion; stupor
0.40	Coma
0.50	Death (usually due to medullar respiratory blocking effects)

diate response. Blood alcohol levels (BALs) are generally obtained to determine the level of intoxication. Table 13.3 lists the symptoms related to blood alcohol levels. Be alert for the problem of mixed addiction. Monitor vital signs frequently. Place the client in a quiet environment to avoid excessive stimulation that could increase agitation. Lighting in the room should be maintained, especially at night, to decrease the possibility of misinterpretation of stimuli and shadows. If there is no one to stay in constant attendance, it may be necessary to restrain the client for protection from injury. However, restraints often increase confusion and agitation. Because seizures may occur, you will have to put the client on seizure precautions, which include an oral airway or bite stick, suction equipment, and padded side rails.

Substance Use Treatment: Drug Withdrawal

Some clients are at high risk for violence related to the psychotic effects of chemicals (hallucinations and delusions), impulsive behavior when intoxicated, and the process of withdrawal from chemicals (agitation, paranoia). Try to determine if there is a history of violence, since that is one of the best predictors of present or future violence. Early intervention with diversional activities can prevent some outbursts by

Text continues on page 342

Critical Pathway for a Client Experiencing Alcohol Withdrawal

Expected length of treatment: 6 days	Date _____ Day 1	Date _____ Day 2	Date _____ Day 3
Daily outcomes	Client will: ■ Have stable vital signs. ■ Remain oriented to time, place, and person. ■ Withdraw from alcohol without injury. ■ Consume 1500 cal and 2000 cc of fluid each day. ■ Verbalize thoughts and feelings. ■ Verbalize commitment to detox program. ■ Maintain stable weight. ■ Demonstrate ability to cope.	Client will: ■ Have stable vital signs. ■ Remain oriented to time, place, and person. ■ Withdraw from alcohol without injury. ■ Consume 2000 cal and 3000 cc of fluid each day. ■ Verbalize thoughts and feelings. ■ Verbalize commitment to detox program. ■ Maintain stable weight. ■ Demonstrate alternate coping mechanisms. ■ Attend AA daily. ■ Identify strategies to promote sleep/rest.	Client will: ■ Be afebrile with stable vital signs. ■ Remain oriented to time, place, and person. ■ Withdraw from alcohol without injury. ■ Remain free of signs and symptoms of delirium tremens. ■ Consume 2000 cal and 3000 cc of fluid each day. ■ Verbalize thoughts and feelings. ■ Begin to verbalize alcohol's negative effects on significant others and lifestyle. ■ Verbalize commitment to detox program. ■ Attend AA daily. ■ Maintain stable weight. ■ Identify strategies to promote sleep/rest. ■ Demonstrate alternate coping mechanisms.
Assessments, tests, and treatments	Vital signs q 4 hr if stable. Intake and output. Blood alcohol level. CBC and urinalysis. Chemistry profile, electrolytes. Serum magnesium. Chest X ray. EKG. PPD. Assess need for HIV testing. Weigh. Assess q 1–2 hr for signs and symptoms of withdrawal, including anxiety, agitation, irritability, tremor, tachycardia, hypertension, diaphoresis, and hallucinations. Assess drinking history and patterns. Establish the date and time of last drink.	Vital signs q 4 hr if stable. Intake and output. Assess q 1–2 hr for signs and symptoms of withdrawal, including anxiety, agitation, irritability, tremor, tachycardia, hypertension, diaphoresis, and hallucinations.	Vital signs q 4 hr and PRN. D/C intake and output if stable. Assess q 1–2 hr for signs and symptoms of withdrawal, including anxiety, agitation, irritability, tremor, tachycardia, hypertension, diaphoresis, and hallucinations. Monitor for delirium tremens. Read PPD. Repeat laboratory studies as indicated.

	Date _____ Day 1 *continued*	Date _____ Day 2 *continued*	Date _____ Day 3 *continued*
Knowledge deficit	Orient client and family to room and routine. Include family in teaching. Review plan of care. Initiate medication teaching. Assess understanding of teaching.	Review plan of care with client and family. Include family in teaching. Assess understanding of teaching.	Review plan of care with client and family. Include family in teaching. Initiate discharge teaching regarding the need for ongoing outpatient therapy and attending a self-help group. Assess understanding of teaching.
Diet	Encourage up to 3000 cc of fluids each day (unless contraindicated). Limit caffeine intake. Provide frequent, small, nutritious feedings, inclusive of all food groups. Nutrition assessment.	Encourage up to 3000 cc of fluids each day (unless contraindicated). Limit caffeine. Dietary consult. Provide frequent, small, nutritious feedings, inclusive of all food groups.	Encourage up to 3000 cc of fluids each day (unless contraindicated). Limit caffeine. Provide frequent, small, nutritious feedings, inclusive of all food groups.
Activity	Assess safety needs and maintain appropriate precautions. Activity as tolerated. Assist with hygiene.	Maintain safety precautions. Activity as tolerated. Prompt and assist with hygiene as needed.	Maintain safety precautions. Self-care/shower.
Psychosocial	Assess level of anxiety. Provide information and ongoing support and encouragement to client and family. Assess sleep patterns and provide measures that promote rest and sleep. Encourage expression of thoughts and feelings. Approach in nonjudgmental manner. Explore availability of support system. Encourage regular aerobic exercise. Explore interests and potential hobbies. Explore attending an AA meeting. Use gentle confrontation strategies. Provide education and set limits. Explore lifestyle changes.	Assess level of anxiety. Encourage verbalization of concerns. Provide information and ongoing support and encouragement to client and family. Assess sleep patterns and provide measures that promote rest and sleep. Encourage expression of thoughts and feelings. Approach in nonjudgmental manner. Explore availability of support system. Choose and begin regular aerobic exercise. Explore interests and potential hobbies. Attend an AA meeting. Use gentle confrontation strategies. Provide education and set limits. Explore lifestyle changes.	Assess level of anxiety. Encourage verbalization of concerns. Provide information and ongoing support and encouragement to client and family. Assess sleep patterns and provide measures that promote rest and sleep. Encourage expression of thoughts and feelings. Approach in nonjudgmental manner. Explore availability of support system. Choose and begin regular aerobic exercise. Explore interests and potential hobbies. Attend an AA meeting. Use gentle confrontation strategies. Provide education and set limits. Explore lifestyle changes.

continued ➤

Critical Pathway for a Client Experiencing Alcohol Withdrawal continued

	Date _____ Day 1 *continued*	Date _____ Day 2 *continued*	Date _____ Day 3 *continued*
Medications	Thiamine 100 mg IM or PO. Routine meds as ordered. Librium as ordered.	Thiamine 100 mg PO. Folic acid 1 mg PO. Multivitamin PO. Routine meds as ordered. Librium as ordered.	Thiamine 100 mg PO. Folic acid 1 mg PO. Multivitamin PO. Routine meds as ordered. Librium as ordered.
Consults and discharge plan	Family assessment if not previously completed. Consult with internist. Refer to neurologist if indicated. Discuss self-help groups. Establish discharge objectives with client and family.	Review discharge objectives and anticipated discharge care with client and significant others. Refer to self-help groups. Refer the family to self-help groups. Complete discharge planning.	Review progress toward discharge objectives and anticipated discharge care with client and significant others. Make appropriate referrals.

	Date _____ Day 4	Date _____ Day 5	Date _____ Day 6 –Discharge
Daily outcomes	Client will: ■ Be afebrile, have stable vital signs. ■ Remain oriented to time, place, and person. ■ Withdraw from alcohol without injury. ■ Remain free of signs and symptoms of delirium tremens. ■ Consume 2000 cal and 3000 cc of fluid each day. ■ Verbalize thoughts and feelings. ■ Begin to verbalize alcohol's negative effects on lifestyle. ■ Verbalize commitment to detox program. ■ Attend AA daily. ■ Maintain stable weight. ■ Establish sleep/rest routine to promote sleep. ■ Demonstrate alternate coping mechanisms.	Client will: ■ Be afebrile, have stable vital signs. ■ Remain oriented to time, place, and person. ■ Withdraw from alcohol without injury. ■ Remain free of signs and symptoms of delirium tremens. ■ Consume 2000 cal and 3000 cc of fluid each day. ■ Verbalize thoughts and feelings. ■ Begin to verbalize alcohol's negative effects on lifestyle. ■ Verbalize commitment to detox program. ■ Attend AA daily. ■ Maintain stable weight. ■ Establish sleep/rest routine to promote sleep. ■ Demonstrate alternate coping mechanisms.	Client is afebrile, has stable vital signs. Client is alert and oriented. Client has withdrawn from alcohol safely and without injury. Client maintains adequate nutrition and fluid intake. Client's weight remains stable. Client verbalizes understanding of hazards of alcohol. Client is independent in self-care. Client verbalizes times and places for AA meetings. Client verbalizes commitment to detox program and regular attendance at AA meetings. Client verbalizes home care instructions including the importance of ongoing counseling. Client has established a sleep/rest pattern and verbalizes understanding of sleep-promoting measures. Client demonstrates ability to cope with ongoing stressors.

	Date _____ Day 4 *continued*	Date _____ Day 5 *continued*	Date _____ Day 6–Discharge *continued*
Assessments, tests, and treatments	Vital signs BID if stable. Assess for signs and symptoms of withdrawal, including anxiety, agitation, irritability, tremor, tachycardia, hypertension, diaphoresis, and hallucinations. Monitor for delirium tremens.	Vital signs BID if stable. Assess for signs and symptoms of withdrawal, including anxiety, agitation, irritability, tremor, tachycardia, hypertension, diaphoresis, and hallucinations. Monitor for delirium tremens.	Vital signs BID if stable. Assess for signs and symptoms of withdrawal, including anxiety, agitation, irritability, tremor, tachycardia, hypertension, diaphoresis, and hallucinations. Monitor for delirium tremens.
Knowledge deficit	Review plan of care. Include family in teaching. Continue discharge teaching regarding the detox program and need for ongoing counseling. Assess understanding of teaching.	Review plan of care with client and family. Continue discharge teaching regarding the detox program and need for ongoing counseling. Assess understanding of teaching.	Client or significant other verbalizes understanding of discharge teaching including wound care, exercise program, strategies to prevent relapse, diet, signs and symptoms to report, follow-up care and MD appointment, medications; name, purpose, dose, frequency, route, dietary interactions, and side effects, and home care arrangements. Assess understanding of teaching.
Diet	Encourage up to 3000 cc of fluids each day (unless contraindicated). Provide frequent, small, nutritious feedings, inclusive of all food groups.	Encourage up to 3000 cc of fluids each day (unless contraindicated). Provide frequent, small, nutritious feedings, inclusive of all food groups.	Encourage up to 3000 cc of fluids each day (unless contraindicated). Provide frequent, small, nutritious feedings, inclusive of all food groups.
Activity	Maintain safety precautions. Self-care/shower.	Maintain safety precautions. Self-care/shower.	Maintain safety precautions. Self-care/shower.
Psychosocial	Assess level of anxiety. Encourage verbalization of concerns. Provide information and ongoing support and encouragement to client and family. Provide measures that promote rest and sleep. Encourage expression of thoughts and feelings. Approach in nonjudgmental manner. Explore availability of support system. Continue regular aerobic exercise.	Assess level of anxiety. Encourage verbalization of concerns. Provide information and ongoing support and encouragement to client and family. Provide measures that promote rest and sleep. Encourage expression of thoughts and feelings. Approach in nonjudgmental manner. Explore availability of support system. Continue regular aerobic exercise.	Assess level of anxiety. Encourage verbalization of concerns. Provide information and ongoing support and encouragement to client and family. Provide measures that promote rest and sleep. Encourage expression of thoughts and feelings. Approach in nonjudgmental manner. Explore availability of support system. Continue regular aerobic exercise.

continued ➤

Critical Pathway for a Client Experiencing *Alcohol Withdrawal* continued

	Date _____ Day 4 *continued*	Date _____ Day 5 *continued*	Date _____ Day 6–Discharge *continued*
Psychosocial *continued*	Explore interests and potential hobbies. Attend an AA meeting. Use gentle confrontation strategies. Provide education and set limits. Explore lifestyle changes. Encourage verbalization of concerns. Provide ongoing support and encouragement to client and family.	Explore interests and potential hobbies. Attend an AA meeting. Use gentle confrontation strategies. Provide education and set limits. Explore lifestyle changes. Encourage verbalization of concerns. Provide ongoing support and encouragement to client and family.	Explore interests and potential hobbies. Attend an AA meeting. Use gentle confrontation strategies. Provide education and set limits. Explore lifestyle changes. Encourage verbalization of concerns. Provide ongoing support and encouragement to client and family.
Medications	Thiamine 100 mg PO. Folic acid 1 mg PO. Multivitamin PO. Routine meds as ordered. Librium as ordered.	Thiamine 100 mg PO. Folic acid 1 mg PO. Multivitamin PO. Routine meds as ordered. Librium as ordered.	Thiamine 100 mg PO. Folic acid 1 mg PO. Multivitamin PO. Routine meds as ordered. Librium as ordered.
Transfer/ discharge plan	Review with client and significant others discharge objectives regarding activity and home care.	Review with client and significant others discharge objectives regarding activity and home care. Complete referrals for home care.	Discharge with referrals for home health care.

channeling energy into other activities. Decrease environmental stimuli or remove the person to a quieter area, as this may decrease the risk. As a last resort, use seclusion or restraints if clients cannot control their behavior. See Table 13.4 for an overview of emergency management of acute alcohol intoxication and drug overdose withdrawal.

Substance Use Treatment

An important nursing intervention is helping clients overcome denial and recognize the significance of the substance dependence. Keep in mind that it is very painful for clients to stop denying that alcohol and drugs are causing problems for themselves and others. Together, you begin to identify the situations in which substance abuse occurs, the type and amount of substances used, and the frequency of the abuse. You can then help the client identify what the nega-

tive consequences of this behavior have been and connect problems in life directly to the drug dependence. Using the one-day-at-a-time philosophy will minimize their feelings of being overwhelmed. Clients must identify a personal motivation for abstinence and then make a commitment to it. You can help them through this process by listening and through active support. Finally, it is very important to help clients identify their strengths and abilities, to decrease their feelings of helplessness and hopelessness.

Teach clients *problem-solving skills*. Many clients who abuse substances have avoided problems in life through the use of drugs. In order to abstain, they will need to develop alternative solutions to a broad range of life situations. (For a detailed discussion on teaching clients how to problem-solve, see Chapter 5.)

In working with clients who have abused alcohol or drugs, you often provide *vocational guidance*. If

Nursing Interventions Classification

CLIENTS WITH SUBSTANCE ABUSE

DOMAIN: Behavioral

Class: *Behavior Therapy*

> **Interventions:** *Substance Use Treatment: Alcohol Withdrawal:* Care of the patient experiencing sudden cessation of alcohol consumption.
>
> *Substance Use Treatment: Drug Withdrawal:* Care of a patient experiencing drug detoxification.
>
> *Substance Use Treatment:* Supportive care of patient/family members with physical and psychosocial problems associated with the use of alcohol or drugs.
>
> *Impulse Control Training:* Assisting the patient to mediate impulsive behavior through application of problem-solving strategies to social and interpersonal situations.

Class: *Coping Assistance*

> **Interventions:** *Spiritual Support:* Assisting the patient to feel balance and connection with a greater power.
>
> *Hope Instillation:* Facilitation of the development of a positive outlook in a given situation.

DOMAIN: Physiological: Basic

Class: *Nutrition Support*

> **Interventions:** *Nutrition Management:* Assisting with or providing a balanced dietary intake of foods and fluids.

there are educational deficiencies, they must be addressed. Clients must determine how to keep the jobs they currently have or how to obtain new jobs. Attaining financial stability is one of the goals of recovery. You can help clients plan short-term and long-range goals related to education and employment. It is often helpful to role-play employment situations such as on-the-job pressures and getting along with peers and supervisors.

You can encourage clients to improve their *physical health and fitness.* Many will benefit from regular exercise programs. Those who get involved in running often describe the natural "high" of running as a replacement for the old "high" of drugs.

Refer clients and their families to *self-help groups.* Mutual support makes people feel useful and valuable. At the beginning of rehabilitation, you may need to monitor client attendance at group meetings. Within each category there are special interest groups, including AA meetings for nurses, AA meetings for gays and lesbians, and women's groups such as Women Reaching Women or Women for Sobriety. Refer to the Self-Help Groups section at the end of this chapter.

Because of enabling behaviors and codependent family members, many families have ineffective coping skills. Encourage the recognition that chemical dependency is a family disease. Help codependent members talk about feelings of pain and anger since they have most likely been prevented from expressing their feelings directly. Help them learn how to respect and take care of themselves, decrease their need for perfectionism, and "own" their full range of feelings. They must become empowered in order to give up codependent behavior. Identify enabling behaviors by nonabusing family members since they are often unaware of their own problematic behaviors. Help family members acknowledge and change overresponsible behaviors such as covering up for and protecting the client. To equalize power in adult relationships, help the family develop a list of responsibilities. Encourage role playing of these new behaviors to reinforce the change in behavior.

Many people have developed a lifestyle revolving around substance abuse. Their social interactions have been largely restricted to drinking or using "buddies." Facilitate clients in developing an appropriate social support system and discuss the importance

Table 13.4 Management of Drug Overdose

Substance	Respiratory Status	Cardiac Status	Neurological Status	Medications	Other
Alcohol	Ventilation may be necessary	BP from ruptured esophageal varices	Possible head injuries		BAL (blood alcohol level); blood glucose—hypoglycemia mimics intoxication
Cocaine	Ventilation may be necessary	Lidocaine and defribrillation may be necessary; hypertension; cardiac arrest	Seizures	Acetaminophen, Dantrium for hyperthermia; propranolol for tachycardia; hydralazine or nitroprusside for hypertension; Valium, phenobarbital for seizures	Cooling blanket-for hyperthermia
Amphetamine	Ventilation may be necessary	Tachycardia hypertension	Seizures; CVA	Diazepam IV for seizures; Hydralzaine or nitrorusside for hypertension; propranolol for tachycardia	Oral ingestion-activated charcoal or gastric lavage. Protective environment to prevent injury/suicide.
Hallucinogen	Ventilation may be necessary		Stupor, coma seizures	Valium if sedation necessary	Reduce sensory stimuli. Tell what is happening to increase contact with reality. Reassure that effect of drug will wear off. Observe closely—prevent injury or suicide. Client may lose control. Dialysis if necessary.
Opioid	Severe respiratory depression pulmonary edema		Coma	Narcan to reverse respiratory depression and coma—may need repeated doses; Lasix for pulmonary edema	Glucose IV to prevent hypoglycemia; dialysis if necessary.
Sedative	Ventilation may be necessary	Hypotension	Sedation, coma	IVs to support BP; sodium bicarbonate to promote excretion	Activated charcoal or gastric lavage.

of regular social contacts. Help clients identify alcohol- and drug-free social activities. Group therapy is a treatment of choice in most programs. Clients learn to accept themselves as recovering individuals and help themselves while helping others. The group provides a sense of belonging and a source of friendships. Realizing that they are not alone, people feel less ashamed and despairing. Group members can also monitor one another for signs of relapse.

Impulse Control Training

Impulse control training is an important part of relapse prevention. The first step is to help clients identify and verbalize feelings and explore the origins of these feelings. Through discussion, you can help them recognize how they used alcohol and drugs to avoid the pain of their emotions. Another step in relapse prevention is having clients identify high-risk situations, such as specific people (friends who also use), places (bars), or specific activities ("coke" parties). Clients must also identify internal as well as external cues that trigger the urge to use chemicals. If possible, help them identify techniques from the past that led to success in avoiding substance abuse. The next step is to help clients anticipate and plan for problem situations by developing strategies for avoiding or actively coping with them when faced with such situations. Active strategies include self-statements to remind oneself of the commitment, assertiveness skills, and relaxation techniques. Provide opportunities to role-play these strategies.

Having a great deal of unstructured time is not helpful to people in early recovery. In the past they spent a great deal of time and energy thinking about and using chemicals. Having to change daily activities can pose a problem for newly sober people who have no substitutes. Give them the task of planning a daily schedule, especially for the days off work. This promotes the creation of a healthy balance of activities and aids in preventing relapse. Finally, clients must learn to identify early warning signals of impending relapse in order to seek support and help as early as possible.

Behavioral: Coping Assistance

Spiritual Support

Most chemical dependency treatment approaches have a strong spiritual basis and stress that people need to feel connected to a greater power. Review the 12 Steps of Alcoholics Anonymous in Box 13.2 in terms of the spiritual focus. Refer clients to spiritual advisors of their choice. Facilitate their use of meditation, prayer, and other religious traditions and rituals.

Hope Instillation

Demonstrate hope by responding to clients' worth and dignity and viewing their substance use disorder as only one facet of each person. Encourage clients to realistically view themselves in the present after sorting through past experiences and to "let go" and move on. Promote anticipated positive experiences and the hope that life will be better without alcohol or drugs. Attitudes to be encouraged are hoping, having faith, trusting, anticipating the positive, looking forward to the future, and believing (Wing, 1996).

Physiological: Basic: Nutrition Support

Nutrition Management

Nutritional interventions have achieved more importance in the past several years. Health care professionals now advocate precursor amino-acid loading in the diet to facilitate the restoration of neurotransmitters. Tryptophan is the precursor for serotonin, and tyrosine is the precursor for epinephrine. Two vitamins, ascorbic acid and folic acid, are necessary for the metabolism of tyrosine. Vitamin and mineral mixtures are added to the diet. Tropamine includes precursors for most of the neurotransmitters as well as substances that inhibit the destruction of neuropeptides. It has been found that tropamine effectively decreases drug and alcohol craving. Nutritional interventions often help achieve the first goal of treatment—keeping the client in the program. As many as 96% of clients can manage their cravings with nutritional support (Kinney, 1996).

Evaluation

While attempting to help clients prevent recurrences of substance use, acknowledge the possibility that slips will occur, and develop strategies to limit the duration and intensity of any relapse episodes. It is believed that it takes 9–15 months to adjust to a lifestyle free of chemical use. Most treatment failures and relapses occur in the first 15 months after abstinence begins. In one study of people who were treated for cocaine abuse, less than 20% had achieved sustained abstinence in the first 6–12 months. There is also a lifelong vulnerability to relapse. Close to half of recovering people fail to maintain abstinence after a year—about the same proportion of people with diabetes and hypertension who fail to comply with their diet, exercise, and medications. With the limitations on the length of intensive treatment programs, clients are often discharged well before the plan of care has been fully evaluated (Am J Psychiatry, 1995).

Recovery is total abstinence from all drugs, not just the drug of choice. Once people have crossed the line from chemical use to chemical dependence, they can never return to controlled use without rekindling the addiction. A reasonably motivated client involved in an effective treatment program can have a better prognosis than previously thought. A variety of factors, such as social support, level of functioning before the addiction, and willingness to accept the need for lifestyle changes, influence the treatment outcome.

The future of drug and alcohol treatment is uncertain; the problems are great and the needs are many. There is increasing reluctance to expend resources on people who may show little gratitude and who seem to have brought their troubles on themselves. Programs often suffer from the burdens of inadequate staff and unreliable funding. Waiting lists are long and the average length of treatment, days to a couple of months, is generally thought to be insufficient.

Clinical Interactions

A Substance-Abusing Client

Jim, age 34, has two daughters who live with his ex-wife. His parents are still living, and he has a twin sister and two older brothers. He has been living with his parents and has maintained a close relationship with all family members until recently, when his cocaine abuse problems worsened. He has recently entered a drug rehabilitation program. In the interaction, you will see evidence of:

- **grandiose thinking**
- **use of cocaine to decrease anxiety about the family's response**

- **denial**
- **deterioration of family relationships**
- **lack of control in the use of cocaine**

NURSE: Would you tell me a little about what led up to your coming into the program?

JIM: Well, I was on my way to work and I had to stop and get more coke before I went in. I was on my bike going about 110 mph. I always push it like that—going real fast. I don't worry about it because I know I'll always get away with it. They all know who I am.

NURSE: Who is "they"?

JIM: The police. All I have to do is show them a picture of my dad and they know right away who it is—he was a fireman and battalion chief for years. I was always getting pulled over when I was a kid, and they would just take the booze and tell me to go home because they knew who I was because of my dad. So, anyway, I'm driving along and my bike runs out of gas, so I'm trying to push it to get some gas and I get too tired and just push it to the side of the road, lay down on it, and go to sleep. It must have been about 2 hours later when one of these roadside helper vans came by and woke me up. They filled my tank and by then it was too late to go to work and I knew I couldn't go home because I think my family had decided they were going to get me to go for some help. So I went into the city, met these guys I deal with all the time, and traded them my bike for an 8-ball [an eighth of an ounce of cocaine] and a little money so I could get something to eat.

NURSE: Are you saying that your family was aware of your drug use and that's why you came in for treatment?

JIM: I don't really have a problem. I could quit any time, but they know there was something wrong. I had gotten to the point I would light up and smoke it in front of my sister.

NURSE: How did she react to that?

JIM: She asked me not to do it in front of her. She didn't like the way it made me act. My mom even told me she didn't like the way I had been acting. She told me the other day that she had gotten to the point she didn't even know who I was anymore. She wanted her Jimmy back. [Hands the nurse a sheet of paper.] I wrote this the other day. I don't know . . . maybe you'd like to read it and maybe not.

NURSE: Do you want me to read it?

JIM: Well . . . yeah.

[This was a poem about cocaine where cocaine is an entity calling out to the victim, promising euphoria, and taking away all his troubles.]

NURSE: You write here about this taking away all your troubles and cares. Is that how you feel about using cocaine?

JIM: When you're high you don't care about anything.

NURSE: How do you feel when you don't have the high?

JIM: Like going and getting more. Not now, though. I'm through. I've given it up and I'm not going to do it anymore.

NURSE: You sound pretty determined.

JIM: I am. I've got to get back to how I was before. My oldest daughter called me and told me she didn't like me the way I had become. She said I wasn't like her dad anymore. But she realized now it was the drugs. She wants me to get better so I'll be more fun than I have been lately. I used to be a pretty friendly guy, smiled a lot, liked to have a good time. Before I came here I usually just stayed at home and got high or was out trying to get more. ■

Self-Help Groups

Clients with Substance-Related Disorders and Their Families

Adult Children of Alcoholics (ACOA)
(213) 534-1815
www.recovery.org

Al-Anon/Alateen
(800) 344-2666
www.Al-Anon-Alateen.org

Alcoholics Anonymous
World Services Office
P.O. Box 459, Grand Central Station
New York, NY 10163
(212) 686-1100
www.alcoholics-anonymous.org

Cocaine Abuse
(800) 553-1694

800 Cocaine Information
(800) 262-2463

Co-Dependents Anonymous
(602) 277-7991
www.ourcoda.org

International Nurses Anonymous
1020 Sunset Drive
Lawrence, KS 66044
(913) 842-3893
www.suresite.com

Mothers Against Drunk Driving
(800) 438-MADD
www.madd.org

National Association for Children of Alcoholics
31582 Coast Highway, Suite B
South Laguna, CA 92677
(714) 499-3889
www.health.org

National Association for the Dually Diagnosed
(800) 331-5362

National Drug and Alcohol Treatment
Routing Service
(800) 622-HELP

Narcotics Anonymous
(800) 992-0401
www.wsoinc.com

Nurses and Recovery
(800) 872-9998

Women for Sobriety, Inc.
(800) 333-1606
www.mediapulse.com

Key Concepts

Introduction

- Chemical dependence is a chronic and progressive disease that can be fatal if untreated.

- Most people who are chemically dependent are poly-drug abusers.

- Substance abuse contributes to other illnesses, fetal syndromes, accidents, suicides, and homicides.

Knowledge Base

- The pattern of dependence on substances varies from person to person. Some abuse daily, some abuse on weekends, and others abuse on periodic binges.

- Blackouts are a form of amnesia for events that occur during the drinking period.

- Wernicke's disease results from thiamine deficiency and is characterized by ataxia, abnormal eye movements, and confusion.

- Korsakoff's syndrome is an inability to retain new information and a disruption in long-term memory.

- Confabulation is the making up of information to fill memory blanks.

- Alcohol withdrawal syndrome usually begins about 6–8 hours after the last drink and is characterized by irritability, anxiety, insomnia, and tremors. Later symptoms, referred to as delirium tremens, include seizures, hallucinations, disorientation, confusion, tachycardia, hypertension or hypotension, diaphoresis, and fever.

- The primary reason people use cocaine is to stimulate the CNS reward center. Cocaine alters DA transmission and affects the endorphins, GABA, and ACH.

- Amphetamines stimulate the CNS by inhibiting the reuptake of DA, 5-HT, and NE. Ice, the smokable form of methamphetamine, may substitute for cocaine as a stimulant because it is more easily available, is less expensive, and produces a much longer high.

- Cannabis, the drug category that includes marijuana and hashish, is the most widely used illegal drug in the United States.

- Hallucinogens can lead to accidents, out-of-control behavior, and a psychotic state.

- Opioids can be abused by prescription or through illegal sources. Withdrawal symptoms may last as long as 1–2 weeks.

- Sedatives, hypnotics, and anxiolytics provide a sense of well-being and relaxation. There is a great risk for addiction and overdose.

- Inhalants produce euphoria and perceptual changes; the use may lead to sudden death.

- Lack of control in using chemicals is the central behavioral characteristic of people who are chemically dependent. They may become loud, hostile, argumentative, and even violent. They may experience work or school problems and may become involved in a drug subculture.

- The overall intention of substance dependence is to decrease negative feelings and increase positive feelings. People who are chemically dependent are emotionally labile and experience guilt and shame.

- Alcoholic denial includes denial of facts, denial of implications, denial of change, and denial of feelings.

- Substance abuse is a family problem, and the most devastating impact occurs when the abuser is a parent. To avoid embarrassment, family members often deny the severity of the problem.

- Codependency may occur in non-substance-abusing partners when they become overresponsible and the substance-abusing partner becomes underresponsible. Codependents engage in enabling behavior, which is any action that facilitates substance dependence.

- Children growing up in a substance-abusing home learn not to talk about the problem, not to talk about their own needs and wants, and not to feel. They become objects whose reason for existence is to please the abusing parent. They are expected to be perfect and always in control. They learn very early not to trust other people.

- Children of alcoholics suffer the consequences of a dysfunctional family. They expect all relationships to be based on power, violence, deceit, and misinformation. Some grow up to repeat the family patterns by either becoming addicted themselves or marrying an addicted person.

- Most Americans view substance dependence as a sin or the result of a weak will. Women are more stigmatized than men, and lesbians suffer the double stigma of being lesbian and being alcoholic.

- Men abuse substances at a higher rate than women. Among women, twice as many European American women drink heavily compared to African American, Hispanic American, Asian American, and Native American women.

- The rate of premature death from the abuse of alcohol is 11 times higher than that from the abuse of other substances.

- Toxic levels of cocaine can cause seizures, cerebral hemorrhage, respiratory collapse, and cardiac arrest.

- People who have used hallucinogens may have dilated pupils, tachycardia, hypertension, muscle rigidity, and seizures. They may be confused, delirious, and psychotic.

- Heroin may cause respiratory depression and sudden, irreversible pulmonary edema.

- Sexually transmitted infections and AIDS are on the rise among people who abuse substances.

- Sexual consequences of substance-related disorders include decreased desire, erection problems, and orgasmic difficulties. Cocaine is linked to sexual acting-out behaviors.

- FAS is the third leading cause of birth defects in the United States. Effects include heart defects, malformed facial features, mental retardation, a slow growth rate, hyperactivity, and learning disabilities.

- Cocaine use during pregnancy is associated with an increased rate of prematurity, growth retardation, microcephaly, cerebral infarction, abnormal sleep patterns, tremors, poor feeding, irritability, seizures, and a tenfold greater risk of SIDS.

- Children who have been exposed to opioids prior to birth have an increased rate of prematurity, irritability, uncoordinated sucking and swallowing reflexes, and a 5–10 times higher risk of SIDS.

- Dual diagnosis indicates that there is a substance abuse problem as well as another coexisting mental disorder.

- Neurobiological theorists believe that an underlying predisposition to substance abuse is the result of genetic defects. Genetic defects lead to deficiencies and imbalance in neurotransmitters, neuropeptides, and receptors. An abnormal mechanism involving the reward center of the brain creates compulsive behaviors involving alcohol and drugs. The primary neurotransmitter involved is DA.

- Behavioral theory considers reinforcement principles that maintain substance dependence. Learning theory states that it is a result of learned maladaptive ways of coping.

- Sociocultural theory considers cultural and family values regarding the use of chemicals, peer group pressure, and the impact of racism in the development of chemical dependence.

- Feminist theory believes that addiction may be a response to an inadequate self-concept. There is often a history of abuse, dysfunctional relationships, or both.

- Medications used during alcohol withdrawal include Librium, Valium, Tranzene, Ativan, and thiamine. Antabuse and naltrexon may be used by some individuals to help avoid the impulse to drink.

- Opioid overdose is a medical emergency and is treated with Narcan intravenously. The client is likely to need repeat doses.

- Drug rehabilitation is the recovery of optimal health through medical, psychological, social, and peer group support. The recovery model is a lifelong, day-to-day process, typically includes 12-step programs, and places the responsibility for recovery on the client.

Nursing Assessment

- The nursing assessment begins with a substance abuse history and the CAGE Questionnaire. This is followed by a focused nursing assessment designed to elicit understanding of the impact of substance abuse on the client and family.

Nursing Diagnosis

- Nursing diagnoses include *Alteration in thought processes, Ineffective individual coping, Social isolation, Ineffective family coping, Powerlessness, Disturbance in self-concept, Ineffective denial,* and *High risk for violence.*

Outcome Identification

- Client outcomes include acknowledging the disorder and its negative consequences, sobriety, rehabilitation, and improved family coping.

Nursing Interventions

- Emergency management of acute alcohol intoxication or drug overdose is vitally important to save the client's life. Common problems include respiratory depression, seizures, and cardiovascular disorders. Clients may need ventilatory support, cardiac monitoring, seizure precautions, medications to support blood pressure, and treatment for hyperthermia.

- Nursing interventions include helping clients overcome denial and recognize the significance of their problem. This must occur before clients can make a commitment to abstinence and recovery.

- Relapse prevention includes self-control training. Clients are taught to identify and manage feelings, high-risk situations, and active coping strategies.

- Most substance-abusing clients need to learn how to solve problems rather than avoid problems through the use of drugs.

- Self-help groups for clients and families are an important part of the recovery process.

- Nutritional interventions can aid in the restoration of neurotransmitters.

- Clients may need vocational guidance such as educational programs and job training.

- A client's history of violent behavior is one of the best predictors of current potential for violence. Clients must be assessed frequently and provided with outlets for anxiety and energy. Other interventions include a quiet environment, PRN medication, and, if absolutely necessary, seclusion or restraints.

- Family members need help in identifying and changing codependent and enabling behaviors. They must learn new ways to respond to the client and how to respect and care for themselves.

- Spiritual support and hope installation promote recovery from substance abuse.

Evaluation

- Recovery is total abstinence from all drugs. The recovering person can never return to controlled use without rekindling the addiction.

Review Questions

1. Of the following people, who would be most likely to have the highest consumption of alcohol?
   a. an African American woman
   b. a European American woman
   c. a Hispanic American woman
   d. an Asian American woman

2. You have determined that your client often cannot remember what he did the night before while he was drinking. You would document this as
   a blackouts.
   b. confabulation.
   c. Wernicke's disease.
   d. Korsakoff's syndrome.

3. Your client, who abuses many substances, has three children. The oldest child acts as the surrogate parent and keeps the family functioning. This role is called the
   a. mascot.
   b. lost child.
   c. scapegoat.
   d. hero.

4. Your client has decided to take Antabuse to help him avoid using alcohol. Which one of the following statements should you include in your teaching?
   a. This medication can cause you to get a severe sunburn if you don't cover up and use sunscreen.
   b. Alcohol can cause a severe reaction as long as 14 days after you stop taking this medication.
   c. You must avoid driving while taking this medication because it will make you very sleepy.
   d. You must have BALs measured frequently because it is easy for blood to become toxic on this medication.

5. Your client in the emergency department has overdosed on cocaine. Which of the following interventions would be most appropriate?
   a. Determine blood pressure since hypotension may result from ruptured esophageal varicies.
   b. Use activated charcoal or gastric lavage.
   c. Reassure the client that he is not losing his mind and that the effects of the drug will wear off.
   d. Treat for hyperthermia and seizures.

References

Alcoholics Anonymous World Services. (1952). AA: 44 Questions. Alcoholics Anonymous World Services.

Am J Psychiatry. (1995). Practice guidelines for the treatment of patients with substance use disorders. *Am J Psychiatry, 152*(11), 5–80.

American Psychiatric Association. (1994). *Diagnostic and Statistical Manual of Mental Disorders,* (4th ed.) Washington, D.C.: American Psychiatric Press.

Baberg, H. T., et al. (1996). Amphetamine use. *Am J Psychiatry, 153*(6), 789–793.

Brown, S. A., et al. (1995). Alcoholism and affective disorder. *Am J Psychiatry, 152*(1), 45–52.

Coleman, P. (1993). Overview of substances. In R. D. Blondell (Ed.), *Primary Care: Substance Abuse* (pp. 1–18). Philadelphia: Saunders.

Crenshaw, T. L. & Goldberg, J. P. (1996). *Sexual Pharmacology.* New York: Norton.

Cummings, J. L., & Trimble, M. R. (1995). *Neuropsychiatry and Behavioral Neurology.* Washington, D.C.: American Psychiatric Press.

Desjarlais, R., et al. (1995). *World Mental Health.* Oxford, England: Oxford University Press.

Diamond, I., & Gordon, A. (1995). In H. Begleiter, & B. Kissin (Eds.), Biochemical phenotypic markers in genetic alcoholism. *The Genetics of Alcoholism.* Oxford, England: Oxford University Press.

Evans, K., & Sullivan, J. M. (1995). *Treating Addicted Survivors of Trauma.* New York: Guilford Press.

Foulks, E. F., & Pena, J. M. (1995). Ethnicity and psychotherapy. *Psychiatr Clin North Am, 18*(3), 607–620.

Freed, P. E., & Nattkemper, L. (1997) Naltrexone: A controversial therapy for alcohol dependence. *J Psychosoc Nurs, 35*(7): 24–28.

George, D. T., et al. (1997). Behavioral and neuroendocrine responses to m-chlorophenylpiperazine in subtypes of alcoholics. *Am J Psychiatry, 154*(1), 81–87.

Hedaya, R. J. (1996). *Understanding Biological Psychiatry.* New York: Norton.

Higuchi, S., et al. (1995). Alcohol and aldehyde dehydrogenase polymorphisms and the risk for alcoholism. *Am J Psychiatry, 152*(8), 1219–1221.

Kearney, R. J. (1996). *Within the Wall of Denial.* New York: Norton.

Kinney, J. (1996). *Clinical Manual of Substance Abuse.* (2nd ed.) St. Louis, MO: Mosby.

Little, K. Y., et al. (1996). Alteration of brain dopamine and serotonin levels in cocaine users. *Am J Psychiatry, 153*(9), 1216–1218.

Mayfield, D. G., McCleod, G., & Hall, P. (1974). The CAGE questionnaire. *Am J Psychiatry, 131,* 1121–1123.

Miller, D. T. (1997). Dual diagnosis: A clinical challenge. *Nurs Spectrum,* 14–15.

O'Brien, C. P. (1997). Progress in the science of addiction. *Am J Psychiatry, 154*(9), 1195–1197.

O'Malley, S. S., et al. (1996). Experience of a "slip" among alcoholics treated with naltrexone or placebo. *Am J Psychiatry, 153*(2), 281–283.

Pace, E. P.(1995). *Achievement and Addiction.* New York: Brunner/Mazel.

Ruden, R. A. (1997). *The Craving Brain.* New York: HarperCollins.

Schuckit, M. A., et al. (1997). Comparison of induced and independent major depressive disorders in 2,945 alcoholics. *Am J Psychiatry, 154*(7), 948–956.

Skinner, W. F. (1994). The prevalence and demographic predictors of illicit and licit drug use among lesbians and gay men. *Am J Public Health, 84*(8), 1307–1310.

Spector, R. E. (1996). *Cultural Diversity in Health & Illness.* (4th ed.) Norwalk, CT: Appleton & Lange.

Streissguth, A. P., & O'Malley, K. D. (1997). Fetal alcohol syndrome/fetal alcohol effects. *Treatment Today, 9*(2), 16–17.

Tiedje, L. B., & Starn, J. R. (1996). Intervention model for substance-using women. *IMAGE, 28*(2), 113–118.

Tsai, G., et al.(1995). The glutamatergic basis of human alcoholism. *Am J Psychiatry, 152*(3), 332–340.

Volavka, J. (1995). *Neurobiology of Violence.* Washington, D.C.: American Psychiatric Press.

Washton, A. M. (1995). Clinical assessment of psychoactive substance use. In A. M. Washton (Ed.), *Psychotherapy and Substance Abuse.* New York: Guilford Press.

Williams, T. G. (1996). Substance abuse and addictive personality disorder. In F. W. Kaslow (Ed.), *Handbook of Relational Diagnosis and Dysfunctional Family Patterns.* New York: Wiley & Sons.

Wing, D. M. (1996). A concept analysis of alcoholic denial and cultural accounts. *Adv Nurs Sci, 19*(2), 54–63.

CHAPTER 14

Personality Disorders

Karen Lee Fontaine

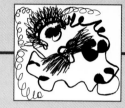

Objectives

After reading this chapter, you will be able to:

- Describe the concept of personality disorder.
- Identify the characteristics of the three clusters of personality disorders.
- Discuss the causative theories of personality disorders.
- Specify assessment criteria for clients with these disorders.
- Identify basic approaches nurses use when working with clients in the three clusters of personality disorders.
- Plan and implement care based on identified priorities.
- Identify your own feelings when caring for these clients.
- Evaluate and modify the plan of care for clients with personality disorders.

Key Terms

antisocial personality disorder
avoidant personality disorder
borderline personality disorder
Cluster A
Cluster B
Cluster C
dependent personality disorder
histrionic personality disorder
narcissistic personality disorder
obsessive-compulsive personality disorder
paranoid personality disorder
schizoid personality disorder
schizotypal personality disorder

To understand the nature of personality disorders, it is helpful to review the concept of personality. Personalities develop as people adapt to their physical, emotional, social, and spiritual environments. *Personality* determines how people cope with feelings and impulses, how they see themselves and others, how they respond to their surroundings, and how they find meaning in relationships and cultural values. These patterns are noticeable in a wide variety of situations. A personality becomes *disordered* when the patterns are inflexible and maladaptive. Some people with personality disorders suffer intense emotional pain, while others seem invulnerable to painful feelings. Some are able to maintain relationships and careers, while others become functionally impaired.

Clients with personality disorders are among the most difficult to treat. Most will never enter a psychiatric hospital, seek or receive outpatient treatment, or even undergo a diagnostic evaluation. Some will enter the mental health system through family pressure or because of a court order. With those who do come into the system, mental health professionals find their expertise tested. In the majority of cases, the personality problems are ego-syntonic. They perceive their difficulties in dealing with other people to be external to them. Incapable of considering that their problems have anything to do with them personally, they will describe being victimized by specific others or by "the system." Some may develop an awareness of their self-defeating behavior but remain at a loss as to how they got that way or how to begin to change.

Personality disorders are diagnosed or coded on Axis II of the *DSM-IV*. There is a high degree of overlap among the personality disorders, and many individuals exhibit traits of several disorders. Typically, personality disorders become apparent before or during adolescence and persist throughout life. In some cases, the symptoms become less obvious by middle or old age (Personality Disorders, 1996).

It is extremely difficult to estimate the incidence of personality disorders. Many people with personality disorders never come to the attention of the mental health system. The best estimate is that 6–13% of the general population suffers from some disruption serious enough to be diagnosed as a personality disorder. Currently, the most commonly diagnosed is borderline personality disorder. This group accounts for 50% of the diagnoses, and all the other disorders together make up the remaining 50%. Of all psychiatric inpatients, 15% are diagnosed with borderline personality disorder (Isometsa et al, 1996).

Knowledge Base

There are ten personality disorders, grouped into three clusters. The disorders within each cluster are considered to have similar characteristics. The clusters and corresponding disorders are:

Cluster A

1. Paranoid

2. Schizoid

3. Schizotypal

Cluster B

4. Antisocial

5. Borderline

6. Histrionic

7. Narcissistic

Cluster C

8. Avoidant

9. Dependent

10. Obsessive-compulsive

People with diagnoses from **Cluster A** usually appear eccentric, and they exhibit much withdrawal behavior. People with diagnoses from **Cluster B** appear dramatic, emotional, or erratic. They tend to be very exploitive in their behavior. People with diagnoses from **Cluster C** are those who appear anxious or fearful. Their behavior pattern is one of compliance. Table 14.1 summarizes these characteristics.

Cluster A Disorders

Paranoid Personality Disorder

Behaviorally, people with **paranoid personality disorder** are very secretive about their entire existence. Confiding in other people is perceived as dangerous and is not likely to occur, even within family relationships. Paranoid people are hyperalert to danger, search for evidence of attack, and become argumentative as a

■ *Table 14.1* Characteristics of Personality Disorders

Cluster	Behavioral	Affective	Cognitive	Sociocultural
A	Eccentric, craves solitude, argumentative, odd speech	Quick anger, social anxiety, blunted affect	Unable to trust, indecisive, poverty of thoughts	Impaired or nonexistent relationships; occupational difficulties
B	Dramatic, craves excitement, wants immediate gratification, self-mutilates	Intense, labile affect; no sense of guilt; anxious; depressed	Considers self special and unique, egocentric, identity disturbances, no long-range plans	Manipulates and exploits others; stormy relationships
C	Tense, rigid routines, submissive, inflexible	Anxious, fearful, depressed	Moralistic, low self-confidence	Dependent on others, avoids overt conflict, seeks constant unconditional love

way of creating a safe distance between themselves and others. They rarely seek help for their personality problems, and they seldom require hospitalization.

Affectively, paranoid people typically avoid sharing their feelings except for a very quick expression of anger. They may never forgive perceived slights and may bear grudges for long periods of time. There is a prevalent fear of losing power or control to others. These individuals experience a chronic state of tension and are rarely able to relax.

Cognitively, paranoid people are very guarded about themselves and secretive about their decisions. They expect to be used or harassed by others. When confronted with new situations, they look for hidden, demeaning, or threatening meanings to benign remarks or events, and they respond by criticizing others. For example, if there is an error in a bank statement, the paranoid person may say the bank did it to ruin his or her credit rating.

Socioculturally, paranoid people have great difficulty with intimate relationships. They interact in a cold and aloof manner, thus avoiding the perceived dangers of intimacy. Because they expect to be harmed by others, they question the loyalty or trustworthiness of family and friends. Pathological jealousy of the spouse or sex partner frequently occurs (Personality Disorders, 1996).

Devin's boss has been critical of Devin's inability to get his work done in a timely fashion. Although Devin is constantly trying to hear what others are talking about and is easily distracted,

he is unable to relate this behavior to his job difficulties. Instead he states, "People at work keep bothering me and talking to each other just to slow me down. They are trying to turn my boss against me. Every little thing I do or say is used against me."

Schizoid Personality Disorder

Behaviorally, people with **schizoid personality disorder** are loners who prefer solitary activities because social situations and interactions increase their level of anxiety. They may be occupationally impaired if the job requires interpersonal skills. However, if work may be performed under conditions of social isolation, such as being a night guard in a closed facility, they may be capable of satisfactory occupational achievement.

Affectively, people with schizoid personality disorder are stable but have a limited range of feelings. Their affect is blunted or flat. Because they do not express their feelings either verbally or nonverbally, they give the impression that they have no strong positive or negative emotions. However, if they are forced into a close interaction, they may become very anxious.

Cognitively, they could be described as having poverty of thoughts. The thoughts they do express are often vague. Some of their beliefs are these: "It doesn't matter what other people think of me" and "Close relationships are undesirable."

Socioculturally, they interact with others in a cold and aloof manner, have no close friends, and prefer not to be in any relationships. They are indifferent to the attitudes and feelings of others, and thus are not influenced by praise or criticism (O'Brien, Trestman, and Siever, 1993).

> Charlie, age 34, lives alone in a residential hotel. He is employed as a night guard in a warehouse. He interacts minimally with the other night guards and always eats his meals by himself. He has no friends and no social contacts outside of work. He describes people as "replaceable." He visits his parents, who live a mile away, once a year.

Schizotypal Personality Disorder

Behaviorally, people with **schizotypal personality disorder** have a considerable disability. With peculiarities of ideation, appearance, and behavior that are not severe enough to meet the criteria for schizophrenic disorder, this disorder appears to be related to schizophrenia. Some studies have shown a greater prevalence of this personality disorder among biological relatives of people suffering from schizophrenia. Under periods of extreme stress and anxiety, they may experience transient psychotic symptoms that are not of sufficient duration to make an additional diagnosis (Millon and Kotik-Harper, 1995).

People with this disorder exhibit odd speech. It is coherent but often tangential and vague or, at times, overelaborate. They prefer solitary activities and often experience occupational difficulties.

Affectively, they are typically constricted, and their affect may be inappropriate to the situation at times. Social situations create anxiety for those with schizotypal personality disorder.

Cognitively, these individuals experience the most severe distortions of any of the personality disorders. The disturbances include paranoid ideation, suspiciousness, ideas of reference, odd beliefs, and magical thinking. They may experience illusions such as seeing people in the movement of shadows. They usually experience difficulty in making decisions.

Socioculturally, they fear intimacy and desire no relationships with family or friends. Thus, they are very isolative and are usually avoided by others (O'Brien, Trestman, and Siever, 1993).

> Carol, a 24-year-old unemployed single woman, lives in a rooming house. She keeps to herself, and most of the other boarders in the rooming house find her to be eccentric. Carol is preoccupied with the idea that her dead father was a movie star who left her a fortune with which her guardian absconded. Carol has a habit of saying odd things like, "So go the days of our lives." Most of the rooming house boarders avoid Carol because of her strange behaviors.

Cluster B Disorders

The three unstable disorders in this category—borderline, histrionic, and narcissistic—can barely be distinguished from one another. More so than with other disorders, the diagnosis may be influenced by personal bias, gender stereotypes, and cultural prejudices on the part of the professional.

Antisocial Personality Disorder

A diagnosis of **antisocial personality disorder (ASPD)** requires that the characteristics appear before the age of 15, and the client is usually given the diagnosis of conduct disorder. The diagnosis of antisocial personality disorder is not applied until after the age of 18. In boys, the behavior typically emerges during childhood, while for girls it is more likely to occur around puberty.

Behaviorally, predominant childhood manifestations are lying, stealing, truancy, vandalism, fighting, and running away from home. In adulthood, the pattern changes to failure to honor financial obligations, an inability to function as a responsible parent, a tendency to lie pathologically, and an inability to sustain consistent appropriate work behavior. People with ASPD conform to rules only when they are useful to them.

Affectively, people with ASPD express themselves quickly and easily but with very little personal involvement. Thus, they can profess undying love one minute and terminate the relationship the next. In addition, they are very irritable and aggressive. They have no concern for others and experience no guilt when they violate society's rules.

Cognitively, people with ASPD are egocentric and grandiose. They are extremely confident that everything will always work out in their favor because they believe they are more clever than everyone else. The disorder is ego-syntonic, and they have no desire to change in any way. They make no long-range plans.

Socioculturally, these individuals are generally unable to sustain lasting, close, warm, and responsible relationships. Their sexual behavior is impersonal and impulsive. They exploit others in a cold and calculating way, while disregarding others' feelings and rights. With their quick anger, poor tolerance of frustration, and lack of guilt, they are often emotionally, physically, and sexually abusive to others (*DSM-IV,* 1994).

> Stephen, a divorced 20-year-old, works as a busperson at a pizza parlor, but he has a new job every other month. Stephen has an arrest record going back to high school. There, he was often truant and was picked up many times by the police for using marijuana and receiving stolen goods. Stephen often took money from his mother's purse, and he once fenced the family silver for drug money. Stephen married when he was 18, but the marriage lasted only 6 months. Stephen liked having women on the side, and his wife wasn't very understanding. When she nagged him about going out, Stephen beat her up. Stephen is working as a busperson to get enough money together to start a marijuana crop. As soon as he has enough money to buy some starter plants, he plans to go into business for himself.

Borderline Personality Disorder

Individuals with **borderline personality disorder (BPD)** exhibit a heterogeneous mixture of symptoms.

Behaviorally, people with BPD are generally impulsive, unpredictable, and manipulative. They engage in such self-destructive behaviors as reckless driving, substance abuse, binge eating, risky sexual practices, financial mismanagement, and violence. Self-mutilation, suicide threats, and attempted suicide are maladaptive responses to intense pain or attempts to relieve the sense of emptiness and gain reassurance that they are alive and can feel pain. (See Chapter 6 for a full discussion of self-mutilation.) They may manipulate others to act against them in a negative or aggressive way. They alternate between periods of competence and incompetence. Although they do not deliberately avoid responsibility, they cannot explain how such avoidance occurs. They may be arrogant and challenging one minute and eager to please and submissive the next (Cowdry, 1997; Greene and Ugarriza, 1995).

Affectively, people with BPD are intense and unstable. They often have difficulty managing anxiety. Some are anxious most of the time, some have recurrent bouts of anxiety, and others experience intermittent panic attacks. People with BPD have difficulty tolerating and moderating strong feelings, which rapidly escalate to intense states of emotion. Irritation jumps to rage, sadness to despair, and disappointment to hopelessness. Their emotions are labile without any apparent reason or stimulus. Anger is often the predominant feeling. Some are incapable of caring for or loving others because of their feelings of inferiority. They might say they don't deserve to exist. In contrast, most have an inability to experience empathy in interactions with others or guilt for personal wrongdoings (Stein, 1996).

Cognitively, people with BPD are characterized by identity disturbance. Their self-descriptions tend to be vague and confusing. These individuals often suffer from changing identity and body image and changing sexual orientation, all of which may be indications of transient dissociative states. Some take on the identity of the people with whom they are interacting. Self-evaluation of abilities and talents alternates between grandiosity and depreciation. At times, they feel entitled to special treatment and, at other times, unworthy of anyone's attention. Believing the world is dangerous and hostile, they feel powerless and vulnerable. Another cognitive characteristic is dichotomous thinking—things are either all good or all bad. For example, people with BPD are unable to see both positive and negative qualities in the same person at the same time. Psychotic episodes are common for some clients with BPD. These episodes may be brief or lengthy and are likely to result in repeated hospitalizations (Gold, 1996).

Socioculturally, people with BPD have a history of intense, unstable, and manipulative relationships. Inside is a deprived, fragile child who grew up in a dysfunctional family. As adults, they desperately seek the love and nurturing they never received as a child. At the same time, they fear they will be abused and abandoned by others. This fear leads to rapid shifts from extremes of dependency to extremes of autonomy. Desperate clinging alternates with accusations and fights, in a frantic effort to avoid abandonment (Gunderson, 1996).

There is a great overlap between BPD and all the other personality disorders. Because symptoms vary in any given client at any given time, the disorder is both difficult to diagnose and difficult to treat. These clients use a large amount of mental health resources, often present themselves in acute crisis, and frequently drop out of treatment programs (Gold, 1996). Two-thirds of people diagnosed with BPD are female. Some professionals believe that the borderline diagnosis has become the negative catch-all of psychiatric diagnoses. There is concern that any female client who is resistant to an authoritarian therapist is labeled BPD. Other explanations for the high rate of occurrence among females include the stresses of being female in a sexist culture, gender differences for "normal" behavior, and differences in the socialization of boys and girls. Many people with BPD have been sexually abused as children. For these individuals a better diagnosis might be atypical posttraumatic stress disorder or severe survivor syndrome, neither of which are standard diagnoses in the *DSM-IV* (Cowdry, 1997; Evans and Sullivan, 1995).

> Julie, a 25-year-old part-time college student, frequently tells her friends how inconsiderate her parents are because they don't take care of her the way they "should" and, conversely, how awful it is because she can't become independent and live on her own. At times she tries to manipulate her friends into doing things for her, and at other times she barely acknowledges that they exist. After dating Greg for only 2 weeks, she has told everyone he is absolutely perfect and they are "madly in love." One afternoon, Greg tells Julie he can't see her that evening because he must study for an exam. Julie flies into a rage, jumps into her car, and goes to a local bar, where she impulsively picks up a stranger and has sex with him in the parking lot. Returning home, she scratches her wrists with a broken bottle and calls Greg to tell him it's all his fault that she slashed her wrists and is going to die.

Histrionic Personality Disorder

Behaviorally, people with **histrionic personality disorder** (HPD) are most prominently characterized by seeking stimulation and excitement in life. Their behavior and appearance focus attention on themselves in an attempt to evoke and maintain the interest of others. They are seen as colorful, extroverted, and seductive individuals who seem always to be the center of attention. When they don't get their own way, however, they believe they are being treated unfairly and may even have a temper tantrum. They

may resort to assaultive behavior or suicidal gestures to punish others.

Affectively, people with HPD are overly dramatic. Even minor stimuli cause emotional excitability and an exaggerated expression of feelings. They often seem to be on a roller coaster of joy and despair.

Cognitively, they are very self-centered. They become overly concerned with how others perceive them because of a high need for approval. Thoughts are, for example: "I need other people to admire me in order to be happy," "People are there to admire me and do my bidding," and "I cannot tolerate boredom." Histrionic people are guided more by their feelings than by their thinking, which tends to be vague and impressionistic. The basic belief is: "I don't have to bother to think things through—I can go by my gut feeling."

Socioculturally, they constantly seek assurance, approval, or praise from family and friends. There is often exaggeration in their interpersonal relationships, with an emphasis on acting out the role of victim or princess. People with HPD commonly have flights of romantic fantasy, though the actual quality of their sexual relationships is variable. They may be overly trusting and respond very positively to strong authority figures, whom they think will magically solve their problems (Millon and Kotik-Harper, 1995).

> Leticia, a 25-year-old hairdresser, is popular with her clients. Leticia is very attractive, with long black hair and elegantly sculptured nails. She always wears the latest fashions and lots of jewelry. Leticia enjoys entertaining her customers with tales of exploits with the many men in her life. Recently, she told of meeting a handsome cowboy in a bar and deciding to go to Las Vegas with him for the weekend. She claimed he treated her like a queen, hiring a chauffeured limo, dining by candlelight, and dancing until dawn. However, Leticia doesn't plan to see the young man again because she lives by the motto, "So many men, so little time!"

Narcissistic Personality Disorder

Behaviorally, those with **narcissistic personality disorder** (NPD) strive for power and success. Failure is intolerable because of their own perfectionistic standards. They do what they can to maintain and expand their superior position. Thus, they may seek wealth, power, and importance as a way to support their "superior" image. They tend to be highly competitive with others they view as also being superior.

Affectively, people with NPD are often labile. If criticized, they may fly into a rage. At other times, they may experience anxiety and panic and short periods of depression. They try to avoid feelings of blame and guilt because of intense fear of humiliation. When their needs are not met, they may react with rage or shame but mask these feelings with an aura of cool indifference.

Cognitively, those with narcissistic personality disorder are arrogant and egotistical. They are even more grandiose than people with HPD. They have a tendency to exaggerate their accomplishments and talents. They expect to be noticed and treated as special whether or not they have achieved anything. Their feelings of specialness may alternate with feelings of special unworthiness. They are preoccupied with fantasies of unlimited success, power, brilliance, beauty, and ideal love. Underneath this confident manner is very low self-esteem.

Socioculturally, people with NPD have disturbed relationships. They have unreasonable expectations of favorable treatment and exploit others to achieve personal goals. Friendships are made on the basis of how they can profit from the other person. Romantic partners are used as objects to bolster self-esteem. They are unable to develop a relationship based on mutuality (Millon and Kotik-Harper, 1995).

> Santo, a 43-year-old attorney, lives in an expensive house and drives a foreign sports car. He thrives on letting others know how successful his law practice is and about all the luxuries it affords him. He pays meticulous attention to his appearance. He has had multiple affairs during his marriage and justifies these by saying that his wife isn't living up to his expectations. He doesn't believe others have a right to criticize him and becomes irate if his wife makes requests of him.

Cluster C Disorders

Avoidant Personality Disorder
Behaviorally, social discomfort is the primary characteristic of people with avoidant **personality disorder (APD)**. Any social or occupational activities that involve significant interpersonal contact are avoided. The belief underlying this behavior is: "If people get close to me, they will discover the 'real' me and reject me."

Affectively, these individuals are fearful and shy. They are easily hurt by criticism and devastated by the slightest hint of disapproval. They are distressed by their lack of ability to relate to others and often experience depression, anxiety, and anger for failing to develop social relationships.

Cognitively, people with APD are overly sensitive to the opinions of others. They suffer from an exaggerated need for acceptance. The thought is: "If others criticize me, they must be right."

Socioculturally, they are reluctant to enter into relationships without a guarantee of uncritical acceptance. Since unconditional approval is not guaranteed, they have few close friends. In social situations, people with APD are afraid of saying something inappropriate or foolish or of being unable to answer a question. They are terrified of being embarrassed by blushing, crying, or showing signs of anxiety to other people (Millon and Kotik-Harper, 1995).

> Eric, a 22-year-old college senior, is considered shy by other students. Eric stays in his room studying and generally avoids parties. He has no real friends at college and spends his time watching television when he has no homework. Eric has a hard time in some of his classes, especially those that require him to speak in front of the group. He frets for hours over being embarrassed by something he might say that will make him look foolish. In class, Eric never sits next to the same person twice because this helps him avoid having to socialize. He has been admiring a girl named Jennie in his philosophy class, but he has never attempted to speak to her. Eric has been trying to find a way to ask Jennie out. However, everything he plans to say seems foolish. He is afraid Jennie will say no.

Dependent Personality Disorder
Behaviorally, dependence and submissiveness are the major features of **dependent personality disorder (DPD)**. People with DPD have difficulty doing things by themselves and getting things done on their own. They go to great lengths not to be alone and always agree with others to avoid rejection. With a strong need to be liked, dependent people volunteer to do unpleasant or demeaning things to increase their chances of acceptance. They avoid occupations in which they must perform independent functions.

Affectively, they fear rejection and abandonment. They feel totally helpless when they are alone. They are easily hurt by criticism and disapproval and are devastated when close relationships end. These fears contribute to a chronic sense of anxiety, and they may develop depression.

Cognitively, people with DPD have a severe lack of self-confidence and belittle their abilities and assets. Unable to make everyday decisions without an excessive amount of advice and reassurance from others, they often allow others to make choices for them. They exercise dichotomous thinking, such as: "One is either totally dependent and helpless or one is totally independent and isolated."

Socioculturally, those with DPD desire constant companionship because they feel helpless when they are alone. Passively resisting making decisions, they often force their spouses or partners into making important choices for them, such as where to live, where to work, with whom to socialize, and in what activities to participate (Millon and Kotik-Harper, 1995).

> Min, a 32-year-old homemaker, married at 18 and moved directly from relying on her parents to relying on her husband. She was unable to go to any stores alone and unable to drive. She relied on her husband to pick out her clothing because she felt she had no taste. She stayed in the marriage for 10 years, even though her husband was verbally abusive and had multiple affairs. When she separated from her husband, she felt devastated, even though it was a terrible relationship. Within a few months, Min remarried and felt very relieved to be taken care of again.

Obsessive-Compulsive Personality Disorder

Behaviorally, people with **obsessive-compulsive personality disorder (OCPD)** exhibit perfectionism and inflexibility. The need to check and recheck objects and situations demands much of their time and energy. They are industrious workers, but because of their need for routine, they are usually not creative. They may fail to complete projects because of the unattainable standards they set for themselves. No accomplishment ever seems good enough.

People with OCPD are polite and formal in social situations, where they can maintain emotional distance from others. They are very protective of their status and material possessions, so they have difficulty freely sharing with other people.

Affectively, they are unable to express emotions. To alleviate the anxiety of helplessness and power-lessness, they need to feel in control. Total control means that emotions, both tender and hostile, must be held in check or denied. Life and interpersonal relationships are intellectualized. The blocking of feelings and emotional distance are attempts to avoid losing control over themselves and their environment.

Because defenses are rarely adequate to manage anxiety, they develop a number of fears. They fear disapproval and condemnation from others and therefore avoid taking risks. They dread making mistakes. When mistakes occur, they experience a high level of guilt and self-recrimination, thus becoming their own tormentors. They also fear losing control. Rules and regulations are an attempt to remain in control at all times. Still fearful that things could go wrong, people with OCPD invent rituals in an attempt to ensure constancy and increase their feelings of security. As they try to control fear with a narrow focus on details and routines, the need for order and routine escalates.

People with OCPD have three types of *cognitive* distortions: perfectionism, a need for certainty, and a belief in an absolutely correct solution for every problem. Procrastination and indecision are common because they would rather avoid commitments than experience failure. Before making a decision, they accumulate many facts and try to figure out all the potential outcomes of any particular decision. When a decision is finally made, they are plagued by doubts and fears that an alternative decision would have been better. Since there is a constant striving to be perfect in all things, doing nothing is often considered better than doing something imperfectly. The underlying belief is: "I must avoid mistakes to be worthwhile."

Questioned as to how they view themselves, they say they are conscientious, loyal, dependable, and responsible—descriptions that conflict with an underlying low self-esteem and belief of inadequacy.

Socioculturally, their need for control extends to interpersonal relationships. Regarding themselves as omnipotent (all-powerful) and omniscient (all-knowing), they expect their opinions and plans to be acceptable to everyone else; compromise is hardly considered. Frequent demands on their families to cooperate with their rigid rules and detailed routines undermine feelings of intimacy within the family system. Because they view dependency as being out of control and under the domination of the partner, they may abuse or oppress their partners so that an illusion of power and control can be maintained.

When interacting, people with OCPD have an overintellectual, meticulous, detailed manner of speaking designed to increase feelings of security. They unconsciously use language to confuse the listener. By bringing in side issues and focusing on nonessentials, they distort the content of the subject, which is a source of great frustration to the listener (Stone, 1993).

> Jim, a 42-year-old mid-level executive for a food-processing plant, is always in trouble with the plant manager because he fails to get reports in on time. Jim blames his secretary for the problem, saying, "I can't get anything done right unless I do it myself." However, Jim's secretary promptly types exactly what he gives her. Jim then adds new details and reorganizes the report, and she has to type a new version. Jim keeps all the drafts of the report and documents the time it takes for the secretary to type them. He stores these in a file that only he is allowed to use. Jim lost his "to do" list one morning and had his secretary help him try to find it for over half an hour. Jim yelled at the secretary when she suggested that he try to remember what was on the list.

Obsessive-compulsive personality disorder (OCPD) must be distinguished from obsessive-compulsive disorder (OCD). In the past, it was thought that OCD was a more severe form of OCPD. Research indicates distinct differences between the disorders, with only 20% of people with OCD exhibiting characteristics of the personality disorder (Stone, 1993). People with OCD do not experience rigid patterns of many behaviors, the restricted affect, nor the excessive passion for productivity. OCD is ego-dystonic, while OCPD is ego-syntonic.

Personality Disorder Not Otherwise Specified

The label *personality disorder not otherwise specified* is used when a person does not meet the full criteria for any one personality disorder, yet there is significant impairment in social or occupational functioning or in subjective distress (*DSM-IV,* 1994).

Concomitant Disorders

There is a high correlation between substance abuse and antisocial personality disorder. In several studies, it has been found that the rate of ASPD is as high as 50% among male opioid addicts and alcoholics. At

---

Critical Thinking

Marty is a 27-year-old client whose problems began during childhood. He was frequently in trouble at school for biting, fighting, or stealing. He also stole money from his parents and siblings and was arrested at the age of 17 for shoplifting. Marty consistently denied any wrongdoing.

Marty had held a series of low-paying jobs. When not terminated because of aggressive behavior or suspicion of stealing, he quit, always blaming someone else for his failure.

Marty has had numerous girlfriends, one of whom became pregnant. Marty coldly told the girl he was sure it wasn't his child, she should have an abortion, and to leave him alone.

When confronted about his behavior, Marty fails to show remorse for having broken the law or for emotionally hurting others. You are the nursing student assigned to care for Marty. You have not cared for a client with Marty's diagnosis, but you have cared for a client with borderline personality disorder.

1. What conclusions can be drawn about Marty based on his past and present behavior?
2. What data support your conclusions?
3. Explain Marty's behavior in light of "social" causative theory?
4. How will your care of a previous client with borderline personality disorder benefit you when planning care for Marty?
5. What nursing interventions would be helpful for the client with a cluster C disorder but could be detrimental to the client with a cluster B disorder?

Suggested answers can be found in Appendix D.

---

times, it is difficult to separate these disorders, as substance abuse is itself an antisocial behavior that causes problems similar to those of the personality disorder. Thus, substance abusers are divided into two groups: *primary antisocial addicts,* whose antisocial behavior is independent of the need to obtain drugs, and *secondary antisocial addicts,* whose antisocial behavior is directly related to drug use (Oldham et al, 1995; Volavka, 1995). Psychotic disorders often co-occur with schizotypal, borderline, and dependent personality disorders. Mood disorders co-occur more often with avoidant and borderline personality disorders, and anxiety disorders co-occur with avoidant, dependent, and borderline personality disorders (Oldham et al, 1995). Suicides among people with personality disorders are often associated with those who are concurrently depressed, abuse substances, or both (Isometsa et al, 1996).

Causative Theories

As with other psychiatric disorders, a number of theories have been offered to identify the causes of personality disorders. With continuing refinement of diagnostic criteria for each cluster of disorders, it will become possible to conduct useful research on specific populations that have been accurately diagnosed. In the past, wide differences in the application of specific diagnostic labels precluded the gathering of reliable data. Since there was so little agreement about whether a person should be included in the category at the outset, it is easy to understand why the search for any common factors—in genetics, early experiences, family patterns, or any other variable—failed to yield results from which general conclusions could be drawn.

Remaining obstacles are the refusal to seek treatment on the part of the client and the relatively infrequent need for psychiatric hospitalization. These obstacles have limited research to those seeking therapy (most often with borderline personality disorder) or those being referred through the criminal system (most often with antisocial personality disorder).

There is no single cause of the personality disorders. Most likely, they arise from an interaction between biological factors and the environment. Just as one's biology or constitution can alter experiences in life, so, too, may experiences alter one's basic biology. The brain constantly changes to absorb new experiences.

Neurobiological Theory

It is thought that abusive experiences have affected the neurological development of people with BPD. BPD is primarily a disorder of impulse control, which most likely occurs from excessive CNS irritability. There may be problems with limbic system regulation. People diagnosed with BPD appear to have lower serotonin (5-HT) activity than control groups. The lower the 5-HT levels, the more likely the client is to self-mutilate, experience intense rage, and behave aggressively toward others. A concurrent high level of norepinephrine (NE) creates hypersensitivity to the environment. Abnormalities in levels of dopamine (DA) may explain the psychotic episodes experienced by some clients with BPD and schizotypal personality disorder (deVegvar and Siever, 1994; Greene and Ugarriza, 1995).

Recent research has found that there may be a relationship between criminal behavior and physiological underarousal to stimulation. This underarousal may contribute to antisocial behavior as these individuals seek stimulating situations. Schizotypal personality disorder may be, in fact, a milder schizophrenia-spectrum disorder. Further research is needed to understand the relationship between these disorders (Raine et al, 1995; Roitman et al, 1997).

Intrapersonal Theory

People with Cluster A personality disorders have been studied minimally because they seldom request or are forced into treatment. Intrapersonal theory suggests that the primary defense mechanism is one of projection; that is, they project their own hostility on others and respond to them in a fearful and distrustful manner. It is also thought that they defensively withdraw from others for fear they will be hurt (Personality Disorders, 1996).

With Cluster B disorders, intrapersonal theorists focus on the child's relationship with the parents. Johnson describes the parental message to the child: "Don't be who you are, be who I need you to be. Who you are disappoints me, threatens me, angers me, overstimulates me. Be what I want and I will love you" (1987, p. 52). Johnson goes on to say that the child is forced to reject the real self and develop a false self. Individuation is prevented when the child is forced to become the idealized person the parents desire. As adults, these individuals become grandiose in an attempt to live up to exaggerated parental expectations. In an attempt to prove the false self to others and compensate for the rejected real self, they focus on having the right clothes, home, car, and career. Perfectionist standards become a defense against unrealistic expectations.

Intrapersonal theory explains ASPD as a developmental delay or failure. It is believed that people with ASPD have an underdeveloped superego, in that authority and cultural morals have not been internalized. Conformity to cultural expectations is situational and superficial, and there is an inability to experience guilt when rules are violated.

Individuals with BPD often think, feel, and behave more like toddlers than adults. When young children experience inadequate parenting, their basic needs and desires remain unsatisfied. Unmet needs lead to hostility toward those upon whom their lives depend. At the same time, these children are terrified by the destructiveness of their anger. They begin to believe that they have been, or will be, abandoned, and the parents are unable to provide good experiences to balance the intense feelings of neglect. All of this contributes to making adults who feel so utterly empty inside that they can never get enough attention and nurturing. At the same time, they are terrified of intimacy because of their fears of abandonment. This constant tension between need and fear leads to acting out feelings of rage and self-destructive behavior to manage the guilt (Personality Disorders, 1996).

Social Theory

A variety of social conditions lead to low self-esteem, negative self-concept, and even self-hatred. When one is on the receiving end of social oppression, it is more difficult to develop self-esteem and a healthy identity.

Cluster B personality disorders may be a response to society's increasing complexity. Some believe that industrialization, for example, has contributed to a changing value system. We have come to recognize values such as these: Personal needs are more important than group needs, expediency is more important than morality, and appearance is more important than inner worth. Believing that survival depends solely on themselves, those with Cluster B personality disorders develop a value system of "Every person for herself or himself" and "Take care of number one first."

Family Theory

People with ASPD are thought to come from families with inconsistent parenting that resulted in emotional deprivation in the children. Because of their own personality or substance abuse problems, parents may be unable to supervise and discipline their children, or they may even model antisocial behavior for the children. Others seem to come from healthy families and had good childhood experiences (Evans and Sullivan, 1995). Family theorists view BPD as a dysfunction of the entire family system across several generations, with similar dynamics of blurred generational boundaries of the incestuous family (see Chapter 19). BPD usually occurs in an enmeshed family system. With a high family value on children's loyalty to parents,

adult children cling to their parents even after marriage. As a result, the marital couple is unable to bond with each other. When children are born, they are encouraged to cling, and normal separation behavior is discouraged. Often the children end up in a caretaking role with parents and must assume a high level of family responsibility. During late adolescence, they are unable to separate from their parents because of an incorporated family theme that separation and loss are intolerable. It is within the third or fourth generation of enmeshed families that borderline traits develop into the personality disorder. Male children with BPD tend not to marry and remain connected with their families of origin. Female children with BPD often marry but tend to pick passive and distant partners who are enmeshed with their own families (Greene and Ugarriza, 1995). It is believed that a chaotic, depriving, abusive, or brutalizing environment is a major factor in the development of BPD. Research shows that up to 80% of clients diagnosed with BPD have a history of abuse. Tentative findings at this point indicate that the abuse began at an early age, that the child was neglected as well as abused, that sexual abuse was often combined with physical abuse, and that there was usually more than one perpetrator. It must be noted that abuse within the family is not a single incident but rather part of a dysfunctional family behavior pattern that is either chaotic or coercively controlling. Dysfunctional families distort all interactions and relationships (Teicher et al, 1994; Zanarini et al, 1997).

Feminist Theory

Girls and boys are socialized very differently in America. Boys are encouraged to be independent, self-sufficient, active, and thinking rather than feeling individuals. Girls are taught to be dependent, submissive, passive, and feeling individuals who are more concerned with the needs of others than with their own needs. Such rigid role expectations can lead to identity difficulties. The same behaviors that may be considered acceptable in men (impulsiveness, expressing anger, argumentativeness, making demands) are labeled pathological in women. It is more likely that men are diagnosed as having antisocial personality disorder and women are diagnosed as having BPD when exhibiting similar behaviors. These differences in diagnoses reflect the real and unfortunate consequences of gender-role stereotyping in American culture (Cowdry, 1997).

Psychopharmacological Interventions

Studies are being conducted on the effectiveness of medications in treating personality disorders. Psychotic symptoms appear to respond to low doses of the antipsychotic agents. These medications are best used for relief of acute symptoms and are typically discontinued when the psychotic features disappear. A number of medications are being tried to decrease the impulsive, aggressive, and self-destructive behavior patterns of BPD. Selective serotonin reuptake inhibitors (SSRIs) diminish rage and rapid mood swings as well as decrease aggression and impulsive and self-destructive behavior. SSRIs are also used to treat obsessive ruminations in people with personality disorders. SSRIs include Prozac (fluoxetine), Paxil (paroxetine), and Zoloft (sertraline). Medications should be viewed as a means of controlling symptoms that are disabling. The overall treatment plan includes individual, group, family, and behavioral therapy. As more is learned about these disorders, improved techniques can be designed to better meet individual client needs (Evans and Sullivan, 1995; Salzman, 1996).

The Nursing Process

Assessment

As with other psychiatric disorders, data collection serves as the starting point for the nursing process for clients with personality disorders. The main obstacle to assessment is the probability that the client will not perceive that a problem exists. If possible, interview family members for their perceptions of the problem. Exercise professional judgment in seeking information from others about their relationships with the client. Although the objective is to obtain a description of the client's functioning within various family and social contexts, you must be certain that the client's rights are protected. By remaining alert to the potential for a breach of confidentiality, you can ensure that neither the legal nor the ethical limits of the professional domain are exceeded. The Focused Nursing Assessment table lists assessment questions for clients with personality disorders.

Nursing Diagnoses

Clients with Personality Disorders

Cluster A

Ineffective individual coping related to inability to trust.

Fear related to perceived threats from others or the environment.

Social isolation related to inadequate social skills, craving of solitude.

Spiritual distress related to lack of connectedness to others.

Cluster B

Impaired social interaction related to manipulation of others, unstable mood, poor impulse control, extreme emotional reactions, extreme self-centeredness, seductive behavior.

High risk for violence, self-directed (suicide or self-mutilation), related to intense emotional pain, poor impulse control.

High risk for violence directed at others or objects related to intense rage, poor impulse control.

Personal identity disturbance related to changing identities, changing body images, dissociation.

Fear related to feelings of abandonment.

Cluster C

Ineffective individual coping related to high dependency needs, rigid behavior/thoughts, inadequate role performance, high need for approval from others, inability to make independent decisions.

Fear related to feelings of abandonment, disapproval, losing control, conflict.

Diagnosis

Probable nursing diagnoses can be identified for each cluster of personality disorders. Remember that no client fits neatly into any theoretically determined diagnostic category and that no standardized list or table can provide a comprehensive description of the problems specific to individual clients. The diagnoses in the Nursing Diagnoses box serve as a framework for nursing care, but they cannot replace a comprehensive, individualized plan for the client.

Focused Nursing Assessment

CLIENTS WITH PERSONALITY DISORDERS

Behavior Assessment	*Affective Assessment*	*Cognitive Assessment*	*Social Assessment*
What is your usual pattern of daily activities?	Describe your usual mood.	Would you describe yourself as independent or dependent?	How do you usually relate to others?
What is your work history?	What happens when you feel frustrated? Angry? Fearful? Happy? Peaceful?	What do you like about yourself?	When do you prefer to be alone? To be with others?
Describe your functioning at work/school.	What causes you to be upset with others?	What would you like to change about yourself?	Describe the differences between your business and social relationships.
Has anyone ever told you your behavior was a problem? If so, what did they tell you?	How do you react to criticism?	What are your expectations for the future?	How many close relationships with others do you have? Describe the relationships.
Describe any problematic behavior you displayed as a teenager.	Do others ever describe you as detached, cool, or aloof? If so, what do they say?		Are other people out to discredit or hurt you?
Describe both successful and unsuccessful attempts you have had in trying to modify your behavior patterns.	How do you feel when you are with groups of people?		Are you able to say "no" to other people?
How do you resolve conflicts with others?	How often are you rejected or do you feel you are rejected by others?		
When did you have your last drink? When did you last use drugs?	Would you consider yourself to be affectionate and empathetic toward others?		

Outcome Identification

Once you have established diagnoses, you and the client mutually identify goals for change. Client outcomes are specific behavioral measures by which you, clients, and significant others determine progress toward goals. The following are examples of some of the outcomes appropriate to people with personality disorders:

- implements behavioral contract to reduce self-destructive activities
- incidents of self-mutilation decrease
- suicidal behavior decreases
- utilizes the problem-solving process
- verbalizes an internal locus of control
- socially interacts with others
- verbalizes decreased anxiety
- decreases perfectionistic behavior

Nursing Interventions

Approach clients with Cluster A personality disorders in a gentle, interested, and nonintrusive manner that is respectful of the client's need for distance and privacy. Clients with Cluster B personality disorders require much more patience and structure from nurses. The approach must be one of consistency. Clients with Cluster C diagnoses will find it helpful when you point out their avoidance behavior and secondary gains. Assertiveness training helps these clients manage their dependency and anger.

Three fundamental beliefs guide your approach in working with persons experiencing personality disorders. The first is self-determination. Clients are partners in treatment and have the right to choose their own course in life. Second, the focus is on role functioning while recognizing that not all symptoms will disappear. Third is maintaining hope. These clients are particularly susceptible to loss of hope for change and giving up on treatment. See the accompanying box for an overview of the nursing interventions classifications (NIC) for people with personality disorders.

Behavioral: Behavior Therapy

Impulse Control Training

The first priority of care is client safety. These clients, especially those with BPD, are often suicidal or they self-mutilate. Take all suicidal thinking seriously. It is an indication they are not feeling safe. (Nursing interventions for clients who are suicidal are covered in Chapter 17.) Intense emotional pain and poor impulse control contribute to self-destructive behavior. The most helpful initial response is to talk in a calm, monotone voice, repeating a phrase such as: "You are with me. I will help you remain safe." Often clients regress to an earlier age and thus your interventions should match the presenting age. For example, if they are acting like 3- or 4-year-olds in a rage, use a kind, soothing approach with simple, firm directions to contain the behavior. Once clients are able to control behavior, there are a number of nursing interventions directed toward the goal of remaining safe and increasing impulse control. Establish an hour-by-hour or day-by-day antiharm contract with clients. This may be either a verbal or a written agreement. Help them identify and label feelings (self-monitoring) in order to learn to recognize that self-destructive behaviors are responses to feelings and that these responses can be changed over time. This is the beginning of the problem-solving process. Next, ask clients to identify triggers to and patterns in their self-destructive behavior. Diaries can be used to track the changes in feelings and to identify the specific stimuli that caused the change. Brainstorm ideas on what other behaviors might be substituted for the harmful ones. Clients decide which response they will implement the next time they feel like hurting themselves. When that has been done, evaluate the effectiveness of the new behavior with the client. Clients need a great deal of support, reminding, and guidance from nurses before they are able to develop any consistency in new behaviors. They need to be encouraged to identify and use sources of support during this time.

Limit Setting

Many of these clients tend to test nurses and behave in a manipulative manner. They respond best to a high level of structure and clear ground rules. You must maintain a careful balance between being an authority figure while not being harsh or judgmental. If you try to be their "friend" you will be open to manipulation. The best approach is straightforward

Nursing Interventions Classification

CLIENTS WITH PERSONALITY DISORDERS

DOMAIN: Behavioral

Class: *Behavior Therapy*

Interventions: *Impulse Control Training:* Assisting the patient to mediate impulsive behavior through application of problem-solving strategies to social and interpersonal situations.

Limit Setting: Establishing the parameters of desirable and acceptable patient behavior.

Behavior Modification: Social Skills: Assisting the patient to develop or improve interpersonal social skills.

Class: *Psychological Comfort Promotion*

Interventions: *Anxiety Reduction:* Minimizing apprehension, dread, foreboding, or uneasiness related to an unidentified source of anticipated danger.

---

and business-like. Together, develop the goals of treatment and behavioral contracts to reduce self-destructive activities. Convey expectations in a clear, direct manner and request clarification from clients of their understanding. This decreases the use of manipulation through misunderstanding.

Pay attention to your own emotional responses to these clients. It is very easy to internalize the client's sense of chaos, anger, and frustration. In a residential home or inpatient unit, power struggles often develop, and the milieu becomes chaotic for everyone. Remaining therapeutic may require supervision or consultation from an unbiased colleague. One staff member may see a client as vulnerable and needy, while another might perceive the same client to be aggressive, provocative, and in need of clear limits. Without outside supervision, debates among staff members can become highly personalized and polarize the staff into several factions.

Behavior Modification: Social Skills

The goal of nursing interventions with clients who are helpless and dependent is to increase their coping skills and encourage independent functioning. The first step is to communicate to clients that you recognize their feelings of helplessness and fears of becoming more independent. This expression of empathy

will help them be more collaborative in the problem-solving process. Explore examples of dichotomous thinking, such as "One is either totally dependent and helpless or one is totally independent and isolated." Often clients view nurses as all-powerful rescuers who will make everything better. But carefully avoid rescuing behavior because it would reinforce the client's feeling of helplessness and the external locus of control. The next step is to help clients identify what would be different, what they would gain, and what they would lose if they were less helpless. Focus on one issue at a time. Begin with a fairly insignificant situation, and help them identify what they would like out of this situation. They can then problem-solve ways to achieve their goals. With each subsequent use of the problem-solving process, their skills will increase, and they will become more confident in their ability to handle problems as they arise.

Interventions designed to decrease socially isolative behaviors and reward socially outgoing behaviors are often accomplished through social skills training and assertiveness training. Be sure to respect a client's need to be distant or isolative, while encouraging and supporting interactions with others. Help clients identify interpersonal problems resulting from social skills deficits. Encourage them to verbalize their feelings associated with these problems, and assist them in identifying alternative ways to relate without seduction or intimidation. Role-play and provide feedback about the appropriateness of their responses. Encourage them to evaluate their behavior in social situations.

Group therapy is often an adjunct to individual therapy. The process of group therapy helps clients focus on interpersonal issues as well as individual issues. Clients not only get feedback from more than one person, they also have the opportunity to be therapeutic with other group members. Since clients with personality disorders have inadequate social skills, group therapy is one way to develop and foster better relationships with others.

Behavioral: Psychological Comfort Promotion

Anxiety Reduction

Some clients avoid making decisions to avoid the anxiety of failure. Whenever possible, encourage them to make their own decisions to reinforce a sense of competence and an internal locus of control. Point out the destructive effects of indecision to further their understanding that an imperfect decision may be less harmful than no decision. Explain that there are no absolute guarantees of the future for any of us. Explore how many decisions in life can be remade, as these clients often believe that decisions are always final. Anxiety is increased when they fear failure if the "perfect" decision is not made. Teach clients the problem-solving process. This increases their skills in decision making and helps them see there are a variety of choices that can be made, tested, and evaluated. Give feedback for decisions they make to reinforce positive changes in behavior.

Some clients become perfectionistic to guard against the anxiety of feeling inferior. To help clients gain insight into the need for perfectionistic behavior, comment upon the link between this behavior and feelings of anxiety and helplessness. Explore their fear of being judged inferior by others and help them evaluate whether this is a realistic appraisal of others' responses. Promote realistic self-appraisal through discussion of abilities and limitations. Some clients benefit from being assigned three purposeful, nonharmful mistakes per day, such as setting the table incorrectly, giving wrong directions, putting postage stamps on upside down, or wearing two different socks. They are to use a journal to record their feelings in response to the mistakes. This exercise serves to increase clients' sense of control over errors and helps them recognize that many mistakes are not serious. Provide feedback for positive changes to reinforce behavior and increase their ability to accurately appraise themselves. Help clients acknowledge that an anxiety-free life is impossible, which may help them give up striving for perfection.

Some clients keep others at a distance and reduce anxiety by the need to always "be right." Do not get caught up in a struggle for control in being right as this will reinforce maladaptive behavior. Facilitate clients' acceptance of responsibility for their own behavior and explore how this affects other people. When they see themselves more realistically, they may be able to behave in more socially effective ways. Use relevant humor and laughter regarding perfectionism as a relief from tension and anxiety. Humor allows clients to risk speaking about the need to be right without fear of ridicule. Teach clients that humor used appropriately is a highly valued attribute in this culture. Humor allows people to experience pleasure and decreases emotional distance from others.

Anxiety prevents some clients from asking for help when it is needed. Have clients identify expectations that will occur should help be sought. They need to recognize that fear of rejection precludes seeking help. Use appropriate self-disclosure regarding situations in which you have sought help, to enable clients to recognize that asking for assistance need not result in rejection. Role-play with clients how to ask for help in a particular situation to increase the use of unfamiliar skills. After seeking help, have clients evaluate the situation in terms of feelings and how others responded. This helps them assess the reality of their anticipated fears.

Evaluation

Personality traits are almost always too ingrained for radical change through therapy.

Because the problems associated with personality disorders have been with most clients for their entire lives, clients respond to intervention strategies very slowly. You must define small steps toward the achievement of therapeutic goals. You can help them most by helping them see how their behavior affects their lives so that they can learn to modify patterns enough to develop a more adaptive lifestyle. Some clients are in enough pain that they wish to grow and change. Others do not see that they have any problems and choose not to be involved in the therapeutic process.

BPD can be as lethal as depression or schizophrenia. The risk of suicide is highest during the 20s, and clients often kill themselves unexpectedly. The first 2 years after discharge from treatment are often the most painful for clients, whereas 2–8 years after discharge, they often get much better. Like clients with antisocial personality disorder, clients with BPD who survive into their 40s often improve. Concomitant disorders such as substance abuse, depression, eating disorders, and anxiety disorders worsen the prognosis. Attributes such as an ability to empathize, an ability to commit to others, and an ability to control aggression and violence make for a better prognosis (Gunderson, 1996).

Clinical Interactions

A Client with Borderline Personality Disorder

Enid, age 34, is an inpatient with a diagnosis of borderline personality disorder. She has been in and out of relationships with many different men and does not stay in a job for more than a year. She has a history of self-mutilation and numerous suicide attempts. During the past year, she has been writing love letters to her psychiatrist. She has just demanded one-to-one contact with her nurse. In the interaction, you will see evidence of:

- attempted manipulation of the nurse
- self-mutilation as a way to decrease anxiety
- labile affect

ENID: First my doctor doesn't see me until after he sees all his other patients. Then you're too busy doing group. I just don't have anyone to talk to.

NURSE: Enid, I do one group per day, and I'm available most of the other hours of my shift. You need

to deal directly with me, but if necessary, there are other staff members available.

ENID: But you are the only nurse who understands me. You are the only one I feel I can really open up to. I can't talk about my issues with anyone but you!

NURSE: Enid, what is making you so upset?

ENID: Do you promise not to tell anyone else if I tell you? You must promise me this! My doctor made me talk about the letters I've written him. They were beautiful. He sat there and read them to me . . . like he was reading the newspaper . . . totally devoid of the emotion they were written with. So I did this [pulls up sleeves to reveal multiple new longitudinal superficial lacerations]. Now you have to promise me not to tell anyone else!

NURSE: I can't promise that. I will need to inform the other members of your treatment team. Any time there is a significant event or change in a client's status, that information needs to be shared. But why don't we talk about it first.

ENID: You are just like all the others. You are going to betray me! How dare you!

NURSE: If I failed to share this information, that would be unfair to you. ■

Self-Help Groups

Clients with Personality Disorders

Alcoholics Anonymous
(212) 686-1100

The Center Post-Traumatic
and Dissociate Disorders Program
(800) 369-2273

CHANGE: Free From Fears
2915 Providence Road
Charlotte, NC 28211
(704) 365-0140

Local suicide-prevention hotline numbers

Narcotics Anonymous
(818) 780-3951

Key Concepts

Introduction

- Personality disorders are inflexible and maladaptive behavior patterns by which certain people cope with their feelings, the way they see themselves and others, how they respond to their surroundings, and how they find meaning in relationships.

- There is a high degree of overlap among the personality disorders, and many people exhibit traits of several disorders. The most commonly diagnosed is borderline personality disorder.

Knowledge Base

- The common characteristics of Cluster A disorders are odd, eccentric behavior and social isolation.

- Paranoid personality disorder refers to clients who are suspicious, secretive, and pathologically jealous.

- Schizoid personality disorder refers to clients who have a restricted range of emotions, are loners, and are not influenced by praise or criticism.

- Schizotypal personality disorder may be related to chronic schizophrenia. People with this disorder have an odd style of speech and their affect is often inappropriate. They may be suspicious and experience ideas of reference and magical thinking.

- The common characteristics of Cluster B disorders are dramatic, emotional, or erratic behavior, and behavior that exploits others.

- Antisocial personality disorder (ASPD) refers to clients who consistently violate the rights of others as well as the values of society. They are unable to experience guilt for their inappropriate behavior. They are more often found in prisons than in hospitals.

- Borderline personality disorder (BPD) sufferers often have other mental disorders such as mood disorders, eating disorders, and substance abuse. Symptoms vary in any given person at any given time. Their behavior is impulsive and manipulative, and they are at high risk for suicide and self-mutilation. Their moods are intense and unstable.

- Histrionic personality disorder (HPD) refers to clients who are overly dramatic and self-centered, and who need people to admire them constantly.

- Narcissistic personality disorder (NPD) refers to clients who strive for power and success, mask their feelings with aloofness, and are extremely grandiose. They exploit others to achieve personal goals.

- The common characteristics of Cluster C personality disorders are anxiety, fear, and overtly compliant behavior.

- Avoidant personality disorder (APD) refers to clients who are shy, introverted, lacking in self-confidence, and extremely sensitive to rejection.

- Dependent personality disorder (DPD) refers to clients who are unable to do things by themselves, fear abandonment, and force others into making their decisions.

- Obsessive-compulsive personality disorder (OCPD) refers to clients who have a high need for routines, are unable to express feelings, fear making mistakes and therefore have difficulty making decisions, and attempt to control all interpersonal relationships.

- Concomitant disorders include substance abuse, chronic anxiety, panic attacks, and depression.

- There is no single cause of personality disorders. They likely arise from an interaction between biological factors and the environment. Neurobiological factors include limbic system dysregulation, low levels of 5-HT, high levels of NE, and abnormal levels of DA.

- Intrapersonal factors include projection of hostility, perfectionistic standards, underdeveloped superego, and fear of abandonment.

- Social oppression and changing value systems may contribute to the development of personality disorders.

- Family factors include an inability to manage conflict, lack of individuation from the parents, and a chaotic and abusive environment.

- Feminist theorists consider rigid sex-role stereotyping to be a factor in personality disorders.

- Medications used for clients with personality disorders include SSRIs and antipsychotic agents.

Nursing Assessment

- Clients typically do not see that a problem exists within themselves. It is often helpful to interview family and friends, if possible.

- You must maintain a sensitivity in the interview process so that the client does not become guarded or defensive.

Nursing Diagnosis

- Based on the typical characteristics, nursing diagnoses can be made for each cluster and individualized for each client.

Outcome Identification

- Outcomes include a decrease in self-destructive behavior, verbalization of less anxiety, utilization of the problem-solving process, and the development of healthy peer relationships.

Nursing Interventions

- You should approach people with Cluster A disorders in a gentle, interested, and nonintrusive manner that is respectful of the client's need for distance and privacy.

- Clients with Cluster B disorders require much more patience and structure on your part. The milieu must be consistent to avoid manipulation and power struggles.

- In clients with Cluster C disorders, it is helpful to point out their avoidance behaviors and secondary gains. Problem solving and assertiveness training help them become more independent.

- The first priority of care is safety from suicide and self-mutilation. Clients must be protected until they can protect themselves.

- Manipulative clients need a highly structured approach. Nurses may need frequent staff reports and supervision to counteract the client's ability to play one staff member against the other.

- Helpless and dependent clients need interventions to increase their coping skills and develop a more independent style of functioning. Problem solving, social skills training, and assertiveness training are effective interventions.

Evaluation

- In evaluating the care of clients with personality disorders, it is important to remember that these disorders are often lifelong and are not likely to yield readily to intervention strategies.

Review Questions

1. A behavioral characteristic common to persons with personality disorders from Cluster A is

   a. social isolation.

   b. manipulation by the use of narcissism.

   c. high sociability.

   d. impulsive antisocial acts.

2. An affective characteristic common to persons with personality disorders from Cluster B is

   a. flat or blunted affect.

   b. intense and changing expression.

   c. passive affect.

   d. minimal expression.

3. A cognitive characteristic common to persons with personality disorders from Cluster C is

   a. indecision.

   b. lack of long-range plans.

   c. inability to trust others.

   d. poverty of thoughts.

4. Which of the following nursing diagnoses is applicable to the client with borderline personality disorder?

   a. *Fear* related to perceived threats from others or the environment

   b. *Social isolation* related to lack of empathy

   c. *Potential for noncompliance* related to denial of problems

   d. *Ineffective coping* related to unstable mood

5. Your client has the diagnosis of *Ineffective individual coping* related to indecision to avoid the anxiety of failure. Which of the following nursing interventions would be most appropriate?

   a. Help client recognize that absolute guarantees of the future are unrealistic.

   b. Keep the environment and routines consistent so decisions do not have to be made.

   c. Explore the fear of being judged inferior by others.

   d. Have client role-play how to ask for help.

References

American Psychiatric Association (1994). *Diagnostic and Statistical Manual of Mental Disorders,* 4th ed. Washington, D.C.: American Psychiatric Press.

Cowdry, R. (1997). Borderline personality disorder. *NAMI Advocate, 18(4),* 8–9.

deVegvar, M. L., & Siever, L. J. (1994). Treatment of impulsivity and serotonin in borderline personality disorder. In K. R. Silk (Ed.), *Biological and Neurobehavioral Studies of Borderline Personality Disorder* (pp. 23–40). Washington, D.C.: American Psychiatric Press.

Evans, K., & Sullivan, J. M. (1995). *Treating Addicted Survivors of Trauma*. New York: Guilford Press.

Gold, J. H. (1996). The intolerance of aloneness. *Am J Psychiatry, 153*(6): 749–750.

Greene, H., & Ugarriza, D. N. (1995). Borderline personality disorder: History, theory, and nursing intervention. *J Psychosoc Nurs, 33*(12), 26–30.

Gunderson, J. G. (1996). The borderline patient's intolerance of aloneness. *Am J Psychiatry, 153*(6), 752–758.

Isometsa, E. T., et al. (1996). Suicide among subjects with personality disorders. *Am J Psychiatry, 153*(5), 667–673.

Johnson, S. M. (1987). *Humanizing the Narcissistic Style*. New York: Norton.

Millon, T., & Kotik-Harper, D. (1995). The relationship of depression to disorders of personality. In E. E. Beckham & W. R. Leber (Eds.), *Handbook of Depression* (2nd ed., pp. 107–146). New York: Guilford Press.

O'Brien, M. M., Trestman, R. L., & Siever L. J. (1993). Cluster A personality disorders. In D. L. Dunner (Ed.), *Current Psychiatric Therapy* (pp. 399–404). Philadelphia: Saunders.

Oldham, J. M., et al. (1995). Comorbidity of Axis I and Axis II disorders. *Am J Psychiatry, 152*(4), 571–578.

Personality Disorders. (1996). *Harvard Mental Health Letter, 12*(8), 1–3.

Raine, A., et al. (1995). High autonomic arousal and electrodermal orienting at age 15 years as protective factors against criminal behavior at age 29 years. *Am J Psychiatry, 152*(11), 1595–1600.

Roitman, S. E .L., et al. (1997). Attentional functioning in schizotypal personality disorder. *Am J Psychiatry, 154*(5), 655–660.

Salzman, C. (1996). What drug treatments are available for borderline personality disorder? *Harvard Mental Health Letter, 12*(8), 8–9.

Stein, K. F. (1996). Affect instability in adults with a borderline personality disorder. *Arch Psychiatr Nurs, 10*(1), 32–40.

Stone, M. H.(1993). Cluster C personality disorders. In D. L. Dunner (Ed.), *Current Psychiatric Therapy*. Philadelphia: Saunders.

Teicher, M. H., et al. (1994). Early abuse, limbic system dysfunction, and borderline personality disorder. In K. R. Silk (Ed.), *Biological and Neurobehavioral Studies of Borderline Personality Disorder* (pp. 177–207). Washington, D.C.: American Psychiatric Press.

Volavka, J. (1995). *Neurobiology of Violence*. Washington DC: American Psychiatric Press.

Zanarini, M. C., et al. (1997). Reported pathological childhood experiences associated with the development of borderline personality disorder. *Am J Psychiatry, 154*(8), 1101–1106.

CHAPTER 15

Cognitive Impairment Disorders

Brenda Lewis Cleary
Karen Lee Fontaine

Objectives

After reading this chapter, you will be able to:

- Differentiate between dementia and delirium.
- Assess clients with dementia and delirium and differentiate these disorders from pseudodementias.
- Intervene with clients suffering from cognitive impairment disorders.
- Assist families in planning care for clients with dementia.
- Evaluate the plan of care based on the outcome criteria.

Key Terms

agnosia
agraphia
alexia
aphasia
apraxia
astereognosia
confabulation
delirium
dementia
hyperorality
hyperetamorphosis
perseveration phenomena
pseudodelirium
pseudodementia
sundown syndrome

The process of mental deterioration related to cognitive impairment disorders has a profound effect on clients, their families, and society as a whole. This chapter presents dementia and delirium, the two most common forms, in which there are diffuse disturbances in cognitive performance. In general, they differ in both symptoms and outcome.

Dementia is a chronic, irreversible brain disorder characterized by impairments in memory, abstract thinking, and judgment, as well as changes in personality. Dementia in old age is most commonly due to Alzheimer's disease, which accounts for 50–75% of dementing illness. Most of the remaining cases in older individuals are caused by vascular accidents; these cases are known as multi-infarct dementia. Another type of dementia, typically affecting younger people, is AIDS Dementia Complex (ADC), caused by HIV infection of the brain. It is estimated that ADC occurs in 30–65% of people with AIDS, with a widely varied but progressively deteriorating course (Price, 1995).

Dementia of the Alzheimer's type (DAT) currently affects about 4.8 million Americans. It strikes 1 out of 12 people over the age of 65, 1 out of 3 over age 80, and almost 1 out of 2 over the age of 85. Onset generally occurs in late life but in rare cases the disorder appears in the 40s and 50s. More women than men are affected, in part because women live longer. The impact of DAT will be felt more severely in the twenty-first century, when the baby boom generation reaches old age. By the middle of the twenty first century, it is estimated that 14 million Americans will experience the destruction of Alzheimer's disease. Alzheimer's disease is the third most expensive disease in the United States, after heart disease and cancer. The average lifetime cost per client is $174,000 (American Journal of Psychiatry, 1997; Cost of Alzheimer's Disease, 1997; Cummings and Trimble, 1995). Approximately 15–20% of Alzheimer's cases are believed to be inherited; this form is known as familial Alzheimer's disease (FAD). Because FAD often begins at a much younger age, it is also referred to as early-onset Alzheimer's disease. For first-degree relatives of a person with FAD, the risk is 50% for developing the disorder (Cutler and Sramek, 1996).

Delirium is an acute, usually reversible brain disorder characterized by clouding of the consciousness (a decreased awareness of the environment) and a reduced ability to focus and maintain attention. The presence of delirium indicates that a medical illness is affecting the brain, and rapid medical intervention is needed to prevent irreversible deterioration or death (Reichman, 1994).

For a comparison of dementia and delirium, see Table 15.1.

Knowledge Base: Dementia

Because multi-infarct dementia and DAT demonstrate many of the same characteristics and the latter is believed to be more prevalent, DAT is used as the model for dementia. The average course of DAT is 5–10 years, but the range may be 2–20 years. People who have early onset often deteriorate more rapidly. The progression is roughly divided into three stages: Stage 1 typically lasts 2–4 years, stage 2 may continue for several years, and stage 3 usually lasts only 1–2 years before death occurs (Cutler and Sramek, 1996).

Behavioral Characteristics

The most notable changes in behavior during stage 1 are difficulties performing complex tasks, related to a decline in recent memory. People suffering from Alzheimer's disease are unable to balance their checkbooks or plan a well-balanced meal. They may have difficulty remembering to buy supplies for the home or responding to different schedules within the home. At work, the ability to plan a goal-directed set of behaviors is seriously limited, resulting in missed appointments and incomplete verbal or written reports. Personal appearance begins to decline, and they need help selecting clothes appropriate for the season or particular event. They remain capable of independent living. During stage 1, these people recognize their confusion and are frightened by what is happening. Fearing the diagnosis, they attempt to cover up and rationalize their symptoms (Klebanoff and Smith, 1997). In stage 2, behavior deteriorates markedly and is often socially unacceptable. Exhibiting poor impulse control, they may have outbursts and tantrums. The most common accidents are falls, followed by injuries resulting from difficulty using sharp objects. Wandering behavior poses a potential danger because DAT sufferers get lost easily and are

■ *Table 15.1* Dementia and Delirium Compared

Dementia	Delirium
Onset	
Onset of impairment generally slow and insidious.	Onset usually sudden. Acute development of impairment of orientation, memory, cognitive function, judgment, and affect.
Essential Feature	
Not based on disordered consciousness; however, delirium, stupor, and coma may occur.	Clouded state of consciousness.
Etiology	
Generally caused by irreversible alteration of brain function.	Caused by temporary, reversible, diffuse disturbances of brain function.
Course	
No diurnal fluctuations. The clinical course usually progresses over months or years, ending in death.	Short, diurnal fluctuations in symptoms. The clinical course is usually brief, although it may last for months. Untreated, prolonged delirium may cause permanent brain destruction and lead to dementia.
History	
Onset: insidious. Duration: months to years. Course: consistent deterioration with occasional lucid moments.	Onset: sudden. Duration: hours to days. Course: fluctuating arousal.
Motor Signs	
None (until late).	Postural tremor, restless, hyperactive or sluggish.
Speech is usually normal in early stages, but word-finding difficulties progress.	Slurred speech, reflecting disorganized thinking.
Mental Status	
Attention generally normal in early stages; inattention progresses.	Attention fluctuates.
Memory	
Memory impairment; recent memory affected before remote.	Impaired by poor attention.
Language	
Aphasia in later stages.	Normal or mild misnaming of objects.

continued ➤

Table 15.1 Dementia and Delirium Compared *continued*

Mental Status *continued*

Perception

Hallucinations not prominent, although cognitive impairment may lead to paranoid delusions.	Visual, auditory, and/or tactile hallucinations.

Pronounced Mood/Affect

Disinterested and/or disinhibited.	Fear and suspiciousness may be prominent; anxiety, depression, anger, irritability, or euphoria may occur.

Review of Systems

Extraneural organ systems usually uninvolved.	History of systemic illness or toxic exposure.

EEG

Normal or mildly slow.	Pronounced diffuse slowing of fast cycles related to state of arousal.

Sources: Cummings and Trimble, 1995; Klebanoff and Smith, 1997.

unable to retrace their steps back home. Lost and confused, they may become victims of street crime.

During stage 2, they need assistance with the sequence of skills for toileting and bathing. They also need help in dressing. The inability to carry out skilled and purposeful movement or the inability to use objects properly is called **apraxia.** Also evident is **hyperorality,** the need to taste, chew, and examine any object small enough to be placed in the mouth. People in this stage need to be protected from accidentally eating harmful substances such as soaps or poisons. Although there may be a sharp increase in appetite and food intake, there is seldom a corresponding weight gain. In contrast, some individuals have limited or no recognition of meal times or even food. Behavior in this stage is characterized by continuous, repetitive acts that have no meaning or direction. These repetitive behaviors—which may include lip licking, tapping of fingers, pacing, or echoing others' words—are referred to as **perseveration phenomena** (Ford, 1996; Lach et al, 1995).

Many long-lived adults, including those suffering from DAT, become disoriented at the end of the day; this is usually referred to as **sundown syndrome.** Orientation seems to decrease as daylight recedes. It

becomes more difficult to distinguish shapes from shadows and to pinpoint the source of sounds in the environment. Sundown syndrome is more pronounced when clients are fatigued. Various behaviors relating to sundown syndrome include wandering, confusion, hyperactivity, restlessness, and aggression (Burney-Puckett, 1996).

In the middle and later stages, psychotic symptoms are common. Aggressive behavior, delusions, and hallucinations are seen. Wandering is another problem at this time. Wandering may be a substitute for social interaction and thus is a way to alleviate loneliness and separation from others. Wandering may also be an expression of agitation, boredom, pain, or discomfort. Within a safe environment, wandering can be beneficial since it stimulates circulation and oxygenation and promotes exercise (Aarsland et al, 1996; Coltharp, Richie, and Kaas, 1996).

In stage 3 of Alzheimer's disease, a syndrome like Klüver-Bucy syndrome develops, which includes the continuation of hyperorality and the development of periodic binge eating. Behavior is also characterized by **hyperetamorphosis,** the need to compulsively touch and examine every object in the environment. There is a sharp deterioration in motor ability that progresses from an inability to walk, to an inability to sit up, and finally to an inability even to smile.

Affective Characteristics

In stage 1 of Alzheimer's disease, anxiety and depression may occur as affected people become aware of and try to cope with noticeable deficits. They frequently experience feelings of helplessness, frustration, and shame in relation to their deficits. Diagnosis of a concomitant depression is important because depression can worsen the symptoms of dementia and for that reason must not be ignored. Those in stage 1 of Alzheimer's lack spontaneity in verbal and nonverbal communication. As a result of chosen or forced withdrawal from social contacts, an apathetic affect may ensue (American Journal of Psychiatry, 1997).

In stage 2, there is an increased lability of emotions from flat affect to periods of marked irritability. Delusions of persecution may precipitate feelings of intense fear. Catastrophic reactions, resulting from underlying brain dysfunction, are common. In response to everyday situations, the person may overreact by exploding in rage or suddenly crying. As the disease progresses through stage 3, response to environmental stimuli continues to decrease until the person is wholly nonresponsive (Gerdner, Hall, and Buckwalter, 1996).

Cognitive Characteristics

The primary cognitive deficit in stage 1 is memory impairment with a decrease in concentration, an increase in distractibility, and an appearance of absentmindedness. The ability to make accurate judgments also declines. People suffering from early Alzheimer's may have difficulty managing their finances or may give away large amounts of money in response to radio and television solicitations. It is difficult to decide when to prevent them from driving. Because they are easily distracted, may forget the meaning of road signs, may confuse the meaning of red and green lights, and may not look to see that no other cars are coming, they are extremely accident-prone.

They may be disoriented about time but remember people and places. Transitory delusions of persecution may develop in response to the memory impairment. The person may make such statements as "You hid my keys. I know you don't want me to be able to get out of the house and drive"; "Where are my shoes? Everybody keeps hiding things to make me crazy"; "Why didn't you tell me there was a party tonight? You just don't want me to go and have any fun." It is difficult for sufferers of DAT and their families to balance the need for independence with situations in which they need help. Caregivers may be accused of treating them like children on the one hand, and not giving them enough attention on the other.

Language skills begin to deteriorate in stage 1 as individuals have problems in thinking of what to say and language processing takes longer. They may have word-finding and object-naming difficulties. They have problems with complex conversations, rapid speech, and speech in noisy and distracting environments. At this stage they may self-correct or apologize for communication problems (Richter, Roberto, and Bottenberg, 1995; Ripich, Wykle, and Niles, 1995).

In stage 2 of Alzheimer's disease there is a progressive memory loss, which includes both recent and remote memory. New information cannot be retained, and there is no recollection of what occurred 10 minutes or an hour ago. Loss of remote memory becomes obvious when there is no recognition of family members or recall of significant past events. This loss may be the most painful aspect of DAT, erasing a whole lifetime of memories for that person (Rentz, 1995).

Confabulation, the filling in of memory gaps with imaginary information, is an attempt to distract others from observing the deficit. Comprehension of language, interactions, and significance of objects is greatly diminished. During this stage, the person becomes completely disoriented in all three spheres of person, time, and place.

Approximately half of people with DAT develop psychotic symptoms associated with agitation, irritability, and aggression. Delusions can occur, especially those involving themes of persecution such as believing that misplaced items have been stolen. Hallucinations can occur in all of the senses, but visual hallucinations are the most common. Misidentification syndrome frequently occurs. Familiar people are seen as unfamiliar and vice versa. They may even believe that people on television are really present (American Journal of Psychiatry, 1997; Cutler and Sramek, 1996).

As the disease progresses, communication breakdowns become more frequent and more severe. Stressful and confusing situations compound the difficulty in understanding others or expressing thoughts. There is increasing **aphasia,** the loss of the ability to understand or use language, which begins with the inability to find words and eventually limits the person to as few as six words. Concurrently, **agraphia,** the inability to read or write, develops. Finally, the inability to recognize familiar situations, people, or stimuli evolves; this is known as agnosia. Auditory **agnosia** is the inability to recognize familiar sounds such as a doorbell, the ring of a telephone, or a barking dog. Tactile agnosia, **astereognosia,** occurs when the person is unable to identify familiar objects placed in the hand, such as a comb, pencil, or paintbrush. Visual agnosia, or **alexia,** occurs when the person can look at a frying pan, a telephone, or a toothbrush and have no idea what to do with these objects (Matteson, Linton, and Barnes, 1996).

The following interchange illustrates the aphasic characteristics of DAT. Pat is able to give a variety of descriptors but cannot think of the one necessary word.

> **Sue called her mother, Pat, to see how she was doing.**
>
> Sue: **It sounds like you are eating, Mom. What are you eating?**
>
> Pat: **I can't tell you.**
>
> Sue: **Is it hot or cold?**
>
> Pat: **It's cold.**
>
> Sue: **Did you get it out of the refrigerator?**
>
> Pat: **No, it's like bread.**
>
> Sue: **Is it a sandwich?**
>
> Pat: **Sort of. I put butter on it.**
>
> Sue: **Is it crackers?**
>
> Pat: **No. I used to buy a lot of it and put it in the freezer.**
>
> Sue: **Is it cookies?**
>
> Pat: **No. Usually I have it for breakfast. I took the last slice.**
>
> Sue: **Is it coffee cake?**
>
> Pat: **Yes, that's what it is.**

In stage 3 of DAT, there is a severe decline in cognitive functioning. Clients may be oblivious to others in the home and may be unable to recognize themselves in the mirror. They may scream or yell spontaneously or be able to say only one word or unable to say anything. In addition, there is no longer any nonverbal response to internal and external stimuli; the person degenerates to a vegetative state.

> **Mr Goldstein, a 67-year-old engineer, began to forget where he placed familiar objects around the house and, as his wife noted, had difficulty balancing the checkbook. His coworkers began to notice impaired judgments in the workplace. Mr Goldstein tended to project on others his increasing inability to handle usual tasks efficiently. Within 2 years, he was in stage 2, and Mrs Goldstein had to label objects in the home so that he could identify them by name. He responded with fear to sounds he could no longer identify. He needed assistance with eating, bathing, and dressing and constant supervision because of his wandering behavior. Mrs Goldstein found that a regular routine was helpful and continually repeated, "My husband is still in there, I just have to go in and draw him out."**

For a comparison of changes in normal aging with changes in Alzheimer's disease, see Table 15.2.

Social Characteristics

There are at least two victims of DAT: the person with the disease and the caregiver(s). Remember that for every client, there is a family in distress. Families

Table 15.2 **Changes in Normal Aging and Changes in Alzheimer's Disease Compared**

Normal Aging	Alzheimer's Disease
Recent memory more impaired than remote memory.	Recent and remote memory profoundly affected.
Difficulty in recalling names of people and places.	Inability to recall names of people and places.
Decreased concentration.	Inability to concentrate.
Writing things down is helpful in stimulating memory.	Inability to write; nothing stimulates memory.
Changes do not interfere with daily functioning.	Changes cause an inability to function at work, in a social relationship, and at home.
Insight into forgetful behavior is preserved.	With progression, the person has no insight into changes that have occurred.

are the primary providers of long-term care for people who suffer from dementia. Most often, the sufferer is elderly. Elderly spouses, who are most likely to provide care, have limited strength and energy to meet the demands of the situation. Middle-aged children, most typically daughters, must manage their own problems as well as the role reversal that occurs with a dependent parent. Caring for a person with dementia is among the most difficult of family responsibilities and the one for which caregivers receive minimal support and training (England, 1995; Gerdner, Hall, and Buckwalter, 1996).

Concerns about intimacy and sexuality are important for most couples, regardless of sexual orientation. They range along a continuum of no interest to active, ongoing interest. Some healthy partners have no interest in continuing a sexual relationship with an ill partner. This may be in response to problems with hygiene, feeling more like a parent to the partner, or feeling insignificant when not recognized by the ill person. Some healthy partners are interested in maintaining sexual intimacy but may be physically exhausted or feel guilty about being sexual with a partner who is unable to clearly consent. Other healthy partners express no interest in genital sex but remain interested in emotional intimacy (loving words) and physical intimacy (holding, kissing, stroking). Others are able to maintain all types of intimacy, including genital sex, and feel satisfied and joyful with the interaction (Davies, Zeiss, and Tinklenberg, 1992).

Communication problems cause more caregiver stress as clients are unable to take part in family conversations and fail to start or sustain conversations, all of which leads to caregivers feeling frustrated, lonely, and isolated. See Box 15.1 for ways to improve communication.

The changes that occur in DAT are frightening to family members, and witnessing the steady deterioration of their loved ones is extremely painful. Many families eventually become exhausted and suffer from emotional, physical, and financial problems. Outside relationships may have to be forfeited. The necessity of drastically altering lifestyles may lead to overwhelming feelings of anger, depression, and hopelessness. These feelings may be displaced onto the ill person, who then may become more vulnerable to elder abuse. (Elder abuse is discussed in Chapter 18.) Research indicates that caregivers who are at high risk for abusing are those who have been in the caregiving role for many years, who have been providing care for

---

Box 15.1

Improving Communications

- Reduce background noise
- Speak only when you can be seen so your facial expression can provide visual cues to the meaning of your words
- Address by name
- Speak slowly to compensate for decreased ability to process information
- Ask only one question at a time and wait for the response
- Give instructions one step at a time
- When possible, demonstrate actions you want the person to take—miming and gestures can increase understanding
- Pictures may increase understanding
- Learn the limits of the person's attention span
- Be quick with praise and encouragement

---

many hours every day, and whose loved one is severely impaired (American Journal of Psychiatry, 1997).

While clients are still able to participate and make their wishes known, family members can seek their guidance regarding long-term plans. A living will or an advance directive may be formulated. A durable power of attorney for health care should be named as well as a durable power of attorney for financial matters.

Physiological Characteristics

Deterioration of the CNS results in physical changes throughout the body. People with dementia may suffer from *hypertonia*, an increase in muscle tone that results in muscular twitchings. While hyperactivity may occur, eventually there is a loss of energy and increasing fatigue with physical activity. The sleep cycle is impaired; there is a decrease in total sleep time and more frequent awakenings. This disruption leads to sleep deprivation, which magnifies the already disturbed cognitive functions.

People suffering from DAT are susceptible to injuries from falls. About half the falls are secondary to medical problems such as orthostatic hypotension, arrhythmias, and impaired vision. Other falls are

■ *Table 15.3* CNS Pathways of Destruction

Area	Function	Symptoms
Limbic system	Memory, interpretation of emotion.	Problems with recent and later remote memory; depression.
Frontal lobe	Cognition, planning; motor aspects of speech; control of movement; control of outbursts; insight into own behavior.	Problems with planning activities; inability to carry out skilled, purposeful movement; catastrophic reactions and emotional outbursts; delusions; inability to walk, talk, swallow.
Parietal lobe	Sensory speech and ability to recognize written words; proprioception; ability to recognize objects and their function.	Inability to recognize familiar places, people, and purpose of common household objects; expressive aphasia; agraphia; agnosia; hallucinations; seizures; falls.
Temporal lobe	Memory, judgment, learning; ability to understand spoken words.	Receptive aphasia; problems with memory and learning new concepts or activities.
Occipital lobe	Ability to understand written words.	Inability to read with comprehension; hallucinations.

related to such factors as poor lighting or loose rugs. Some people will fall because of poor judgment, as in putting a chair on top of a table and climbing up to reach something. Because of changes in the CNS, these people have a decreased reaction time. Thus, it is more difficult to regain balance when beginning to fall.

As the disease progresses, incontinence of both urine and stool occurs. In the final stage, anorexia leads to an emaciated physical condition. Death usually occurs from pneumonia, urinary tract infection leading to sepsis, malnutrition, or dehydration (Klebanoff and Smith, 1997).

Pathophysiological changes associated with Alzheimer's disease are degenerative and result in gross atrophy of the cerebral cortex. As the disease destroys brain cells, two types of abnormalities occur. *Tangles* are thick, insoluble clots of protein inside the damaged brain cells or neurons. *Plaques,* found on the outside of dead and damaged neurons, consist of bits of dying cells mixed with beta-amyloid protein.

Refer to Chapter 4 for a review of normal brain function. There is a specific pattern in the death of neurons in Alzheimer's disease. The first nerves to die are in the limbic system, the center for emotion and memory. The limbic system interprets emotional responses coming from the cerebral cortex, and the hippocampus, a part of the limbic system, is involved in memory storage. Destruction of the hippocampus results in recent memory loss. Remote memory loss is slower to occur, possibly because the memories are stored in more than one location in the brain. Alzheimer's disease often brings on depression related to limbic system damage, as well as damage to the locus ceruleus, which is responsible for the production of dopamine. Decreased serotonin (5-HT) in the brain is associated with increased aggressive behavior. Dopamine (DA) and the balance between DA and acetylcholine (ACH) may also influence aggression in persons with DAT (Aarsland et al, 1996; Cutler and Sramek, 1996).

The destruction of neurons spreads toward the surface of the brain, killing off nerve cells in the cerebral cortex. A wide variety of symptoms appear as the destruction spreads throughout the four lobes. The relationship between symptoms and specific areas of destruction is covered in Table 15.3. CAT scans may demonstrate brain atrophy, widened cortical sulci, and enlarged cerebral ventricles. PET scans can detect Alzheimer's-related abnormalities by the way certain sugars are processed in the brain, especially in the temporal and parietal lobes.

Concomitant Disorders

It is estimated that 20–50% of long-lived adults suffering from dementia experience mental deterioration related to vascular accidents or cerebral arteriosclerosis. Narrowing of arteries in the brain leads to multiple infarctions, thus the term *multi-infarct dementia*. Less common forms of dementia stem from degenerative nervous system disorders such as Parkinson's disease, Huntington's chorea, multiple sclerosis, Pick's disease, and Creutzfeldt-Jakob disease. Dementia may also occur secondarily to some other pathological process such as AIDS dementia complex (ADC), drug intoxication, Korsakoff's syndrome, CNS neoplasms, and head injuries.

There are several reversible disorders that simulate or mimic dementia. Referred to as **pseudodementias**, these include drug toxicity, metabolic disorders, infections, and nutritional deficiencies. Chronic lung disease and heart disease can lead to cerebral hypoxia and symptoms of dementia. The most common cause of pseudodementia is depression, which is often overlooked by health care professionals. It is imperative that such disorders be recognized and differentiated from irreversible dementia. Only through recognition can appropriate treatment measures be initiated. For a comparison of depression and dementia, see Table 15.4.

Causative Theories

The cause of Alzheimer's disease is unknown but is likely to be a combination of aging and genetic and environmental factors. Research continues in an effort to understand the biochemical events responsible for the destruction of brain cells and is currently focusing on the role of chromosomes 1, 14, 19, and 21. People with Down syndrome, an abnormality on chromosome 21 including the amyloid precursor protein gene, are at high risk for developing lesions in the brain similar to those seen in Alzheimer's disease. Seventy-five percent of persons with Down syndrome over the age of 60 have dementia, with neurobiological changes postmortem that are indistinguishable from those of DAT (Pietrini et al, 1997).

It is not yet known how the genes and their various mutations cause DAT, but scientists are looking for some link between genes and the production of apolipoprotein E (apo E). It comes in three varieties: apo E2, E3, and E4. The E2 version of the gene protects people from getting DAT, while E4 makes it start at a younger age. The risk from E3, the most common apo E gene, falls in between. It is thought that apo E somehow changes the form of a substance called amyloid in the brain, the principal component

Table 15.4 Depression and Dementia Compared

Depression	Dementia
Relatively rapid onset.	Insidious onset.
Symptoms progress rapidly.	Symptoms progress slowly.
Able to recall recent events.	Has difficulty recalling recent events.
Has long-term memory.	As disease progresses, loses long-term memory.
"Don't know" answers are common.	Uses confabulation rather than admitting "don't know."
Attention span normal.	Impaired attention span.
Affect is depressed.	Affect is shallow and labile.
Oriented to person, time, and place.	Unable to recognize familiar people and places; becomes lost in familiar environments; disoriented as to time.
Apathetic in relationship to ADLs.	Struggles to perform ADLs and is frustrated as a result.

of the plaques associated with Alzheimer's disease (Cutler and Sramek, 1996; Filley, 1995).

Psychopharmacological Interventions

No known treatment can stop or reverse the mental deterioration of DAT. Researchers are looking for ways to increase the amount of ACH in the brain. Because it is digested in the GI tract, ACH cannot be taken orally. Two medications increase the availability of ACH in the synapses: Cognex (tacrine) and Aricept (donepezil). One study involving clients with mild to moderate DAT found that those taking Cognex regained about 6 months' worth of the mental functioning they had lost. Cognex and Aricept do not cure DAT but may slow the progression of the disorder. They are not effective for those in stage 3. Some researchers are investigating nerve growth factor, a normal protein that nurtures and restores nerve cells (American Journal of Psychiatry, 1997). Because a concomitant depression may increase functional disability, antidepressant medications are prescribed for people with depressive symptoms. Antipsychotic medications may decrease agitation, aggression, paranoid thinking, and poor impulse control. The half-life of these agents is also extremely prolonged when they are administered to long-lived adults. Medication should not be overused to sedate and calm clients. For those experiencing sleep problems, the use of hypnotics is contraindicated because the medication does not improve sleep patterns and often increases confusion and sedation during awake periods. However, Haldol, 0.5 mg at bedtime, may help regulate sleep (Aarsland et al, 1996; Marchello, Boczko, and Shelkey, 1995). Researchers have found that vitamin E modestly slows the progression of DAT. Others have found that Eldepryl (selegiline), a drug for Parkinson's disease, works about as well as vitamin E; both seem to slow the rate of functional decline. Research also suggests that women can reduce their risk of DAT by taking hormones during and after menopause. It is thought that estrogen may protect the brain by keeping nerve cells healthy and by increasing neurotransmitters (American Journal of Psychiatry, 1997; Cutler and Sramek, 1996).

Multidisciplinary Interventions

The most effective approach to DAT occurs with the coordinated efforts of the multidisciplinary team. Speech therapists may be able to slow down the aphasic process as well as restore partial swallowing function. Physical therapists can maintain or increase range of motion, improve muscle tone, improve coordination, and increase endurance for exercise. Occupational therapists can provide additional sensory stimulation and self-care training programs. Social workers can provide individual or group therapy for families of people with DAT; moreover, they can help with community resources or institutional placement. Pastoral counselors can help clients and families meet religious and spiritual needs.

Knowledge Base: Delirium

Delirium, an acute disorder of cognition and attention, has become increasingly recognized as a common and serious problem for hospitalized individuals. Delirium occurs in 15–56% of hospitalized elderly clients and 30–40% of hospitalized people with AIDS. In the general hospital population the rate is 10–30%. Delirium develops quickly and usually lasts about 1 week unless the underlying disorder is not corrected. Prompt medical attention is vital in order to prevent permanent brain damage or death. If the cause is not found and treated, death may occur in a matter of days or weeks. The course of the disorder is one of fluctuation; that is, periods of coherence alternate with periods of confusion (Breitbart et al, 1996; Inouye and Charpentier, 1996).

Behavioral Characteristics

People suffering from delirium generally display an alteration in psychomotor activity and poor impulse control. Some are apathetic and withdrawn, others are agitated and tremulous, and still others shift rapidly between apathy and agitation. Hyperactivity is typical of a drug withdrawal state, whereas hypoactivity is typical of a metabolic imbalance. Speech patterns may be limited and dull, or they may be fast, pressured, and loud. There may be a constant picking at clothes and bed linen as the result of an underlying restlessness. This combination of restlessness and cognitive changes interferes with the person's ability to complete tasks. Bizarre and destructive behavior, which worsens at night, may occur as they attempt to protect themselves or escape from frightening delusions or hallucinations. This behavior may take the form of calling for help, striking out at others, or even attempting to leap out of windows (Sullivan-Marx, 1994).

> Over the course of the past 2 days, Mary has exhibited abrupt behavioral changes. Sometimes she seems apathetic and withdrawn, barely responding to questions or environmental stimuli. Most of the time, however, particularly at night, she becomes agitated and calls out loudly. She vacillates between being verbally aggressive and abusive and being very vulnerable and frightened, asking for help and whimpering like a small child. Much of the verbal content of her messages has to do with snakes that are in bed with her. She desperately keeps trying to remove these snakes from her bed linens.

Affective Characteristics

In the state of delirium, a person's affect may range from apathy to extreme irritability to euphoria. Emotions are labile; they can change abruptly and fluctuate in intensity. A person may be laughing and suddenly become extremely sad and tearful, reflective of the CNS insult. The predominant emotion in delirium is fear. Illusions, delusions, and hallucinations are vivid and extremely frightening (Tune and Ross, 1994). Mary is terrified by the visual hallucinations of snakes on her bed. She perceives her safety to be threatened and cries for help in removing the snakes. During a family interview, the nurse in charge learns that Mary has always been extremely frightened of snakes, which increases the impact of her hallucinations.

Cognitive Characteristics

The primary cognitive characteristics of delirium are disorganized thinking and a diminished ability to maintain and shift attention. Disorganized thinking is evidenced by rambling, bizarre, or incoherent speech. Lack of judgment and reason severely impairs the decision-making process. Delirious people have difficulty focusing their attention and are easily distracted by environmental stimuli; therefore, interactions are difficult, if not impossible. Attention problems result in an impairment in recent memory. Remote memory problems may result from changes in the neurotransmitters, making the retrieval of information difficult.

Another cognitive disruption is disorientation, which often results from attention deficits. Disorientation as to time and place is common, whereas identity confusion is rare. Almost all people suffering from delirium misperceive sensory stimuli in the environment. The result is usually visual or auditory illusions. For example, the person may believe that spots on the floor are insects. Visual hallucinations are also common and may involve people, animals, objects, or bright flashes of light or color. Delusional beliefs exist, supporting the illusions and hallucinations. These changes often extend into sleep, which may be accompanied by vivid and terrifying dreams (American Journal of Psychiatry, 1997).

> **Marie is an 18-year-old, extremely thin, anorexic client. Laboratory analysis reveals her blood glucose level to be 40 mg/dL. She is agitated and incoherent. Owing to her inability to think logically and also to the fact that she is trying to communicate to others not actually present, she is unable to give a history. She is completely disoriented as to time and place. In terms of orientation to people, she is able to state her own name but does not recognize the boyfriend who brought her to the hospital. In fact, she is convinced that Ron, a nurse, is her boyfriend.**

Sociocultural Characteristics

Because of the sudden and often unexplained onset of delirium, families are usually anxious and frightened. They may not know how to respond to the agitation, pressured speech, destructive behavior, and labile moods. Equally confusing to families are the disorientation, illusions, hallucinations, and delusions. Because delirious individuals are unable to make decisions, family members must temporarily assume that responsibility.

Physiological Characteristics

People with delirium experience a disturbance in the sleep cycle. Some have hypersomnia and sleep fitfully throughout the day and night. Others have insomnia and sleep very little, day or night. There are obvious signs of autonomic activity, including increased cardiac rate, elevated blood pressure, flushed face, dilated pupils, and sweating. Respiratory depth or rhythm may be altered as a result of brain stem depression, or in an attempt to correct an acid-base imbalance that results from the underlying disorder.

Delirious individuals may experience irregular tremors throughout the body. Those in a resting position may have myoclonus, a sudden, large muscle spasm. Although they occur most frequently in the face and shoulders, these spasms, which are a result of irritation of the cerebral cortex, can happen anywhere in the body. If the hand is hyperextended, there will be an involuntary palmar flexion called *asterixis*. Generalized seizures may also occur (Tune and Ross, 1994).

Concomitant Disorders

Delirium occurs in people of all ages. However, the incidence increases with age because of the accompanying illnesses and medication use. Physiological changes of aging such as decreased blood flow to the liver and kidneys predispose long-lived adults to delirium. People with DAT are also predisposed to delirium because their CNS function is already compromised. Other groups at high risk include people with terminal cancer and those with AIDS.

The term **pseudodelirium** is used to describe symptoms of delirium that occur without any identifiable organic cause. The symptoms may occur from sensory deprivation or from the effects of psychosocial stress. Those most vulnerable to pseudodelirium have some pre-existing cerebral disease such as a mood disorder, anxiety, schizophrenia, and dementia (Inouye and Charpentier, 1996).

Causative Theories

By affecting the CNS, many conditions may lead to delirium. Cerebral metabolism is dependent on sufficient amounts of oxygen, glucose, and metabolic cofactors. Brain hypoxia may result from pulmonary disease, anemia, or carbon monoxide poisoning. A decreased cerebral blood flow leads to ischemia of the CNS. Ischemia may result from cardiac arrhythmias or arrest, congestive heart failure, pulmonary embolus, decreased blood volume, systemic lupus erythematosus, or subacute bacterial endocarditis. A lack of adequate glucose for cerebral metabolism occurs during a state of hypoglycemia. Certain metabolic cofactors are essential for cerebral enzyme actions. Cofactor deficiencies involve thiamine, niacin, pyridoxine, folate, and vitamin B_{12} (Inouye and Charpentier, 1996). Endocrine disorders of the thyroid, parathyroid, and adrenal glands are associated with delirium. Hepatic and renal failure may be contributing disorders. Fluid and electrolyte imbalance—particularly acidosis, alkalosis, potassium, sodium, magnesium, and calcium imbalances—are additional causes of delirium. Toxicity from substances such as alcohol, sedatives, antihistamines, parasympatholytics, opioids, cerebral stimulants, digitalis, antidepressants, and heavy metals may also lead to a delirious state. (See Chapter 13 for a discussion of alcohol and drug abuse.) Other likely offenders include anticholinergics and analgesics, which induce CNS depression. Any direct or primary CNS disturbance—trauma, infection, hemorrhage, neoplasm, or a seizure disorder—is likely to trigger delirium. In addition, drugs used for the treatment of hypertension and Parkinson's disease have been implicated in causing delirium (Cummings and Trimble, 1995). The use of physical restraints may be a contributing factor to delirium. The use of restraints with older adults is often said to be for their personal safety and avoidance of harm. Yet restraint use has many negative affects, such as decreased mobility, skin breakdown, cardiac stress, agitation, confusion, and lowered self-esteem. Physical restraints can precede the onset of delirium, thus precipitating this acute disorder (Inouye and Charpentier, 1996; Sullivan-Marx, 1994).

Psychopharmacological Interventions

The medical treatment of delirium involves the swift identification of the organic cause. Appropriate treatment requires removal of an offending substance, stabilization in the presence of trauma, administration of antibiotics for infection, or re-establishing of nutrition and metabolic balance. Medications used in managing substance withdrawal delirium are discussed in Chapter 13.

Controlling the symptoms of delirium may be accomplished through the administration of Haldol intravenously over a period of 1–3 minutes. When combined with Ativan, there is often a rapid reduction of delirium and severe agitation. IM administration of Haldol has an unpredictable rate of absorption and is more likely to produce extrapyramidal side effects. Because Haldol has not yet been approved for intravenous use, each hospital's human studies committee must approve its use for each client. The usual dose is 2–5 mg. Doses may be repeated every 20–30 minutes but should not total more than 5 mg every 15 minutes, with a maximum of 240 mg in a 24-hour period. The desired clinical effect is a person who is drowsy but arousable. Once the person is calm, 0.5–3 mg of Haldol may be administered orally. If a client develops extrapyramidal symptoms, 25–50 mg of Benadryl (diphenhydramine) may be given intravenously (Breitbart et al, 1996).

▌*The Nursing Process*

Assessment

Assessing clients with cognitive impairment disorders—and, specifically, DAT—can be a challenge to a nurse's ingenuity and patience. Some clients can respond appropriately when questions are asked simply and enough time is given. Others are so disoriented and confused that they are unable to answer questions; in these situations, you must rely on family members to provide the necessary assessment data.

See the Focused Nursing Assessment table for clients with cognitive impairment disorders and their family members.

Hamdy and colleagues (1990) developed a *differential diagnosis tool* based on the word "dementia." It is critical that all other disease processes be identified and treated before a person is diagnosed with Alzheimer's disease.

D   Drugs and alcohol. Long-lived people often purchase many OTC medications, have many medications prescribed, and sometimes borrow medication from friends.

E   Eyes and ears. People who cannot hear or see well often appear confused.

M   Metabolic and endocrine diseases. Disruptions such as electrolyte imbalance, hypothyroidism, and uncontrolled diabetes may mimic dementia.

E   Emotional disorders. Mood and schizophrenic disorders may be mistaken for DAT.

N   Nutritional deficiencies. These may mimic dementia.

T   Tumors and trauma. Disorders of the CNS may be confused with DAT.

I   Infection. Infections of the urinary tract and pneumonia in long-lived people may lead to confusion. Clients may not have an elevated temperature.

A   Arteriosclerosis. A decreased blood flow to the brain, CVAs, and multi-infarct dementia often mimic DAT.

Diagnosis

The most common nursing diagnoses for clients with cognitive impairment disorders include:

- *Impaired home maintenance management* related to disorientation, wandering behavior, poor impulse control.
- *Bathing/hygiene/dressing/grooming/feeding self-care deficit* related to an inability to sequence these skills.
- *Anxiety* related to an awareness of cognitive and behavioral deficits.
- *Altered thought processes* related to distractibility, decreasing judgment, memory loss, confabulation.

- *Impaired verbal communication* related to aphasia, agraphia, agnosia.
- *Altered sexuality patterns* related to change in desire for sexual activity.
- *Ineffective family coping* related to changing roles, physical exhaustion, financial problems.
- *High risk for violence directed at others* related to labile emotions, aggressive behavior.

Outcome Identification

Once you have established diagnoses, you and the family, and client (if possible) mutually identify goals for care. Client outcomes are specific behavioral measures by which you and significant others determine progress toward goals. The following are examples of some of the outcomes appropriate to people (and their caregivers) with cognitive impairment disorders:

- orientation improves as delirium clears
- participates in appropriate social activities
- participates in a gentle exercise routine
- establishes routines to decrease confusion
- remains safe from harm
- utilizes support groups and respite care

See also the Critical Thinking Pathway for a Client with Dementia: Outpatient Treatment on pages 388–390.

Nursing Interventions

Most clients with delirium will be in the acute care setting. In caring for these clients, all measures must be taken to ensure that permanent brain damage or death does not occur. Because delirium is acute and short-term, plans of care are directed toward short-term goals, with the long-term medical and nursing goal of correcting the underlying disorder.

Over 50% of people with DAT live in the community. Home care can be a great challenge to families and health care professionals. The role of the nurse is to build therapeutic alliances with significant others and teach specific skills for caregiving. All of the following nursing interventions are skills to be taught to caregivers. In caring for clients with DAT,

Text continues on page 391

Focused Nursing Assessment

CLIENTS WITH COGNITIVE IMPAIRMENT DISORDERS

Behavior Assessment	Affective Assessment	Cognitive Assessment	Social Assessment
How much assistance is needed in bathing? Toileting? Dressing? Eating?	What kinds of things make you feel anxious?	What month is it?	How close do you feel to your family members?
Describe any difficulties in performing complex tasks at home and at work.	When do you feel sad?	What year is it?	How do you handle disagreements?
Give me an example of something that has confused you recently.	How often do you feel irritable?	Who is the President of the United States?	
Have you ever become lost when you went out for a walk?	What are your major frustrations in life?	What is your telephone number (or address)?	
	How do you feel about growing older?	Where are you right now?	
		Tell me your complete name.	
		What did you do for activity this morning?	
		What is the purpose of (show the objects to the client) a comb? Toothbrush? Pencil? Telephone book? Shoe?	
		What is the meaning of the proverb "People in glass houses shouldn't throw stones"?	
		What would you do if someone shouted "Fire!" right now?	

FAMILIES OF CLIENTS
WITH COGNITIVE IMPAIRMENT DISORDERS

Behavior Assessment	Affective Assessment	Cognitive Assessment	Social Assessment
How much assistance is needed in activities of daily living?	Describe the degree of spontaneity to verbal and non-verbal stimuli.	Have there been changes in her/his ability to concentrate?	Is there a family history of organic brain disorder?
Tell me about her/his wandering away from home.	How anxious does she/he seem to you?	Describe any confusion about person, time, or place.	What are previous hobbies/interests? Family activities?
Is there difficulty in carrying out psychomotor activities?	How depressed does she/he seem to you?	Describe any suspicious thinking.	Who has been the primary caregiver?
Is she/he picking up and putting things in the mouth?	In what way is irritability increasing?	Describe any recent memory loss.	Describe the stresses in caregiving (emotional, physical, financial).
Does she/he touch everything in sight?	Does she/he have wide mood swings? Describe.	Describe any remote memory loss.	Describe the positive aspects of caregiving.
What kinds of repetitive movements does she/he make?		Does she/he make up answers when facts cannot be remembered?	What kinds of support systems are you able to use? Family? Friends? Religious? Self-help groups?
Describe her/his interactions with other people.		Is there difficulty in finding the right word for objects?	What kinds of discussions have taken place regarding placement?
Is she/he withdrawn? Agitated? Aggressive?		Has she/he lost the ability to read and write?	What other kinds of living arrangements are possible?
Are the behavior problems worse at night?		Is there an inability to identify familiar sounds?	Who is involved in making these decisions?
		Give me examples of irrational decision making.	How united is the family in providing care?
		Has she/he thought that strangers were family members? Please give examples.	

Critical Pathway for a Client with Dementia: Outpatient Treatment

	Date _____ Day 1	Date _____ Days 2–10	Date _____ Days 11–30	Date _____ Ongoing: Days 31–
Daily outcomes	Client will: ■ Maintain stable vital signs. ■ Remain free of injury. ■ Consume 1500 cal and 2000 cc of fluid each day. ■ Verbalize thoughts and feelings. ■ Sleep 6–8 hr/night. ■ Participate in self-care activities to ability. ■ Demonstrate trust with family caregivers. Family caregivers will: ■ Verbalize ability to cope with responsibilities.	Client will: ■ Maintain stable vital signs. ■ Remain free of injury. ■ Consume 1500 cal and 2000 cc of fluid each day. ■ Verbalize thoughts and feelings. ■ Sleep 6–8 hr/night. ■ Participate in self-care activities to ability. ■ Demonstrate trust with family caregivers. ■ Establish regular urine and bowel elimination pattern. ■ Spend short intervals with diversional activity. ■ Demonstrate increasing attention span. Family caregivers will: ■ Verbalize ability to cope with responsibilities.	Client will: ■ Maintain stable vital signs. ■ Remain free of injury. ■ Maintain stable weight. ■ Verbalize thoughts and feelings. ■ Sleep 6–8 hr/night. ■ Participate in self-care activities to ability. ■ Demonstrate trust with family caregivers. ■ Establish regular urine and bowel elimination pattern. ■ Spend increasing intervals with diversional activity. ■ Demonstrate increasing attention span. Family caregivers will: ■ Verbalize ability to cope with responsibilities.	Client will: ■ Maintain stable vital signs. ■ Remain free of injury. ■ Maintain stable weight. ■ Verbalize thoughts and feelings. ■ Sleep 6–8 hr/night. ■ Participate in self-care activities to ability. ■ Demonstrate trust with family caregivers. ■ Maintain regular urine and bowel elimination pattern. ■ Spend increasing intervals with diversional activity. ■ Demonstrate increasing attention span. ■ Stay focused on simple task for 10–15 minutes. Family caregivers will: ■ Verbalize ability to cope with responsibilities.
Assessments, tests, and treatments	Obtain and review copies of pertinent medical records. Assess for co-occurring health conditions. Initiate nursing assessment. Include family caregivers in admission process.	Assess and document advanced directives, code status, client and family goals. Determine treatment plan and objectives with client and family.	Evaluate effectiveness of treatment plan. Revise treatment plan as indicated.	Evaluate effectiveness of treatment plan. Revise treatment plan as indicated.
Diet	Assess: ■ Intake and output. ■ Weight. ■ Dietary preferences.	Assess: ■ Intake and output. ■ Weight weekly. ■ Dietary preferences.	Assess: ■ Intake and output. ■ Weight weekly. ■ Dietary preferences.	Assess: ■ Intake and output. ■ Weight monthly. ■ Dietary preferences.

	Date _____ Day 1 *continued*	Date _____ Days 2–10 *cont.*	Date _____ Days 11–30 *cont.*	Date _____ Ongoing: Days 31–*cont.*
Diet *continued*	■ Chewing and swallowing ability. ■ Caloric intake if indicated. Limit caffeine intake. Encourage frequent, small, nutritious feedings, inclusive of all food groups.	■ Chewing and swallowing ability. ■ Caloric intake if indicated. Limit caffeine intake. Encourage frequent, small, nutritious feedings, inclusive of all food groups.	■ Chewing and swallowing ability. ■ Caloric intake if indicated. Limit caffeine intake. Encourage frequent, small, nutritious feedings, inclusive of all food groups.	■ Chewing and swallowing ability. ■ Caloric intake if indicated. Limit caffeine intake. Encourage frequent, small, nutritious feedings, inclusive of all food groups.
Elimination	Assess bowel and urine elimination patterns. Encourage family caregivers to toilet client q 2–3 hr while awake and PRN.	Assess bowel and urine elimination patterns. Encourage family caregivers to toilet client q 2–3 hr while awake and PRN. Initiate bowel routine if indicated. Initiate continence program if indicated.	Assess bowel and urine elimination patterns. Encourage family caregivers to toilet client q 2–3 hr while awake and PRN. Initiate bowel routine if indicated. Initiate continence program if indicated.	Assess bowel and urine elimination patterns. Encourage family caregivers to toilet client q 2–3 hr while awake and PRN. Initiate bowel routine if indicated. Initiate continence program if indicated.
Activity	Assess safety needs and assist caregivers to maintain appropriate precautions and frequent observations. Activity as tolerated. PR evaluation if indicated. Assess self-care abilities.	Assess family caregivers' abilities to maintain safety. Activity as tolerated. Encourage caregivers to prompt and assist with hygiene as needed. OT evaluation if indicated. Assess caregivers' abilities to assist with self-care activities.	Assess family caregivers' abilities to maintain safety. Activity as tolerated. Encourage caregivers to prompt and assist with hygiene as needed. OT evaluation if indicated. Evaluate caregivers' abilities to assist with self-care activities.	Assess family caregivers' abilities to maintain safety. Activity as tolerated. Encourage caregivers to prompt and assist with hygiene as needed. OT evaluation if indicated. Assess caregivers' abilities to assist with self-care activities.
Psychosocial	Assess level of anxiety. Approach client in calm, quiet, nonjudgmental manner. Provide information and support and encouragement to client and family caregivers.	Assess level of anxiety. Approach client in calm, quiet, nonjudgmental manner. Provide information and support and encouragement to client and family caregivers.	Assess level of anxiety. Approach client in calm, quiet, nonjudgmental manner. Provide information and support and encouragement to client and family caregivers.	Assess level of anxiety. Approach client in calm, quiet, nonjudgmental manner. Provide information and support and encouragement to client and family caregivers.

continued ➤

Critical Pathway for a Client with Dementia: Outpatient Treatment continued

	Date _____ Day 1 *continued*	Date _____ Days 2–10 *cont.*	Date _____ Days 11–30 *cont.*	Date _____ Ongoing: Days 31–*cont.*
Psychosocial *continued*	Encourage expression of thoughts and feelings. Explore availability of support system.	Encourage expression of thoughts and feelings. Identify interests. Discuss availability of community resources. Make appropriate referrals.	Encourage expression of thoughts and feelings. Identify and involve client in activities related to interest. Assess effectiveness of support systems and community resources.	Encourage expression of thoughts and feelings. Continue to encourage involvement in activities related to interests. Continue to assess effectiveness of support systems. Make additional referrals as indicated.
Medications	Routine meds as ordered. Assess need for PRN meds for agitation. Assess for side effects. Assess medication compliance. Assess caregivers' knowledge of medications.	Review medication regime with caregivers. Routine meds as ordered. Assess need for PRN meds for agitation. Assess for side effects. Assess medication compliance. Provide caregivers with teaching related to medications.	Routine meds as ordered. Assess need for PRN meds for agitation. Assess for side effects. Assess medication compliance. Reinforce teaching related to medications.	Routine meds as ordered. Assess need for PRN meds for agitation. Assess for side effects. Assess medication compliance. Reinforce teaching as needed.
Sleep and rest	Assess sleep and rest routines, including hours awake and asleep, time of rising, naps, dreams/nightmares.	Provide measures that promote rest and sleep, such as warm milk, guided imagery, relaxation techniques.	Provide measures that promote rest and sleep.	Provide measures that promote rest and sleep.
Cognitive/ knowledge	Mental status exam. Orient client and family to outpatient care and community resources. Include client and family caregivers in teaching. Assess understanding of teaching.	Mental status exam weekly and PRN. Orient client and family to outpatient care and community resources. Include client and family caregivers in teaching. Assess understanding of teaching.	Mental status exam weekly and PRN. Orient client and family to outpatient care and community resources. Include client and family caregivers in teaching. Assess understanding of teaching.	Mental status exam monthly and PRN.

Nursing Interventions Classification

CLIENTS WITH COGNITIVE IMPAIRMENT

DOMAIN: Safety

Class: *Risk Management*

> **Interventions:** *Delirium Management:* Provision of a safe and therapeutic environment for the patient who is experiencing an acute confusional state.
>
> *Dementia Management:* Provision of a modified environment for the patient who is experiencing a chronic confusional state.
>
> *Environmental Management: Safety:* Monitoring manipulation of the physical environment to promote safety.

DOMAIN: Behavioral

Class: *Cognitive Therapy*

> **Interventions:** *Reality Orientation:* Promotion of patient's awareness of personal identity, time, and environment.

DOMAIN: Family

Class: *Life Span Care*

> **Interventions:** *Family Involvement:* Facilitating family participation in the emotional and physical care of the patient.

patience and compassion are the guiding principles, with innovation and flexibility as the key elements. What works today may not work tomorrow. Because cognition underlies and directs behavior, clients' cognitive abilities guide the selection of appropriate nursing interventions. Even though the disorder is progressive and eventually terminal, it is important to support and encourage clients to remain at the highest possible level of functioning. See the accompanying box for a summary of the nursing interventions classifications (NIC).

Safety: Risk Management

Delirium Management

Management of clients who are experiencing delirium includes initiating therapies to reduce or eliminate the factors that are causing the delirium. The neurological status of clients must be monitored on an ongoing basis. Clients benefit from nursing interventions designed to prevent or manage agitation, anxiety, and perceptual or cognitive disturbances. (For nursing care of clients who have hallucinations and/or delusions, see Chapter 6). Frequent contact, repeating of information, and reassurance will increase the client's orientation. Brief, simple statements are better understood than lengthy explanations. Give the client and family information about what is happening and what can be expected to occur in the future. Orient the client as necessary and avoid frustration through quizzing with questions that cannot be answered. Since both sensory deprivation and sensory overstimulation can worsen symptoms, you will need to adjust the environment according to the client's response. This is often a process of trial and error. In general, you will want enough light at all times to minimize shadows that may contribute to illusions (McCloskey and Bulechek, 1996).

Dementia Management

Communication with clients is an extremely important nursing intervention. Attempts to communicate are more likely to be successful when environmental distractions and noise are kept to a minimum. Begin each conversation by identifying yourself and addressing clients by name to orient them and get their attention. Speak slowly and distinctly, in a low tone or voice, conveying a sense of calm. Because these clients may not be able to comprehend complex language, use clear, simple sentences. Do not demean the person or use baby talk; clients can often comprehend the emotional tone of speech even when they can no longer understand the words. Closed-ended questions are easier to respond to than open-ended questions;

ask only one question at a time. Pronouns are often misunderstood, and clients may respond more appropriately to direct address, as in "Mary, it is time to eat now." Using nonverbal communication such as smiles, hugs, and hand-holding will reinforce verbal communication. Above all, remember that these clients are adults and should be treated with respect and dignity.

Involvement with their environment is important for clients with DAT. Caregivers should plan regular social activities. Clients are often more capable than either they or their families realize, and there may be any number of simple tasks they could do by themselves. Performing simple tasks around the home keeps them busy and helps them feel good about themselves. It is important that they be provided with regular exercise such as walking, group exercise, or dancing. Studies have shown that exercise decreases disruptive behaviors and increases appropriate interactions with others. The rhythmic motions of exercise may be a way to meet the need for the repetitive behavior that occurs in Alzheimer's clients. They may participate in exercise more willingly if others exercise with them. Having a regular routine (same time, same exercises) will minimize confusion. If the client is unsteady, a supportive person should be nearby to prevent falls and injuries. Consistent, low-impact exercise will increase the oxygenation of the brain, slow the loss of motor function, and increase energy and feelings of well-being and accomplishment.

Because many clients suffering from DAT experience sleep problems, actions to improve sleep will benefit both clients and families. Encourage clients and family members to keep a sleep journal to establish baseline data. The journal should answer such questions as: How many daytime naps are being taken? How many times a night does the client awaken? What medications are being taken? Several factors may exacerbate sleep problems. Pain, as from arthritis, can make sleep more difficult. Caffeine intake, eating rich foods near bedtime, fluid intake in the evening, and exercising too close to bedtime can be detrimental. Interventions include minimizing napping during the daytime, regular exercise but not too close to bedtime, modifying the environment by decreasing noise, and providing comfort measures such as back rubs.

Instruct caregivers to maintain a regular schedule of mealtimes to prevent confusion that is caused by change. Limit the number of foods in front of clients since they may have difficulty deciding which food to eat. Provide utensils with large built-up handles or use finger foods when lack of coordination interferes with eating. Try using bowls rather than plates and offer soup in a mug. This is easier because food is not pushed off a plate and liquid is not spilled from a spoon. Remove other distractions from the eating area to maintain the focus on eating. Do not rush eating, since people with DAT often eat slowly.

Encourage ADL skills that are still present to maintain independence and provide opportunities for clients to feel a sense of competence. Try to follow old routines as much as possible, such as time of day for a bath or preference for a bath or a shower. Clients should be encouraged to make as many decisions as possible in ADLs. This increases their sense of control and prevents the disengagement that occurs when all responsibility is taken away. Lay out clean clothes in the order to be put on. Velcro tape instead of buttons and zippers is often helpful.

Environmental Management: Safety

Even first-stage Alzheimer's disease can impair driving to some extent, and the risk of accidents increases with increasing severity of the dementia. Discuss the risks of driving with clients and caregivers. Explore clients' current driving patterns, transportation needs, and possible alternatives. These issues should be reassessed frequently. At some point, caregivers will need to prevent clients' driving. Encourage them to lock the car keys in a cabinet, hide the garage door controller, and learn easily reversible ways to disable the car.

Caregivers must minimize specific hazards in the home because people with DAT suffer from poor judgment. Objects that may be potentially dangerous must be locked up or removed, including irons, power tools, paints, solvents, stove knobs, and cleaning agents. The hot water heater should be turned to a lower temperature to prevent accidental burning. Paint hot water faucets and knobs red. Remove footstools, extension cords, and throw rugs that can lead to tripping, as well as table lamps, vases, and other breakables that are easily knocked over.

The client should be prohibited from smoking or be provided with supervision in order to prevent burns or fires. Prescribed medications can become a hazard when clients take the wrong medication, too much medication, or the right medication at the wrong time. Since memory loss interferes with correct self-administration, it is often appropriate for caregivers to administer the medications. Rid the home of firearms and poisonous plants and put safety locks on cabinets containing harmful substances.

Family members and/or institutional staff members need to be taught measures to reduce potential injury from wandering or becoming lost. Provide clients with an ID bracelet and ID card. Have the family register with the Safe Return program through the Alzheimer's Association (1-800-621-0379). If the client can still read and comprehend, a family member can write out simple directions home, along with the home phone number. Family members should assess the neighborhood for potentially dangerous areas such as busy streets, swimming pools, rivers, and bridges. Other people living in the neighborhood can be alerted to the situation, which will increase protection for the client. If the client is wandering away from the home, the yard can be fenced in with locked gates. The doors to the house should be kept locked, and an alarm system can be connected to the doors. This will prevent the person from slipping out unnoticed. Wandering is often decreased in clients who are provided regular outlets for exercise.

Many clients will require safety measures regarding impaired physical mobility, which might be evidenced by stiffness, awkwardness, and unsteadiness. Keep furniture in the same places, and provide good lighting. Pad sharp corners, and discard throw rugs to minimize the likelihood of falls. If the client is unsteady, a supportive person should be nearby to help maintain balance. Handrails on staircases and in bathrooms provide additional support. If the client is unable to sit unassisted, posey restraints or a posey chair may be helpful.

As many as 33% of clients with DAT become physically abusive to their caregivers. Steps should be taken to ensure the safety of client, family, and staff. Catastrophic reactions may occur when clients feel overwhelmed. They may respond with anger, stubbornness, agitation, and combativeness. The first step is to respond calmly and not retaliate with anger. Remember that the client's anger is often exaggerated and displaced. Remove objects in the environment that may be used to harm self or others. Try to understand what precipitated the aggressive behavior. Some clients may perceive that they are being threatened, and the aggressive behavior may be an attempt to defend themselves. Determine whether the client behaves this way toward everyone in the environment or only to specific people. Some clients become aggressive when they have pain and believe nothing is being done to help them. Accurately identifying

precipitating events increases one's ability to prevent or minimize recurrence. Finally, clients should be removed from the upsetting situation or environment. Distractions are often effective because impaired memory makes them forget what caused the immediate anger. Catastrophic reactions can be avoided by:

- keeping requests relatively simple to avoid frustration
- avoiding confrontation and deferring requests if client becomes angry
- being consistent and avoiding unnecessary change
- providing frequent reminders, explanations, and orientation cues
- ignoring inappropriate behavior that is not harmful
- avoiding crowds, strangers, confusion, and noise

Behavioral: Cognitive Therapy

Reality Orientation

Use the name clients prefer to reinforce their identity. Provide aids that assist with orientation, such as large-print calendars, clocks, and labels on objects in the environment. Be selective regarding media and avoid programs with intricate plots or frightening content. If clients are using confabulation to reduce their shame or embarrassment about memory losses, give cues to help them remember reality and gently remind them of what actually occurred by filling in information gaps. Routinely and frequently orient clients to who, where, and what is happening, which allows them to become oriented without shame. Do not argue or persist in trying to convince clients of actual reality. When confusion is irreversible this will only increase confusion and frustration. Discuss topics meaningful to clients, such as work, hobbies, children, or significant life events, as these topics promote their identity.

Caregivers can establish measures to decrease agitation and disorientation. The physical environment should be kept stable to increase comfort and decrease frustration and agitation. ADLs should be scheduled at a regular time. As much as possible, encourage clients to participate in decisions regarding their care. If appropriate, you should make certain that clients are wearing their glasses and hearing aids. Poor vision and hearing deficits will increase the potential for confusion.

Family: Life Span Care

Family Involvement

As a nurse, you must be an advocate for family caregivers. Families are often in need of teaching and counseling, support groups, and respite care. Help them locate local resources and develop support networks (see Self-Help Groups/Resources). By decreasing caregiver burden, these groups may improve the quality of life for clients and their families. Other resources that might help include social service agencies, home health agencies, cleaning services, Meals on Wheels, transportation programs, geriatric law specialists, and financial planners. Caregivers need breaks from a very stressful job. They may need assistance in developing coping strategies that deal directly with specific problems, as well as the multitude of emotions they are experiencing. Respite care provided by other family members or through adult day care programs may limit the sense of being overwhelmed by the combination of hard work and personal loss associated with caring for a person with DAT. Discuss the need for periods of rest and recreation to prevent total emotional and physical fatigue of caregivers. Since clients are unable to provide positive feedback to caregivers, discuss how they might seek rewards and recognition apart from clients.

Families need to keep their expectations realistic. Their loved ones with DAT will not get better, but with good caregiving, clients can maintain independence and dignity for a long time.

Evaluation

Evaluation is conducted according to the outcome criteria. You must continually evaluate whether the criteria are being met, and modify the plan accordingly. In relation to DAT, you must evaluate whether clients are reaching their maximum potential and whether their families have the support they need to deal with the disorder. The following are evaluative questions for the family:

1. Are caregivers experiencing stress-related symptoms?
2. How supportive is the family system?
3. Has the family been able to adapt by providing relief for the caregiver in terms of cleaning, shopping, and time away from the home?
4. Has the family been able to discuss feelings of helplessness, embarrassment, guilt, and grief?
5. Has the family been able to support the optimal level of functioning for the client?

Clinical Interactions

A Client with Dementia of the Alzheimer's Type

Ray, 72 years old, has been experiencing symptoms of DAT for the past several years. For the past year he has been attending a day program for persons with DAT. His daughter drops him off on her way to work and picks him up on her way home. If outside appointments need to be scheduled during that time, the staff of the day program provides transportation. Ray's daughter has forgotten to inform the staff about Ray's appointment to have his hair cut. In the interaction, you will see evidence of:

- confusion with pronouns; he uses "we" to mean "I."
- difficulty comprehending even small changes in schedule.
- loss of short-term memory.
- an inability to remember the word "barber."

NURSE: Ray, we are going to have lunch 30 minutes earlier today because it is the day for the music therapist to be here with us.

RAY: We go to lunch at 12.

NURSE: It is necessary to have lunch now.

RAY: We don't want to go now.

NURSE: Please come with me. It is time to go to lunch.

RAY: We won't go now.

NURSE: It's time to go to lunch.

RAY: We go at 12!

NURSE: It's time for lunch.

RAY: [Throwing up his hands.] Okay, okay.

[Ray eats and returns to the day room.]

RAY: We have an appointment at 2 PM.

NURSE: Can you tell me what that appointment is for?

RAY: It's at 2 PM.

NURSE: Do you know where you are supposed to go for the appointment?

RAY: Main Street.

NURSE: Do you know where you are supposed to go on Main Street?

RAY: Main Street. That's where we have to go.

NURSE: Can you give me any other hints as to where you are supposed to go?

RAY: We need the wallet.

NURSE: You need your wallet. Is it a store?

RAY: We need the wallet.

NURSE: Do you need to buy something?

RAY: Hair.

NURSE: Hair. Did you make an appointment at the barber shop?

RAY: Yes.

NURSE: I need to take you to your barber shop on Main Street at 2 PM.

RAY: We have an appointment at 2 PM.

NURSE: I will make certain that you get to your hair appointment by 2 PM. ■

Self-Help Groups/Resources

Clients with DAT

Alzheimer's Disease Association
919 North Michigan Avenue
Chicago, IL 60611-1676
(800) 272-3900
www.alz.org

The 36-Hour Day: A Family Guide to Caring for Persons with Alzheimer's Disease, revised edition. Johns Hopkins University Press, 1991.

Key Concepts

Introduction

- Dementia is a chronic, irreversible brain disorder characterized by impairments in memory, abstract thinking, and judgment, as well as changes in personality. Dementia of the Alzheimer's type (DAT) accounts for 50–75% of dementing illnesses. Familial Alzheimer's disease (FAD) begins at a much younger age, and first-degree relatives have a 50% risk of developing the disorder.

- Delirium is an acute, usually reversible brain disorder characterized by clouding of the consciousness and a reduced ability to focus and maintain attention. It may be the result of a wide variety of pathophysiological conditions.

Knowledge Base: Dementia

- Behavioral characteristics of dementia include a decline in personal appearance, socially unacceptable behavior, wandering, apraxia, hyperorality, perseveration phenomena, hyperetamorphosis, and a deterioration in motor ability. Psychotic symptoms may occur with hallucinations, delusions, and aggressive behavior.

- Affective characteristics of dementia include anxiety, depression, helplessness, frustration, shame, lack of spontaneity, and irritability. Moods are often labile, and catastrophic reactions are common.

- Cognitive characteristics of dementia include memory loss, poor judgment, disorientation, language problems, delusions of persecution, confabulation, aphasia, agraphia, and agnosia.

- Families are typically the primary caregivers for people with dementia. As such, they risk emotional and physical fatigue and financial hardship. They need to be encouraged to use supportive resources.

- Deterioration of the CNS results in physical changes such as hypertonia, impaired sleep cycles, injuries from falls, slowed reaction time, and incontinence.

- As the disease progresses, tangles and plaques develop in the brain. The first cells to die are in the limbic system. The destruction of neurons then spreads throughout the four lobes of the cerebral cortex. Symptoms correlate with destruction of various parts of the brain.

- Other forms of dementia result from multiple infarctions in the CNS and from degenerative nervous system disorders, and are secondary to other disorders such as AIDS, drug intoxication, Korsakoff's syndrome, CNS neoplasms, and head injuries.

- There are several reversible disorders that can masquerade as dementia. Referred to as pseudodementias, these include depression, drug toxicity, metabolic disorders, infections, and nutritional deficiencies.

- FAD has a stronger genetic link. It appears that chromosomes 1, 14, 19, and 21 may play a role in the development of this disease. Apo E, produced in the brain, changes the form of amyloid, the principal component of the plaques associated with DAT.

- The drugs Cognex (tacrine) and donepezil slow the breakdown of ACH, thereby increasing the amount available for neurotransmission. Vitamin E and Eldepryl (selegiline) slow the rate of functional decline.

Knowledge Base: Delirium

- Behavioral characteristics of delirium include apathy and withdrawal, agitation, and bizarre and destructive behavior.

- Affective characteristics of delirium may range from apathy to irritability to euphoria, and they may change abruptly.

- The main cognitive characteristics are disorganized thinking, difficulty focusing attention, and easy distractibility. Additional characteristics include recent memory difficulties, disorientation, illusions, hallucinations, and delusions.

- Because of the sudden and often unexplained onset of delirium, families are usually anxious, frightened, and confused.

- Physiological characteristics of delirium include disturbance in sleep cycles, increased autonomic activity, and irregular tremors throughout the body.

- Delirium occurs in people of all ages, but the incidence increases with age. Any physical illness has the potential to cause delirium.

- Concomitant disorders that increase the risk of delirium include decreased blood flow to the liver and kidneys, DAT, terminal cancer, and AIDS. The use of physical restraints can contribute to the onset of delirium.

- Pseudodelirium describes symptoms of delirium that occur without any identifiable organic cause.

- Intravenous Haldol is the most effective method of controlling the symptoms of delirium.

Nursing Assessment

- Client assessment must include the family's perception of changes because the client is not considered a reliable source of accurate information.

- Nurses must assess for other disorders that may mimic dementia. These include drug and alcohol abuse, visual or hearing problems, metabolic and endocrine diseases, emotional disorders, nutritional deficiencies, CNS tumors or trauma, infections, and arteriosclerosis.

Nursing Diagnosis

- Nursing diagnoses relevant to caring for clients with cognitive impairment disorders range from *Impaired home maintenance* to *Altered thought processes* to *Ineffective family coping*.

Outcome Identification

- Since dementia is a progressive disorder, outcomes are developed to maintain the highest level of functioning that is possible at any given time.

Nursing Interventions

- In caring for clients with delirium, all measures must be taken to ensure that permanent brain damage or death does not occur.

- Keeping the client safe is a priority. Interventions include measures to reduce potential injury from wandering or becoming lost, measures to decrease agitation and disorientation, measures to manage aggressive behavior, safety measures regarding impaired physical mobility, and steps to minimize specific hazards in the environment.

- Finding ways to communicate with clients is an extremely important nursing intervention. You will be most successful when you decrease environmental distractions, identify yourself and clients by name, speak slowly and distinctly, use simple sentences, give instructions one step at a time reinforced with demonstrations, and use touching and smiling to reinforce verbal communications.

- Develop plans to include clients in regular social activities and exercise routines. Many clients can be responsible for simple daily tasks.

- Interventions to improve sleep patterns will benefit both clients and families.

- Encourage clients and families to seek legal guidance early in the disease process, when clients are still able to make their wishes known.

- The overall goal of nursing intervention is to help maintain the quality of life in spite of impairments. Nurses must also function as advocates for family caregivers.

- For the client who is experiencing delirium, the environment must be adapted according to the client's response.

Evaluation

- Evaluation of nursing care is based on progress toward the outcome criteria by the client and family.

Review Questions

1. LaVon is in stage 2 of DAT. When the family told her to get dressed to go out to dinner, she appeared at the doorway wearing purses on her feet instead of shoes. This behavior is best described by which of the following terms?

   a. agnosia

   b. apraxia

   c. aphasia

   d. agoraphobia

2. Marc relies on confabuation to fill in his memory gaps. Which approach would be most helpful to teach the family to use with Marc when this occurs?

   a. Label objects in the environment with the correct name.

   b. Put necessary objects in his hand, such as a fork or spoon.

   c. Help Marc locate the lost object with minimal fuss.

   d. Gently remind Marc of what has occurred.

3. Osama, who has DAT, often wanders out of her house during the night in search of her infant children. What safety suggestions would be best for the family to implement?

   a. Put an alarm system on all exit doors.

   b. Put Osama in a waist restraint at night.

   c. Alert neighborhood people to the problem.

   d. Have family members alternate staying awake at night.

4. Which one of the following evaluation statements by the family would indicate that the family is feeling fulfilled by caring for Moshe in his home?

   a. "It's wonderful when he has flashes of memory and we can all share the joy."

   b. "Every day we ask ourselves how much longer we can go on."

   c. "We remind ourselves that our past life has been rewarding even if the present is not."

   d. "It's very frustrating not to be able to communicate with him. It's like talking to a dummy."

5. The most effective way to communicate with a person with DAT is to

   a. use open-ended questions.

   b. use general leads.

   c. offer interpretations.

   d. use closed-ended questions.

References

Aarsland, D., et al. (1996). Relationship of aggressive behavior to other neuropsychiatric symptoms in patients with Alzheimer's disease. *Am J Psychiatry, 153*(2), 243–247.

American Journal of Psychiatry. (1997). Practice guideline for the treatment of patients with Alzheimer's disease and other dementias of late life. *Am J Psychiatry: Supplement, 154*(5), 1–39.

Breitbart, W., et al. (1996). A double-bind trial of haloperidol, chlorpromazine, and lorazepam in the treatment of delirium in hospitalized AIDS patients. *Am J Psychiatry, 153*(2), 231–236.

Burney-Puckett, M. (1996). Sundown syndrome: Etiology and treatment. *J Psychosoc Nurs, 34*(5), 40–43.

Coltharp, W., Richie, M. F., & Kaas, M. J. (1996). Wandering. *J Gerontol Nurs, 22*(11), 5–10.

Cost of Alzheimer's Disease. (1997). *J Psychosoc Nurs, 35*(9), 8.

Cummings, J. L., & Trimble, M. R. (1995). *Concise Guide to Neuropsychiatry and Behavioral Neurology.* Washington, D.C.: American Psychiatric Press.

Cutler, N. R., & Sramek, J. J. (1996). *Understanding Alzheimer's Disease.* Jackson, MS: University Press of Mississippi.

Davies H. D., Zeiss, A., & Tinklenberg, J. R. (1992). Til death us part: Intimacy and sexuality in the marriages of Alzheimer's patients. *J Psychosoc Nurs, 30*(11), 5–10.

England, M. (1995). Crisis and the filial caregiving situations of African American adult offspring. *Issues Ment Health Nurs, 16*(2), 143–163.

Filley, C. M. (1995). Alzheimer's disease: It's irreversible but not untreatable. *Geriatrics, 50*(7), 18–23.

Ford, G. (1996). Putting feeding back into the hands of patients. *J Psychosoc Nurs, 34*(5), 35–39.

Gerdner, L. A., Hall, G. R., & Buckwalter, K. C. (1996). Caregiver training for people with Alzheimer's based on a stress threshold model. *IMAGE, 28*(3), 241–246.

Hamdy, R. C., et al. (1990). *Alzheimer's Disease: A Handbook for Caregivers.* St. Louis, MO: Mosby.

Inouye, S. K., & Charpentier, P. A. (1996). Precipitating factors for delirium in hospitalized elderly persons. *JAMA, 275*(11), 852–857.

Klebanoff, N. A., & Smith, N. M. (1997). *Behavior Management in Home Care.* Philadelphia, PA: Lippincott.

Lach, H. W., et al. (1995). Alzheimer's disease: Assessing safety problems in the home. *Geriatric Nurs, 16*(4), 160–164.

Marchello, V., Boczko, F., & Shelkey, M. (1995). Progressive dementia: Strategies to manage new problem behaviors. *Geriatrics, 50*(3), 40–43.

Matteson, M. A., Linton, A. D., & Barnes, S. J. (1996). Cognitive developmental approach to dementia. *IMAGE, 28*(3), 233–240.

McCloskey, J. C., & Bulechek, G. M. (1996). *Nursing Interventions Classification.* St. Louis, MO: Mosby.

Pietrini, P., et al. (1997). Low glucose metabolism during brain stimulation in older Down's syndrome subjects at risk for Alzheimer's disease prior to dementia. *Am J Psychiatry, 154*(8), 1063–1069.

Price, N. (1995). The role of the consultation-liaison nurse. *J Psychosoc Nurs, 33*(12), 31–34.

Reichman, W. E. (1994). Nondegenerative dementing disorders. In C. E. Coffey & J. L. Cummings (Eds.), *Textbook of Geriatric Neuropsychiatry* (pp. 370–388). Washington, D.C.: American Psychiatric Press.

Rentz, C. A. (1995). Reminiscence. *J Psychosoc Nurs, 33*(11),15–26.

Richter, J. M., Roberto, K. A., & Bottenberg, D. J. (1995). Communicating with persons with Alzheimer's disease. *Arch Psychiatr Nurs, 9*(5), 279–285.

Ripich, D. N., Wykel, M., & Niles S. (1995). Alzheimer's disease caregivers: The FOCUSED program. *Geriatric Nurs, 16*(1), 15–19.

Sullivan-Marx, E. M. (1994). Delirium and physical restraint in hospitalized elderly. *IMAGE, 26*(4), 295–300.

Tune, L., & Ross, C. (1994). Delirium. In C. E. Coffey & J. L. Cummings (Eds.), *Textbook of Geriatric Neuropsychiatry* (pp. 352–365).Washington, D.C.: American Psychiatric Press.

PART IV

Crisis

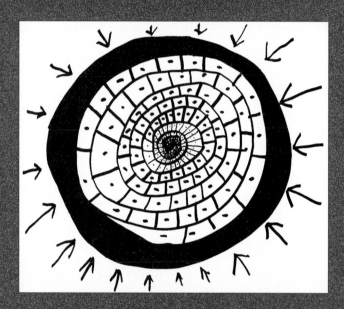

HOW I SEE MY ILLNESS: *Engulfed in Darkness Spiraling inward, wearing a web that is ultimately devastated by a darkness whose victim I always have been but always hope to never be.*

CHAPTER 16

Grief and Loss

Patriciann Brady

Objectives

After reading this chapter, you will be able to:

- Define loss, grief, bereavement, and mourning.
- Discuss the influence of culture on the process of mourning.
- Describe the impact of death on the family unit.
- Assess people who are vulnerable to disenfranchised grief.
- Differentiate between uncomplicated and complicated grieving.

Key Terms

bereavement
mourning
grieving

*L*ife is a series of experiences and challenges. Loss is a human experience and a challenge we all must face. Loss requires that we give up something familiar, comfortable, and personal. The more intense the attachment, the more deeply felt the sense of loss. Loss of a person includes death, separation, divorce, moving, and changes in mental or physical status. We can also lose aspects of ourselves such as self-esteem, health, roles in life, and dreams. We are vulnerable to loss of objects such as possessions or pets. As we go through our life span we experience developmental losses associated with life transitions, such as grown children leaving the home or retirement from a career (Klebanoff and Smith, 1997).

The meaning of loss is subjective, as is the process of responding to a loss. The more significant the loss, the more intense the reaction we experience. Unresolved losses in the past influence how we manage current losses. Factors such as guilt, financial issues, ambivalence, age, culture, number of current stressors, and available support systems determine how we react to loss and express our grief (Gorman, Sultan, and Raines, 1996).

Bereavement is the feelings, thoughts, and responses that loved ones experience following a death of a person with whom they have shared a significant relationship. **Mourning** or **grieving** is the active process of learning to adapt to the loved one's death. Mourning is a progression through a series of phases that include recognition and acceptance of the death, the experience of emotional and physical pain, and the rebuilding of a life without the loved person. Grieving also occurs with any significant loss experience, as mentioned above, and is a process of learning to live with our feelings as we struggle to re-establish our self-esteem or self-confidence in the face of these personal losses. The process of grieving is essential for our mental and physical health as it allows us to cope with the loss gradually and to accept it as part of reality. Mourning and grieving are influenced by our families, our religious beliefs, and our cultural customs. It is a social process and is best shared and carried out with the help of others. None of us grieves predictably or uniformly. As caring nurses, we must always respect individuality in the way persons grieve and mourn (Attig, 1996).

Culture and the Grieving Process

The culture in which each of us is raised and the culture in which each of us lives partially determine what is acceptable in terms of the grieving process. Each culture has grieving rules that tell members who, when, where, how, how long, and for whom people should grieve. Stated more specifically (Shapiro, 1994), each culture:

- describes the nature of life after death
- explains the meaning of the death
- defines the relationship between the dead and the living
- designates the processes of bereavement
- establishes symbolic rituals
- delineates the appropriate expression of feelings
- determines patterns of behavior specific to age and gender
- assigns social roles to survivors

Death is a choiceless event that leads to chaos and disorder for survivors. Our culture tells us how to behave in response to death, which helps us stabilize and cope when we are feeling confused and chaotic. In North America as a whole, death is a taboo topic, a subject that is not spoken of openly. We are socialized to think of death as the worst occurrence in life. We do our best to avoid thinking or talking about death. Dominant cultural values include independence, personal mastery over adversity, and a belief in letting go and moving on. Grief is thought to be a private matter to be endured internally. Therefore feelings tend to be repressed and may remain unidentified. As a result of these cultural values, bereaved people often feel profoundly isolated with very little preparation for this experience (Moos, 1995).

Ethnic minorities in the United States and Canada are not static groups with unchanging traditions and values. It is important for nurses to understand the diverse cultural milieu of mourning but not to stereotype an extremely complex process. Some groups value social support and the expression of loss. The expression of grief through wailing, crying, physical prostration, and other outward demonstrations are acceptable and encouraged as part of the resolution of grief. Other groups may frown on this demonstration as a loss of control, favoring a more quiet and stoic expression of grief. Whatever your own cultural values, it is important that you respect other's ethnic rituals and rules concerning death and grieving. Even when families appear acculturated to the dominant American culture, under circumstances of life cycle transitions, stress, or death, they are more likely to draw on traditional customs and beliefs (Shapiro, 1994).

Families and the Grieving Process

Cultural expectations and reactions to death are closely related to family expectations and history. We live, die, grieve, and survive within a family context. Prior experiences with death and loss in the family influence how we grieve. Families teach us how to behave and the way we should express our feelings when a significant death occurs. Family gender roles also affect reactions at times of loss. In North America, women are often the ones who grieve outwardly in the form of tears and sorrow, while men are expected to "be strong" and show minimal emotion during grief. Men may choose strategies such as logical reasoning or diversional activities to manage their unacknowledged feelings. Our families' spiritual beliefs and religious practices influence how we react to loss and death and our resulting behavior. Most religious groups have customs and practices which can help survivors with the process of grieving (Moos, 1995).

Family systems, like individuals, experience symptoms of grief including changes in communication patterns, changes in family structure and changes in relationships outside the family. Some families experience an increase in communication while others experience a decrease. Some families avoid communicating about certain content areas. There may be a change in the pattern of communication, such as who talks to whom. Some families cut off or reject certain members, while others may reconnect with distant family members.

In response to death, family structure often changes temporarily. There may be role confusion which contributes to turmoil in the family's hierarchy. Relationships with people outside the family often change as the family overprotects some or all members, effectively isolating people. Some families are able to reach out to others, but some withdraw from

their friends and other support networks (Moos, 1995). See Chapter 2 for further information on family functioning.

The death of a family member radically disrupts the family system. The first priority in managing the crisis of grief is to re-establish a stable equilibrium that is necessary to support ongoing family development. This requires the resources of the individual, extended family, friends, and community. Family members need to be able to talk with one another about their emotions concerning the death and its circumstances. A family's ability to communicate about death is partially determined by its members' previous patterns of communication. If individuals are unable to talk about the death, any misconceptions about the cause or circumstances cannot be corrected. For example, in some families the cause of death is never told to children, who then grow up with questions or distorted ideas.

All family members play roles both within and outside the family. Realignment of roles is a necessary function of grieving. Roles may be reassigned on the basis of achievement and interest or on the basis of gender and age. Individuals must adapt and adjust to the new roles and the absence of the deceased member. The more flexible family will typically be more successful. Like individuals, families are unique in their mourning process. What is effective for one family may not be effective for another (Moos, 1995).

Children experience the same emotions of grief as adults but are less likely to show acute grief in the initial phase and more likely to experience the process over a much longer period of time. At each developmental level, children rework the meaning of a family member's death from more mature cognitive and emotional functioning. Preverbal children understand death as a separation, not as a finite end to life. They are often convinced the deceased person could come back if she or he really wanted to. When children develop language skills at 2–3 years they can begin the process of comprehending death and its causes, although they still believe death to be reversible. School-age children tend to be more avoidant in speaking of their grief than either preschoolers or teens, resulting in an appearance of unconcern. Because they equate death with abandonment, this age group is especially vulnerable to reacting with depression, self-blame, and low self-esteem for some months. Adolescents cognitively can understand death in adult terms. They may associate the tragedy with their age-appropriate search for independence. Some teens may become closer to the family and may even feel responsible for their family's survival. Others may begin acting out as their attempts to become their own person are complicated with grief (Shapiro, 1994).

Disenfranchised Grief

Every culture establishes grieving norms and denies such emotions to people who are deemed to have insignificant losses. These losses are not acknowledged or validated by others and the survivors are deprived of their right to grieve. Disenfranchised grief means that the loss cannot be openly acknowledged, socially validated, or publicly mourned. Typically, there are three categories of disenfranchised grief: the relationship is not recognized, the loss is not recognized, or the griever is not recognized.

Often relationships are not recognized when there are no kin ties. These would include close friendships, lovers, neighbors, or caregivers. Other unrecognized relationships are those which are not socially sanctioned, such as nontraditional relationships, extramarital affairs, or same-gender relationships. Relationships that existed primarily in the past are often not recognized as needing to be grieved, such as former friends, past lovers, or ex-spouses. There are some losses that cultures do not socially recognize. These include elective abortions, perinatal deaths, giving up a child for adoption, and even the loss of a beloved pet. The third category are grievers who are not recognized. In this instance, the person is not socially defined by the culture as capable of grief. The very old, who are thought to be too frail and fragile to cope with loss, and the very young, who are thought to be oblivious to loss, are often excluded from discussions and rituals. Sometimes it is assumed that people who are developmentally disabled are incapable of understanding death and have no need to mourn.

As nurses, we must remember that people exist in multiple relationships and form meaningful and significant attachments in different kinds of relationships. The dominant culture often ignores these in favor of the nuclear family, who is given a monopoly on mourning. Past relationships, such as those of ex-spouses, may still hold a degree of attachment and thus there may be grief. When the promise of unborn children is terminated, parents experience grief. In our

> ### Box 16.1
>
> ## Factors Influencing Outcomes in Mourning
>
> **Increased Psychological Distress**
> - Predeath psychiatric disorder—coping with changes is especially difficult
> - Manner of death—sudden, unexpected death more difficult to manage
> - Family life cycle—loss of spouse for young parent with children
> - Dysfunctional relationship with deceased person
> - Constricted capacity to express feelings
> - Financial problems
>
> **Increased Ability to Cope**
> - Good health prior to death
> - Sense of optimism
> - Belief system that helps deal with death
> - Self-sufficient
> - Experience with loss
> - Functional family interactions
> - Supportive social network
> - Adequate financial resources

society, significant pet-human bonds develop and there is grief when the pet dies. People are capable of a great capacity for attachments, so they are vulnerable to grief when these attachments are ended. The problem results when that fact is forgotten and the grief is minimized or ignored.

Complicated Grief

The boundaries between normal and complicated grief are unclear. The judgment that a person's grief reaction is complicated is based not only on the individual but also on the range and tolerance of differences in grieving allowed by the culture. See Box 16.1 for factors that contribute to increased distress or to a good outcome during mourning.

Complicated grief may include symptoms such as intrusive images, severe feelings of emptiness, and

Table 16.1 Differences Between Depression and Grief

Trait	Depression	Grief
Trigger	Specific trigger not necessary.	Trigger usually loss or multiple losses.
Active/Passive	Passive behavior tends to keep them "stuck" in sadness.	Actively feel their emotional pain and emptiness.
Emotions	Generalized feeling of helplessness, hopelessness.	Experience a range of emotions that are generally intense.
Ability to laugh	Likely to be humorless and incapable of being happy or even temporarily cheered up; likely to resist support.	Sometimes will be able to laugh and enjoy humor; more likely to accept support.
Activities	Lack of interest in previously enjoyed activities.	
Self-esteem	Low self-esteem, low self-confidence; feels like a failure.	Can be persuaded to participate in activities, especially as they begin to heal.
Feelings of failure	May dwell on past failures; catastrophize.	Self-esteem usually remains intact; does not feel like a failure unless it relates directly to the loss.
		Any self-blame or guilt relates directly to the loss; feelings resolve as they progress toward healing
Grief to depression		Grief can turn into serious depression when grieving process is blocked.

Sources: Klebanoff and Smith, 1997; Silverstein and Perlick, 1995.

neglect of activities at home and at work. Other symptoms include preoccupation with thoughts of the deceased person, yearning and searching for her or him, inability to accept the death, auditory and visual hallucinations of the person, bitterness and survivor guilt over the death, and symptoms of identification such as having pain in the same part of the body as the deceased person (Horowitz et al, 1997; Prigerson, 1997).

Individuals who experience complicated grief are at a higher risk for a variety of health problems. In American culture, grief is considered to be complicated when there is enormous social, psychological, and medical morbidity. Psychiatric complications include depressive episodes, anxiety-related symptoms and disorders, suicidal ideation, or psychotic denial of the death. See Table 16.1 for a comparison between depression and grief. Medical problems include hypertension, cardiac problems, impaired immune function, and cancer. Some people develop chronic illness behavior and hypochondriasis, which leads to a preoccupation with health and an inability to reinvest energy or interest in social relationships (Prigerson, 1997).

Life Transitions as Loss

When considering life transitions that include loss, often the older population is the first that comes to mind. There is no question that life becomes a series of adaptation to loss for older adults. However, as people move through developmental states they encounter a number of losses. Examples have been selected to illustrate loss during major developmental stages.

Childhood

The rearing and socialization of children is one of the most important functions of the family. Thus the major significance of divorce is not that husbands and wives break up but that parents break up. Separation and divorce may be the child's first significant loss. Children's adaptation to divorce varies on a continuum from healthy to unhealthy. At the onset of separation it is difficult to predict what, if any, long-lasting changes will occur. Change from a nuclear to a binuclear family produces situational stress. Initially, the custodial parent may experience role overload and be unable to meet the emotional needs of the children. The out-of-home parent may struggle with ways to stay involved in child care. This situational stress often results in temporary emotional distress in the children. Typically these issues are resolved within 1 year, and the children return to the previous or an improved level of functioning.

The formation of binuclear families demand psychological, social, and economic reorganization by all family members. The picture they once had of the future is gone, and a new future must be designed. If parental conflict was high prior to the divorce, the children may experience relief from stress with the new family structure. Children's adjustment to the binuclear family is correlated to the parents' adjustment. When parents cope well by living in the present and designing a new future, children are able to adapt and cope better.

Adolescence

One of the major tasks of adolescence is individuation and separation from the family. Adolescents must give up their dependence on their parents, develop more independence, and form interdependent relationships with their peer group. The peer group becomes the source of learning and evaluating the skills necessary for responsible adult behavior. The peer group is the means of promoting the adolescent's adjustment to the adult world. As such it is a necessity—not a luxury—of the teen years. Peers become idealized and serve as replacements for the formerly idealized parents. As the number of acquaintances increases during early adolescence, teens become aware of the importance of belonging to a group. New people and new events expand their worlds, and peer interactions help them test their self-concepts, values, and social identities. They develop the social skills necessary to manage competition and aggression within the group. Adolescents certainly do participate in the larger society, but the peer subculture is extremely influential in determining behavior, beliefs, and values.

The majority of adolescents work through this maturational crisis and develop into mature young adults. A small percentage of teens are unable to develop meaningful peer relationships and become isolated and lonely young adults. Another small percentage find their peer group within the gang structure and exchange dependence on the family for the dependence on the gang. Remaining in the gang prevents growth toward social responsibility apart from the peer group.

Middle Adulthood

The middle adulthood period presents unique challenges to each person. Generally, the middle-aged adult is considered to be at the apex of life and is expected to achieve maturity during this time. This is the period when one is to be most productive in the work setting. This peak of life frequently stimulates a period of self-assessment. The person begins to recognize the limits of physical and psychological abilities and realizes that achievement of life goals may not be possible.

The response to the physiological limitations and health risks associated with the aging process may bring about changes in behavior. The person no longer has the physical endurance of the younger adult and must adapt to a decrease in activity level, a decreased metabolic rate, and obvious physical changes within the body. The effects of dietary practices, smoking, alcohol or drug consumption, and other lifestyle habits are explored. Attempts at altering certain "unhealthy" behaviors may occur. As individuals age, loss occurs and awareness of these changes requires adjustment to a new image of their bodies. If they have placed a great investment on their young body image, their reaction can be seen as a grieving response (Barry, 1996; Behler, Tippett, and Mandle, 1994).

The middle adult may also be in the "middle" in other ways. At a time when they are being freed from parental responsibility and expect greater independence and more social mobility, middle adults may find that their dependent parents restrict their leisure time. Although most older adults wish to be independent of their adult children, it is primarily their offspring, especially female adult children, to whom they turn in the time of need.

Late Adulthood

The developmental stage that most reflects change and transition is late adulthood. Philosophers and poets have written extensively about the later years as the "season of loss." Loss of work roles with retirement, loss of body image, and loss associated with mortality are both expected and unexpected events for the older adult. Dealing with immortality and death is perhaps the most significant psychosocial stressor of late adulthood. Death is frequently viewed as the ultimate loss. It involves not only the loss of all significant relationships but also the loss of oneself.

Older adults constantly face loss. Loss of significant others can occur not only by death, but also by relocation. Placing a loved one in a nursing home or having children move away can leave a void in the older person's life. Other losses include loss of control and competence, loss of some life experiences, loss of material possessions, and loss of dreams. The goal for the older adult who has confronted loss is to use adaptive mechanisms to understand and accept the inevitability of those losses and live the remaining years to the maximum potential.

Psychiatric Disability as a Loss

Individual Loss

People who are psychiatrically disabled experience many losses. These losses are often in the following areas: activities of daily living, social interactions, school, employment, housing, and community participation. The Americans with Disabilities Act defines disability as "a physical or mental impairment that substantially limits one or more of the major life activities" of a person (ADA, 1990, Section 3(2)). Emotional or mental disabilities may be less visible than physical disabilities and are therefore often ignored. Additionally, a strong cultural stigma attached to these individuals interferes with attempts to respond to the needs of this population. The stigma surrounding people with mental disorders is painful and frustrating and all too evident in their daily lives. The linkage of violence and mental disorders by the media perpetuates the myth that most individuals who are psychiatrically disabled are dangerous and

must be avoided. Lack of knowledge and lack of empathy contribute to unrealistic fear in the general population (Wasserbauer, 1997).

People who are psychiatrically disabled struggle to meet their needs in communities that do not want them. They face stigma and discrimination both in public housing and in the private rental market, which results in loss of their freedom to live where they would like. Although many were successfully employed prior to their illnesses, they typically experience job discrimination after the onset of their mental disorder. To obtain employment protection under the American with Disabilities Act, the disabled person must be otherwise qualified and able to perform the essential functions of the job. Many psychiatrically disabled persons are unable to compete for existing jobs because they lack job training, education, or rehabilitation. Some are unable to manage the stress of the daily requirements of a job or may require flexible work hours to manage their illness. Thus, suffering from psychiatric disability often means losing hopes and dreams of meaningful work or a career (Chafetz, 1996; Perese, 1997; Wasserbauer, 1997).

People with severe mental disorders also experience losses in their relationships with others. Often they have few relationships with people who are not connected to the mental health system. Their small networks may be restricted to family members and other mental health clients. Thus, many live very isolated lives.

The goal of mental health care in North America has been one of community integration. The belief is that all people, including people with psychiatric disabilities, have the right to full community participation. The objective is to ensure that individuals live fulfilling lives within their communities. At this time real integration has not happened. Psychiatrically disabled individuals do not live and work side by side with those who are more fortunate, and the disabled population is treated as fringe community members at best.

In the future, community integration will be achieved only through peer support, self-help, and vocational and social programs that help people into mainstream housing and jobs. The professional role in community integration is not to "fix" problems but to support consumers. Consumers need to be empowered to control their own lives and make choices about which supports to use. In addition, communities must be mobilized to welcome and support consumers (Carling, 1995).

Family Loss

People are both individuals and family members, simultaneously independent of and part of families. Psychiatric disability is stressful, not only for individuals but for their families. Only 15% of consumers participate in mental health programs. Therefore, families are often forced to compensate for the deficiencies of the mental health system as they become the major source of support and rehabilitation. Of clients discharged from acute care, 65% return to their families. At any given time, 40–50% of the 48 million Americans with mental disorders live with their families on a regular basis. Even when consumers do not live at home, their families are often the only source of support. The emotional and economic stress on families can be overwhelming (Carling, 1995; Saunders, 1997).

Caregiver burden may lead to loss of independence and increased responsibility as families try to cope with day-to-day living. Deficit behaviors such as lack of motivation, difficulty in completing tasks, isolation from others, inability to manage money, poor grooming and personal care, and poor eating and sleeping behavior can be of great concern to families. Intrusive or acting-out behaviors such as lack of consideration for others, excessive arguing, conflicts with neighbors and friends, damaging material possessions, inappropriate sexual behavior, suicide attempts, and substance abuse are very disturbing to family members. These behaviors may be more episodic than the deficit behaviors but may have more severe immediate consequences. Some families cope fairly well while others are easily exhausted and give up.

Badger (1996) describes the process of family transformation when living with a person experiencing a mental disorder. Three stages have been identified: acknowledging the strangers within, fighting the battle, and gaining a new perspective.

During the first stage, acknowledging the strangers within, individuals and their family members recognize that family functioning has changed. When people become psychiatrically disabled they often find they cannot carry out their family roles and responsibilities. Thus, other family members must assume those role functions and come to terms with an altered family lifestyle. As the family attempts to explain the altered lifestyle to others, they may attribute the changes to something more socially acceptable than mental illness. For example, they might tell others that the person is suffering from exhaustion or an endocrine problem or that stress at school or work is causing the difficulties. This avoidance of stigma and prejudice of the part of others can lead to family isolation and loss of extrafamily relationships. As it becomes more evident that there is a significant problem, the family begins to search for reasons and solutions by gathering available information. Families begin to develop their own image of the disease process and expectations of mental health professionals. Many families also hope for what was in the past and for what might be in the future. It is very sad to lose a close family member to the world of mental illness. Many people do not believe that mental illness is a brain disease. If the disorder begins in childhood, it is easier to think that it is a result of bad parenting because that means good parenting should fix it. That is like telling parents of a child with leukemia that if they were better parents they could stop those white cells from growing. When a person experiences a mental disorder, the loss of ideal family dreams occurs. The expectation of a meaningful and productive individual and family life is shattered. All must be supported as they grieve the loss of their hopes and dreams (Badger, 1996).

The second stage, fighting the battle, includes the day-to-day efforts to cope with all the changes that occurred during the first stage. Family members develop cognitive, emotional, and behavioral coping strategies to be able to live with their loved one who is experiencing a mental disorder. Coping strategies protect the affected family member and maintain the stability of family functioning. Some of these strategies include expressing affection, suggesting alternative choices, reducing conflict, seeking social support, and trying to make the best of their experiences by focusing on the positive parts of the relationship with the ill family member. Fighting the battle also involves working with the mental health system to obtain treatment. Family members want to be seen as partners in treatment and do not want to be excluded from discussions and treatment recommendations. Ideally, professionals, clients, and families all work together in joint problem solving. At times the issue of client confidentiality is raised. Family members generally respect confidentiality but do need information about treatments, medications, and ways to cope with certain behaviors (Badger, 1996; Sveinbjarnardottir and de Casterle, 1997).

In the third stage, gaining a new perspective, the intense focus on the ill family member lightens up as other members being to focus on taking care of them-

Critical Thinking

Mr. King is a 71-year-old widower. Nine months ago his wife of 48 years died suddenly of a stroke. The Kings owned their own business and worked together for over 30 years, retiring just 6 months prior to her death. Three months ago Mr. King was diagnosed with colon cancer for which he underwent surgery to have the tumor removed.

Currently Mr. King is living with his daughter and her family. He has his own room and bathroom in the basement of their home. His family is very supportive and is happy to have him nearby. In spite of this, Mr. King occasionally feels that he is intruding on their privacy and prefers to spend the majority of his time watching TV alone. At night he has difficulty sleeping. He lies awake thinking about his wife, the life they had together, and the home he had to give up. Sometimes he thinks he hears her talking to him or he sees her in the shadows. He cries for her frequently. In spite of encouragement and support from his daughter, Mr. King seldom leaves the house, visits with friends or family members, or participates in activities he previously enjoyed.

1. What are the most obvious conclusions about Mr. King's grief process? What data support your conclusions?
2. What factors placed Mr. King at risk for this type of grieving?
3. What aspects of Mr. King's grieving signal that he may be developing depression?
4. What positive factor is present in Mr. King's life that will help him cope with his wife's death?
5. How does Mr. King's grief differ from disenfranchised grief?
6. What is the possible relationship between Mr. King's grief and his development of cancer?
7. As a nurse working with Mr. King, how might you intervene to help him cope with his grief and move toward healing?

Suggested answers can be found in Appendix D.

---

selves and reconnecting with others outside the family as they move through the process of grief. The family adapts to their changed circumstances and continues to function successfully (Badger, 1996).

See Chapter 2 for more information on families and mental disorders.

The Nursing Process

Assessment

Assessment of clients in the grieving or mourning process includes an accurate perception of the loss from their viewpoint. You begin by identifying the loss, be it a person or a relationship or a change in health status, roles in life, or dreams and aspirations for the future. Seek to understand the nature of the attachment to the lost person, object, or expectation. Assess past experiences with loss and the impact those have on the present experience. Assess cultural rituals and rules about mourning to understand the unique experience of grieving individuals.

Diagnosis

Possible nursing diagnoses for survivors of a family member who has died include *Anticipatory grieving, Dysfunctional grieving, Social isolation, Altered role performance, Risk for altered parenting, Ineffective family coping: compromised,* and *Family coping: potential for growth.* Nursing diagnoses for children of divorce include *Altered family processes, Risk for caregiver role strain,* and *Family coping: potential for growth.* For adolescents who lack a peer group, nursing diagnoses might be *Impaired social interaction* and *Self-esteem disturbance.* Nursing diagnoses for middle adults experiencing loss might be *Impaired adjustment, Self-esteem disturbance,* and *Health-seeking behaviors.* Nursing diagnoses in late adulthood include *Spiritual distress, Social isolation,* and **Hopelessness.** Nursing diagnoses for families experiencing loss through mental illness include *Impaired* *social interaction, Social isolation, Caregiver role strain, Ineffective family coping: compromised, Family coping: potential for growth,* and *Ineffective community coping.*

Nursing Interventions

Behavioral: Coping Assistance

Grief Work Facilitation

Assisting individuals and families to progress through the grief process is an important nursing intervention. Encourage people to express their feelings about the loss and help them identify their greatest fears concerning the loss. Help them recognize that all these feelings are a normal part of grieving. Discuss the active process of grieving as they meet new challenges in coping. Let them know that you understand grieving takes a great deal of time and energy.

As new skills are identified and implemented, support those which are most effective. If appropriate, suggest alternative ways of dealing with challenges while supporting them in following their own choices. An important aspect of grieving is establishing autonomy and direction in their own lives (Attig, 1996; McCloskey and Bulechek, 1996).

Discuss potentially difficult times such as holiday seasons or anniversary dates. Role playing may be helpful as they anticipate these painful events. Assist survivors to identify goals that are unattainable because of the loss while encouraging realistic goal setting. Explore the ways in which social support systems have changed as a result of the loss or death. Refer to appropriate self-help groups for survivors of death, families of mentally ill persons, and individuals who are psychiatrically disabled (Klebanoff and Smith, 1997).

Spiritual care includes helping grieving persons to seek new meanings in both life and death. Encourage them to implement religious beliefs and rituals surrounding death. Guide them through the process of self-reflection as they think about what has happened to them. As grieving progresses, you can provide a listening ear while they recover old and discover new goals and purposes in life (Attig, 1996; McCloskey and Bulechek, 1996).

If children are involved in the grieving process, answer their questions associated with the loss. Use clear words, such as dead or died, rather than euphemisms, such as passing on or gone to sleep. Clear up any misunderstandings the children may have. Use play, art, or journal therapy to help children identify and work through their feelings. Refer to community resources designed to help children cope with the loss of a family member (McCloskey and Bulechek, 1996).

Families have specific needs as they address losses associated with having a member who is psychiatrically disabled. Assist them in redefining roles, responsibilities, and functions within the family. Teach them how to navigate the mental health system to obtain treatment and locate sources of emotional and financial support. If necessary, help them locate respite care to prevent caregiver burnout. Teach them ways to cope with deficit behaviors and intrusive or acting out behaviors by their loved one. Discuss stigma and ways to respond to prejudice from individuals, from communities, and from state and federal legislative branches as health care resources are allocated. Act as an advocate in preventing family exclusion and fostering family inclusion as a member of the team, all of whom work together to support the individual in living the fullest life possible. See Chapter 2 for more detailed information on family interventions.

Evaluation

Living with losses is a normal but very stressful part of life. When coping with loss through grieving or mourning, people may respond in adaptive or maladaptive ways. Some never lose their sense of despair. In the face of this overwhelming negativism, family and friends often avoid the despairing person. Others are able to move through the process and focus on positive achievements and celebrate the relationship that was or is now. Family and friends find delight in sharing this positive process.

Some nurses have difficulty dealing with loss and death since they view the essence of caring as supporting life processes. To accept death as a process of life enables other nurses to support people through this final stage of growth. To be effective caregivers, nurses must be willing to talk openly about death as well as accept their own mortality. As Hoff (1989, p. 418) states: "A healthy attitude toward our own death is our most powerful asset in assisting the dying through this final life passage and comforting their survivors."

Key Concepts

Introduction

- Loss includes loss of a person, parts of ourselves, our possessions and pets as well as developmental losses.
- Bereavement is the feelings, thoughts, and responses that happen to us when a person dies. Grief and mourning are active processes of learning to adapt to the death or loss.

Culture and the Grieving Process

- The culture in which each of us is raised and the culture in which each of us lives partially determine what is acceptable in terms of the grieving process.
- Families also have general rules of behavior and expressions of feelings during grief.
- Family coping strategies include re-establishing a stable equilibrium, realigning family roles, and communicating clearly.
- Disenfranchised grief means that the loss cannot be openly acknowledged, socially validated, or publicly mourned.
- Complicated grief occurs when there is enormous social, psychological, and medical morbidity.

Life Transitions as Loss

- Separation and divorce may be a child's first significant loss.
- Adolescents must give up their dependence on their parents and form interdependent relationships with their peer group.
- Middle adults must respond to losses in physical status as well as managing dependent parents.
- Older adults deal with many losses, such as the loss of work roles, body image, relationships, control, material possessions, and death.

Psychiatric Disability as Loss

- Individuals who are psychiatrically disabled experience many losses in areas such as ADLs, social interactions, school, employment, housing, and community participation.

- Families of people with mental illness experience losses such as family roles, expectations of an ideal family life, and social stigmatization.

Nursing Interventions

- Nursing interventions for survivors of death include helping them express feelings, meet new challenges, establish autonomy, anticipate difficult times, find support systems, and self-reflect, as well as helping children cope.
- Nursing interventions for individuals and families coping with mental illness include helping them redefine roles and responsibilities, navigate the mental health system, locate respite care, cope with inappropriate behaviors, and work as a team with mental health professionals.

Review Questions

1. Each culture influences grieving by
   a. ignoring inappropriate grieving behaviors.
   b. tolerating any expressions of grief.
   c. establishing symbolic rituals.
   d. supporting all individual responses.

2. The first priority in managing the crisis of grief within a family is to
   a. establish a stable equilibrium.
   b. reassign family roles.
   c. clarify children's misperceptions.
   d. establish contact with supportive others.

3. Which of the following is an example of disenfranchised grief? The death of a
   a. two-year-old son.
   b. father-in-law.
   c. great uncle.
   d. former spouse.

4. Which of the following is a symptom of complicated grief?
   a. psychotic denial of the death
   b. longing to see the person again
   c. experiencing intense emotions
   d. self-esteem remains intact

5. When people are psychiatrically disabled, they experience which of the following losses? The loss of

   a. liberty.

   b. voting privileges.

   c. freedom to live where they choose.

   d. legal competency.

References

Americans with Disabilities Act. 1990. Public Law 101–336.

Attig, T. (1996). *How We Grieve.* New York: Oxford Univ. Press.

Badger, T. A. (1996). Living with depression. *J Psychosoc Nurs, 34*(1), 21–29.

Barry, P. (1996). *Psychosocial Nursing: Care of Physically Ill Patients and Their Families* (3rd ed.). Philadelphia: Lippincott.

Behler, D., Tippett, T., & Mandle, C. L. (1994). Middle adults. In C. L. Edelman & C. K. Mandle (Eds.), *Health Promotion Throughout the Lifespan* (3rd ed.) (pp. 607–631). St. Louis, MO: Mosby.

Carling, P. J. (1995). *Return to Community.* New York: Guilford Press.

Chafetz, L. (1996). The experience of severe mental illness. *Arch Psychiatr Nurs, 10*(1), 24–31.

Gorman, L. M., Sultan, D. F., & Raines, M. L. (1996). *Davis's Manual of Psychosocial Nursing for General Patient Care.* Philadelphia: F. A. Davis.

Hoff, L. A. (1989). *People in Crisis* (3rd ed.). Reading, MA: Addison-Wesley.

Horowitz, M. J., et al. (1997). Diagnoistic criteria for complicated grief disorder. *Am J Psychiatry, 154*(7), 904–910.

Klebanoff, N. A., & Smith, N. M. (1997). *Behavior Management in Home Care.* Philadelphia: Lippincott.

McCloskey, J. C., & Bulechek, G. M. (1996). *Nursing Interventions Classification* (2nd ed.). St. Louis, MO: Mosby.

Moos, N. L. (1995). An integrative model of grief. *Death Studies, 19*(4), 337–364.

Perese, E. F. (1997). Unmet needs of persons with chronic mental illnesses: Relationship to their adaptation to community living. *Issues Ment Health Nurs, 18*(1), 19–34.

Prigerson, H. G. (1997). Traumatic grief as a risk factor for mental and physical morbidity. *Am J Psychiatry, 154*(5), 616–623.

Saunders, J. (1997). Walking a mile in their shoes . . . Symbolic interactionism for families living with severe mental illness. *J Psychosoc Nurs, 5*(6), 8–13.

Shapiro, E. R. (1994). *Grief as a Family Process.* New York: Guilford Press.

Silverstein, B., & Perlick, D. (1995). *The Cost of Competence.* New York: Oxford Univ. Press.

Sveinbjarnardottir, E., & de Casterle, B. D. (1997). Mental illness in the family: An emotional experience. *Issues Ment Health Nurs, 18*(1), 45–56.

Wasserbauer, L. I. (1997). Mental illness and the Americans with Disabilities Act. *J Psychosoc Nurs, 35*(1), 22–26.

CHAPTER 17

Suicide

Karen Lee Fontaine

Objectives

After reading this chapter, you will be able to:

- Identify people who are at high risk for suicide.
- Discuss some of the reasons people have for committing suicide.
- Assess individuals who are at risk for suicide.
- Implement a plan of care for clients who are suicidal.

Suicide is a worldwide, national, local, and familial problem. While the definitions of suicidal behavior and suicide overlap, there are slight differences. Suicidal behavior can be defined in two ways:

- The behavior and thoughts leading up to the act of suicide.
- The act of taking one's own life.

The word "suicide" is used in the following three ways:

- The act of taking one's own life.
- A person who takes his or her own life.
- The end result—survival or death—described as either attempted or successful.

Worldwide, there are 360,000 suicides every year. Every 15 minutes, another American commits suicide. The reported numbers are actually low because many suicides are reported as accidental deaths. The real rate may be three to five times higher. Even with the underreporting, suicide remains the eighth-leading cause of death in the general population. The impact of these statistics becomes even greater when we recognize that for every successful suicide, there are 10–20 unsuccessful attempts (Fine, 1997; Hendin, 1995).

For people with mental disorders, 1 out of 1000 dies from suicide each year. The highest rate occurs among individuals suffering from substance use disorders, mood disorders, and schizophrenia. In the general population, women attempt suicide 2–3 times as often as men, though twice as many men carry out successful suicides.

Although suicide occurs at all stages throughout life, people continue to be surprised when they learn about suicide in a child younger than 12. The fact is, children as young as age 3–5 have been known to commit suicide. Suicide is the sixth leading cause of death for children ages 5–14 and the second leading cause of death for teenagers 15–19 years old. Every year, about 2000 teenagers commit suicide in the United States. In one study of high school students, 27% had seriously thought about attempting suicide, 16% had made a specific suicide plan, and 8% had actually attempted suicide in the past year. People who are 65 and older have the highest suicide rate of all age groups. They make up only 13% of the population, but they account for 25% of all suicides. Men account for 81% of suicides among persons age 65 and older. With the increasing number of older adults in the United States, this fact has serious implications for future health care planning (Brown, 1996; Brown and Lempa, 1997; Moscicki, 1995).

Knowledge Base

There are various philosophies about suicide, ranging from believing it is wrong to believing it has a positive value. See Box 17.1 for these philosophies.

People commit suicide for hundreds of reasons. Here are a few:

- Some are driven by delusions or command hallucinations.
- Because of depressed feelings related to a chronic or terminal illness, some see no hope for the future.
- For some, suicide is a relief from intolerable and inescapable physical or emotional pain.
- Some have experienced so many losses that life is no longer valuable.
- Some have been beset with multiple crises, which have drained their internal and external resources.
- For some, suicide is the ultimate expression of anger toward significant others.

Suicide can be precipitated by many factors. It carries a great variety of meanings to the victims as well as the survivors. Despite this variety, potential suicide victims have a number of characteristics in common that can alert you to the danger.

Behavioral Characteristics

Suicide is not a random act. It is a way out of a problem, dilemma, or unbearable situation. Suicidal individuals suffer intensely, and people contemplating suicide often make subtle or even overt comments that indicate as much. They may mention all the pressure and stress they are experiencing and how helpless they feel. Some may discuss beliefs concerning life after death. Verbal cues are such statements as:

- "It won't matter much longer."
- "Will you miss me when I'm gone?"
- "I can't take this much longer."
- "The pain will be over soon."
- "I won't be here when you come back on Monday."
- "You won't have to worry about the money problems much longer."
- "The voices are telling me to hurt myself."

Certain behaviors may indicate suicidal intentions. Obtaining a weapon such as a gun, a strong rope, or a collection of pills is a high indicator of impending suicide. Often people contemplating suicide begin to withdraw from relationships and become more isolative. There may be a change in school or work performance. An increased tendency toward accidents might indicate initial suicidal behavior. Some may show a sudden interest in their life insurance policy, whereas others may make or change their will and give personal belongings away. Signs of substance abuse may also be present (Chiles and Strosahl, 1995).

> Willis, 16, was the youngest of four children and had enjoyed a stable family life. Two years earlier, he cut himself just enough to draw a little blood following a breakup with a girlfriend. There was no follow-up to this incident. His friends described Willis as very tense on some days and his relationship with his current girlfriend as "rocky." The day before he killed himself, Willis gave his music collection to his older brother, saying that where he was going, he would no longer need it. He told his girlfriend that if she would not see him anymore, he would be watching her from above. At the time, she didn't understand what he meant. The next day, Willis took the gun his family kept for protection, put it to his head, and pulled the trigger.

Behavioral characteristics also include choosing a method for suicide. Lethality is measured by four factors:

1. The degree of effort it takes to plan the suicide.
2. The specificity of the plan.
3. The accessibility of the weapon or method.
4. The ease by which one may or may not be rescued.

Box 17.1

Philosphies About Suicide

Suicide is wrong
- Suicide does violence to the dignity of human life.
- Suicide is an irrevocable act that denies future learning or growth.
- It is only for God to give and to take away human life.
- Suicide does violence to the natural order of things.
- Suicide adversely affects the survivors.

Suicide is sometimes permissible
- Suicide is permissible when the person's life is unbearable.

Suicide is not a moral or ethical issue
- Suicide is a fact of life that can be studied like other life events.
- Suicide is a morally neutral act in that every person has a free will and the right to act according to that will.

Suicide is a positive response to certain conditions
- When life ceases to be enjoyable, people have the right to end their lives.
- There are certain times in life when death is less an evil than dishonor.
- Some suicides are demanded by society as a way of dispensing justice.

Suicide has intrinsic positive value
- Suicide has a positive value when it is the way people can enter a meaningful afterlife that they desire.
- Suicide has a positive value because it is a way in which people can be immediately reunited with valued ancestors and loved ones.

Source: Chiles and Strosahl, 1995.

More people kill themselves with guns than by all other methods combined. More than half of the teenagers who commit suicide shoot themselves with a gun kept at home. An important social issue is the alarming increase in the number of guns purchased in the United States. Those who are most vulnerable to impulsive suicide are clearly the most affected by availability of guns. The dramatic increase in suicide in children and adolescents is almost solely due to guns. In one study of home gun deaths the following individuals were victims (Hendin, 1995):

- 0.5% intruders
- 3% accidental gunshot deaths
- 12.6% adult homicides during a quarrel
- 83.2% adolescent or adult suicide

The next most commonly used methods are hanging and poisoning by liquids, solids, and gases such as carbon monoxide. The methods most often chosen by younger children are hanging and jumping from a window or in front of a car (Hendin, 1995).

Affective Characteristics

All the affective characteristics indicative of depression may be associated with people who are suicidal. These include feelings of desolation, guilt, failure, shame, and loss of emotional attachments. A pervading sense of hopelessness has the highest association with suicide. Life is seen as intolerable, with no hope for change or improvement. Fifteen percent of people suffering from depression commit suicide (Chiles and Strosahl, 1995).

People have a high degree of ambivalence before making the final decision to commit suicide. An internal conflict exists between the wish to die and the wish to live. If the part that wants to live can be adequately supported during this struggle, the balance may shift in favor of life. Once the decision has been made to commit suicide, conflict and anxiety cease, and the person may appear calm and untroubled. Others may interpret this change in the affective state as an improvement. What appears to be a change for the better may in fact be an indication of the decision to die.

Some people who are suspicious, or who are prone to violence as a method of coping with feelings, may combine suicide with homicide. These people usually kill someone they know, a relative or friend, and then commit suicide; less commonly, they will kill a stranger before killing themselves (Hendin, 1995).

Cognitive Characteristics

Suicidal behavior has a variety of cognitive components. Suicidal people tend to think dichotomously, that is, all-or-none reasoning such as good or bad, right or wrong. This rigid cognitive style makes it difficult for people who are suicidal to problem-solve. Recurring thoughts of self-blame, negative self-evaluation, and dire expectations of the future contribute to a hopeless outlook. When people choose to die, they are so distorted by pain—physical, mental, or emotional—that the world is reduced to a solitary alternative. There seems to be only one answer: to die (Rickelman and Houfek, 1995).

Another cognitive component involves fantasies. Unable to see the finality of death, suicidal people sometimes have fantasies about continuing on after their own death. They may talk about being able to see how people will react to their death or how their children will grow up. Others have expectations about meeting up with departed loved ones after death. Many people eagerly look forward to this reunion with family and friends.

A smaller percentage of people hope or believe a suicide attempt will force a solution to interpersonal problems. For some, it is a cry for help. In either case, the suicidal behavior is a form of manipulation. They are so desperate that they can see no other method to resolve problems or get the necessary help.

People with sensory or thought disorders may be potentially suicidal. Command hallucinations are common and may often direct the person to commit suicide. At first, the person may be frightened by the voices, but later the person may be compliant and carry out the command. People with delusions of control or persecution may also be at risk for suicide. If these delusions cannot be managed with treatment, they may believe the only way to escape those who are controlling or persecuting them is to die. It is the ultimate method of getting relief from their extremely painful thoughts.

Kendall had a 15-year history of delusions of control. His delusional system was fixed, and he had responded poorly to a variety of interven-

tions. His system centered on the belief that there was an electrode in his ear by which his family controlled him. They woke him up, they put him to sleep, they thought for him, and they talked for him through this electrode. Three weeks before his suicide, he expressed feelings of desperation. He said the doctors had done everything, but they either couldn't or wouldn't remove the electrode from his ear. He said he couldn't go on this way, not being himself and being controlled by hateful family members. His final solution was to kill himself to escape the total control that had plagued him for 15 years.

For those rescued from their suicidal behavior, there is often a change of mind. Either they return to the ambivalent state of thought, or they decide they do want to live. Throughout their lives, however, they remain at higher risk for suicide than the general population. It seems that once the decision to die was made in the past, that decision may be easier to make again.

Social Characteristics

People who attempt or commit suicide are often in periods of high stress in their lives. They often have a limited social network, and when their attempts to get support fail, their level of distress increases. When people either have not developed their coping skills or have exhausted their ability to cope, suicide may be a last, desperate attempt to cope with stress and resolve problems.

When teenage suicides are publicized by the news media or when there are television dramas about suicide, the rate of adolescent suicide increases several weeks following the event. Suicides that are inspired by suicides in this way are called *copycat suicides*. Copycat suicide seems to be an adolescent phenomenon, with girls more susceptible than boys. The potential copycat appears to be a troubled adolescent who empathizes with the pain of the suicidal person and is easily influenced by the media.

Whatever way the act of suicide is committed, it has a traumatic effect on the family and friends of the victim. In addition to the grief, these people must cope with the stigma and cultural taboos associated with suicide. Family and friends are frequently unaware of the danger signs and respond to the suddenness of the death with shock and bewilderment.

Some people respond with anger toward the victim and the event. Others feel betrayed and abandoned. Because society assumes that all survivors must feel guilty and responsible for the suicidal behavior, those who do not experience guilt may wonder why and may feel guilty about not feeling guilty. Some survivors experience a sense of relief when a suicide ends the physical or mental suffering of a loved one. Other survivors blame themselves with such thoughts as "If only I had done [had not done] . . ., this would not have happened." Shame and guilt cast family members in the role of murderers, when in truth they, too, are victims. The death of a child, in particular, puts extreme strain on the parents. Because they were unable to protect their child, they may be overwhelmed with feelings of guilt and powerlessness (Fine, 1997).

Many survivors are plagued with real or imagined images of the death scene. Families must also cope with other people seeking details about the death, with others' inability to acknowledge the death, or others even blaming them for the death. Some people develop obsessions about their own suicide. Family survivors enter a higher risk category for suicide; about 20% of them will exhibit suicidal behavior themselves. Having a loved one die is traumatic at any time, but having a loved one die as a result of suicide can be overwhelming (Fine, 1997).

Culture-Specific Characteristics

Suicide continues to be an urgent problem in all countries of the world, especially among the youth, where suicide is the second or third leading cause of death. Acts of suicide relate to a range of social, political, and psychological factors. Philosophies about suicide are deeply rooted in cultural traditions. Because it is highly stigmatized and illegal in many places, it is thought to be severely underreported (Desjarlais et al, 1995).

Reported rates throughout the world are consistently higher among men than women regardless of age group. China is the only exception, where more women than men kill themselves. Hungary has the highest suicide rate, followed by Sri Lanka, Russia, China, Japan, Germany, Australia, Singapore, Canada, and the United States. Means of suicide include self-immolation (sacrifice) in Hindu and Buddhist cultures; pesticides or toxic plants in agrarian societies; and leaping from high places such as bridges, mountain tops, or waterfalls. In the United States, guns are the most common method (Desjarlais et al, 1995).

European Americans have the highest rates of suicide in the United States. The peak for females is around age 50. For males, the suicide rate continues to increase throughout life, with those over 65 having the highest suicide rate of all groups.

Native Americans are not a culturally homogeneous population. There are wide variations in the suicide rates of different Native American tribes. For example, the Chippewa have the lowest rate, with 6 suicides out of 100,000 people, and the Black Feet have the highest rate, at 130 out of 100,000. The suicide rate for Alaskan natives is twice that of the general population of the United States. Tribes that have maintained traditions have the lowest rates. High rates of suicide are related to multiple factors such as the breakdown of traditional values, enforced residence on reservations, geographic isolation, inadequate housing, high unemployment, extreme poverty, and a high incidence of alcoholism (Desjarlais et al, 1995; Gregory, 1994). Hispanic Americans are at highest risk for suicide during young adulthood. This is thought to be related to the stress of acculturation because the rates are higher in the United States than in their countries of origin. Stressors include the language barrier, discrimination, poverty, and educational disadvantages (Desjarlais et al, 1995).

Asian Americans are one of the fastest-growing ethnic groups in the United States. Having never been treated with the same courtesy given to immigrants from Europe, they have suffered a long history of discrimination. Typically, the suicide rate increases with age among Asian Americans (Desjarlais et al, 1995).

African Americans experience the highest rate of suicide between the ages of 25 and 34, after which there is a general decline to low levels in old age. Among African Americans, older adults have more purposeful roles, higher status, and much lower rates of suicide than European Americans of the same age group. The very low rate of suicide among African American women is attributed to their participation in community activities, including church, and to the strong psychosocial support they share, which contributes to positive self-esteem and minimal need for approval from the dominant culture (Hendin, 1995). For an overview of suicide rates according to ethnicity and gender, see Table 17.1.

Table 17.1 Suicide Rates According to Ethnicity and Gender Group

Ethnic Group	Sex	Number per 100,000 Population
Native American	Male	24.2
European American	Male	19.4
Hispanic American	Male	17.8
Japanese American	Male	11.1
African American	Male	10.8
Chinese American	Female	8.0
Chinese American	Male	7.9
European American	Female	6.2
Japanese American	Female	5.0
Native American	Female	4.6
Hispanic American	Female	4.0
African American	Female	2.1

Source: Committee on Cultural Psychiatry, 1989.

Assisted Suicide

Physician-assisted suicide has received increased attention over the past decade. Among the general public, support for the "right to die" has grown steadily, with 64% of the population supporting assisted dying for people with terminal illness. At issue is whether the dying should have the right to request and receive aid-in-dying from physicians. Legal safeguards include multiple requests from the person over a 2-week period, witnessed and documented discussion of treatment options and hospice care, a confirmation of the terminal condition by another physician, and psychiatric assessment that the person is not impaired by a mental illness.

Those who are against the issue believe that the greater good for the society demands keeping the prohibitions in place. It is seen as a form of medical killing in violation of social, ethical, and medical traditions which would turn physicians from healers into killers. There is concern that it will be applied in an involuntary way against the elderly, poor, handicapped, or otherwise disadvantaged people. A further concern is that some individuals will be pressured to end their lives as an economic sacrifice for their families.

Those who support assisted suicide believe a change in the law is necessary based on reasons of compassion and freedom of choice in the face of intolerable suffering. The desire to have medical help in ending one's life is seen as an extension of the right to refuse to be sustained on life support systems or to request not to be resuscitated. It must be remembered that many people with life-threatening illnesses are already taking matters into their own hands and ending their lives, with or without help and regardless of laws. Most people have no one with whom they can discuss these issues and no place to turn for advice. Proponents believe everyone has the right to open dialogue, counseling, and involvement of family, partners, and friends regarding the wish to die when further living is intolerable (Hendin, 1995; Jamison, 1995).

Concomitant Disorders

Among people with schizophrenia, 10% commit suicide; for those with mood disorders, the rate is 10–13%. People with borderline personality disorder and concomitant depression may be at very high risk. Alcohol and cocaine are frequently involved in suicide completion. Typically, a younger age at death is associated with substance use disorders and psychotic illness, and an older age at death is associated with mood disorders (Conwell et al, 1996; Fenton et al, 1997). See Box 17.2 for a list of factors contributing to suicidal behavior.

People with chronic diseases are more likely to commit suicide than those with acute illnesses or no illness. At highest risk are people suffering from progressive diseases such as cardiovascular disease, multiple sclerosis, and cancer. Moreover, people who take a large number of medications may, as a direct result of the chemical effects on the body, experience a depressive episode leading to suicide. Substance abuse is a contributing factor for some suicidal people, particularly older men who live alone and have few or no support systems. The use of chemicals may be an attempt to self-medicate to control the symptoms of depression, or it may be a way to overcome inhibitions over the actual act of suicide.

Box 17.2

Factors Contributing to High Suicidal Risk

- European American
- Elderly people, especially men, followed by adolescents and college students
- People who are isolated without support systems
- Individuals who are recently unemployed
- Recent loss of a significant relationship
- Separated, divorced, or widowed people
- Presence of a substance use disorder
- Presence of a mental disorder
- Feelings of failure and hopelessness
- Presence of a gun in the home
- Previous suicide attempts
- Positive family history of completed suicide

Causative Theories

Suicide is a complex act, and a variety of factors contribute to the behavior. The degree of influence of each factor varies from individual to individual.

Neurobiological Theory

Recent research indicates that the primary neurobiological factor in suicide is a disturbance related to serotonin (5-HT) dysfunction. There is a significant decrease in 5-HT in both attempted and successful suicides, irrespective of their primary psychiatric diagnosis. 5-HT may be related to the person's tolerance for adversity, the ability to resist impulsive urges, and the means to find solutions to problems. Interestingly, 5-HT levels rise during pregnancy and pregnant women are at very low risk for suicide. The fetus produces much of the excess 5-HT, which may be self-protective by inhibiting self-destructive behaviors by the mother.

The final decision to commit suicide may be an impulsive act that is the result of a powerful biological process (Chiles and Strosahl, 1995; Marzuk et al, 1997).

Genetic Theory

Adoption studies in the United States and Denmark indicate that there may be a genetic factor in suicidal behavior. Individuals who were adopted at birth and later committed suicide were found to have significantly more biological relatives who had committed suicide than the control group. In one study of twin pairs in which one or both twins had committed suicide, in 11% of the monozygotic pairs both twins committed suicide compared to 2% of the dizygotic twins.

It is believed this possible genetic factor may be an inability to control impulsive behavior, and that either environmental stress or a mental illness may drive the impulsive behavior toward suicide (Roy, Segal, and Sarchizpone, 1995).

Sociocultural Theory

Suicide may result when people experience social isolation, alienated from society, family, and friends. Another sociocultural factor is rapid social change resulting in the loss of previous patterns of social integration. People who have difficulty adapting to the demand of new roles are more likely to view suicide as a solution to their problems.

Loss is another factor closely related to suicide. Certainly, the impact of any loss depends on the significance the person attributes to that loss. Whenever the most important and significant aspects of a person's life are threatened or destroyed, suicide is likely to be considered. Women's motives tend to be interpersonal, that is, related to painful or lost relationships. Men's motives tend to be intrapersonal, that is, related to financial problems or the loss of a job.

Behavioral Theory

Behavioral theorists believe that suicide is often a learned problem-solving behavior. They consider the reinforcements prior to and following attempted suicidal behavior. The internal reinforcement is that the behavior itself serves to decrease anxiety. Following the suicidal behavior, the external reinforcement is that the person is removed from the stressful environment and freed from daily pressures. Significant others who were critical may now become supportive. These types of reinforcement are essential in the repetition of suicidal behavior (Chiles and Strosahl, 1995).

Developmental Theory

In addition to these general causes of suicide, there are more specific causes for the various age groups. Some of the reasons children commit suicide are to escape from physical or sexual abuse, a chaotic family situation, feeling unloved or constantly criticized, anticipation of disciplinary action, humiliation in school, and the loss of significant others.

Adolescents may commit suicide for the same reasons children do. Additional age-specific causes include the absence of meaningful relationships, difficulties in maintaining relationships, sexual problems, and acute problems with parents. Additional suicidal factors for college students include competition for success, anxiety over academic work, and academic failure signifying a loss of parental love or esteem. Of the high achievers in *Who's Who in American High Schools*, 31% have considered suicide and 5% have made an attempt. Compared to adults, suicidal teens are less depressed but much more desperate (Newton, 1995).

Social pressures and a lack of resources often result in depression in adolescents who are lesbian, gay, or bisexual. They feel ostracized from the dominant culture because of an absence of role models and distorted media presentations. They may suffer intimidation ranging from ridicule to threats and physical violence from beatings to rape. For reasons of acceptance and personal safety, gay, lesbian, and bisexual youth remain hidden from their families and the community in which they live. Given this type of social climate, it is no surprise that lesbian and gay youths are six times more likely to commit suicide than heterosexual youths (Richardson, 1995).

Suicide among older adults may be related to a change in status from autonomy to dependency, accompanied by decreased participation in social activities. Many of the changes experienced by older adults may contribute to a higher incidence of suicide. Those who experience illness that results in a lower level of functioning may become suicidal. Other factors include loneliness and social isolation, loss of partner and friends, loss of work deemed important by the culture, and outliving resources.

The Nursing Process

Assessment

You may be apprehensive about assessing people who are at risk of attempting or committing suicide. Your reasons may include fear of giving the person the idea of suicide, fear of being incorrect, fear of the person's reaction, and reluctance to discuss a taboo subject. It is important for you to recognize that *you cannot give the idea of suicide to anyone*. By late childhood or early adolescence, every person knows that suicide is one alternative to solving problems. Most youngsters, without being actively suicidal, have thoughts of suicide in times of stress. An example is the child who is angry at his parents and thinks, "If I went out and got run over by a car, they'd be sorry they were so mean to me!" Many adults have considered what method they would choose if they were to commit suicide. Thus, even though the topic is taboo under most social conditions, the majority of people have thought about and formed an opinion about suicide.

Remember that people who are suicidal are afraid. They fear that no one cares. They may not introduce the topic because they fear being judged or considered weak or "crazy." When confronted with your own fears about discussing suicide, remember that no nursing intervention will be effective unless the suicide threat is assessed. If the person is not suicidal, no damage will be done by asking the questions. But if the person is suicidal and the topic is *not* discussed, the person has been abandoned while in a dangerously vulnerable position.

You may find yourself struggling with ambivalence about suicide. The conflict centers on the issue of people's right to choose their own time and method of dying. Many of us have thought about the conditions under which we would choose not to live, such as with a chronic or terminal illness. Having considered suicide as an option, you may question whether you have the right to prevent another person's suicide. Or, you may not experience this conflict at all because you believe that all suicides should be prevented.

You and the families of clients should not expect that an accurate assessment will prevent all suicides. This expectation would contribute to unrealistic guilt when a person does successfully commit suicide. Not all victims exhibit cues before their death; many people cannot be correctly identified before they kill themselves. This is not intended to minimize the importance of a suicide assessment; rather, it is to establish realistic professional expectations. If a person is intent on suicide, it is difficult to intervene effectively. However, if a person is still ambivalent, intervention may save that person's life. Therefore, it is always vital that, for those at risk, a suicide assessment be done. See the Focused Nursing Assessment table for specific questions to ask when assessing a person's potential for suicide.

Diagnosis

For a person who is actively suicidal, the most obvious nursing diagnosis is **High risk for violence, self-directed,** related to acute suicidal state. Other nursing diagnoses to consider are **Ineffective individual coping** related to a desire to kill oneself as a solution to problems; and **Impaired home maintenance management** related to an increased risk of suicide in the future. If a person has successfully committed suicide, the family may become your client—in the short term, as in the emergency department, or for a longer period, in a community or home setting. Possible nursing diagnoses may be **Ineffective family coping, compromised,** related to the suicide of a family member; and **Spiritual distress** related to questions regarding the death, anger at the deceased, or a struggle with the sense of life's injustices.

Outcome Identification

Once you have established diagnoses, you and the client mutually identify goals for change. Client outcomes are specific behavioral measures by which you, clients, and significant others determine progress toward goals. The following are examples of some of the outcomes appropriate to people who are suicidal:

- remains safe from self-injury
- utilizes the problem-solving process
- discusses personal philosophy of death
- develops an anti-suicide contract

Nursing Interventions

Safety: Crisis Management

Suicide Prevention
In planning nursing care, use the following questions to guide the process:

- Is the client actively suicidal?
- What is the degree of lethality of the plan?
- Does the client need to be in a protected environment?
- What is the extent of the supportive network system?

Focused Nursing Assessment

CLIENTS WITH SUICIDE POTENTIAL

Behavior Assessment	Affective Assessment	Cognitive Assessment	Social Assessment
Are you thinking about suicide?	How would you describe your overall mood?	What will your suicide accomplish for you?	What kinds of losses have you sustained during the past year? Relationships? Separations? Divorce? Deaths? Jobs? Roles? Self-esteem?
By what method would you commit suicide?	What kinds of things make you feel guilty?	What will your suicide accomplish for others?	
Do you have the means on hand?	In what areas of life do you feel like a failure?	What would have to change for you to decide to live?	
Have you done a practice session of the suicide?	What does the future look like to you?	What are your thoughts about death?	What kinds of stress have you been under during the past 6 months?
When do you plan to commit suicide?	To what degree do you feel hopeless or out of control of your life?	Is there a way for you to continue on in life after death?	Which people are able to provide support for you?
Have you tried to kill yourself before?	What part of you wishes to die?	Do you hope to meet dead loved ones after you die?	Have any of your friends or family members committed suicide? What is the anniversary date? What thoughts and feelings do you have about this suicide?
How have things been going at school/work for you?	What part of you wishes to live?	Do you hear voices that others say they do not hear?	
Are you still interested in visiting with friends?		What do the voices say to you?	
How much have you been drinking lately?		Is suicide a way for you to escape control or persecution by others?	Who will benefit from your suicide? How?
How often do you use street drugs?			
Have you made or changed your will recently? Have you checked your life insurance policy?			
What kinds of personal belongings have you given away?			
Have you planned your funeral?			

When clients are acutely or actively suicidal, the first priority of care is client *safety*. If clients are not in the hospital, someone must remain with them at all times until they can be moved to a safe environment. They should be transported to the hospital by family members, friends, or police to ensure accurate evaluation and possible admission. Upon admission, all dangerous objects will be removed, such as pocket knives, glass articles, belts, razors, and pills. If the client is on medication, be certain that all medication is swallowed, not stockpiled for a future suicide attempt. Suicidal precautions include checking clients' whereabouts and status every 10–15 minutes on an irregular schedule of observation. If the client is acutely suicidal, constant observation is necessary. Seclusion can be a terrifying experience for the client and constant observation is usually demoralizing and dehumanizing. It is important that you gently explain to clients that the protection is necessary until they are able to resist suicidal impulses. Clients should never be lectured about the negative consequences of suicide.

The main goal is to protect clients who are suicidal until they are able to protect themselves. Through active intervention, it is hoped that clients will be able to develop alternative solutions to the difficulties fostering their suicidal intentions. The role of the nurse is one of active participation in *problem solving*. The first step is to have clients write a list of reasons to live and reasons to die, to help them conceptualize the conflict more clearly. The next step is to have them describe the goal they hope to achieve with suicide. At this time, remind them that suicide is only one of several possible alternatives. Together, you and the client develop a list of alternatives for meeting the stated goal. Discussion of the potential outcomes of suicide is the next step in the problem-solving process. The following questions are appropriate: "What is the likelihood that you will injure yourself seriously if your attempt is not successful?" "Will death be the most successful method of meeting your goal?" Clients have often not considered the negative outcomes, such as permanent bodily damage and failure to achieve the goal. Next, focus the discussion on potential outcomes of other alternatives. The rationale for this phase is to support the part of the client that wishes to live.

People who are suicidal may not have thought past the act of self-injury, that is, the reality and finality of death. It is appropriate to discuss death: what it means, feelings about death, and what they think it

will be like. The next step is reviewing the reasons to continue living and a list of meaningful supportive network systems. This focus on available support systems will decrease feelings of isolation and helplessness. Some clients have not considered the impact of their suicide on family members. It may be helpful to discuss the impact on survivors: grief, anger, shame, guilt, and the increased risk for family members to commit suicide themselves. This external focus and concern may reduce the possibility of impulsive behavior.

Clients are often asked to write their own anti-suicide contract and sign it. Your signature on the contract indicates that you will help them keep their contract. The purpose is to formalize their agreement not to act on suicidal impulses and evoke a commitment to life. Assist clients in developing a crisis card to enable them to use existing support systems and community resources. Names and phone numbers of competent and willing family and friends are written on the card as well as numbers of community resources such as hotlines, mental health center emergency services, and local emergency departments.

When clients are successful with suicide, you must quickly intervene to *support the family* through the crisis. Provide opportunities for family members to discuss the death; many of their friends will avoid the topic because of discomfort. Most have a desperate need to talk in an environment of acceptance and understanding. The family should be allowed to express anger at the victim for abandonment and anger at themselves for not being able to prevent the suicide. This will normalize anger as an important part of the grieving process. Offer information on literature, community resources, and available support groups. Anticipatory guidance, as in foreseeing the stress of holiday times and the anniversary of the death, will decrease the impact of these situations. If family issues remain unresolved, those involved should be referred for family therapy. The Self-Help Groups/Resources list at the end of this chapter provides resource information for clients with suicide potential and surviving family members.

Evaluation

The most successful outcome of interventions is that clients remain safe from self-harm. The next evaluation criteria are that clients can identify what they are doing in life that is effective, and that they can build on these coping behaviors. As clients increase their skills in problem solving, they may be able to decrease the factors contributing to suicidal thoughts, as well as implement solutions other than suicide to cope with their problems.

When clients are successful at suicide, ask yourself several questions to resolve any unnecessary self-blame and guilt:

- Did I take the client's suicidal intentions seriously?

- Did I provide as safe an environment as possible?

- Was the client willing to find alternative solutions?

- Do I have a right to prevent all suicides?

- Does the client have a right to determine her or his own death?

- Am I the only one who is blaming myself?

- What do I need to do to feel less guilty about this death?

It is necessary for staff members to discuss their feelings and responsibilities in regard to a client's suicide. They will find it helpful to explore concepts of death and cure, as well as their moral obligations. If feelings of guilt and failure are not thought about and expressed, individual staff members may project anger and blame onto others or even onto the dead client.

Self-Help Groups/Resources

Clients with Suicide Potential and Surviving Family Members

Crisis Line
(800) 521-4000

Suicide Prevention Hotline
(800) 882-3386

Associations
American Association of Suicidology
(202) 237-2280

SPAN
Suicide Prevention Advocacy Network
5034 Odius Way
Marietta, GA 30068
(888) 649-1366
www.spanusa.org

Suicide Prevention Center, Inc.
184 Salem Avenue
Dayton, OH 45406

Contact Teleministries, USA, Inc.
900 South Arlington Avenue
Harrisburg, PA 17109

Support for Survivors
Friends for Survival
(800) 646-7322

Heartbeat
(719) 596-2575

SAVE
Suicide Awareness
Voices of Education
P.O. Box 24507
Minneapolis, MN 55424-0507
(612) 946-7998
www.save.org

Newsletters/Pamphlets

After Suicide: A Unique Grief Process
Ray of Hope, Inc.
1518 Derwen Drive
Iowa City, IA 52240

The Ultimate Rejection
Suicide Prevention Center, Inc.
184 Salem Avenue
Dayton, OH 45406

Afterwords: A Letter For and About Suicide Survivors
A. Wrobleski (editor)
5124 Grove Street
Minneapolis, MN 55436-2481

Key Concepts

Introduction

- The highest rate of suicide for people with mental disorders occurs among individuals suffering from substance use disorders, schizophrenia, and mood disorders.

- People who are 65 and older have the highest rate of suicide of all age groups. European Americans have the highest suicide rate of all ethnic groups.

Knowledge Base

- Suicide can be precipitated by delusions, hallucinations, hopelessness, intractable pain, multiple crises, and/or unexpressed anger.

- Behavioral cues to potential suicide are verbal comments, obtaining a weapon, social isolation, giving away belongings, and substance abuse.

- Affective cues to potential suicide are ambivalence, desolation, guilt, failure, shame, hopelessness, and helplessness.

- Cognitive cues to potential suicide are verbalizations about death, interpersonal problems, and command hallucinations.

- At issue in assisted suicide is whether the dying should have the right to request and receive aid-in-dying from physicians.

- The act of suicide has a traumatic effect on the family and friends of the victim.

- They must cope with grief, guilt, anger, and the cultural stigma associated with suicide.

- Suicide may be caused by many factors, including serotonin dysfunction, genetics, rapid social change, interpersonal or intrapersonal losses, a learned method of problem solving, and developmental crises.

Nursing Assessment

- Suicide assessments must be initiated by health care professionals. If the topic is not discussed, the person will have been abandoned while in a dangerously vulnerable position.

Nursing Diagnosis

- Nursing diagnoses include *High risk for violence, Ineffective individual coping, Impaired home maintenance management, Ineffective family coping,* and *Spiritual distress.*

Outcome Identification

- The main outcome is that the client remain safe from self-harm.

Nursing Interventions

- The first priority of care is to keep the client safe. Clients may need to be on suicide precautions or under constant observation.

- Encourage clients to implement the problem-solving process for alternative solutions to the difficulties fostering their suicidal intentions.

- If the suicide is successful, families will need active and supportive intervention.

Evaluation

- The most successful outcomes of the plan of care are that clients remain safe from self-harm, and that they improve their problem-solving skills.

Review Questions

1. Which of the following people is at highest risk for suicide?

   a. male, African American, 65 years old

   b. male, European American, 70 years old

   c. female, Hispanic American, 30 years old

   d. female, African American, 16 years old

2. Your client states that voices are telling him to hang himself. You document that he is at risk for suicide on the basis of

   a. an intractable sense of hopelessness.

   b. intolerable emotional pain.

   c. delusions of grandeur.

   d. command hallucinations.

3. Which of the following statements is most indicative of the potential for suicide?

   a. "I know you've been worried about me. You won't have to worry too much longer."

   b. "I think I've found a solution to my problem. I'm going to check it out with my doctor."

   c. "I'm looking forward to the holiday season and the kids coming home from school."

   d. "The voices have been decreasing in intensity and frequency over the past weeks."

4. Susan has been admitted to the psychiatric unit after spending 24 hours in the intensive care unit. Before her admission, she overdosed on 10 of her antidepressant tablets. All of the following are nursing goals. Which one is the priority goal on admission?

   a. assuring her that someone is concerned about her

   b. protecting her until she can protect herself

   c. teaching her how to problem-solve

   d. discussing the meaning of death

5. While talking to you, Susan becomes very dejected and states that life is not meaningful and no one really care what happens to her. Your best response would be:

   a. "Of course people care. Your parents stayed with you in ICU."

   b. "Let's not talk about sad things. Why don't we go for a walk."

   c. "Tell me, Susan, exactly who does not care for you?"

   d. "I care about you, and I am concerned that you feel so down."

References

Brown, A. (1996, Winter). Mood disorders in children and adolescents. NARSAD Research Newsletter, pp. 11–14.

Brown, A., & Lempa, M. (1997, Spring). Late life depression. *NARSAD Research Newsletter,* pp. 10–15.

Chiles, J. A., & Strosahl, K. (1995). *The Suicidal Patient.* Washington, D.C.: American Psychiatric Press.

Committee on Cultural Psychiatry: *Suicide and Ethnicity in the United States.* New York: Brunner/Mazel, 1989.

Conwell, Y., et al. (1996). Relationships of age and Axis I diagnoses in victims of completed suicide. *Am J Psychiatry, 153*(8), 1001–1008.

Desjarlais, R., Eisenberg, L., Good, B., & Kleinman, A. (1995). *World Mental Health.* New York: Oxford Univ Press.

Fenton, W. S., et al. (1997). Symptoms, subtype and suicidality in patients with schizophrenia spectrum disorders. *Am J Psychiatry, 154*(2), 199–204.

Fine, C. (1997). *No Time to Say Goodbye.* New York: Doubleday.

Gregory, R. J. (1994). Grief and loss among Eskimos attempting suicide in western Alaska. *Am J Psychiatry, 151*(12), 1815–1816.

Hendin, H. (1995). *Suicide in America* (2nd ed.). New York: Norton.

Jamison, S. (1995). *Final Acts of Love.* New York: G. P. Putnam's Sons.

Marzuk, P. M., et al. (1997). Lower risk of suicide during pregnancy. *Am J Psychiatry, 154*(1), 122–123.

Moscicki, E. K. (1995). Sucide in childhood and adolescence. In F. C. Verhulst, H. M. Koot (Eds.), *The Epidemiology of Child and Adolescent Psychopathology* (pp. 291–308). New York: Oxford Univ. Press.

Newton, M. (1995). *Adolescence.* New York: Norton.

Richardson, J. (1995). The science and politics of gay teen suicide. *Harvard Rev Psychiatry, 3,* 107–110.

Rickelman, B. L., & Houfek, J. F. (1995). Toward an interactional model of suicidal behaviors. *Arch Psychiatr Nurs, 9*(3), 158–168.

Roy, A., & Segal, N. L., & Sarchiapone, M. (1995). Attempted suicide among living co-twin suicide victims. *Am J Psychiatry, 152*(7), 1075–1076.

CHAPTER 18

Domestic Violence

Karen Lee Fontaine

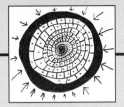

Objectives

After reading this chapter, you will be able to:

- Identify people who are at high risk for domestic violence.
- Assess all clients for evidence of domestic violence.
- Identify multidisciplinary treatment interventions.
- Evaluate the short-term and long-term effectiveness of the plan of care.

Domestic violence—violence within the family—occurs at all levels of society. The myth is that violence occurs only among the poor and undereducated, but the reality is that violence occurs also among the middle and upper classes and professional elite. See Box 18.1 for myths and facts about domestic violence. In the past, these problems among wealthy or prominent people were kept hidden from the general public. With an increase in national concern, however, more publicity is being given to cases of domestic violence at all socioeconomic levels.

In this chapter, the word "family" refers to any one of these three categories: those who are related by birth, adoption, or marriage; those in an intimate relationship; and those who are in a domestic relationship, that is, sharing the same household. Although the image of the American family is one of happiness and harmony, this ideal is often in conflict with the underlying reality of domestic violence. The home is the most frequent place for violence of all types.

Abuse, interchangeable with violence in this chapter, refers to a pattern of behavior that dominates, controls, lowers self-esteem, or takes away freedom of choice. It is systematic persecution of another individual ranging from subtle words or actions to violent battering—acts of commission. Abuse also includes various types of neglect—acts of omission. See Box 18.2 for definitions of types of abuse.

The incidence of domestic violence can only be estimated. Studies often include only those people who are willing to respond to surveys. Typically underrepresented in such studies are those who do not speak English, the very poor, the homeless, and those who are hospitalized or incarcerated at the time of the survey. The actual rates of domestic violence are probably much higher than reported.

In all 50 states, nurses are required by law to report suspected incidents of child abuse, and in every state, there is a penalty—civil, criminal, or both—for failure to report child abuse. State laws vary for reporting the abuse of adults and the elderly. In 1994 the Violence Against Women Act made it a federal crime to cross state lines to assault a spouse or domestic partner. Domestic violence is now considered to be a violent crime against which the victim has the right to be protected and for which the perpetrator can be arrested and prosecuted.

Box 18.1

Myths and Facts About Domestic Violence

Myth: Family violence is rare.

Fact: Every year, 10 million Americans are abused by a family member.

Myth: Family violence is confined to mentally disturbed or sick people.

Fact: Fewer than 10% of all cases involve an abuser who is mentally ill. The vast majority seem totally normal and are often charming, persuasive, and rational.

Myth: Violence is trivial—a joking matter.

Fact: A woman is beaten every 15 seconds in the United States, and 2,000–4,000 women are murdered by their husbands or boyfriends every year. Every year, 2.5 million children are abused, and 1,200 die from the abuse. There are 1 million cases of elder abuse annually.

Myth: Family violence is confined to the lower classes.

Fact: Social factors are not relevant. There are doctors, ministers, psychologists, and nurses who beat their family members. Violence occurs at least once in two-thirds of all marriages.

Myth: All members of the family participate in the family dynamics; therefore, all must change in order for the violence to stop.

Fact: Only the perpetrator has the ability to stop the violence. A change in the victim's behavior will not cause the abuser to become nonviolent.

Myth: Family violence is usually a one-time event, an isolated incident.

Fact: Violence is a pattern, a reign of force and terror. It becomes more frequent and severe over time.

Myth: Abused women like being hit; otherwise, they would leave.

Fact: Abused women are forced to stay in the relationship for many reasons. The perpetrator dramatically escalates the violence when a woman tries to leave.

Box 18.2

Types of Abuse

Emotional Abuse

Frequent belittling or demeaning; words or behaviors that undermine sense of self, competence, safety; psychological intimidation; accusations; demand obedience to every order; destruction of property, pets.

Physical Abuse/Battering

Hitting, punching, grabbing, shoving, slapping, kicking, biting, hit with objects, use of weapons.

Sexual Abuse

Inappropriate sexual behavior, including peeping, touching, rape, use of objects, forced sex with animals.

Social Abuse

Isolation from actual and potential support systems; controlling use of time and space; continual watching/spying.

Economic Abuse

Little or no access to assets; minimal input into family expenditures.

Neglect

Physical

Failure to provide adequate food, shelter, sleeping arrangements, clothing, and general physical care.

Emotional

Failure to nurture, love, support; failure to validate self-worth.

Medical

Failure to provide adequate medical care, especially when serious or life-threatening.

Educational

Failure to enroll child in school or alternative means of education; failure to get child to school; failure to assist child in completing educational tasks. Generally applied to child under age 11.

Abandonment

Leaving child alone without adequate supervision; abandoning child, throwing child out of home, not allowing a runaway to return home.

Sibling Abuse

The most common and unrecognized form of domestic violence occurs between siblings. Many people assume it is natural and even appropriate for children to use physical force with one another. Parents say things like "It's a good chance for him to learn how to defend himself," "She had a right to hit him; he was teasing her," and "Kids will be kids." With these attitudes, children learn that physical force is an appropriate method of resolving conflict among themselves. Children who are hit by their parents have more than double the rate of violence against siblings than children whose parents did not hit them. Hitting children increases the probability that they will be violent. Parents should not be complacent about sibling aggression; 3% of all child homicides in the United States are caused by siblings. Even though violence decreases with age, studies indicate that 63–68% of adolescent siblings use physical violence to resolve conflict (Straus, 1994).

Child Abuse

Each year, approximately 2.5 million American children experience at least one act of physical violence. Younger parents are more likely to physically abuse children than older parents. For many, hitting begins when they are infants and does not end until they leave home. Younger children are spanked, punched, grabbed, slapped, kicked, bitten, and hit with fists or objects. Adolescents are more likely to be beaten up and have a knife or gun used against them. Both men and women are equally likely to abuse young children. During adolescence, however, the abuser is more likely to be male. Shaken baby syndrome is one of the most serious yet frequently overlooked forms of child abuse. It involves vigorous shaking of the babies who are being held by the extremities or shoulders that causes whiplash-induced intracranial and intraocular bleeding. It is estimated that one-third of those seen for medical attention have no long-term effects; another one-third have significant and permanent brain damage; and one-third of the victims die. Not recognizing the dangers, many parents shake rather than hit the child, mistakenly believing it is less violent (Butler, G. L., 1995).

In the United States, homicide is one of the five leading causes of death before the age of 18. Some 72% of children killed between the ages of 1 week and 1 year are killed by a parent. Between age 1 and 17, 23% of homicides are caused by parents, 3% by step-parents, and 6% by other family members (Straus, 1994).

Although it is a very rare event, adolescents have been known to kill their parents. The most frequent situation, 90% of cases, is one in which the teen has been severely abused and/or the mother is a victim of abuse. The adolescent's attempts to get help have failed and the family situation becomes increasingly intolerable prior to the murder. A critical factor is the easy availability of guns in the home. The other 10% of cases involve either a severely mentally ill child who experiences hallucinations and delusions or the dangerously antisocial child who has extreme conduct problems (Heide, 1995) (see Chapters 14 and 21).

Partner Abuse—Heterosexual

Female partner abuse in heterosexual relationships is the most widespread form of family violence in the United States. It is thought that 1 woman in 6 is physically abused by her partner, and that 2–3 million women are severely assaulted every year. If verbal and emotional assaults were included, the numbers would be much higher. Violence is the single largest cause of injury to women in the United States, with 20% of emergency department visits resulting from physical abuse. As many as 50% of female homicide victims are killed by their husbands or lovers. Of men who are violent toward their partner, 53% are also violent toward their children (Garske, 1996; Stark and Flitcraft, 1996). Overwhelmingly, the first acts of partner violence occur in dating relationships. Physical abuse occurs among as many as 30–40% of adolescent and college students who are dating. Sadly, more than 25% of victims and 30% of offenders interpret violence as a sign of love (Riggs and Caulfield, 1997). For early warning signs of teenage dating violence, see Box 18.3.

Half the women who are abused suffer beatings several times a year. The other half may be beaten as often as once a week. The intensity and frequency of

---

Box 18.3

Early Warning Signs of Teenage Dating Violence

The teenage boy:

- Believes that men should be in control and women should be submissive.
- Is jealous and possessive of his girlfriend, won't let her have friends, and checks up on her.
- Tries to control his girlfriend by giving orders and making all the decisions.
- Threatens his girlfriend with violence.
- Uses or owns weapons.
- Has a history of losing his temper quickly and fighting.
- Brags about mistreating others.
- Blames his girlfriend when he is violent; says she provoked him and made him do it.
- Has a history of abusive relationships.

---

attacks tend to escalate over time. Compared to nonabused women, abused women are 5 times more likely to attempt suicide, 15 times more likely to abuse alcohol, and 9 times more likely to abuse drugs (Stark and Flitcraft, 1996).

Partner Abuse—Homosexual

Until very recently, there has been a public minimization or denial of physical abuse in lesbian and gay relationships. This denial has been supported by the myths that women are not violent people and that men can defend themselves. In reality, violence does occur in some gay and lesbian families, for the same reasons as in heterosexual families: to demonstrate, achieve, and maintain power and control over one's partner. In addition to physical or emotional abuse, the violent partner may use homophobic control—the threat of telling family, friends, neighbors, or employers about the victim's sexual identity.

In the United States, domestic violence is the third-largest health problem for gay men, following substance abuse and AIDS. It is estimated that 11% of coupled gay men are victims. Men rarely talk about being victims for fear of being considered feminine if they admit that their partners are hurting them. Homophobia and hatred of homosexuals in the United States contributes to difficulties of battered lesbians and gays. They are cut off from the usual support systems available to heterosexual victims such as specialized counseling services and shelters. Fear of being identified as gay or losing custody of children adds to the silence about the violence. Members of lesbian and gay communities are currently making an attempt to intervene with and support victims (Island and Letellier, 1991; Loring, 1994).

Elder Abuse

Elder abuse takes many forms. Some older adults may have their basic physical needs neglected and suffer from dehydration, malnutrition, and oversedation. Families may deprive them of necessary articles such as glasses, hearing aids, and walkers. Some older people are psychologically abused by verbal assaults, threats, humiliation, and/or harassment. Families may violate an older person's rights by refusing appropriate medical treatment, forcing isolation or unreasonable confinement, denying privacy, providing an unsafe environment, or demanding involuntary servitude. Some are financially exploited by their relatives through theft or misuse of property or funds. Others are beaten and even raped by family members.

A number of factors contribute to abuse of older adults. Perpetrators may have personal problems such as lack of support in caring for the older family member, alcohol or drug addiction, and a family history of violence. Family factors include unresolved previous conflicts and power struggles. When the culture devalues older people, abuse is more likely to occur. There are similarities with child abuse in that in both situations, the perpetrator is usually a family member and the victim is dependent on the perpetrator (Whittaker, 1996).

Abuse of Pregnant Women

Pregnancy is a time of increased risk for abuse. There are more incidents of violence during pregnancy than of either gestational diabetes or placenta previa, both of which are screened for regularly. Indeed, 16 to 22% of women report abuse during pregnancy. A past history of abuse is one of the strongest predictors of abuse during pregnancy. Nonpregnant women are usually beaten in the face and chest. But pregnant women tend to be beaten in the abdomen, which can lead to miscarriage, placenta abruptio, fetal loss, premature labor, fetal fractures, pelvic fractures, rupture of the uterus, and hemorrhage. Physical abuse during pregnancy may be related to ambivalent feelings about the pregnancy, competition for attention with the developing fetus, increased vulnerability of the woman, increased economic pressures, and decreased sexual availability. Unfortunately, abuse of pregnant women is often overlooked by health care professionals even when the victim appears in the emergency department with bruises, cuts, broken bones, and abdominal injuries (Butler, J. B., 1995; McFarlane, Parker, and Soeken, 1996).

Stalking

Domestic stalking occurs when a former partner, spouse, or family member threatens or harasses a person. The stalker is usually motivated by a desire to continue the relationship, which can evolve into an attitude of "If I can't have her/him, no one can." Frequently there is a history of domestic violence and the stalking often ends in a violent attack on or killing of the victim (Wright et al, 1995).

Knowledge Base

As a nurse, you must be involved in the prevention, detection, and treatment of domestic violence. Development of the knowledge base and the ability to identify factors that contribute to family violence will help you arrive at early detection and an accurate diagnosis of the problem.

Behavioral Characteristics

Domestic violence often happens without warning and without a buildup of tension. A pattern of violence usually develops. The first incident may be precipitated by frustration or stress. If the victim immediately refuses to accept the violence and seeks outside help, there are often no further episodes. If the victim submits to the violence, then physical force, without the stimulus of frustration or stress, becomes a way of relating, and the pattern becomes resistant to change. A typical cycle occurs when conflict escalates into a violent episode, after which the perpetrator begs for the victim's forgiveness. The victim stays in the system because of promises to reform. With the next episode of conflict, the cycle of violence begins again and becomes part of the family dynamics. Perpetrators are not out of control, as is commonly assumed. They may be enraged or cool and calculating, but in either case they have made a choice. The victim cannot "make them do it." Generally, perpetrators of domestic violence are law-abiding and are dangerous only to their loved ones (Dutton, 1995).

Acts of violence against children range from a light slap to severe beating to homicide. Hitting or spanking children is condoned and even approved of as being necessary and good for the child. Many parents, however, do not realize the underlying messages they are giving to the child by hitting (Straus, 1994):

- If you are small and weak, you deserve to be hit.
- People who love you, hit you.
- It is appropriate to hit people you love.
- Violence is appropriate if the end result is good.
- Violence is an appropriate method of resolving conflict.

See Box 18.4 for myths that surround the use of spanking.

Parental violence often becomes chronic in that it occurs periodically or regularly. In extreme cases, it ends in the death of the infant or child. Child victims are helpless captives because they are dependent on the adults in the family. Abused children often try to please the abusing parent and may become overly compliant to all adults. They may avoid peers and withdraw from outside contacts. It is not unusual for child victims to act out with aggressive behavior later, during adolescence.

Among adult family members, women commit fewer violent acts than men. Women do more hitting, kicking, and throwing of objects, while men are more likely to push, shove, slap, beat up, and even use knives or guns against their partner. The acts that men commit against women are more dangerous and result in more severe injuries. While the victim is being beaten, she is also being verbally abused, often by being called a slut, a bad housekeeper, or a rotten mother. The abuser attacks aspects of life that women use to measure their success: homemaking, child care, attractiveness, sex appeal, and sexual fidelity.

The abuser is the most powerful person in the life of the victim. The abuser's purpose is to enslave the

---

Box 18.4

Myths that Surround the Use of Spanking

Myth: Spanking is harmless.

Fact: Spanking makes parenting more difficult because it reduces parents' ability to influence their children, especially when the children are teens and are too big to control by physical force. Also, authority figures should be trusted and respected, not feared.

Myth: I was spanked, and I'm okay.

Fact: You made it despite being hit; hitting increases the probability that you are more likely to use aggression to handle conflicts.

Myth: If you don't spank, your children will be spoiled or run wild.

Fact: Nonspanked children are better behaved than children of parents who spank. Non-spanking parents tend to pay more attention to their children's behavior and tend to do more explaining and reasoning, which helps children develop internal controls.

Myth: Spanking is needed as a last resort.

Fact: If spanking is done at all, "last resort" may be the worst since parents are usually very angry and act impulsively. It teaches children that being extremely angry justifies hitting.

Myth: Parents spank rarely or only for serious problems.

Fact: Parents who spank tend to use this method for almost any misbehavior; many do not even give the child a warning—they spank before trying other things.

Myth: It is unrealistic to expect parents to never spank.

Fact: It is no more unrealistic to expect parents to not hit a child than to expect that husbands not hit their wives or that a supervisor never hit an employee.

Source: Straus, 1994.

victim, while simultaneously demanding respect, gratitude, and love. Control over the victim is established by repetitive emotional abuse that instills terror and helplessness. Threats of serious harm or threats against other family members keep the victim in a constant state of fear. In order to have complete domination, the abuser isolates the victim. She often is forced to give up work, friends, and family. He may stalk her, eavesdrop, and intercept letters and phone calls. Control and scrutiny of the victim's body and bodily functions further destroy her sense of autonomy. She is shamed and demoralized when told what to eat, when to sleep, what to wear, when to go to the bathroom, and so on. For a victim who has been deprived long enough, the hope of a meal, a bath, or a kind word can be a powerful reward. All this abusive behavior alternates with unpredictable outbursts of physical violence. Such domestic captivity of women, along with traumatic bonding to the batterer, often goes unrecognized.

Homicide is the ultimate expression of male control over females. Of women who are murdered, 50% are killed by a past or present husband or lover. At least two-thirds of these women have been abused by their murderer prior to their death. Women sometimes kill their husbands or lovers, almost invariably in response to years of abuse. They most often murder their partners in self-defense, fearing for their lives and the lives of their children. In the case of a joint homicide-suicide, the perpetrator is almost always male and the victim is almost always female (Campbell, 1995; Stark and Flitcraft, 1996).

Affective Characteristics

Violent people are often extremely jealous and possessive. They view other family members in terms of property and ownership. Abusers use violence in an attempt to prove to themselves and others that they are superior and in control. The use of physical force temporarily obliterates their sense of inadequacy and compensates for a lack of internal resources.

Victims may be immobilized by a variety of affective responses to the abuse such as anxiety, helplessness, and depression. Feelings of self-blame may be expressed in such statements as "If I hadn't talked back to my mother, she wouldn't have hit me," and "If I were a better wife, he wouldn't beat me." Guilt can contribute to depression, which further immobilizes victims and keeps them from leaving or seeking help for the family system.

Fear contributes to women's inability to leave abusive relationships. Often threatened with death at the idea of leaving, they live in fear of physical reprisal. Fearing loneliness, some women may believe that being in a bad relationship is better than being alone. Also, leaving the relationship does not necessarily ensure the end of the abuse. The abuser is often most dangerous when threatened with or faced with separation. Some choose to kill when they believe that death is better than divorce (Stark and Flitcraft, 1996). See Box 18.5 for reasons why people stay in or return to abusive relationships.

Fear also contributes to the inability to leave for a partner in an abusive gay or lesbian relationship. Because many couples share close friends within the same community, victims may fear shaming their partners. They may also fear friends will either deny the problem or take the abuser's side. Homophobia contributes to the victim's reluctance to seek help. Calling the police may result in ridicule or hostile responses from the officers. Victims may not seek help from family members to avoid reinforcing negative stereotypes about homosexuality, which might exacerbate the family's homophobia (Island and Letellier, 1991).

Cognitive Characteristics

Many abusive people have perfectionistic standards for family members. An unrealistically high standard results in rigidity and an obsession with discipline and control. Inflexibility hinders the abuser's ability to find alternative solutions to conflict. Some abusers have a self-righteous belief that they have a prerogative to use physical force to make others comply with their wishes. Many abusers lack an understanding of the effect of their behavior on the victims and may even blame their abusive behavior on the victims, evidence of the use of denial, projection, and an external locus of control. See Box 18.6 for examples of how people "explain" their violent behavior.

Many parents who abuse their children suffered emotional deprivation or abuse when they themselves were children. As parents, they may lack information about the normal growth and development of children and therefore have unrealistic expectations. Anger may turn to violence when a child is unable to meet the parent's unreasonable demands.

Victims of abuse often begin with or develop low self-esteem. They begin to believe the violence itself is evidence of personal worthlessness. Some victims

■ *Box 18.5*

Why Do They Stay? Why Do They Go Back?

Fear

Of physical reprisal if they resist, of being found and beaten again, of their children being hurt; those who attempt to leave risk suffering worse violence and even death.

Learned Helplessness

They believe they have no choices and no control; they have come to believe that violence is an accepted way of life.

Traumatic Bonding

Results from alternating good and bad treatment; they have no sense of autonomy.

Emotional Dependency

They are convinced that they are weak and inferior, and do not deserve better treatment; they are insecure over potential autonomy.

Financial Dependency

They may not have a source of income; if the abuser is arrested, he may lose his job and the family will have no income; they have been taught that they have to be submissive in exchange for financial support.

Guilt/Shame

They have been convinced that they provoked the abuse; guilt over failure of the relationship; family/religious/cultural values against divorce or separation; shame about remaining in the abusive relationship.

Isolation

They have few, if any, friends; little support from family; no phone, no mail, no car.

Children

They may believe two parents are better than one; they may be threatened with loss of custody; the abuser may threaten to harm or kidnap the children.

Hope

They hope that if they change in the way the abuser wants them to, the abuse will stop; hope that the abuser will keep promises and stop the assaults.

---

even absolve the abuser from responsibility by blaming violent behavior on a high level of stress or too much alcohol.

Social Characteristics

The abuser's family history is an important factor in understanding domestic violence. Much of adult behavior is determined by childhood experiences within the family system. The experience of violence in the family of origin teaches that the use of physical force is appropriate. Children may cope with exposure to abuse by identifying with either the aggressor or the victim. Often these children grow up to become another abuser or adult victim. In addition, the media provide ample opportunity for children to see violence and learn to identify with and tolerate violent behavior (Fortin and Chamberland, 1995).

The violent family is often socially isolated. In some families, the isolation precedes the violence. In others, the isolation is in response to the violence. Family members, ashamed of what is occurring, withdraw from interactions with others to avoid the humiliation that might occur if the violence became known (Stark and Flitcraft, 1996).

Culture-Specific Characteristics

Violence is a complex behavior, and like all behaviors it occurs in the context of culture. Severe and ongoing domestic violence has been documented in almost every country in the past 20 years. The vast majority of victims are females. In a study of 90 societies throughout the world, wife beating was present in 75. There appear to be four cultural factors that are strong predictors of wife abuse. The strongest factor

Box 18.6

How Perpetrators Explain Violent Behavior

Denial

Denial of all or part of their violent behavior. "It never happened."

Forgetting

Blanking out their behavior. "I can't remember."

Minimization

Minimizing the extent, frequency, and effects. "It was just . . ." or "It was only . . . "

Removal of Self

Separation of the sense of self from the abusive behavior. "I'm not a violent person."

Event Without Intention

Abuse has an independent dynamic of its own. "If she hadn't ducked down, she wouldn't have been hit in her face. She would have only been hit in her belly."

Excuses

Accepts the blame but not the responsibility. "I was abused as a kid, that's why I do it," or "I couldn't help it, I had too much to drink."

Justifications

Accepts the responsibility but not the blame. "You're a lousy mother—I'll teach you to keep these kids quiet."

Confessions

These can be with or without remorse. Confessions become normalized as part of a violent way of life. "I didn't mean to hit you so hard."

is gender economic inequality, followed by male authority and decision making in the home, divorce restrictions for women, and a pattern of using physical violence for conflict resolution. The more completely women are dependent on men, the more vulnerable they are to violent action with no options for escape. The following are some examples of violence against women (Desjarlais et al, 1995; Schuler, 1992):

- Papua, New Guinea—56–62% of women are beaten
- Bangladesh—50% of all murders are husbands killing their wives
- Sri Lanka—60% of women are beaten
- Mexico—60% of women are physically abused
- Kenya—42% of wives say they are beaten regularly
- Chile—80% of women have suffered abuse by male partner or relative
- Thailand—more than 50% of married women are beaten regularly
- Peru—33% of women who come to the emergency department are victims of domestic violence

- Norway—25% of women have been physically and/or sexually abused
- Italy—The highest court has ruled that it is not a crime to beat your wife, as long as you do it only once in a while.

Domestic violence resulting in death is a serious problem in some parts of the world. In India, the illegal "dowry death" or "bride-burning" occurs in some areas. The relatives of married sons demand large sums of material goods from the families of daughters-in-law. If this is not provided, they may kill the young woman. Female infanticide has increased in parts of Asia over the past decade. Not only is this a tragic loss of life, but it also has a tremendous impact on the mental health of mothers and other family members. Women are forced from family pressures and agonizing circumstances to make desperate moral choices. These choices are not easily made nor ever forgotten (Desjarlais et al, 1995).

The United States has a higher rate of intrafamily homicide than the overall rate of homicide in European countries such as England, Germany, and Denmark. There have been some studies on domestic violence in ethnic minorities. African American women are twice as likely to experience severe violence compared to European American women. Risk factors include young age, low socioeconomic status, and unemployment/underemployment of men. Domestic violence often arises out of dysfunctional adaptation to extreme economic pressure. Among Hispanic American couples the rates vary according to immigration status. Mexican Americans born in the United States report rates 2.5 times higher than those born in Mexico (Hampton and Yung, 1996).

Domestic violence is not traditional in Native American life but has evolved in modern times. The sanctions and protections against battering have decreased and women are increasingly vulnerable to violence. As with other minority groups, family tension is increased by unemployment, undereducation, and financial strain. Elders believe the long-term solution is to return to traditional values that nurture children, give them self-esteem, and teach boys to love and respect women (Spector, 1996).

Causative Theories

Domestic violence is easy to describe but difficult to explain. There is no single cause of this type of violence. It results from an interaction of neurobiological, personality, situational, and societal factors that have an impact on families.

Neurobiological Theory

Neurobiological theorists propose that genes and neurotransmitters may contribute to causing violent behavior. Although a genetic predisposition may make certain behaviors more likely, it does not make them inevitable. Serotonin (5-HT) exhibits inhibitory control over aggression. Low levels of 5-HT are implicated in a lack of control, loss of temper, and explosive rage (Volavka, 1995).

Intrapersonal Theory

Intrapersonal theory suggests that the cause of violence lies in the personality of the abuser. It is thought that people who are violent are unable to control their impulsive expressions of anger and hostility. As many as 80% of male abusers grew up in homes in which they were abused or observed their mothers being abused. With these family dynamics, the child sees the father as frightening and intimidating and sees the mother as helpless and nonprotective. This early emotional deprivation contributes to an adult who is very needy of nurturance and support. He

comes to adult relationships with unrealistic demands for time and attention. As the relationship develops, he discourages his partner's relationships with other people because of his low self-esteem and fear of abandonment (Blue and Griffith, 1995).

Social Learning Theory

Social learning theory proposes that violence is a learned behavior and people are conditioned to respond aggressively and violently. Children learn about violence from observation, from being a victim, and from behaving violently themselves. If the use of violence is rewarded by a gain in power, the behavior is reinforced. If there is immediate negative reinforcement within the family, a decrease in violent behavior will result. Parents who abuse their children often have inappropriate expectations of themselves and their children. They may have inadequate parenting skills and a lack of resources. Often they lack empathy toward children's needs and there may even be role reversal between parent and child.

In addition to family models, the media provide many models of violence to which children are exposed. Some movies and television shows demonstrate that "good" people use force to achieve "good" ends. Many of the stories make no attempt to justify the use of force for "good" ends; they simply present endless, senseless acts of cruelty by one human being upon another. With these types of family and media examples, children develop values that tolerate, and even accept as normal, everyday violence between people.

Feminist Theory

Feminist theory describes the sexist structure of the family and society as an important factor in domestic violence. The cultural value is that men have a right to keep women subordinate through power and privilege. Men abuse because they believe they have a right to do so and because they can get away with it. Domestic violence is both a gender issue and a power issue. Victims are sometimes labeled as codependent in the abusive relationship, but such labeling is just another way of blaming the victim for the abuse. Women are sexualized as objects, restricted in state and federal participation in decision making, dehumanized with labels, controlled over the rights to their own bodies, and demeaned in value (Garske, 1996).

The sexist economic system helps entrap women, who often are forced to choose between poverty and abuse. It is difficult for women to find advocates and solutions within the male-dominated legal, religious,

Critical Thinking

Branko and Drenko, a Serbian/American couple, dated for 9 months prior to their marriage, during which time Branko was attentive and adoring of Drenko but often jealous and possessive. Following their marriage Branko insisted that Drenko quit her job and stay home even though Drenko enjoyed working and feared becoming bored. Drenko became pregnant right away. During her pregnancy, Branko became totally possessive of Drenko, keeping her from family or friends. After the birth of their daughter, Branko began criticizing Drenko for her care of the baby, her care of the house, and the time she devoted to him. Drenko always felt that Branko's criticism was justified because she didn't enjoy being a housewife. Eventually Branko's criticism gave way to pushing, shoving, hitting, and threatening Drenko's life. He maintained that she forced him to be violent because she didn't perform her duties as well as he expected. After each violent episode, Branko would vow his undying love for Drenko and promise that he would never hit her again. Drenko feels frightened and ashamed but does not report Branko's violence because she believes that if she works harder, Branko's behavior will change.

Suggested answers can be found in Appendix D.

1. What affective and cognitive characteristics in Branko's behavior may have forewarned of his abusive tendency?
2. Based on data about domestic violence, what social characteristic was likely present in Branko's past that predisposed him to becoming violent?
3. What is the fallacy in Drenko's belief that if she works harder, Branko's behavior will change?
4. What is the prediction based on the interaction between Drenko and Branko if he seriously injured her and she had to be cared for in a health care setting?
5. Based on your understanding of domestic violence and spousal abuse, what are the greatest dangers to Drenko if she does not seek help?
6. As a mental health nurse, if you were Drenko's friend and she confided in you that she was in an abusive relationship, how might you respond?

mental health, and medical systems. Society sanctions male violence by neglecting female victims. What remains unacknowledged is that women are being murdered on a regular basis, not by strangers but by husbands and lovers (Stark and Flitcraft, 1996).

The Nursing Process

Assessment

Given the incidence of abuse, it is logical to assume that you will encounter victims in a variety of clinical settings. Although one-third of all women's visits to emergency departments are caused by domestic violence, fewer than 10% are identified. There are clues that you need to recognize that would indicate the possibility of domestic violence. One of the behaviors to look for is the man speaking for the woman in response to questions about the injury. She may seek his approval before answering questions. He may criticize or correct her answers. Often, he may not want health care professionals to talk to the woman alone (Bicehouse and Hawker, 1995).

During the assessment of every client, one or two introductory questions should be asked. In assessing a child, say, for example, "Moms and dads try to help their children learn how to behave well. What happens to you when you do something wrong?" Or ask, "What is the worst punishment you ever received?" In assessing adults, you may begin with this approach: "One of the sources of stress in our lives is family disagreement. Could you describe how disagreements affect you? What happens when you disagree?" If the responses to these questions are indicative of violence, a focused nursing assessment must be conducted; see the Focused Nursing Assessment table. Obviously, the assessment questions must be adapted to the client's age, gender, and family situation.

Text continues on page 440

Focused Nursing Assessment

VICTIMS OF DOMESTIC VIOLENCE

Behavior Assessment	Affective Assessment	Cognitive Assessment
What types of things cause conflict within your family? How is this managed or resolved?	Who do you view as responsible for the use of physical force within the family?	Do you believe or hope the violence will not recur?
Who in your family loses control when angry?	How much guilt are you experiencing at this time?	What are your beliefs about keeping the family together?
Have you been slapped? Hit? Punched? Thrown? Shoved? Kicked?	Tell me about your fears: Financial problems? Child care problems? Loneliness? Further physical injury?	Describe your personal strengths and abilities.
Have you attempted to leave the relationship in the past? What occurred then?	How hopeless do you feel about your situation?	What are the rules about using physical force within your family?

Social Assessment

How did your parents relate to each other?

What type of discipline was used when you were a child?

Describe your relationships with people outside your basic family unit.

Who can you turn to for support in times of stress?

What types of contact have you had with the legal system: Phoned police? Restraining order? Obtained a lawyer? Court cases? Protective services?

Physiological Assessment

Is there evidence of trauma such as bruises, burns, and old scars?

Are there any fractured bones or dislocated joints?

Does the client have problems with mobility?

Is there any evidence of internal injuries?

Does the client complain of abnormal sensations, numbness, or pain?

Is growth and development normal for the client's age?

Diagnosis

Priority must be given to critical and serious physical injuries. The severity and potential fatality of the situation must be considered, as well as the needs of dependent children and legal issues surrounding the case. Consider the following nursing diagnoses when analyzing your assessment data:

- *Ineffective family coping, disabling,* related to an inability to manage conflict without violence
- *Ineffective individual coping* related to being a victim of violence
- *Altered parenting* related to the physical abuse of children
- *Powerlessness* related to feelings of being dependent on the abuser
- *Self-esteem disturbance* related to feeling guilty and responsible for being a victim
- *Social isolation* related to shame about family violence
- *High risk for violence, directed at others,* related to a history of the use of physical force within the family

Outcome Identification

Once you have established diagnoses, you and the client mutually identify goals for change. Client outcomes are specific behavioral measures by which you, clients, and significant others determine progress toward goals. The following are examples of some of the outcomes appropriate to people who are victims of domestic violence:

- remains safe and free from harm
- develops an escape plan
- manages conflict appropriately
- verbalizes an internal locus of control
- verbalizes an understanding of normal growth and development of children
- implements appropriate and safe parenting techniques
- utilizes community resources

Nursing Interventions

Most victims of domestic violence would like it to end, but they may not know how to seek the help they need. It is extremely important that you be nonjudgmental in your interactions with all family members. Initially, clients may be unwilling to trust you because of family shame and fears of being accused for remaining in the violent situation. It is vital that you not impose your own values by offering quick and easy solutions to the very complicated problem of domestic violence. See the accompanying box for the nursing interventions classification (NIC).

Treatment of families experiencing violence requires a multidisciplinary approach, with a broad range of interventions. Nurses, social workers, physicians, family therapists, vocational trainers, police, protective services personnel, and lawyers must coordinate to intervene effectively in a domestic violence situation.

Safety: Risk Management

Abuse Protection

In the initial contact with family members, assure their physical safety as much as possible. It is critical to assess the level of danger for the victim; homicide may be a real possibility if previous threats have been made. If an adult is being abused, there is a likelihood that children are being abused. Even if the children are not being physically abused, witnessing domestic violence can be devastating. It is also important to assess the level of danger for the abuser. The severity and duration of the violence are the factors that contribute the most directly to victims killing their abusers in self-defense. If the level of danger is high, protective services or the police should be contacted for emergency custody placement or removal to a shelter.

You should help women develop a "safe plan" or "escape plan" to use when their safety is threatened. You may suggest that they have all important documents such as birth certificates and orders of protection, some money, a list of important phone numbers, and a couple days' clothing gathered in one secure location. They should have a second set of car keys so they can leave quickly if they need to.

Families experiencing violence often have poor communication skills. Nursing interventions can be designed to improve the family members' effective

---

Nursing Interventions Classification

VICTIMS AND PERPETRATORS OF DOMESTIC VIOLENCE

DOMAIN: Safety

Class: *Risk Management*

> **Interventions:** *Abuse Protection:* Identification of high-risk, dependent relationships and actions to prevent further infliction of physical or emotional harm.
>
> *Abuse Protection: Child:* Identification of high-risk, dependent child relationships and actions to prevent possible or further infliction of physical, sexual, or emotional harm or neglect of basic necessities of life.
>
> *Abuse Protection: Elder:* Identification of high-risk, dependent elder relationships and actions to prevent possible or further infliction of physical, sexual, or emotional harm; neglect of basic necessities of life; or exploitation.

DOMAIN: Behavioral

Class: *Behavior Therapy*

> **Interventions:** *Impulse Control Training:* Assisting the patient to mediate impulsive behavior through application of problem-solving strategies to social and interpersonal situations.

---

communication. The skills you can teach include active listening with feedback, clear and direct communication, and communication that does not attack the personhood of others. Identify the normality of conflict within all families by discussing how disagreements are inevitable. From there, discuss the use of the democratic process in conflict resolution and decision making. It is best to practice with minor, unemotional family problems at first.

Family interventions also include helping identify methods to manage anger appropriately. All family members must assume responsibility for their own behavior. They can learn and practice talking out anger as it occurs. Make suggestions for appropriate expression, such as relaxation, physical exercise, and striking safe, inanimate objects (a pillow, a couch, or a punching bag). Guide the family in establishing limits and defining consequences if violence recurs. Emphasize that violence within the family will not be tolerated.

Feminist-sensitive therapy can and should be practiced by all professionals, female and male, who are involved with victims of domestic violence. This might also be called a survivor-centered approach—not specific techniques, but rather a perspective or way of seeing and understanding the context in which women and children live, recognizing the cultural values that underlie domestic violence. Using this approach, you speak up and say that violence is wrong and will not be tolerated.

One of the primary goals of feminist-sensitive therapy is the empowerment of victims. The process of violence removes all power and control from a person, resulting in low self-esteem, anxiety, depression, and somatic problems. The following principles are basic to the empowerment of victims:

- A commitment to the belief that women and men are inherently equal.

- An egalitarian approach to the nurse-client relationship in which the client is viewed as an equal partner rather than a helpless recipient of nursing interventions.
- Interventions that focus on the enhancement of the victim's power.
- An emphasis on the victim's strengths and abilities.
- Respect for the victim's ability to understand her or his own experiences.
- Family interventions that change destructive roles and expectations within the family system.
- A willingness to state clear value positions about domestic violence.

Through this approach, clients can become aware that they have choices in, and control over, their lives. Avoid trying to convince adult victims to leave their abuser. As difficult as it may be, you must be willing to support clients in their pain, rather than telling them what to do about their problems. For the most positive adaptive outcome, adult victims must be their own rescuers and take charge of their own safety and protection plan. If they need help with this process, they must be taught to ask for that help directly. This is not meant to imply in any way that you would abandon clients; rather, you stand by, support, and affirm the positive choices and decisions they make.

Adult clients must begin identifying ways in which they are dependent on their abusers. High levels of dependency make it difficult for victims to leave abusers without intense support. You can help them identify intrapersonal and interpersonal strengths to decrease their feelings of powerlessness. From there, clients can move on to identifying aspects of life that are under their control. Offer assertiveness training to help them develop new skills for relating to others in the future. But caution them, if they are still in the abusive relationship, that assertive behavior may escalate the violence.

Abuse Protection: Child

Parents who are physically abusive need help in developing and improving their parenting skills. Begin by recognizing their current positive parenting skills, to increase their self-worth and help them engage in the learning process. Share your understanding that the use of violence is a desperate attempt to cope with their children. Confirming that they care about their

children will increase the likelihood of their active participation in the treatment process. Because domestic violence is often transgenerational, discuss with the parents how they were punished as children. Teach them about the normal growth and development of children. Unrealistic demands for children to comply beyond their developmental ability often result in violence. The first step in the problem-solving process is helping parents identify specific problems they experience with raising children. They can then go on to identify solutions, other than physical force, that are age-appropriate for their children. They need support in implementing, practicing, and evaluating these new skills. See the Self-Help Groups list at the end of this chapter for community resources for referring both victims and perpetrators of domestic violence.

Abuse Protection: Elder

Support the elder person and caretakers in identifying and expanding social support networks. These outside individuals may be able to help with ADLs, transportation, financial advice, and assistance with personal problems. Assist the caretakers in exploring their feelings about the older person in their care. Help them identify factors that are disturbing to them and which may contribute to neglect or abuse. Determine the caretakers' ability to meet their loved one's needs, and provide appropriate teaching. Provide community resource information, including addresses and phone numbers of agencies that offer senior service assistance. See the Self-Help Groups list at the end of this chapter, as well as Chapter 15, for a list of community resources.

Behavioral: Behavior Therapy

Impulse Control Training

Most abusers do not seek treatment unless it is court-ordered or there are custody issues involved. It is frustrating to intervene with abusers who deny the reality of or the responsibility for the violence. Group therapy for abusers is sometimes helpful. The group setting is more effective than individual therapy because interactions with a number of people more successfully address the anger and control problems. The responsibility for aggression is always placed on the aggressor. Issues regarding the patriarchal and power views of relationships are discussed in great depth. Types of abuse are examined as well as the underlying belief systems. Participants are asked to specify their abusive behaviors, identify the intentions behind those behaviors, and examine the effects of the abuse on their victims. The goal is to establish new skills and techniques of coping with life's problems. Abusers learn that anger *can* be controlled and that violence is always a *choice*.

Evaluation

Nurses in acute care settings may not have the opportunity for long-term evaluation of the family system. Stark and Flitcraft (1996) state that short-term evaluation focuses on:

1. The identification of domestic violence.
2. The family's ability to recognize that a problem exists.
3. The willingness of the family to accept assistance by following through with referrals.
4. The removal of the victim from a volatile situation.

Nurses in long-term settings or within the community have an opportunity to evaluate the effectiveness of the multidisciplinary treatment plan over an extended period of time. When violence no longer exists within the family system, the plan has succeeded. Sharing in the process of family growth and adaptation can be a tremendous source of professional satisfaction.

Achievement of the following outcome criteria is evidence that the plan of intervention was successful. The victims have:

1. Recognized that they are not to blame for the violence of others.
2. Ended the denial and minimization of domestic violence.
3. Demonstrated an awareness of strengths, skills, and competence.
4. Re-established a sense of power over their own lives.
5. Verbalized their right to express their own needs and to satisfy them.
6. Established social networks to decrease isolation and secrecy.

All nurses should evaluate their professional obligations and practice in counteracting those aspects of society that foster domestic violence. Domestic violence is a mental health problem of national and international importance, and nurses should be leaders in helping prevent it in future generations.

Primary prevention includes educating the general population on the existence of domestic violence and its devastating effects. Nursing interventions include parent education, family life education and conflict resolution programs in schools, referral for appropriate child or elder care, establishment of support groups, and education of fellow nurses about the problem of domestic violence. As a professional you can monitor the media and keep the pressure on to decrease the amount of violence that is portrayed. Similar to the seat belt campaign, state and federal campaigns should be developed for zero tolerance against domestic violence.

Secondary prevention includes working with children who are victims or who have seen their mothers beaten, and making referrals for multidisciplinary intervention. Nurses must be community advocates in supporting hotlines, crisis centers, and shelters for victims of domestic violence. On the political level, nurses must make their voices heard in regard to policies and laws affecting children, women, and older people. Questions to guide the evaluation of nursing practice include the following:

- What action have I taken to decrease violence in the media?
- Have I been an advocate for gun control?
- Have I confronted the use of physical punishment within families?
- Have I volunteered to teach parenting classes at grade schools and high schools?
- Have I written to legislators to protest funding cuts in programs designed to help children, women, and older people?
- Have I spoken out on the need to increase the number of bilingual/bicultural counselors, lawyers, nurses, and physicians to attend to the needs of ethnic families?

Self-Help Groups

Victims and Perpetrators of Domestic Violence

Victims

American Association for Protecting Children
(800) 227-5242

Bridgework Ministries, Inc.
1226 Turner Street, Suite C
Clearwater, FL 34616
(813) 530-1499

Child Abuse Prevention—Kids Peace
(800) 257-3223

Child Help
(800) 422-4453
www.childhelpusa.org

Domestic Violence Hotline
(800) 799-SAFE
hearing impaired
(800) 787-3224

KIDS USA
(800) 543-7025

National Council on Child Abuse
and Family Violence
(800) 222-2000

National Gay and Lesbian Task Force
1517 U Street, NW
Washington, DC 20009
(202) 332-6483
www.ngltf.org

National Organization for Victim Assistance
(NOVA)
717 D Street, NW
Washington, DC 20004
(202) 393-NOVA

National Victim Center
307 West 7th Street
Fort Worth, TX 76102
(817) 877-3355
www.nvc.org

Parents Anonymous
(800) 421-0353

Perpetrators

Brother to Brother
1660 Broad Street
Providence, RI 02905
(401) 467-3710

Men Stopping Violence
1020 DeKalb Avenue, NE
Atlanta, GA 30307
(404) 688-1376

Key Concepts

Introduction

- Although the image of the ideal American family is one of happiness and harmony, in reality there is a great deal of domestic abuse and violence.

- Nurses are required by law to report suspected incidents of child abuse.

- The most common and unrecognized form of domestic violence occurs between siblings.

- Each year, 2.5 million American children experience at least one act of physical violence. Shaken baby syndrome causes permanent brain damage or death to many children.

- In the United States, 72% of children killed under age 1 are killed by a parent.

- In most cases of adolescents killing their parents, the teens have been severely abused.

- In heterosexual partner abuse, 95% of the batterers are men. Violence is the single largest cause of injury to women in the United States.

- The first acts of partner violence usually occur in dating relationships.

- Domestic violence occurs in some gay and lesbian relationships, for the same reasons as in heterosexual relationships.

- Elder abuse includes neglecting basic physical needs, psychological abuse, violation of rights, financial abuse, and physical abuse.

- Pregnancy is a time of increased risk for abuse, and a past history of abuse is one of the strongest predictors of the likelihood that pregnant women will be abused.

Knowledge Base

- Domestic violence can happen without warning and without a buildup of tension. A pattern or cycle develops, consisting of begging for forgiveness, hope on the part of the victim, and a return to violence.
- Abused children often try to please the parent in order to stop the violence.
- The abuser has total control over the victim, who lives in a constant state of fear.
- Some 50% of the women who are murdered are killed by a past or present husband or lover.
- Violent people are extremely jealous and possessive and view others in terms of property and ownership.
- Victims may be immobilized by anxiety, helplessness, depression, self-blame, and guilt.
- The abuser is often most dangerous when threatened with or faced with separation.
- Anger may turn to violence when children are unable to fulfill the unrealistic expectations of parents.
- Severe and ongoing domestic violence has been documented in almost every country.
- Risk factors related to ethnicity in the United States include financial strain, unemployment/underemployment, and undereducation.
- There appears to be a genetic-environmental link to violence involving low levels of serotonin (5-HT).
- Domestic violence is frequently transgenerational; as many as 80% of male abusers have grown up in violent homes.
- If the use of violence is rewarded by a gain in power, the behavior is reinforced.
- The cultural values and economic system help entrap women, who are often forced to choose between poverty and abuse.

Nursing Assessment

- Clients in all clinical settings should be routinely assessed for evidence of violence.
- Assessment questions should be adapted to the client's age, gender, and family situation.

Nursing Diagnosis

- The most important outcome of nursing assessment is identifying the existence of domestic violence. Priority must be given to critical and serious physical injuries.
- The severity and potential fatality of the situation must be considered, as well as the needs of dependent children and legal issues surrounding the case.

Outcome Identification

- The most important outcome for victims of domestic violence is remaining safe and free from harm.

Nursing Interventions

- The treatment of families experiencing domestic violence requires a multidisciplinary approach.
- The priority for care is assuring the victim's physical safety.
- Victims need to develop an escape plan to use when their safety is threatened.
- Families must learn to use effective communication.
- Family members must identify methods to manage anger appropriately.
- Parents need help in developing and improving their parenting skills.
- Feminist-sensitive therapy is a survivor-centered approach. Adult victims are supported and empowered to take charge of their own lives.
- Most abusers do not seek treatment unless it is court-ordered or there are custody issues involved. Group therapy is more helpful than individual therapy for abusers.

Evaluation

- Short-term evaluation focuses on the identification of domestic violence, the family's ability to recognize that a problem exists, the willingness of the family to follow through with referrals, and the removal of the victim from a volatile situation.
- Long-term evaluation focuses on the victim's recognition of blamelessness, ending denial of the problem, awareness of competence, sense of power over his or her own life, recognition of personal rights, and decreased isolation and secrecy.
- Evaluation of nursing practice focuses on actions taken to combat violence both within families and in society, preventive teaching strategies, and advocating for increased bilingual/bicultural professionals to intervene with families.

Review Questions

1. Tom, 15 years old, has been accused of killing his parents. You know it is most likely that Tom

   a. was born with criminal tendencies.

   b. was severely abused by his parents.

   c. is a member of a gang.

   d. is mentally retarded.

2. If a child is hit or spanked, what is the underlying message that is given?

   a. Effective communication can prevent violent outbursts.

   b. Conflict can be resolved through the democratic process.

   c. Strangers are more dangerous than family members.

   d. Violence is appropriate if the end result is good.

3. Which of the following is a fact about the use of spanking?

   a. Spanking increases the probability that the child will use aggression to handle conflict.

   b. Spanking makes parenting much easier.

   c. It is unrealistic to expect parents never to spank.

   d. Spanking is needed as a last resort.

4. You are assessing Bill, a perpetrator of violence against his girlfriend. Bill states that he couldn't help it because he was drunk. You point out to him that he is using which one of the following to explain his violent behavior?

   a. justification

   b. excuses

   c. minimization

   d. denial

5. The purpose of empowering victims of violence is to

   a. help clients become aware that they have control over their lives.

   b. convince victims to leave their abusers.

   c. tell them how to solve their problems.

   d. develop safety escape plans for them.

References

Bicehouse, T., & Hawker, L. (1995). Domestic violence: Myths and safety issues. *J Holistic Nurs, 13*(1), 83–92.

Blue, H. C., & Griffith, E. E. H. (1995). Sociocultural and therapeutic perspectives on violence. *Psychiatr Clin North Am, 18*(3), 571–587.

Butler, G. L. (1995). Shaken baby syndrome. *J Psychosoc Nurs, 33*(9), 47–50.

Butler, J. B. (1995). Domestic violence. *J Holistic Nurs, 13*(1), 54–69.

Campbell, J. C. (1995). Prediction of homicide of and by battered women. In J. C. Campbell (Ed.), *Assessing Dangerousness* (pp. 96–113). Newbury Park, CA: Sage.

Desjarlais, R., et al. (1995). *World Mental Health.* New York: Oxford Univ. Press.

Dutton, D. G. (1995). *The Batterer.* New York: Basic Books.

Fortin, A., & Chamberland, C. (1995). Preventing the psychological maltreatment of children. *J Interpersonal Violence, 10*(3), 275–295.

Garske, D. (1996). Transforming the culture. In R. L. Hampton, P. Jenkins, & T. P. Gullotta (Eds.), *Preventing Violence in America* (pp. 263–285). Newbury Park, CA: Sage.

Hampton, R. L., & Yung, B. R. (1996). Violence in communities of color. In R. L. Hampton, P. Jenkins, & T. P. Gullotta (Eds.), *Preventing Violence in America* (pp. 53–83). Newbury Park, CA: Sage.

Heide, K. M. (1995). *Why Kids Kill Parents.* Newbury Park, CA: Sage.

Island, D., & Letellier, P. (1991). *Men Who Beat the Men Who Love Them: Battered Gay Men and Domestic Violence.* Haworth Press.

Loring, M. T. (1994). *Emotional Abuse.* Lexington, MA: Lexington Books.

McFarlane, J., Parker, B., & Soeken, K. (1996). Abuse during pregnancy. *Nurs Res, 45*(1), 37–41.

Riggs, D. S., & Caulfield, M. B. (1997). Expected consequences of male violence against their female dating partners. *J Interpersonal Violence, 12*(2), 229–240.

Schuler, M. (1992). *Freedom from Violence: Women's Strategies From Around the World*. New York: United Nations Development Fund for Women.

Spector, R. E. (1996). *Cultural Diversity in Health & Illness* (4th ed.). Norwalk, CT: Appleton & Lange.

Stark, E., & Flitcraft, A. (1996). *Women at Risk*. Newbury Park, CA: Sage.

Straus, M. A. (1994). *Beating the Devil Out of Them: Corporal Punishment in American Families*. Lexington, MA: Lexington Books.

Volavka, J. (1995). *Neurobiology of Violence*. Washington, D.C.: American Psychiatric Press.

Whittaker, T. (1996). Violence, gender, and elder abuse. In B. Fawcett, B. Featherstone, J. Hearn, & C. Toft (Eds.), *Violence and Gender Relations* (pp. 147–160). Newbury Park, CA: Sage.

Wright, J. A., et al. (1995). Investigating stalking crimes. *J Psychosoc Nurs, 33*(9), 38–43.

CHAPTER 19

Sexual Violence

Karen Lee Fontaine

Objectives

After reading this chapter, you will be able to:

- Explain the factors contributing to sexual violence.
- Assess a survivor's behavioral, affective, and cognitive responses to assault.
- Participate in a multidisciplinary intervention for child or adult victims of assault.
- Refer clients to appropriate community resources.

Key Terms

acquaintance rape
anger rape
date rape
gang rape
power rape
rape
rape-trauma syndrome
ritual abuse
sadistic rape
spiritual recovery

Sexual violence includes criminal behaviors such as sexual harassment, rape, and child sexual abuse. Sexual violence is, first and foremost, an act of violence, hatred, and aggression. Like other acts of violence (assault and battery or murder), there is a violation of and injury to the victims. The injuries may be psychological and/or physical. Victims are overwhelmed and overpowered and are violated as human beings. During the harassment, attack, or abuse, victims are not only out of control of their situation, but they are also assaulted in the most vulnerable dimension of the self. Sexual violence is not an occasional, isolated incident experienced by people in extraordinary situations. Sexual violence is a widespread problem taking place in a broad social context which allows and even encourages it to occur. When we encourage gender role differences that accentuate masculine aggression and feminine passivity and when we confuse sexual activity with sexual violence, we create a climate of tolerance of sexual violence in our society.

Sexual Harassment

Sexual harassment of women in the workplace and in schools has always existed as a hidden crime. Only recently has it been recognized for what it is—discrimination against and violation of women. Prevalence rates reported by women range between 30–55%. However, women frequently do not report harassment because they do not expect to be believed and fear that they will be accused of contributing to the problem (Rutter, 1996; Wyatt and Riederle, 1995). Behaviors include:

- sexual teasing, jokes, remarks, or questions
- pressure for dates
- letters, telephone calls, or e-mail of a sexual nature
- sexual gestures
- deliberate touching, cornering, or pinching
- pressure for sexual favors
- actual or attempted rape

The United States Equal Employment Opportunity commission (EEOC) is the government agency that interprets and enforces employment laws. In 1980, the EEOC issued a position statement clearly stating that sexual harassment is considered a form of sexual discrimination and, therefore, an unlawful employment act. Although most cases of sexual harassment have traditionally involved a male harasser and a female victim, the EEOC also determined that the sexual harasser, as well as the victim, can be either a man or a woman.

There are two distinctive categories of sexual harassment: quid pro quo and hostile environment. Quid pro quo (translated as "this for that") means that an employer or other person of authority suggests that he will give her this job, or promotion, or salary, in return for that sexual favor. This form of sexual harassment is the most well-known. Hostile environment sexual harassment is unwelcome sexual conduct that has the purpose or effect of creating an intimidating, hostile, or offensive working environment. This type of sexual harassment can involve supervisors, coworkers, and even customers or vendors. The intent of the law is to give people the opportunity to work in an environment that is free from sex-based discrimination, taunts, jeers, and insults.

Sexual harassment can lead to severe stress in the victims. Many experience depression, isolation, feelings of powerlessness, helplessness, fear, restlessness, inability to concentrate, somatic complaints, sexual problems, and loss of self-esteem. At its most severe, harassment resembles the other sexual traumas of rape and child sexual abuse and may result in post-traumatic stress disorder. Filing a complaint of sexual harassment is never easy. Regardless of the outcome, the investigation can be extremely stressful for all people involved. See Box 19.1 for the steps toward harassment response.

Rape

Rape is a crime of violence. It is second only to homicide in its violation of a person. The issue is not one of sex but rather one of force, domination, and humiliation. If you think rape is about sex, you have confused the weapon with the motivation. **Rape** refers to any forced sexual activity; the key factor is the absence of consent.

There is no typical rape victim. Of reported rapes, however, 93% of the victims are female and 90% of the perpetrators are male. One can be a victim of rape

Box 19.1

Steps Toward Harassment Prevention and Response

- Give verbal notice to the offender. Respond directly and simply, eg, " I don't like . . . and I want you not to do it again."

- Give stronger warnings and notice that you will report the behavior, eg, "If this happens again, I'm going to discuss this with human resources."

- Issue a written warning.

- Keep a detailed record of the behavior you find objectionable, when it occurred, and what you did in response.

- Make an informal harassment inquiry—discuss the situation with your supervisor or human resources person. The goal is not punishment but problem solving, education, and conscious-ness raising.

- File a formal complaint within the organization. At this point the harasser faces serious personal and professional damage. The situation cannot be kept completely confidential and the company or school is obliged to investigate.

- File with the EEOC in the United States: (800) 669-4000.

- In Canada, file with the Canadian Human Rights Commission: (613) 995-1151. It is highly advisable to have an attorney at this point.

- Go to court. This tends to be a long, painful battle. It may be settled before trial.

Sources: Rutter, 1996; Wyatt and Riederle, 1995.

Box 19.2

Minimizing the Risk of Date Rape

Be cautious in relationships based on dominant-male, submissive-female stereotypes. Date rapists usually have macho attitudes and believe women to be inferior.

Be cautious when a date tries to control your behav-ior—who you can meet, where you can go, what you can do. This indicates a need to dominate and con-trol and increases your vulnerability by isolating you.

Be very clear in your communication. If a simple *no* is not respected, leave or insist he leave. Speak forcefully.

Avoid giving mixed messages. For example: Do not say no and then continue petting.

Do not go to a place that is so private that help is not available.

---

at any age, from childhood through old age. Police records indicate that a woman is raped every 6 min-utes in the United States. Experts believe that 70% of rapes are unreported. It is believed that 1 out of every 3 women will be raped or sexually assaulted at least once in her lifetime; 40–60% of victims are raped by a spouse, partner, relative, or friend (Wiehe and Richards, 1995). Of all women raped on college cam-puses, 50% are date rapes. In surveys of college men, 10–15% admitted that they had committed date rape on at least one occasion, and another 22% admitted they had used verbal coercion and deception to pres-sure a date into having sex. Women very rarely report

rapes when they know their attackers, especially if they are or were in a dating relationship with the attacker. The victim is often blamed, by herself and others, for being naive or provocative. A cultural value, slow to die, is: If a woman accepts a date and allows the man to pay all the expenses, she somehow "owes" him sexual access and has no right to refuse (Wiehe and Richards, 1995). For ways to minimize the risk of date rape, see Box 19.2.

Traditionally, husbands have not been charged when they raped their wives. It was not until 1974 in the United States and 1991 in Great Britain that the first cases of marital rape were prosecuted. In 1993, marital rape became a crime in all 50 states. However, 33 states still have some exemptions from prosecuting husbands for rape. Marital rape is the most prevalent and underreported form of rape, with estimates of 2 million instances per year in the United States. Between one-third and one-half of bat-tered women are raped by their partners. The attacks range from assaults that are relatively quick to those that involve sadistic, torturous episodes that last for hours. In some instances, wives are forced to have sex with other people while their husbands watch (Bergen, 1996).

Some men who rape their wives see the rape as punishment for perceived wrongs. Others believe they have a right to sex on demand and that when sex is refused they have a right to take it. For other perpetrators, rape is a way to assert power and control. Some may even try to impregnate their wives to ensure that they will not leave the relationship. Others become angered over pregnancy and increase the level of violence in an attempt to abort the fetus (Bergen, 1996).

The myth of male rape has been that it occurs only where heterosexual contact is not possible, such as in prisons or in isolated living conditions. As more male rape victims report the crime, however, this myth is being exploded. It is estimated that 5–10% of all sexual assault victims are men. Male victims as a group are more likely to have been beaten and are more reluctant to reveal the sexual component of their assaults. Male rape is not a homosexual attack. Just as in female rape, the issue is one of violence and domination rather than one of sex. Some perpetrators are gay males who coerce partners or dates into sexual activity by use of threats or intimidation, as in date rape. Other perpetrators are heterosexual males who rape other males as a way of punishing and degrading them; this can occur among prison inmates or as part of gay bashing. Inmates who are sexually assaulted are often viewed by the public as deserving of their fate because of the crimes they have committed against society. Similarly, many people believe that gay men deserve to be raped as punishment for their "perverse" lifestyle (Stermac et al, 1996; Struckman-Johnson, 1996).

Childhood Sexual Abuse

Childhood sexual abuse is a major health problem in the United States. The majority of cases are probably unreported. Health care professionals, as well as families, have used denial to cope with ambiguous evidence of the cultural taboos of incest and sex with children. In order to respond appropriately to cues that signal sexual abuse, you must understand the characteristics and dynamics of the families involved. A note of caution must be added, however. With the recent increased publicity, there is a real danger of a witch-hunt developing; any hint or accusation of sexual abuse may be interpreted as absolute proof of guilt. Individuals and families have been destroyed by rumors and false accusations. You must assess carefully and maintain a balance between the extremes of denial and automatic belief of guilt.

Sexually abused children and adult survivors of childhood sexual abuse (hereafter referred to as adult survivors) are crying out for help. A few cry out loudly in protest, but the majority cry inwardly in silence. It is thought that as many as 1 in 3 girls and 1 in 7 boys are abused sexually before the age of 18. Boys are more frequently molested outside the family system than are girls. The period of abuse tends to begin and end at a younger age in boys (Evans and Sullivan, 1995; Fink et al, 1995).

Sexual abuse occurs in all ethnic, religious, economic, and cultural subgroups. Affinity systems—immediate family, relatives, friends, neighbors, clergy members, scout leaders—account for 75–80% of the abusers. Male perpetrators account for 92–98% of the reported cases; however, reports are now acknowledging more female perpetrators (Evans and Sullivan, 1995).

Sexual abuse is defined as inappropriate sexual behavior, instigated by an adult, whose purpose is to sexually arouse the adult or the child. Behavior ranges from exhibitionism, peeping, explicit sexual talk, touching, caressing, masturbation, oral sex, vaginal sex, and anal sex, to forcing children to engage in sex with one another or with animals.

Types of Offenders

Some offenders prefer girls, others prefer boys, and some abuse both, as long as the victim is a child. Some are interested in adolescents or preteens, some in toddlers, and some in infants. Some offenders do not abuse until they are adults, but more than half start in their teens.

Juvenile Offenders   Many, if not most, of these cases are unreported. Family members often want to protect and shield the young offender. At other times, the behavior is rationalized as adolescent male experimentation. Most juvenile offenders were sexually abused as children; they gradually develop offending behaviors as they reach adolescence. Juvenile offenders may seek victims within or outside the family system. The type of sexual offense often parallels their own experiences of abuse. The most frequent offense is sexual touching, which often escalates to rape and other sex crimes.

Male Offenders One research project that studied fathers who abused their daughters established five types of incestuous fathers. *Sexually preoccupied abusers* (26% of the fathers) have a conscious and often obsessive sexual interest in their daughters. Many of them regard their daughters as sex objects, in some cases as early as birth. *Adolescent regressors* (33% of the fathers) become sexually interested in their daughters when they begin puberty. These men sound and act like adolescents around their daughters. *Self-gratifiers* (20% of the fathers) are not sexually attracted to their daughters per se, and during the abuse, they fantasize about someone else. In effect, they are simply using their daughters' bodies. *Emotional dependents* (10% of the fathers) see themselves as failures and feel very lonely and depressed. They see their daughters as romantic figures in their lives. *Angry retaliators* (10% of the fathers) abuse out of anger, either at the daughter or at the mother. This type of offender is most likely to have a criminal history of assault and rape (Vanderbilt, 1992).

Female Offenders Female perpetrators have been largely overlooked but commit between 3% and 13% of sexual abuse cases. The most common types of sexual abuse by women are fondling, oral sex, and group sex.

Female sex offenders fall into four major types. *Teacher-lovers* are older women who teach children about lovemaking. *Experimenter-exploiters* are often girls who have had no sex education growing up. Baby-sitting is often an opportunity to explore younger children. Many of the girls in this group do not even realize what they are doing or that it is inappropriate. *Predisposers* usually come from a family with a long history of physical and sexual abuse. These families have been dysfunctional over many generations. *Women coerced by males* are those who abuse children because men have forced them to abuse. Usually they have been victims as children and are easily manipulated and intimidated (Kaufman et al, 1995).

Ritual Abuse **Ritual abuse** is emotional, physical, and sexual abuse that occurs in a ceremonial or systematic form by a specific group. Children are frequently victimized and forced to participate in the abuse of other children. Types of abuse include drugging; brainwashing; leaving victims in total darkness for extended periods of time; temporary burial in graves or coffins; rape; bestiality; force-feeding of urine, feces, or blood; animal mutilating and sacrifice; and human torture and sacrifice. Victims are programmed to remain silent, and the thought of breaking the silence is terrifying. They are often programmed to commit suicide if they ever speak about what was done to them (Shirar, 1996).

Knowledge Base: Rape

Rape is a violent act against an innocent person. It changes lives forever because once people become victims, they never again feel completely safe. The victim's response to this act of violence is referred to as **rape-trauma syndrome.** Some rape survivors do not develop major symptoms in response to the trauma, while as many as 25% continue to have signs of impairment a year after the assault. A variety of factors contribute to the response, including age or developmental state, a history of prior victimization, the relationship to the offender, precrisis coping abilities, and the ability to use support resources. Response factors related to the rape itself include the severity of the rape, the duration, the frequency, the number of offenders, and the degree of violence. Environmental factors contributing to a rape victim's response are the quality and continuity of social supports, and community attitudes and values (Wiehe and Richards, 1995).

Behavioral Characteristics

Many victims of rape do not report the crime. Sometimes this is due to guilt or embarrassment about what has occurred. Other victims are fearful of how their families or the police will react. Some perpetrators threaten victims by saying they will return to rape them again if the police are notified. Because many of the crimes are committed by acquaintances, friends, dates, or husbands, victims fear they will not be believed.

Some victims respond immediately with agitated and nonpurposeful behavior. They are brought to the emergency department emotionally distraught and unable to respond to questions about what has occurred. Their level of anxiety may be so high that they may not be able to follow simple directions. Some rape victims may shower or bathe before notifying the police or going to the hospital. This cleaning-up behavior is often an attempt to regain control of oneself and counteract the feelings of helplessness induced by the rape.

The majority of victims appear in good control of their feelings and behavior immediately after the rape. This appearance of outward calmness usually indicates a state of numbness, disbelief, and emotional shock. They may say such things as "This whole thing doesn't seem real," "I must be dreaming. This couldn't have happened," and "I just can't believe this has happened to me." You must recognize that underneath the calmness is acute distress. If you assume that the calmness implies no distress, you will overlook the person's need for emotional support and intervention.

There may be long-term behavioral characteristics of the rape-trauma syndrome. Some survivors are prone to crying spells that they may or may not be able to explain. Some may have difficulty establishing or maintaining personal relationships, especially with people who remind them of the perpetrator. Many develop problems at work or school. Some report nightmares and have difficulty sleeping. Others develop secondary phobic reactions to people, objects, or situations that remind them of the rape. A woman who is a survivor of marital rape suffers additional problems. Often, she must continue to interact with her rapist because she is dependent on him. She may be forced to pretend, to herself and to family members and friends, that the rape never occurred. Until it becomes more socially acceptable and legally feasible to report marital rape, many of these survivors will suffer in silence.

Affective Characteristics

Victims of rape suffer immediate and long-lasting emotional trauma. After a period of shock and disbelief, many experience episodes of fear. Fear can result from a stimulus directly associated with the attack, such as a penis, the act of oral sex, or a person who looks like the offender. There are also fears of rape consequences such as pregnancy; sexually transmitted infections, especially HIV; talking to the police; and testifying in court. In addition, there are fears related to potential future attacks, which underlie fears of getting close to men, of being alone, and of being in a strange place. Typically, the level of fear peaks around the third week, but it may take a long time for the

level to decrease. Depression frequently develops within a few weeks of the assault. This posttrauma depression usually lasts about 3 months, and it is not unusual for the survivor to experience suicidal ideation. For some, the depression will develop into a major depressive disorder requiring medical intervention (Wiehe and Richards, 1995).

Rape victims feel physically and emotionally violated, as well as unclean and contaminated. The loss of control over their bodies and their autonomy leads to feelings of helplessness and vulnerability. They may feel alienated from friends and family, particularly if there is not a strong supportive network. Anger is a healthy response to the violation that has occurred, but the energy of anger must be appropriately discharged so the person does not later become obsessed with fantasies of revenge.

Cognitive Characteristics

During the actual rape, some victims use the defense mechanism of depersonalization or dissociation to cope with the attack. By perceiving the attack as "not really happening to me," a victim protects her sense of integrity. Other victims rely on denial to block out the traumatic experience. The use of these defense mechanisms may continue through initial treatment and should be supported until the person is able to face the reality of the attack.

If victims are in a state of emotional shock, they will have great difficulty making decisions. Uncertain of how their significant others will react to the situation, they may hesitate telling family or friends. They need a great deal of support in using the problem-solving process to make decisions.

There may be a period during which victims blame themselves for the rape. This self-blame may be heard in such statements as "If only I had taken a different way home," "I should have been able to escape because he didn't have a gun," and "If I were a better wife, he wouldn't have raped me." Remember that the victim is *never* to blame for this violent crime.

Some survivors develop obsessional thoughts about the rape, which may be severe enough to interfere with daily functioning. Some experience flashbacks, some have violent dreams, and others may be preoccupied with thoughts of future danger. Rape profoundly affects a person's beliefs about the environment. If the assault occurred in the home, the normal feeling of safety within the home will most likely be destroyed. Belief in an inability to protect themselves in the future may lead to social withdrawal or phobic avoidance. Young female survivors, especially, may generalize their fear to the point that it applies to all men or all strange men. Women who have been raped by their husbands often state that their ability to trust the husband or any other man has been destroyed. Box 19.3 describes the phases of response to rape.

Social Characteristics

Families of rape survivors experience many of the same thoughts and emotions as the victims themselves. They may talk about guilt, doubts, fear, anger, hatred of the perpetrator, and feelings of helplessness. They need to be educated about the nature and trauma of rape and the immediate and potential long-term reactions of the survivors. They require direction in how to best support the survivor so that they neither overprotect nor minimize the impact of the rape.

Many cultural myths have surrounded the crime of rape for a long time. Some of these myths are the following:

- "Good girls" don't get raped.
- Women ask to be raped by the clothes they wear.
- The average healthy woman can escape a potential rapist if she really wants to.
- Women cry rape after they have consented to sex with a friend.
- Among males, only homosexuals get raped.
- Any man could resist rape if he really tried.

Changing the misconceptions of the general public has been a slow process. Many people continue to believe the myths that blame the victim rather than the perpetrator. Steps have been taken to abolish these myths from the legal system and to treat rape as the crime of violence it is. However, there is still much work to be done.

Culture-Specific Characteristics

Statistics reveal that the United States leads the Western countries in the number of rapes committed per capita. The United States has 41.2 rapes per 100,000 citizens per year. Contrast this with the following countries: Holland, 8.9; Germany, 8.2; France, 8;

Box 19.3

Phases of Response to Rape

Anticipatory Phase

Begins when the victim realizes the situation is potentially dangerous.

The victim may think about how to get away, may reason or argue with the offender, and recall advice people have given about rape.

Use of dissociation, suppression, or rationalization to preserve the illusion of invulnerability.

Possible physical action.

Impact Phase

The period of actual assault and immediate aftermath.

Intense fear of death or serious injury.

Expressive styles.

- Open expression of feelings—crying, sobbing, pacing.
- Controlled style—numbness, shock, disbelief.
- Compound reaction—reactivated symptoms of previous conditions, eg, psychotic behavior, depression, suicidal behavior, substance abuse.

Somatic reactions—tension headache, fatigue, increased startle reaction, nausea, gagging.

Reconstitution Phase

Outward appearance of adjustment with an attempt to restore equilibrium.

Life activities are renewed, but superficially and mechanically.

Periods of anxiety, fear, nightmares, depression, guilt, shame, vulnerability, helplessness, isolation, sexual dysfunctions.

Resolution Phase

Anger at the assailant, at society, and at the judicial system.

The need to talk to resolve feelings.

The survivor seeks family and professional support.

England, 6.7; Switzerland, 6.3, and Poland, 5.9 (U.S. Has Most Rapes, 1996). Attitudes toward rape vary across cultures. The following numbers of students agreed with the statement "a healthy woman can successfully resist a rapist if she really tries": United States, 20%; Germany, 7%; England, 8%; Turkey, 45%; India, 50%, and Malaysia, 56%. In addition, more than half of students in the United States, Canada, Barbados, Turkey, Malaysia, Zimbabwe, and Mexico believed that women, not men, are responsible for rape. People cling to stereotyped and prejudicial views of victims of sexual violence (Ward, 1995).

The consequences of rape in societies where young women's worth is equated with their virginity are especially disastrous. Their ruined reputation cannot be revised. In some countries women are forced to marry their rapist to erase the stigma of "spoiled goods." Others turn to prostitution to survive, and some commit suicide. Women victims are blamed rather than perpetrators punished. In some instances women may even be killed by male family members to cleanse the family (Desjarlais et al, 1995).

Throughout history, rape has been a part of war and civil strife. The right to rape women and children has been seen as the booty of war for the victors. Recent events in Mozambique, Bosnia, Somalia, South Africa, and El Salvador give evidence of many cases of systematic and repeated rape of civilian and refugee women. Data from the United Nations High Commission on Refugees indicate that 40% of Vietnamese boat women are abducted and/or raped while at sea. These statistics likely underestimate the problem, given women's reluctance to admit violation. Involuntary prostitution or female sexual slavery has a long history and recent attention has been drawn to this problem in the Philippines, Thailand, Nepal, Burma, and India (Desjarlais et al, 1995; Schuler, 1992). Sexual violence is influenced by traditional gender roles that force women to play a submissive role and allow men to construct attitudes viewing sexual behavior as a right tied to masculinity and power.

Physiological Characteristics

Rape usually results in a number of physical injuries. The victim may be beaten, stabbed, or shot. Profuse bleeding and trauma to vital organs may be critical problems. Most likely, the vagina or rectum will be sore or swollen. There may be tearing of the vaginal or rectal wall from forceful insertion of the penis or a foreign object. The throat may be traumatized from forced oral sex.

Female victims of childbearing age may become pregnant as a result of the rape. Victims of all ages and both sexes may contract a sexually transmitted infection from the perpetrator, via any mucous membrane area such as the vagina, rectum, mouth, or throat.

Sexual dysfunction is one of the longest-lasting effects of rape. Nearly all adult rape survivors feel the need to withdraw from sexual activity for a period of time. For some, a period of celibacy is necessary to re-establish control and autonomy. Others may choose abstinence because they feel unclean or contaminated. Both the survivor and the sex partner must understand that the need for closeness and nondemanding physical contact continues. Expressing caring and affection through nonsexual touching minimizes the partner's feelings of rejection and reduces the survivor's feelings of self-blame and uncleanliness.

Causative Theories

Theorists in many disciplines have studied the crime of rape in an effort to understand the causes and develop preventive measures. Most agree that rape is a crime of violence generated by issues of power and anger rather than by sex drive.

Intrapersonal Theory

The intrapersonal perspective views rapists as emotionally immature individuals who feel powerless and unsure of themselves. They are incapable of managing the normal stresses of everyday life. The causes of rape are many, but the dynamics of the act are that perpetrators abuse their own and others' sexuality as a method of discharging anger and frustration. From this perspective, there are five types of rape: anger rape, power rape, sadistic rape, gang rape, and date/acquaintance rape.

An **anger rape** is distinguished by physical violence and cruelty to the victim. Believing that he is the victim of an unjust society, the rapist takes revenge on others by raping. He uses extreme force and viciousness to debase the victim. The ability to injure, traumatize, and shame the victim provides an outlet for his rage and temporary relief from his turmoil. Rapes occur episodically as the rage builds up and he strikes out at others to relieve his pain.

In a **power rape,** the intent of the rapist is not to injure someone but to command and master another person sexually. The rapist has an insecure self-image, with feelings of incompetency and inadequacy. The rape becomes the vehicle for expressing power and strength. Seeing his victim as a conquest, the rapist temporarily feels omnipotent.

A **sadistic rape** involves brutality, bondage, and torture as stimulants for the rapist's own sexual excitement. For the rapist, the assault is an erotic experience. He plans very carefully, and the process of rape may be ritualized. The victims are often murdered after being raped.

A **gang rape** involves a number of perpetrators and may be part of a group ritual that confirms masculinity, power, and authority. The perpetrators may range in age from 10 to 30, but they are most typically adolescents. Victims are usually the same age as the gang members (Holmes, 1991).

A **date rape,** or **acquaintance rape,** is forced sexual activity by a perpetrator who is known to the victim. Typically, there is less physical violence and more coercion and deception involved. Even during the high school years, it is estimated that 30% of female students are sexually or physically abused in their dating relationships (Holmes, 1991).

Not all rapists are alike. Their motives and expectations vary. The majority of convicted sex offenders do not suffer from major mental disorders. Many do meet the criteria for sociopathic, schizoid, paranoid, and narcissistic personality disorders. Rapists are typically young; 80% are under the age of 30, and 75% are under age 25. The majority report having been sexually and physically abused as children or adolescents (Holmes, 1991).

Interpersonal Theory

Most rapists do not have normal interpersonal involvements. Preoccupied with their own fantasies, they want to control and dominate others rather than engage in mutually satisfying relationships. With this model in mind, a rapist sees no need for consent to sexual activity, particularly from his wife. The husband may view the rape as merely a disagreement over sexual behavior. If the wife has said she does not want to engage in sex and the husband uses force, her control and autonomy have been violated. When sex occurs without consent, it is, in fact, rape (Holmes, 1991).

Social Learning Theory

The acceptance of interpersonal violence in a culture contributes to a higher incidence of rape. Society's approval of the use of intimidation, coercion, and force to achieve a goal promotes an excessive level of violence. Violent behavior is an expression of power and strength, and individual rights are disregarded.

Aggression is learned through three primary sources: family and peers, culture/subculture, and the mass media. The modeling effect occurs when potential offenders see rape scenes and other acts of violence against women in real life or in the media, in slasher and horror films, and in violent pornography. The media contribute to the process of desensitization; with repeated exposure, viewers become numb to the pain, fear, and humiliation of sexual aggression (Weisz and Earls, 1995).

Feminist Theory

From the feminist perspective, rape is the result of long and deeply rooted socioeconomic traditions. Men dominate most political and economic activities, and women are viewed as subservient and relatively powerless. At the furthest extreme, women are viewed as property. Sexual gratification is not the prime motive in rape; rather, sex is used to establish or maintain control of one person by another. When women are considered inferior to men, tacit approval is given for coercion and force. These stereotypes support the false beliefs that at times women deserve to be raped, that they may want or need to be raped, and that rape does not cause them much physical or emotional damage.

Sexist values affect people of all ages, both female and male. When 1700 middle school children were asked questions about rape, 65% of the boys and 57% of the girls replied that it was acceptable for a man to force a woman to have sex if they have been dating more than 6 months. College students responded in the following ways to the question of when forced sex is acceptable: It is acceptable if the woman agrees and then changes her mind, 13%; while dating exclusively, 24%; if the woman allows him to touch her genitals, 24%; if she touches his genitals, 29%; and if both partners willingly have their clothes off, 35% (Wiehe and Richards, 1995).

The Nursing Process

Assessment

Rape victims must be assessed physiologically from head to toe for any serious or critical injuries that may have resulted from the assault. With the victim's permission, a vaginal or rectal examination is performed to determine necessary treatment and to provide evidence for legal action. With permission, photographs of the injuries may be taken for legal documentation. The physiological assessment process must be carefully documented in writing to assist with possible prosecution of the perpetrator.

Victims who respond to rape in a controlled manner may be able to answer assessment questions, but those in a state of emotional shock and disbelief may find it difficult to engage actively in the assessment process. The method by which you complete the assessment depends on the person's response to the trauma.

Before the assessment process, clients must be informed of their rights, which include the following:

- A rape crisis advocate present in the emergency department.
- Their personal physician notified.
- Privacy during the assessment and treatment process.
- Family, friends, or an advocate present during the questioning and examination.
- Confidentiality maintained by all members of the staff.
- Gentle and sensitive treatment.
- Detailed explanations of, and giving consent for, all tests and procedures, including photographs.
- Referrals for follow-up treatment and counseling.

As a nurse, you must respect the victim's autonomy in order to prevent revictimization. Give the client as much control as possible through every step of the assessment and treatment process. See the Focused Nursing Assessment table for guidance in the assessment process of people who have been raped.

Diagnosis

The assessment process provides the data from which you develop your nursing diagnoses. Physical and mental status priorities must be quickly established by the health care team. Attention must then be given to the long-range physical, emotional, social, and legal concerns of the survivor.

The nursing diagnosis for clients who have been raped is **Rape-trauma syndrome.** If clients suffer from reactivated symptoms of a previous physical illness or mental disorder, or if they rely on alcohol or drugs to manage their trauma, they are given the more specific nursing diagnosis of **Rape-trauma syndrome: compound reaction.** The nursing diagnosis of **Rape-trauma syndrome: silent reaction** is applied when the client experiences high levels of anxiety, an inability to discuss the trauma, abrupt changes in relationships with men and/or changes in sexual behavior, and the onset of phobic reactions.

Outcome Identification

Once you have established diagnoses, you and the client mutually identify goals for change. Client outcomes are specific behavioral measures by which you, clients, and significant others determine progress toward goals. The following are examples of some of the outcomes appropriate to victims of rape:

- identifies immediate concerns
- utilizes the problem-solving process to make own decisions
- utilizes community resources

Nursing Interventions

The accompanying box lists the nursing interventions classification (NIC) for victims of rape.

Safety: Crisis Management

Rape-Trauma Treatment

It is important to support *defense mechanisms* until clients are able to cope with the reality of the assault. Give them ample time to respond to simple questions;

Nursing Interventions Classification

VICTIMS OF RAPE

DOMAIN: Safety

Class: *Crisis Management*

> **Interventions:** *Rape-Trauma Treatment:* Provision of emotional and physical support immediately following an alleged rape.

DOMAIN: Behavioral

Class: *Coping Assistance*

> **Interventions:** *Support Group:* Use of a group environment to provide emotional support and health-related information for members.

Source: McCloskey and Bulechek, 1996.

anxiety will decrease their ability to perceive input, thereby slowing down their response time. If clients are unable to express feelings, acknowledge the difficulty by saying, "I understand that it's difficult for you to describe your feelings right now. That's okay. You may be able to talk about them later." Communicate your knowledge and understanding of the usual emotional responses to rape. Statements such as "People usually experience a number of feelings, like anxiety, fear, embarrassment, guilt, and anger" will reassure clients that their feelings are a normal reaction to rape.

Encourage the client to *talk about the rape*. Many clients will have a compulsive need to recount the assault. The emotional arousal of the trauma contributes to this intense pressure to talk. Listen patiently and supportively, understanding that compulsive retelling is a natural way by which the victim is gradually desensitized to the trauma.

Identify specific *coping behaviors* clients used during the rape such as screaming, fighting, talking, blacking out, and/or remaining passive. Initially, clients may experience distortions related to self-blame or guilt. Recognizing that their behavior was an adaptive mechanism for survival will raise their self-esteem and decrease their feelings of guilt. Repeatedly tell clients it was not their fault. It is critical to *stress that survival is the most important outcome*. Reassure them that their responses were all that was possible under the degree of fear that rape induces. A helpful statement might be, "I know you handled the situation right because you are alive."

The next step is to help the clients *identify immediate concerns* and prioritize them. Focusing on immediate problems lessens the client's confusion and feelings of being overwhelmed. Next, help the client use the *problem-solving process*. Clients need to be empowered to make their own decisions and act on their own behalf. Restoring personal choice is a primary antidote to rape trauma. Informed choices help clients regain control and autonomy, both of which were violated during the rape.

Rape is both a personal and a family crisis. Clients may need help in *identifying who to tell* about the rape. Victims often fear how family and friends will respond to the situation. Anticipatory guidance on your part will help them take advantage of available support systems. When significant others are involved, prepare them before they join the victim because they may not know how to best support their loved one.

Discuss beliefs about postcoital contraception and abortion if appropriate. Pregnancy may result from the rape, and clients must have information about available options. The most common medical intervention is a course of hormonal treatment. Elevated doses of oral contraceptive or DES (diethylstilbestrol) may be administered if the woman chooses to prevent conception (Krueger, 1988). Clients should be informed about the need for follow-up medical evaluation and treatment for sexually transmitted infections, including a test for HIV.

A *written list of referrals* of community resources should be provided before clients are discharged from the emergency department. Crisis intervention

Text continues on page 462

Focused Nursing Assessment

CLIENTS WHO HAVE BEEN RAPED

Behavior Assessment	*Affective Assessment*	*Cognitive Assessment*
Nursing observations: Is the client able to respond verbally to questions? Is the client able to follow simple directions?	Could you explain ways in which you are experiencing any of the following emotions?	Nursing observations: Is there any evidence of the use of defense mechanisms? Describe the client's attention span.
Have you bathed, douched, changed clothes, or done any self-treatment before coming to the hospital?	Disbelief	Can you tell me where you are? What is today's date?
	Shame	Can you describe what occurred?
	Embarrassment	Have you been informed of your rights?
	Humiliation	Who have you informed about the rape? Family? Friends? Police?
	Helplessness	Do you need help in telling others about the rape?
	Vulnerability	In what way, if any, do you feel responsible for the attack?
	Anxiety	
	Fear	
	Guilt	
	Anger	
	Depression	

Social Assessment	Physiological Assessment
Who do you think are your most available support systems? Family? Friends? Clergy? Rape advocate?	Have physical injuries such as scratches, bruises, and cuts been recorded and photographed?
Are you in need of temporary shelter?	Have fingernail scrapings been taken and preserved?
May I provide you with information about available counseling?	Has blood typing been done?
	Have smears been taken of the mouth, throat, vagina, and rectum for detection of sexually transmitted infections?
	Have combings been made of the pubic hair and preserved?
	Has genital trauma been recorded and photographed?
	Has rectal trauma been recorded and photographed?
	Have semen specimens been preserved?
	If applicable, when was the client's last menstrual period?
	Has the clothing been inspected and preserved?

*All questions in this column are nursing observations; they are not asked of the client.

counseling can help minimize the long-term emotional impact of rape. See the Self-Help Groups section at the end of this chapter for a list of national resources that can provide local referrals.

Behavioral: Coping Assistance

Support Group

Support groups provide an opportunity for victims to meet with other survivors of rape in a safe, supportive, and egalitarian setting. In this therapeutic environment, clients have their feelings validated as normal reactions to the assault and receive confirmation of their survival behaviors. Support groups may help moderate depression by providing an opportunity to speak openly and network with other survivors and supportive people. Individuals may be able to redirect the energy that is often spent on anger and pain into compassionate acts of supporting others. The long-term goal of support groups is to help survivors understand their distress and take charge of their own recovery. Recovery is accomplished by counteracting self-blame, sharing grief, and affirming self and life.

Evaluation

The long-term goal of intervention is to help rape victims return to their precrisis level, or achieve a higher level, of functioning. The following outcome behaviors demonstrate that the crisis has been resolved in an adaptive fashion:

- Control over remembering—can elect to recall or not recall the rape; decreased flashbacks and nightmares.
- Affect tolerance—feelings can be felt, named, and endured without overwhelming arousal or numbing.
- Symptom mastery—anxiety, fear, depression, and sexual problems have decreased and are more tolerable.
- Reconnection—increased ability to trust and attach to others.
- Meaning—has discovered some tolerable meaning to the trauma and to self as a trauma survivor; feels empowered.

As a nurse, you must challenge cultural values and beliefs that promote and condone sexual violence. Myths that support rape in any way must be confronted, and a new understanding of rape and rape victims must be developed. Changing the stereotypes of gender roles and the inequality of power inherent in heterosexual relationships can decrease the prevalence of sexual violence. It is only through this process that long-term changes will occur.

Knowledge Base: Childhood Sexual Abuse

Childhood sexual abuse is a process, not just an event. Sexual abuse affects almost every aspect of the life of the victims. The effects of sex abuse are most severe when the incidents are frequent and occur over a long period of time, the activities are wide-ranging and extensive, there is more than one perpetrator, the relationship to the perpetrator is close, and when sex abuse is combined with physical and emotional abuse. There are behavioral, cognitive, and physical problems, as well as difficulties with emotional stability and interpersonal relationships during childhood, adolescence, and adulthood (Evans and Sullivan, 1995).

Abuse disrupts the smooth progression of development in several ways. For some there is an intensification and fixation of the current developmental stage. Others regress to an earlier stage. And some prematurely accelerate and develop a pseudo-maturity. The earlier the abuse, the more profound the damage (Evans and Sullivan, 1995).

Behavioral Characteristics

Typically, adult perpetrators believe in extreme restrictiveness and domination. There is a characteristic enforcement of petty rules with intermittent rewards. Often the adult coerces the child and misrepresents the abuse as a game or "fun" activity. The behavior usually follows a progression of sexual activity, from exposure and fondling to oral, vaginal, and/or anal sex. Secrecy is imposed on the child by persuasion or threat. The abuser may say such things as "If you tell, you'll be sent away," "If you tell, I won't love you anymore," "If you tell, I will kill you," and "If you tell, I'll do the same thing to your baby brother." Children know adults have absolute power over them, so they obey. When they have been threatened with abandonment or harm, they frequently choose to protect others. When asked, "Why didn't you tell sooner?" the answers are, "I didn't know who to tell," "I was scared," or "I did tell and no one believed me."

Some children who have been sexually abused form a clinging attachment to one or both parents. Some become extremely affectionate both inside and outside the family system, while others have problems with impulse control and aggression toward others. Some children isolate themselves at school or in the neighborhood and limit most of their interactions to family members. They may act out sexually, by initiating oral or genital sex with other children or adults, for example. In addition, sexually abused children often engage in self-destructive behaviors such as head-banging, self-mutilation, and suicide (Glod, 1993).

Adolescent victims may run away from home to escape an intolerable situation. Because they have learned, at home, that sexual behavior is rewarded by affection, love, and attention, some turn to prostitution. Others are forced into prostitution as a way to support themselves while living on the streets.

Some adult survivors engage in self-mutilation, as in cutting, slashing, or burning themselves. It is important to understand the meaning of such behavior. For some, the pain of self-mutilation proves their existence and reassures them that they are alive and real. Self-mutilation may be a plea for nurturance, as they come to the emergency department seeking care. Others nurture them by cleaning up the wounds after self-mutilating. For those who dissociate, self-mutilation may be a way to stop the dissociation with physical pain. Others self-mutilate as a form of self-punishment and a way to decrease feelings of guilt. And finally, some self-mutilate as a way to reduce emotional pain through the feeling of physical pain. It is important to understand the function of the behavior in order to replace it with healthier behaviors that satisfy the same need. See Chapter 6 for further information on self-mutilation.

There are a number of possible sexual effects for adult survivors. Some have a very strong aversion to sex and are filled with terror in sexual situations. Some are sexually inhibited and experience discomfort with sexual thoughts, feelings, and behaviors. Some engage in compulsive sexual behavior, perhaps as an unconscious way to validate their shame and guilt or a way to feel powerful. Many adult survivors go through a period of celibacy as they try to manage fear, anger, and distrust.

Affective Characteristics

Behind a facade of dominance, perpetrators often feel weak, afraid, and inadequate. They inappropriately view the child as a safe and less-threatening source of caring than an adult. They are unable to distinguish between nonsexual and sexual affection for children. Lack of empathy for the victim is typical of perpetrators.

Child victims experience many fears. They fear if they tell another adult, they will not be believed, and they fear that they themselves will be blamed. If the abuse is occurring within the family, they may have fantasies of being rejected by family members. They may fear the family will be separated, especially if this threat was made by the abuser.

Children often feel responsible for the adult's behavior and ashamed that they have not been able to stop the abuse. Secrecy and guilt keep these children isolated, causing them to feel alienated from their peers. The feeling of powerlessness is extremely prevalent because what the victim says and does makes no difference. The associated rage typically does not emerge until adolescence. When the suppressed rage comes to the surface, it may be directed against the self in self-defeating and self-destructive ways.

Many adult survivors continue to believe that they were to blame for the abuse and should have been able to resist the adult. This self-blame often contributes to depression and anxiety and to panic attacks. Distrusting and fearing men, many have multiple fears relating to sexual interactions. For some, anger is the only emotion experienced and expressed, all other feelings being severely repressed. Many adult survivors continue to hate their perpetrators, as well as nonabusing significant adults for not protecting them (Posttraumatic stress disorder, 1996).

Cognitive Characteristics

Cognitive distortions are self-statements perpetrators use to deny, minimize, justify, and rationalize their behavior. In addition, they have an impaired capacity for empathy or bonding with children. They view their victims as objects and they focus primarily on their own pleasure and satisfaction (Hayashino, Wurtele, and Klebe, 1995).

Secrecy and silence are used by perpetrators to escape accountability. When secrecy fails and the child victims or adult survivors begin to talk to others about the abuse, perpetrators usually attack the credibility of the victims and try to make sure no one will listen. Perpetrators make such statements as "It never happened, she's lying," "He's exaggerating some innocent touching," and "Even if it did happen, it's time to forget the past and move on." Other perpetrators acknowledge the abuse but minimize the impact with statements such as "Better for her to learn about sex from her father than from some horny teenager" and "She didn't really mind; in fact, we have a very close relationship." Others use the defense mechanism of projection and blame the child for the abuse, as evidenced by such statements as "She's a very provocative child, and she seduced me" and "If he hadn't enjoyed it so much, I wouldn't have continued."

Some child victims use denial to cope with the trauma. Acknowledging the abuse would mean acknowledging that the world is dangerous and that those who are supposed to protect and nurture failed and caused harm. Other victims minimize the impact and say it was not important, saying things like "It's not so bad; it only happens once a month" and "It's all right because it stopped when I was 11 years old."

Frequently, dissociation is the victim's major defense. The mind is "separated" from the body so the victim is not emotionally present during the sexual attack. Dissociation is evidenced by such statements as "I put myself in the wall, where he couldn't reach all of me" and "When he would come into my room, I would close my eyes and go to my favorite place. Only my body stayed on the bed; the rest of me wasn't there." When sexual abuse is severe and sadistic, the victim may develop dissociative identity disorder (DID) (Shirar, 1996). See Chapter 9 for a discussion of DID, formerly MPD. It is not unusual for adult survivors to have total amnesia for the childhood sexual abuse. In such a case, amnesia is considered a defense mechanism in response to the trauma and is more likely to occur when the abuse began at a very young age. Recall of the abuse may be triggered by a significant life event such as marriage or pregnancy, or during the process of psychotherapy.

Self-blame contributes to low self-esteem in adult survivors. They feel worthless and different from other people. They may believe they are only sex objects to be used and abused by others. They may suffer from flashbacks and nightmares.

Confusion about sexuality is very common among male survivors. Sexual victimization of a male carries a hidden implication of being less than a man. Heterosexual survivors fear that the abuse has made, or will make, them homosexual. Intense homophobia and/or hypermasculine behavior may be an effort to disprove their fears. Gay survivors worry that their sexual preference may have caused the abuse. It must be remembered that childhood sexual abuse is *not* related to adult sexual identity.

Social Characteristics

Male survivors are affected by different social values than women. Men are expected to be powerful, active, and competent. They often equate being abused with being weak, female, or gay. Society believes that men are always sexually willing and eager and therefore sex cannot be abusive. The general thought is that he must have sought it or at least welcomed the sexual activity (Draucker and Petrovic, 1996).

Many adult survivors have difficulties with relationships. Superficial relationships are usually much easier than intimate relationships. As children, these adults learned that those who love you are the ones who hurt you, and that living in a family is not safe. As adults, they may be incapable of trusting others and feel trapped by intimate relationships. Adult survivors also struggle with control issues. Anyone who has been raised in an environment that was out of control or dangerous grows up with a strong need to control the environment as much as possible. Such a need for control can contribute to conflict in relationships.

There is a significant connection between being sexually abused as a child and being revictimized as an adult. This in no way implies, however, that an adult survivor is responsible for being abused, as there is never a legitimate excuse for emotional or physical violence. Adults who were sexually abused as children become victims again in adulthood for many reasons. One thing a person learns from sexual abuse is how to be abused. In order to survive, children teach themselves to endure assaults. They learn they cannot protect themselves. They learn to keep the abuse a secret and to "forgive and forget" each violent incident. All of these survival techniques make them vulnerable to abuse in adulthood (Mendel, 1995).

Culture-Specific Characteristics

The aspects of culture relating to child sexual abuse include family structures, moral and religious principles, and child-rearing practices. Other aspects include the relative value of interdependence, treatment of sexuality, gender roles, and interpersonal boundaries. The ways in which the communities view violence and sexual assault, and the action that is taken when these occur, reflect cultural values. It is only when we understand cultural diversity that we are able to develop effective prevention programs.

There is no such thing as a generic African American, Asian American, Hispanic American, or member of any other minority group. There are differences not only between groups but among members of the same group. These differences are based on gender, socioeconomic status, and level of acculturation to European American norms. The cultural solidifying factor is the experience of racism perpetrated by the majority culture. Box 19.4 gives some culture-specific information on child sexual abuse.

Physiological Characteristics

The obvious physical signs of sexual abuse in a child are the presence of a sexually transmitted infection, irritated or swollen genitals or rectal tissue, or both. Chronic vaginal or urinary tract infections with no known medical cause may be indicators that the child is being sexually abused. Among female victims, 12–24% become pregnant as a result of the abuse (Evans and Sullivan, 1995).

Some children will, consciously or unconsciously, attempt to abuse their bodies to either prevent or stop the sexual abuse. The child may gain a great deal of weight, hoping to become so unattractive that the abuser will leave the child alone. If an older child is being abused, a younger sister may become anorexic in an attempt not to mature and experience the same abuse. This lack of care for the body may continue into adult life in an unconscious attempt to maintain distance and avoid intimate relationships (Vanderbilt, 1992).

Concomitant Disorders

Having suffered sexual abuse in childhood is often a hidden feature of adult mental disorders. As many as 60–70% of psychiatric clients have a history of abuse. Repeated trauma in childhood distorts the personality. Since child victims cannot protect themselves, they must adapt to the trauma as well as they can. Behaviors that were originally adaptive become symptoms in adulthood. These people have a bewildering combination of symptoms, including anger, depression, anxiety, insomnia, suspicion, eating disorders, substance abuse, and self-mutilation. Adult survivors often collect many different diagnoses before the underlying problem of PTSD is correctly identified (Stein et al, 1996). See Table 19.1 for an overview of cues to sexual abuse.

Causative Theories

There is no single cause of childhood sexual abuse. Rather, the abuse results from a combination of personality, family, and cultural factors.

Intrapersonal Theory

There are many types of perpetrators of childhood sexual abuse. Some traits are contradictory, and there is no agreement on a composite personality. Certain characteristics apply to many people, not just abusers. The descriptions are guidelines for assessment, not proof that the person actually committed sexual abuse.

Perpetrators usually have low self-esteem and feel more secure in interactions with children than with adults. Some were emotionally deprived as children and thus have a great need for constant, unconditional love, which is more easily obtained from children than from adults. Some perpetrators are described as lacking impulse control and the ability to experience feelings of guilt. Others are described as rigid and overcontrolled, while others are dominant and aggressive.

If perpetrators were themselves sexually abused as children, they may have learned to associate all feelings of love with sexual behavior. Most people who were sexually abused as children do *not* go on to sexually abuse others. However, some victimized children develop offending behavior in late childhood, adolescence, or adulthood. Most likely, there are a number of factors involved in why some abuse and

Box 19.4

Culture-Specific Characteristics of Sexual Abuse

European Americans

- The keeping of family secrets is a traditional value.
- Sex is a taboo subject.
- Many believe that satisfying one's own needs at the expense of others is a moral right.
- Sexual domination may be a manifestation of power.

African Americans

- Prevalence appears to be the same as for European Americans.
- More likely to be abused by an acquaintance or stranger.
- Many have had negative encounters with the criminal justice system and/or social service agencies, which impedes reporting of child sexual abuse.
- May be reluctant to identify an African American perpetrator and turn him over to a system that administers harsher legal consequences to African Americans for criminal behavior.

Puerto Ricans

- The reaction to sexual abuse is often geared toward maintaining the family's homeostasis; family loyalty is very important.
- If the daughter is a victim, the mother is perceived as being responsible.
- The popular beliefs are that sexually abused males become homosexuals and sexually abused females are considered promiscuous.

Mexican Americans

- There is a tendency for perpetrators to be more closely related to the victim.
- Both boys and girls are more likely than African American children to report rectal penetration.
- Boys are less likely to report abuse than girls.

Asian, Pacific Island, and Filipino Americans

- Sexuality seldom discussed openly.
- Family structure is authoritarian and children are expected to be obedient to all authority figures.
- When child discloses, the family often directs its anger at the child and intervening adults; family will deny the abuse to save the family's reputation.
- Children may recant stories of sexual abuse, thus sacrificing their individual needs for family integrity.

American Jews

- Often have traditional gender roles.
- Believe that family togetherness provides a safe haven from inevitable persecution.
- Sexual abuse is seen as "the way of the gentiles," which burdens victims who anguish about revealing the family secret.

Sources; Abney and Priest, 1995; Comas-Diaz, 1995; Featherman, 1995; Huston et al, 1995; Okamura, Heras, and Wong-Kerberg, 1995; Schmidt, 1995.

others do not. The world of abuse is comprised only of victims (powerless) and perpetrators (powerful). Victims become perpetrators in an unconscious attempt to master the trauma of their own experiences and take over the power. The move from victim to offender may also result when anger and hostility are externalized and projected onto new victims (Shirar, 1996).

Family Systems Theory

Family systems theory considers structure, cohesion, adaptability, and communication patterns of families in which children are being sexually abused.

Family structure is usually hierarchical according to age, roles, and distribution of power. Typically, the adults, who are older, assume the parental roles and are the most influential. The structure of incestuous families, however, is often quite different. An adult

Table 19.1 Cues to Sexual Abuse

	Perpetrator	Child/Adolescent	Adult Survivor
Behavioral cues	Dominating, coercive, inappropriate affection, poor impulse control.	Extremely affectionate, sexual acting-out, isolative, self-destructive, running away, prostitution, suicide.	Sexual dysfunction, compulsive sexual behavior, self-mutilation, substance abuse.
Affective cues	Feelings of weakness, inadequacy; inability to distinguish between nonsexual and sexual affection; lack of empathy.	Multiple fears, guilt, powerlessness, rage.	Anxiety, panic attacks, rage, distrust, fear of men.
Cognitive cues	Denial, minimization of impact, projection.	Denial, minimization of impact, dissociation.	Amnesia for events, self-blame, worthlessness, flashbacks/nightmares, confusion about sexual orientation.
Mental disorders	Impulse control disorders.	Dissociative disorders, including DID; anxiety disorders; mood disorders.	Dissociative disorders, including DID; anxiety disorders; mood disorders; substance abuse; personality disorders; PTSD.

may move "down" in the structure or a child may move "up" in terms of roles and influence. If the father moves downward, he assumes a childlike role and is cared for and nurtured like a child in the family. In this position, the father assumes little parental responsibility. He may then turn to the daughter, as a "peer," for sexual and emotional gratification. As another example, the daughter may move upward and replace the mother in the hierarchy. The mother does not usually move downward but rather moves out of the structure by distancing herself emotionally or physically from the family. As the daughter assumes the parental role and responsibilities, the father may turn to her for fulfilling his emotional and sexual needs (Mendel, 1995).

Family cohesion refers to the degree of emotional bonding that occurs within a family. At one end of the cohesion continuum is the family system that is disengaged; that is, the family members are isolated and alienated from one another. At the other end of the continuum is the enmeshed family system, in which the members are immersed in and absorbed by one another. The healthiest family systems function between these two extremes. Sexual abuse in families usually occurs in an enmeshed family. The need to be overinvolved in each other's lives is accompanied by intense fears of abandonment. See also Chapter 2.

Family system adaptability is also described along a continuum. At one extreme is the rigid family system and at the other end, the chaotic family system. Families involved in sexual abuse tend to function at either end of the continuum. Rigid family systems have strict rules and stereotyped gender-role expectations, with minimal emotional interaction. Children have no power and authority, even over their own bodies. They are not allowed to question or protest inappropriate sexual behavior. In contrast, chaotic family systems have either no rules or constantly changing rules. Within the chaotic system, there may be no assigned roles or no rules regarding appropriate sexual behavior, which may contribute to the incidence of sexual abuse. See also Chapter 2.

Communication patterns within the family system may contribute to the occurrence of sexual abuse. Incest depends on keeping the secret within the family. In family systems that avoid conflict, accusations of sexual abuse are not tolerated. Peace must be kept at all costs.

The Nursing Process

Assessment

It is vitally important that you acknowledge the reality of childhood sexual abuse. Nurses who deny the existence of the problem will miss the cues and fail to complete a detailed assessment. If you are knowledgeable about the incidence and the characteristics of the problem, you will be alert for cues that demand nursing assessment. See the Focused Nursing Assessment table for the types of questions to ask of both child victims and adult survivors.

When assessing children, remember that some will exhibit most of the characteristics presented in this chapter, others will exhibit only some, and still others will exhibit none of the characteristics. Also remember that these same behavioral, affective, and cognitive characteristics may be symptoms of other emotional problems in children. Once it has been discovered that one child in a family is a victim of sexual abuse, suspect the abuse of siblings, both boys and girls, as well. Sometimes entire families are sexually abused before someone "tells."

You must appreciate the power of secrecy and how difficult it is for adult survivors to disclose such information, especially for men, who, in our society, are expected to be anything other than victimized. Routine questions on nursing histories may provide an opportunity for survivors to share their pain and obtain treatment as adults. As a nurse, you are responsible for initiating the topic, as shame and confusion may keep the adult survivor from doing so. If you avoid the topic, you will be contributing to pathology by supporting the client's denial of reality. Failure to initiate a discussion of sexual abuse sends a message to clients that such abuse does not occur or does not matter. Now that childhood sexual abuse has been identified as a major health problem, nurses in every clinical setting must be alert for cues from both individuals and families. When working with adult survivors, you must continuously assess the client's comfort level with the physical setting. Closed doors will increase anxiety in some clients, while others will request that doors never remain open. Some will be uncomfortable in a room with a couch or a bed rather than chairs. How close you sit can be an issue for some clients. Even normally appropriate physical contact, such as a handshake, may increase anxiety. Always ask permission before touching a client.

Diagnosis

Based on assessment data, nursing diagnoses are formulated for the individual child victim, the family members, and/or the adult survivor. Possible diagnoses for the child victim include:

- *Ineffective individual coping* related to being a victim of sexual abuse
- *Powerlessness* related to being a victim of sexual abuse
- *Post-trauma response* related to being a victim of sexual abuse
- *Social isolation* related to keeping the family secret of sexual abuse

For families that are experiencing sexual abuse, some possible diagnoses are:

- *Ineffective family coping, disabling,* related to a child being sexually abused
- *Ineffective family coping, disabling,* related to an enmeshed family system that is either rigid or chaotic
- *Altered parenting* related to being a perpetrator of sexual abuse
- *Altered family process* related to disruption of the family unit when abuse is discovered

For adult survivors of childhood sexual abuse, some possible diagnoses are:

- *Post-trauma response* related to being an adult survivor
- *Spiritual distress* related to asking questions about fairness and justice in life or not being protected by a supreme being
- *Chronic low self-esteem* related to self-blame for the abuse
- *Ineffective denial* related to amnesia for childhood events
- *Social isolation* related to difficulty in forming intimate relationships, mistrust of others

- *Sexual dysfunction* related to the trauma of abuse
- *High risk for injury* related to being revictimized as an adult

Outcome Identification

Once you have established diagnoses, you, the client, and the family mutually identify goals for change. Client outcomes are specific behavioral measures by which you, clients, and significant others determine progress toward goals. The following are examples of some of the outcomes appropriate to people who have experienced childhood sexual abuse:

- remains safe and free from harm
- utilizes a variety of therapies to express feelings about the sexual abuse
- verbalizes improved self-esteem
- manages negative emotions in an appropriate manner
- verbalizes a feeling of connectedness to significant others
- utilizes community resources

Nursing Interventions

The box on page 472 lists the nursing interventions classification (NIC) for victims of childhood sexual abuse.

Safety: Risk Management

Abuse Protection: Child

The first priority of care with child victims is to *ensure the safety of the child*. Nurses are mandated by law to report any suspected child sexual abuse. Protective services will implement one of four plans if the abuse is occurring within the family system. (1) The most frequent option is one in which the abuser is removed from the family. The nonabusing parent must be able to protect the child from any contact with the abuser. (2) When the nonabusing parent is unable to protect the child, both the child and the abuser are removed from the home. This option maximizes the safety of the child and decreases the child's

feelings of responsibility. (3) In a few cases where families have not used physical violence, where there is no substance abuse, and there is someone who can ensure the child's safety, the family may be allowed to remain intact while participating in intensive therapy. (4) In a few instances, the child may be removed from the family when that appears to be the safest option. Unfortunately, this decision may place additional guilt on the child.

When families are enmeshed and either rigid or chaotic, you help family members move to a *moderate position between the extremes*. With a rigid family, you will problem-solve ways in which the members can increase their flexibility of roles and rules. With a chaotic family, you will problem-solve ways to organize appropriate roles and formulate consistent rules. Throughout this approach, you are teaching the family the problem-solving process.

Behavioral: Behavior Therapy

Play Therapy; Art Therapy; Music Therapy

An important goal of nursing intervention is to facilitate the child's ability to talk and to think about the abuse with decreasing anxiety. It is up to you to create a safe and predictable environment in which the child feels supported. Make it clear to the child that you understand that talking about the abuse is difficult. Plan interventions that will encourage affective release in a supportive environment. Child victims must be able to experience a range of emotions. *Play therapy* helps these children play out traumatic themes, fears, and distorted beliefs. It is a nonthreatening way to process thoughts and feelings associated with the abuse, both symbolically and directly. *Art therapy* provides an opportunity to express feelings for which there are no words. *Therapeutic stories* present the traumatic issues of abuse, link victims' feelings and behavior, and describe new coping methods. *Journal writing* can help children over age 10 cope with intrusive thoughts and feelings. They often choose to bring their journal into the one-to-one sessions with their therapist. (Working with children and adolescents is covered in detail in Chapter 20.)

Art therapy helps adults in the healing process. Making group murals to express both individual progress and a sense of unity among clients can be very effective. Sitting and looking at soothing art works may be effective in reducing anxiety. Music therapy, combined with movement or dance, may be

Text continues on page 472

Focused Nursing Assessment

VICTIMS AND SURVIVORS OF CHILDHOOD SEXUAL ABUSE

Behavior Assessment	Affective Assessment	Cognitive Assessment

Behavior Assessment

Child Victim

Are there signs of regressive behavior in the child?

Is the child exhibiting clinging behavior?

Does the child have friendships with other children?

Has there been any sexual acting-out on the part of the child?

Has the child ever run away or threatened to run away?

Has the child ever attempted suicide?

Adult Survivor

When growing up, who had which type of responsibilities in the home?

How were family secrets kept within the family?

When you were young, who was (were) the closest family member(s) with whom you had any sexual activity?

Describe any self-mutilating behavior.

Describe your present state of sexual functioning.

Affective Assessment

Child Victim

Do you get enough love from other family members?

Tell me about the fears you may have if any family secrets are told: Not being believed? Being blamed for the problems? Your parents will not love you? Your parents will be taken away? You will be moved to a foster home? Physical punishment?

Adult Survivor

Describe the relationships in your family of origin.

In what ways do you continue to blame yourself for the childhood abuse?

Describe those people in your life who you are able to trust.

In what situations do you feel angry and out of control?

Cognitive Assessment

Child Victim

How would you describe the family's problems?

Who do you believe is responsible for these problems?

What happens or might happen when you tell the family secrets?

Are you able to separate your mind from your body while you are being hurt?

Adult Survivor

Have you always remembered the abuse or was there a period of amnesia?

What are the things you value most about yourself?

Do you have concerns about your sexual orientation?

*Assessment data is based on your observations plus family, community, or school reporting.

Social Assessment	*Physiological Assessment*

Child Victim

Who are your friends? Do they come over to play at your home?

Who are the people in your life who hurt you?

Adult Survivor

Describe the most important relationships in your life.

Has it been easier for you to maintain superficial relationships as opposed to intimate relationships?

In what ways do you need to be in control in relationships?

In what ways have you been abused as an adult? Emotionally? Physically? Sexually?

Child Victim

Smears of mouth, throat, vagina, and rectum for sexually transmitted infections.

HIV testing.

Throat irritation.

Genital irritation or trauma.

Rectal irritation or trauma.

Chronic vaginal and/or urinary tract infections.

Pregnancy.

Adult Survivor

Weight and nutritional status.

Sleeping problems.

Evidence of substance abuse.

Evidence of self-mutilation.

*N*ursing *I*nterventions *C*lassification

VICTIMS OF CHILDHOOD SEXUAL ABUSE

DOMAIN: Safety

Class: *Risk Management*

    Interventions: *Abuse Protection: Child:* Identification of high-risk, dependent child relationships and actions to prevent possible or further infliction of physical, sexual, or emotional harm or neglect of basic necessities of life.

DOMAIN: Behavioral

Class: *Behavior Therapy*

    Interventions: *Art Therapy:* Facilitation of communication through drawings or other art forms.

    Music Therapy: Using music to help achieve a specific change in behavior or feeling.

    Play Therapy: Purposeful use of toys or other equipment to assist a patient in communicating his/her perception of the world and to help in mastering the environment.

Class: *Coping Assistance*

    Interventions: *Guilt Work Facilitation:* Helping another to cope with painful feelings of responsibility, actual or perceived.

    Self-Esteem Enhancement: Assisting a patient to increase his/her personal judgment of self-worth.

    Coping Enhancement: Assisting a patient to adapt to perceived stressors, changes, or threats which interfere with meeting life demands and roles.

    Spiritual Support: Assisting the patient to feel balance and connection with a greater power.

    Support Group: Use of a group environment to provide emotional support and health-related information for members.

Class: *Psychological Comfort Promotion*

    Interventions: *Simple Relaxation Therapy:* Use of techniques to encourage and elicit relaxation for the purpose of decreasing undesirable signs and symptoms such as pain, muscle tension, or anxiety.

Source: McCloskey and Bulechek, 1996.

---

a way for clients to experience very early memories. Anxiety may be lessened by singing or humming a song, or playing a musical instrument. Journal writing is used more than any other expressive therapy and can be expanded to include poetry, songs, and plays.

Behavioral: Coping Assistance

Guilt Work Facilitation

Feminist-sensitive therapy can and should be practiced by all professionals dealing with sexual abuse. Because the process of sexual abuse is disempowering, it is important to empower survivors. The focus on *traumatic stress therapy* treats the trauma while acknowledging the process and result of victimization. *Developmental therapy* focuses on the "gaps" in the personality that occurred during the abuse process, such as trust issues, identity issues, and relationship issues. *Loss therapy* focuses on helping survivors identify and grieve over things lost during childhood sexual abuse, such as innocence, trust, nurturing, and memories.

Self-Esteem Enhancement

In working with adult survivors, remember that they have been robbed of a sense of power and feel detached from others. Recovery includes *restoring power and control*. Be sure to avoid becoming a "rescuer," as that might send the message that clients are not capable of acting for themselves. Also be careful not to set yourself up as a powerful authority because that might recreate the type of relationship in which the abuse occurred. The most helpful approach is being ally, collaborator, and supporter as clients struggle through the healing process. Point out ways they have taken control of their lives, and help them identify situations in which they are able to make self-respecting choices.

Interventions are designed to *increase self-esteem*. Adult survivors have a continuous internal monologue of negative statements like "You're weak, stupid, incompetent, unlovable, and unattractive." Negative statements become self-administered abuse and keep the survivor weak and powerless. You can help clients become aware of the frequency and intensity of these negative thoughts. Teach them to consciously replace negative thoughts with positive ones. Often difficult at first, it becomes easier with practice. Self-esteem is enhanced through the use of assertive skills. Survivors need to learn how to state their own opinions, interests, and needs directly and clearly. They need to calmly and rationally set limits of others' demands on them. As these new skills increase, so does self-esteem.

Coping Enhancement

Adult survivors also need to learn skills for managing negative emotions, thoughts, and memories. You can instruct them to do simple breathing exercises while focusing their attention on something in the room. Teach them to say to themselves: "Take the next few minutes to let go of the past and let go of your worries about the future. Come into this time and place." Sensory counting is another skill you can teach clients. Ask them to name one thing they can see in the room, then one thing they can hear, then one thing they can sense in their bodies. Continue on with two things they can see, hear, and sense. They can decide if they want to repeat observations or try to find new things. Repeat this process again and again, increasing the number each time. Usually by the time they reach four or five they are back in the here and now. This is a very powerful self-help technique for managing memory flooding and dissociation.

You can also ask clients to imagine a safety "container" in their minds. This container then becomes a receptacle in which they can "put and lock away" unpleasant thoughts. You can teach them to do the same process with a safe place—somewhere they can go to "get away and rest."

Spiritual Support

Betrayal by abusing adults is a spiritual issue. As nurses, we sometimes ignore a client's need for spiritual healing. Especially with adult survivors, you must support *spiritual recovery*. The sense of purpose in life is disrupted for victims and survivors. They also experience a loss in faith in a divine being as well as in other people. They are consumed with spiritual questions like "Why did it happen to me?" "What's wrong with me?" and "Am I some evil person?" When people are sexually abused, they must struggle with questions of a God or some higher power who either overlooked their pain and did not respond or did not even see their pain at all. It is not unusual for survivors to be angry with the Divine and hold God responsible for the abuse. This anger may in turn trigger fear and guilt for hating someone so powerful.

To recover from sexual abuse, survivors must place responsibility for the abuse where it belongs—100% with the offender. If they fail to do this, they will continue to be paralyzed by self-blame and guilt. The adult self needs to reach out and care for the hurt inner child by breaking down the walls that have isolated that child. Fully experiencing the rage and grief enables the survivor to move on to self-forgiveness and more complete healing. Spirituality includes a sense of connectedness to others. Survivors must begin the long journey of developing trusting relationships. They need to experience human contact and the warmth of the nurse-client relationship. Approach each client individually and remember that the paths of human spirituality are as varied as the people on them. Life events often shape belief systems in dramatic ways. The crisis and trauma of sexual abuse challenges victims and survivors to reflect on their values, beliefs, and their search for meaning. Approach each person with a sense of compassion and encourage this spiritual reflection. When requested, refer clients to religious/spiritual counselors who understand the emotional issues surrounding sexual abuse and who are sensitive to the need of survivors to work slowly through their spiritual struggles.

Support Group

Support groups allow survivors to share their feelings and experiences with others who believe their stories. The group setting fosters mutual understanding and decreases the sense of isolation. Many adult survivors find self-help groups to be very supportive in the process of healing. They are given a better idea of how their behavior affects others while helping others makes them feel more competent. They are reassured by seeing others recover. The Self-Help Groups section at the end of this chapter lists national groups designed for survivors as well as perpetrators of child sexual abuse.

Behavioral: Psychological Comfort Promotion

Simple Relaxation Therapy

Because adult survivors are often anxious, interventions to reduce anxiety are also necessary. Clients who learn progressive relaxation and controlled breathing are often able to avoid full-blown panic attacks. Teach the process, and talk clients through the stages of relaxation until they are able to reduce anxiety by themselves. When they are relaxed, instruct them to imagine a scene in which they feel safe and comfortable. Any time they need to, they can return to this safe scene where they are in total control. Daily practice facilitates the usefulness of these techniques.

Evaluation

Nurses in the acute care setting may not have the opportunity for long-term evaluation. Short-term evaluation focuses mainly on identifying child victims and adult survivors and referrals to appropriate community resources.

Nurses in long-term or community settings have the opportunity to evaluate the effectiveness of the multidisciplinary treatment plan over an extended period. Questions to guide the evaluation of the child victim and family include the following:

1. Has the child remained safe from further harm?
2. Has the child returned to functioning at an appropriate developmental level?
3. Is the child able to express feelings either verbally or through play or art therapy?
4. Is the child verbalizing decreasing feelings of guilt and/or responsibility?
5. Is the child developing peer friendships?
6. Has the family structure become more flexible and adaptable?
7. Are there fewer secrets within the family?

As a nurse, you have the opportunity to influence the care of adult survivors of childhood sexual abuse. Explain to others that the survivors' behavior is a post-trauma response that makes sense as an adaptation to trauma and perhaps a dysfunctional family. Intervene if staff members recreate the abuse by assuming a position of power and control. It is very rewarding to share the growth of clients toward making self-respecting choices in their lives. Questions to guide the evaluation of adult survivors include the following:

1. Has the person remained safe from further harm in adult relationships?
2. Is the client able to talk about the childhood trauma? If not, is art therapy, music therapy, movement therapy, or journal writing effective?
3. Is the client able to identify situations in which he or she has been able, or hopes to be able, to make self-respecting choices?
4. Is the client verbalizing increased spiritual comfort regarding the trauma?
5. Is the client verbalizing less self-blame?
6. Is the client verbalizing improved self-image?
7. Is the client no longer fixated on the trauma and able to live in the present and think about the future?

Although as a culture we say that we protect our children, we do not in reality live out this value. We do not invest many of our energies—time, caring, and money—in the prevention of childhood sexual abuse. Our present approaches to treatment and to the social control of sexual abuse are not yet effective enough that we can be assured of the long-term safety of children. As nurses, we must all become active in the battle to stop child sexual abuse.

Self-Help Groups

Victims, Survivors, and Perpetrators of Childhood Sexual Abuse

Children and Adult Survivors
Center for Constitutional Rights
606 Broadway, 7th Floor
New York, NY 10012
(212) 614-6464

Incest Survivors Anonymous
P.O. Box 5613
Department P
Long Beach, CA 90805-0613

Incest Survivors
Resource Network International
(505) 521-4260
www.zianet.com/ISRNI/

International Cult Education Program
P.O. Box 1232
Gracie Station
New York, NY 10028
(212) 439-1550

National Association of Working Women
(800) 522-0925

National Coalition Against Sexual Assault
c/o Volunteers of America
8787 State Street, Suite 202
East St. Louis, IL 62203

National Organization for Victim Assistance
717 D Street, NW
Department P
Washington, DC 20004
www.access.digex.net\~nova\

National Resource Center on Child Sexual Assault
(800) 542-7006

Rape, Abuse, and Incest National Network
(800) 656-4673
www.feminist.com/rainn.htm
e-mail: RAINNmail@aol.com

SNAP (Survivors Network for People Abused by Priests)
8025 South Honore
Chicago, IL 60620
(312) 483-1059

VOCAL (Victims of Clergy Abuse Linkup)
P.O. Box 1268
Wheeling, IL 60090
(708) 202-0242

VOICES (Victims of Incest Can Emerge Survivors)
P.O. Box 14309
Chicago, IL 60614
(800) 786-4238
www.voices-action.org

Perpetrators

Amend
1445 Cleveland Place, Room 307
Denver, CO 80202

Commence
9656 Sycamore Trace Court
Cincinnati, OH 34242

RAVEN
665 Delmar Street, Suite 301
St. Louis, MO 63130

Key Concepts

Sexual Harassment

- Sexual harassment includes a number of behaviors and can be either quid pro quo or hostile environment.

- Sexual harassment can lead to severe stress in the victims.

Rape

- Rape is a crime of violence perpetrated against innocent victims of all ages.

- Date rape and marital rape are often unreported because victims may feel responsible or fear the disbelief of others.

- Rape-trauma syndrome is characterized by symptoms of, or specific responses to, the experience of being raped.

Childhood Sexual Abuse

- Sexual abuse occurs in all ethnic, religious, economic, and cultural subgroups in the United States. The vast majority of victims know their abusers.

- Most juvenile offenders were sexually abused as children; they then develop offending behaviors as they reach adolescence.

- There are five types of incestuous fathers: sexually preoccupied abusers, adolescent regressors, self-gratifiers, emotional dependents, and angry retaliators.

- There are four major types of female offenders: teacher-lovers, experimenter-exploiters, predisposers, and women coerced by males.

- Ritual abuse is emotional, physical, and sexual abuse that occurs in ceremonial or systematic form by a specific group.

Knowledge Base: Rape

- Behavioral characteristics of rape victims include agitation, outward calmness, crying, nightmares, sleep problems, phobias, and relationship difficulties.

- Affective characteristics of rape victims include shock, anxiety, fear, depression, violation, and anger.

- Cognitive characteristics of rape victims include depersonalization, dissociation, denial, an inability to make decisions, self-blame, obsessions, and concerns for future safety.

- Families of rape victims experience many of the same thoughts and emotions as the victims themselves. They must be educated about rape and the immediate and potential long-term reactions of the victims.

- The United States has the highest number of rapes among Western countries.

- In some countries women are forced to marry their rapist or go into prostitution so they may survive, or they may even be put to death by their families to cleanse the family name.

- Physiological characteristics include trauma and injuries, pregnancy, STIs, and difficulties with sexual functioning.

- Most theorists agree that rape is a crime of violence generated by issues of power and anger. Theories relating to rape include revenge, dominance, eroticized assault, gang rituals, inadequate relationships, acceptance of violence within a culture, and sexist cultural values.

Nursing Assessment

- Clients must be immediately assessed for any serious or critical injuries. Prior to any further assessment, clients must be informed of their rights.

Nursing Diagnosis

- The nursing diagnosis is *Rape-trauma syndrome,* which may be further classified as *compound* or *silent reaction.*

Nursing Interventions

- Nursing interventions include supporting defense mechanisms, encouraging clients to talk about the rape, helping clients recognize that survival was the most important outcome, identifying immediate concerns, implementing the problem-solving process, identifying who to tell about the rape, discussing beliefs about possible pregnancy, and providing a written list of referrals.

Evaluation

- Nursing interventions are evaluated as effective when clients return to their precrisis level, or achieve a higher level, of functioning.

Knowledge Base: Childhood Sexual Abuse

- Adult perpetrators believe in extreme restrictiveness and domination. They often feel weak, afraid, and inadequate. They use secrecy and silence to escape accountability. If confronted by others, they will often deny the abuse.

- Child victims are at the mercy of adult perpetrators. Some become extremely affectionate, while others have problems with impulse control and aggression toward others. They may act out sexually with other children or adults.

- Child victims are filled with fears of not being believed, being blamed, and/or being rejected by the family.

- Child victims often feel responsible for the abuse. Secrecy and guilt often keep them isolated from their peers.

- In order to survive the trauma, child victims may use denial, minimization, or dissociation.

- Adolescent victims may run away from home and may turn to prostitution for a variety of reasons.

- Some adult survivors engage in self-mutilation for a number of reasons: to prove their existence, as a plea for nurturance, as a way to self-nurture, to stop dissociation, to punish the self, and/or to reduce emotional pain through physical pain.

- Many adult survivors have sexual problems such as aversion, inhibition, and compulsive sexual behavior. Others suffer from confusion about their sexual orientation.

- Many adult survivors continue to believe that they were to blame for the abuse. They suffer from low self-esteem, depression, anxiety, and rage.

- Some adult survivors have total amnesia about the abuse.

- Intimate relationships are often difficult for adult survivors. Survivors of childhood sexual abuse remain vulnerable and may be revictimized as adults.

- Physiological characteristics of sexual abuse include STIs, trauma to the genitals, chronic vaginal or urinary tract infections, and pregnancy.

- Having suffered sexual abuse in childhood is often a hidden feature of adult mental disorders. Adult psychiatric clients with a history of abuse have a bewildering combination of symptoms, including anger, depression, anxiety, insomnia, suspicion, eating disorders, substance abuse, and self-mutilation.

- There is no single cause of childhood sexual abuse. Perpetrators may lack impulse control, or they may be rigid and overcontrolled. Many of them were sexually abused as children.

- In incestuous families, hierarchical lines are crossed; for example, the father moves down to the child's level, or the child moves up to replace the mother. These families are often enmeshed, and the family system is either chaotic or rigid.

Nursing Assessment

- It is very difficult for both child victims and adult survivors to break the silence and respond to nursing assessment questions.

- When it is discovered that one child in a family is a victim of sexual abuse, all other children in the family must also be assessed for abuse.

- You must continually be aware of the client's comfort level with the physical environment during the assessment process.

Nursing Diagnosis

- Nursing diagnoses are formulated for the child victim, the family members, and the adult survivor.

Nursing Interventions

- The priority of care with child victims is to ensure the safety of the child.

- Nurses help families move toward a moderate position between the extremes of rigid and chaotic; they learn to increase their flexibility of roles or implement consistent rules.

- Child victims learn to manage their feelings through verbalization, play therapy, art therapy, and journal writing.

- Types of therapy useful with adult survivors include feminist-sensitive therapy, traumatic stress therapy, developmental therapy, and loss therapy.

- The most helpful approach with adult survivors is being ally, collaborator, and supporter as they struggle through the healing process.

- It is important to restore power and control to adult survivors.

- Spiritual recovery is part of the healing process.

- Both child victims and adult survivors must place responsibility for the abuse where it belongs—100% with the offender.

- Interventions are designed to help the adult survivor increase self-esteem and reduce anxiety.

- Adult survivors heal through the use of art therapy, music therapy, journal writing, group therapy, and self-help groups.

Evaluation

■ Evaluation questions are related to safety, level of daily functioning, emotional responses, thinking patterns, and relationships with others.

■ As nurses, we all need to become active in assuring the long-term safety of children.

Review Questions

1. Which of the following is an example of hostile environment in terms of sexual harassment?

   a. Your boss suggests that your raise is dependent on having sex with him.

   b. Your supervisor makes masturbatory gestures every time you walk past.

   c. The personnel manager hints that the job will be yours if you cooperate sexually.

   d. The boss assures you of a big promotion if you go out on a couple of dates with him.

2. Your client, who is an adult survivor, states: "Why couldn't I make him stop the abuse? If I were a stronger person, I would have been able to make him stop. Maybe it was my fault he abused me." Based on this data, which would be the most appropriate nursing diagnosis?

   a. *Ineffective family coping*

   b. *Anxiety*

   c. *Social isolation*

   d. *Chronic low self-esteem*

3. In response to the statements in question 2, which would be the most appropriate nursing intervention?

   a. Ask her if she is willing to discuss her relationship with her parents to determine family patterns of ineffective coping.

   b. Connect her feelings of low self-esteen to feelings of guilt and anger, since she is unrealistically blaming herself for the abuse.

   c. Help her identify areas of life she has control over to help her begin to shift from external to internal locus of control.

   d. Refer her to an adult survivors of incest group to decrease her feelings of isolation.

4. One of the ways to cope during an actual rape is through thinking, "This can't possibly be happening to me." This defense mechanism is called

   a. depersonalization.

   b. displacement.

   c. identification.

   d. projection.

5. A rape victim has just been admitted to the emergency department. It has been determined that she does not have any critical injuries from the sexual assault. The next step in the assessment process is to

   a. perform a vaginal examination.

   b. take combings of her pubic hair.

   c. inform her of her rights.

   d. take swabs for diagnosis of sexually transmitted infections.

References

Abney, V. D., & Priest, R. (1995). African Amercians and sexual child abuse. In L. A. Fontes (Ed.) *Sexual Abuse in Nine North American Cultures* (pp.11–30). Newbury Park, CA: Sage.

Bergen, R. K. (1996). *Wife Rape.* Newbury Park, CA: Sage.

Comas-Diaz, L. (1995). Puerto Ricans and sexual child abuse. In L. A. Fontes (Ed.), *Sexual Abuse in Nine North American Cultures* (pp. 31–66). Newbury Park, CA: Sage.

Desjarlais, R., et al. (1995). *World Mental Health.* New York: Oxford Univ. Press.

Draucker, C. B., & Petrovic, K. (1996). Healing of adult male survivors of childhood sexual abuse. *IMAGE, 28*(4), 325–330.

Evans, K., & Sullivan, J. M. (1995). *Treating Addicted Survivors of Trauma.* New York: Guilford Press.

Featherman, J. M. (1995). Jews and sexual child abuse. In L. A. Fontes (Ed.), *Sexual Abuse in Nine North American Cultures* (pp. 128–155). Newbury Park, CA: Sage.

Fink, L. A., et al. (1995). Initial reliability and validity of the childhood trauma interview. *Am J Psychiatry, 152*(9), 1329–1335.

Glod, C. A. (1993). Long-term consequences of childhood physical and sexual abuse. *Arch Psychiatr Nurs, 7*(3), 163–173.

Hayashino, D. S., Wurtele, S. K., & Klebe, K. J. (1995). Child molesters. *J Interpersonal Violence, 10*(1), 106–116.

Holmes, R. M. (1991). *Sex Crimes.* Newbury Park, CA: Sage.

Huston, R. L., et al.(1995). Characteristics of childhood sexual abuse in a predominantly Mexican American population. *Child Abuse & Neglect, 19*(2), 165–176.

Kaufman, K. L., et al. (1995). Comparing female and male perpetrators' modus operandi. *J Interpersonal Violence, 10*(3), 322–333.

Krueger, M. M. (1988). Pregnancy as a result of rape. *J Sex Ed Ther, 14*(1), 23–27.

McCloskey, J. C., & Bulechek, G. M. *Nursing Intervention Classification (NIC),* 2nd ed. St. Louis, MO: Mosby, 1996.

Mendel, M. P. (1995). *The Male Survivor.* Newbury Park, CA: Sage.

Okamura, A., Heras, P., & Wong-Kerberg, L. (1995). Asian, Pacific Island, and Filipino Americans and sexual child abuse. In L. A. Fontes (Ed.) *Sexual Abuse in Nine North American Cultures* (pp. 67–96) Newbury Park, CA: Sage.

Posttraumatic stress disorder. (1996). *Harvard Mental Health Letter, 13(*1), 1–4.

Rutter, P. (1996). *Sex, Power, and Boundaries.* New York: Bantam Books.

Schmidt, M. (1995). Anglo Americans and sexual child abuse. In L. A. Fontes (Ed.) *Sexual Abuse in Nine North American Cultures* (pp. 156–175). Newbury Park, CA: Sage.

Schuler, M. (1992). *Freedom for Violence: Women's Strategies From Around the World.* New York: UN Development Fund for Women.

Shirar, L. (1996). *Dissociative Children.* New York: Norton.

Stein, M. B., et al. (1996). Childhood physical and sexual abuse in patients with anxiety disorders and in a community sample. *Am J Psychiatry, 153*(2), 275–276.

Stermac, L., et al. (1996). Sexual assault of adult males. *J Interpersonal Violence, 11*(1) 52–64.

Struckman-Johnson, C. (1996). Sexual coercion reported by men and women in prison. *J Sex Res, 33*(1), 67–76.

U.S. has most rapes. (1996). *Contemp Sexuality, 30*(1), 6.

Vanderbilt, H. (1992). Incest: A chilling report. *Lear's.*

Ward, C. A. (1995). *Attitudes Toward Rape.* Newbury Park, CA: Sage.

Weisz, M. G., & Earls, C. M. (1995). The effects of exposure to filmed sexual violence on attitudes toward rape. *J Interpersonal Violence, 10*(1), 71–84.

Wiehe, V. R., & Richards, A. L. (1995). *Intimate Betrayal.* Newbury Park, CA: Sage.

Wyatt, G. E., & Riederle, M. (1995). The prevalence and context of sexual harassment among African American and White American women. *J Interpersonal Violence, 10*(3), 309–321.

PART V

Special Populations
and Topics

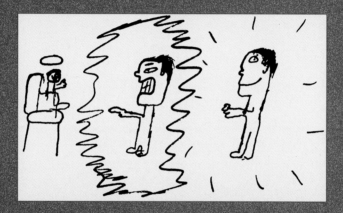

*My picture represents the child in me who can never
be happy and have positive attitudes because the adult
in me keeps criticizing and feeding the negative input
to it and other aspects of life.*

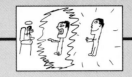

CHAPTER 20

Disorders of Children and Adolescents

Mary J. Roehrig

Objectives

After reading this chapter, you will be able to:

- Differentiate among the mental disorders that occur during childhood and adolescence.
- Communicate effectively with children and adolescents.
- Describe interventions specific to children and adolescents.

*C*hildren and adolescents are not miniature adults. Although they may experience some of the same mental disorders as adults, their symptoms are often determined by their developmental level. Many brain disorders begin in childhood and adolescence and are not diagnosed until adulthood.

Knowledge Base

Anxiety Disorders

It is common for children to experience anxiety. This experience is usually temporary and requires no professional intervention. Very young children fear strangers, being left alone, and the dark; preschoolers fear imaginary creatures, animals, and the dark. Anxiety about physical safety and storms are common among young school-age children. During the middle-school years, the focus of anxiety changes to academic, social, and health-related issues. This focus continues into adolescence.

Many of the disorders discussed in previous chapters have an onset during childhood or adolescence. They are not specified as Axis I disorders (usually first diagnosed in infancy, childhood, or adolescence); rather, characteristics of children and adolescents are described under the adult disorders. Table 20.1 describes some of the common anxiety disorders as they are manifested by children and adolescents. Estimates for the presence of any anxiety disorder range from 6% to 18%. Anxiety disorders are 3–4 times higher in children who also suffer from depression and 2–3 times higher in children with oppositional or conduct disorders (Costello and Angold, 1995).

Separation Anxiety Disorder

A mild form of separation anxiety is fairly common in young children. Most children fear losing their parents. Separation anxiety disorder may develop at any age, although it is more common in children than in adolescents, with the peak onset between 7 and 9 years. The child may follow the parent around the house, needing to be in close proximity at all times. Their worries may focus on separation themes like getting kidnapped and being killed, or the parents being killed. The school-age child may refuse to go to school, although not all refusals are due to separation anxiety. Physiological manifestations include nausea, vomiting, stomach ache, and sore throat. Older children may have palpitations, respiratory distress, and dizziness (Black, 1995).

Separation anxiety disorder may have either an acute or insidious onset. Many children recover without any further problems, while others may have periodic exacerbations. Some may have symptoms into adulthood, especially when attachments are threatened or disrupted.

Selective Mutism

Selective mutism is the steady failure to speak in specific social situations where speaking is expected. The onset is usually between 3 and 6 years and occurs more frequently among girls. The extent to which the child speaks varies greatly. Some children speak loudly and freely at home but never say a word at school. Some speak to strangers in public, while others do not. Some are unable to speak to others face-to-face but may be able to speak to these same individuals on the phone. As is obvious, this disability interferes with education and social relationships. The majority of the children "outgrow" the disorder, although it may persist for several years (Leonard and Dow, 1995).

Mood Disorders

Major Depression

The incidence of depression in children is often underestimated. The cultural norm is that childhood is a carefree and happy time and that there is no reason for children to be depressed. However, about 2–6% of children and adolescents in the United States suffer from significant depression. Children who have a parent with a mood disorder are at the greatest risk for developing a similar disorder (Emslie, 1997; Goodyer, 1995).

Depression is often manifested through negativism, acting-out behavior, and/or unexplained physical complaints. Symptoms are often related to the developmental level. See Box 20.1 for problem behaviors associated with mood disorders. Gender roles may determine some depressive symptoms since depressed girls tend to "internalize" problems and

Table 20.1 Axis II Anxiety Disorders in Children and Adolescents

Disorder	Age	Description
Obsessive compulsive disorder (OCD)	As young as 2; mean age 10 years	Most common behaviors are washing and cleaning, followed by checking, counting, repeating, touching and straightening, and hoarding. Fears include contamination, harm to self, and harm to familiar person. Many are embarrassed and secretive, and the disorder is often unrecognized.
Posttraumatic stress disorder (PTSD)	Related to traumatic event	Traumatic events prior to age 11 are three times more likely to result in PTSD. Younger children may repeatedly act out specific themes of the trauma. Some engage in high motor activity in effort to keep minds off recurring thoughts.
Generalized anxiety disorder (GAD)	5–17 years	Formerly referred to as overanxious disorder of childhood. Affects about 3–15% of children and adolescents. Variety of worries such as future events, performance, personal safety, and the social environment. Often have somatic complaints. Self-conscious and frequently seek reassurance from others. Perfectionistic, eager to please, hypermature.
Specific phobia	Childhood, adolescence	Common phobias include heights, small animals, doctors, dentists, darkness, noises, thunder and lightning. Behaviors include screaming, crying, or running to loved one for safety. There is a common belief that confrontation with phobic stimulus will result in personal harm.
Social phobia	As young as 8; early to mid-adolescence	Persistent fear of one or more situations such as formal speaking, eating in front of others, going to parties, writing in front of others, using public restrooms, speaking to authority figures. Fear is of criticism or failure. 60% of distressing events occur at school.

Sources: *DSM-IV,* 1994; March, 1995.

Box 20.1

Problem Behaviors Associated with Mood Disorders

Infants

- When separated from parent, may have weepy and withdrawn behavior
- Frozen facial expression
- Weight loss
- Increased incidence of infections

One to Three Years

- Delays or regression in toileting, eating, sleeping, intellectual growth
- Increase in nightmares
- May appear sad or expressionless
- Apathetic or more clingy

Three to Five Years

- Loss of interest in newly acquired skills
- Nightmares with themes of annihilation
- Enuresis, encopresis, anorexia, or binge eating may occur
- May also experience separation anxiety
- Frequent negative self-statements and thoughts or impulses of self-harm

Six to Twelve Years

- Depressed mood, irritable, aggressive
- Academic difficulties
- Eating and sleeping disturbances
- Severe self-criticism and guilt
- Suicidal ideation and plans

Adolescents

- Intense mood swings
- Academic difficulties
- Argumentative and/or assaultive
- Risk taking or antisocial behavior
- Hypersomnia
- Very low self-esteem

Sources: Brown, 1996; Speier et al, 1995.

depressed boys tend to "externalize" or act out their problems. Psychotic symptoms (such as auditory hallucinations) may be present in 25–30% of the cases, and many of these individuals will go on to develop bipolar disorder. In adults, depression eventually evolves into bipolar disorder about 5–10% of the time. In children diagnosed with major depression, about 20–30% will develop bipolar disorder (Brage, 1995; Johnston and Fruehling, 1996; Speier et al, 1995; Wilens, 1997).

It is believed that children and adolescents with major depression have brain abnormalities similar to those of adults. There appears to be underactivity of neurotransmitters such as serotonin (5-HT) and norepinephrine (NE). Circadian rhythms are disrupted and there is a reduction of melatonin, a hormone secreted during sleep (Brage, 1995).

> Rachel, age 16, is being seen by her school counselor for depression. Her mother died when she was 10 years old and she has never known her father. She lived with various relatives and is now living with an aunt and uncle. For the past several months she has been tearful, irritable, and unable to concentrate. She is talking about dropping out of school because she is failing all her classes. She has been defiant with her aunt and uncle. At home she has been playing with a butane lighter, burning paper and pencils, and they are afraid she will burn the house down. She thinks about suicide but at this time states that she is too afraid to kill herself.

Seasonal Affective Disorder

Seasonal affective disorder is a form of recurrent major depression affecting 4–6% of adults in the United States. One-third of adult sufferers report onset of the symptoms during childhood. One study found that over 3% of children aged 10 to 18 years suffer from seasonal affective disorder. There appears to be a relationship with puberty, especially in girls. It is thought that perhaps sex hormones increase the brain's vulnerability to changing seasons and light levels (Swedo et al, 1995).

Bipolar Disorder

The first manic episode of bipolar disorder may occur during childhood or adolescence and is characterized by marked instability of behavior and intense turmoil. The diagnosis is often difficult since there is not enough time to establish a history of the cyclic changes of bipolar disorder. It is often mistaken for attention-deficit/hyperactivity disorder (ADHD), conduct disorder, or schizophrenia (Brown, 1996).

There are several differences in bipolar symptoms in younger people compared to adults. Children often experience intense mood swings typically lasting only an hour or two as opposed to at least five days in adults. Adults in a manic state usually increase their involvement in goal-directed, pleasurable activities such as spending sprees or sexual acting out. In addition, adults demonstrate an inflated sense of self-esteem. Conversely, children with bipolar disorder usually do not have inflated self-esteem and often are less involved with goal-directed activities, perhaps because those activities are simply not available to a child (Johnston and Fruehling, 1996).

Attention-Deficit and Disruptive Behavior Disorders

Attention deficit/hyperactivity disorder, oppositional defiant disorder, and conduct disorder are behavioral disorders that sometimes occur during childhood and adolescence. Socially disruptive and inappropriate behaviors are often more of a problem for others than for those who have the problem.

Attention Deficit/Hyperactivity Disorder (ADHD)

Attention deficit/hyperactivity disorder is a chronic disorder that is estimated to affect 6–9% of school-age children. As early as the first few weeks of life and as late as the age of 7, a child may demonstrate signs of hyperactivity. Infants sleep little, are active in the crib, cry frequently, and develop rapidly. Sometimes an infant manages to escape the confines of the crib to begin a journey of rapid, impulsive activity. Toddlers cannot sit still, and they leave a trail of destruction. The degree of activity may be comparable to that of peers, but the child who is hyperactive is unable to stop being active even when appropriate, as in not being able to sit down to eat. Children have difficulty waiting for their turn and cannot tolerate delayed gratification. Impulsive behavior leads to frequent accidents (Milberger et al, 1996).

Before long, children with ADHD begin to recognize that they cannot conform to the expectations of parents and teachers. Some children accept that these expectations are "correct," and their inability to achieve them results in loss of self-esteem, helplessness, and depression. This is more typical of girls and is less disruptive to society. Others, more frequently boys, decide that parents and teachers are "wrong" and develop an antisocial attitude and may act out their frustrations in a hostile manner (Hedaya, 1996).

An interesting perspective on ADHD has been proposed by Thom Hartman (1993). He suggests that persons with ADHD are hunters among farmers. This analogy serves to explain the "roaming" characteristics. The hunter thinks visually, is excited by the hunt, but becomes easily bored with mundane tasks. The hunter constantly monitors the environment and readily changes strategies at a moment's notice. Hunters are often very creative. While they appear disruptive in the school and frustrate many parents, it is good to remember the many hunters who have made positive changes in the world.

Inattention is a hallmark of ADHD. An extremely short attention span and distractibility are sometimes accompanied by learning disabilities. The ability to think abstractly, conceptualize, and generalize are disturbed, as is the ability to assimilate, retain, and recall. Altered visual or auditory perceptions may increase distractibility. In about 50% of cases, symptoms persist into adolescence and adulthood (Wilens et al, 1996).

The exact cause of ADHD remains unknown, but it is likely that it involves genetic factors, anatomical abnormalities, neurotransmission problems, and environmental factors. Twin studies demonstrate that there is a genetic factor in some cases of ADHD. In 50–80% of monozygotic twins, both twins have ADHD. Among dizygotic twins, both twins have the disorder 30% of the time. Structural abnormalities of the frontal cortex are associated with impulsive behavior, socially inappropriate behavior, irritability, euphoria, hyperactivity, and emotional lability. Some studies have shown reduced glucose metabolism in areas of the cortex associated with concentration and motor activity. In some cases it is thought that there are dopamine (DA) abnormalities in the frontal lobe. Others believe that the basic difficulty is related to the balance between DA and NE. One environmental factor may be maternal smoking during pregnancy, which is thought to cause damage to the developing brain. Another environmental factor may be the effect of foods, preservatives, and artificial colors in one's diet. Food additives and salicylates are thought to bind to norepinephrine receptors, while food allergies may change the number of postsynaptic neurons. These changes in neurotransmission can result in a wide range of behavioral symptoms (Boris and Mandel, 1994; Hedaya, 1996; Sherman et al, 1997). Further information can be obtained from the Feingold Association on their web site (www.feingold.org).

Oppositional Defiant Disorder (ODD)

Children with oppositional defiant disorder are frequently disruptive, argumentative, hostile, and irritable. They often deliberately defy adult rules but tend to blame others for their own mistakes and difficulties. Such disruptive behavior occurs at a more frequent rate, at greater intensity, and for longer periods of time than the usual behavioral problems of peers. Disturbances in behavior lead to social problems with peers and adults, and impaired academic functioning.

Conduct Disorder (CD)

Children and adolescents with conduct disorder engage in severe and persistent antisocial behavior that violates the rights of others at home, in school, and in the community. Antisocial behavior may be solitary in nature, or it may occur in a peer group such as a gang. Physical aggression is common, and cruelty to other people and animals may occur. Youths with CD may destroy other people's property, set fires, steal, and rob.

Anger resulting from self-hatred, depression, and helplessness is directed outward. These youths lack guilt or remorse over their deviant behavior. Maladjustment to school, truancy, and dropping out of school are common. Social alienation is brought about by the unacceptable behavior and lack of social controls. Relationships with peers and adults are manipulative and used for personal advantage (Roberts, 1995).

Antisocial childhood behaviors predict multiple problems in adulthood. These problems include substance abuse, criminal behavior, occupational problems, lowered educational level, higher rates of divorce/separation, and less contact with supportive others (Kazdin, 1995).

> Ruben, 15 years old, has been admitted to a residential setting for aggressive behavior. His mother was raped when she was 15 and Ruben is the result of the rape. His mother has been married and divorced twice. He has three younger siblings ages 11, 9, and 5 years. For the past several months, Ruben has been cutting school and getting into gang fights. He has been expelled for truancy and fighting. His mother was disciplining him by making Ruben go to work with her. He recently told his mother that if she continued to make him go to work, he would kill her. His younger siblings are afraid of him and his friends. He becomes very angry with anyone who doesn't agree with his views. He states that he is only in the residential placement because his mother is "crazy and a bitch." When asked about future expectations, he states, "to hang with friends and not go back to school."

Substance-Related Disorders

Adolescent substance abuse is related to many factors. If parents are alcoholics, there may be a genetic influence as well as a modeling influence. Alcohol and drug use is often accepted in the teen peer group. Developmentally, adolescents may abuse substances as a means of rebelling against parents, in a search for identity, and in an effort to separate from the family. Some teens experiencing family dysfunction, problems in school, problems with peers, and/or emotional or physical trauma may feel overwhelmed and attempt to escape through the use of substances. Some adolescents suffering from mental disorders try to self-medicate with alcohol or drugs.

Substance-related disorders progress more rapidly in adolescents than in adults. Adults may take from 2 to 7 years from the first use to full dependency. Teens often make this progression in 6 to 18 months. The use of denial is often stronger since teens do not have years of negative consequences. They often experience developmental delays: growth and development slows down, they fall behind in academics, their social skills stagnate, they experience poor impulse control, and they are intolerant of delayed gratification. They typically shift to a peer group composed solely of other drug-using adolescents. In a two-parent home, the roles may be polarized, with one parent being the enabler and the other parent the enforcer. This creates much family conflict and distress (Margolis, 1995; Zealberg and Santos, 1996).

Critical Thinking

You are the nurse working in a mental health community clinic. Guadalupe, your client, complains that her 10-year-old son, Jorge, has become unmanageable, and she no longer knows how to cope with his behavior at home or the frequent complaints from his teacher at school.

At home Jorge is a bully, insisting on having his way. He takes toys from his siblings, causing arguments and crying, but seldom plays with the toy more than a few minutes. He has difficulty staying in his chair at school, misses important information, and disrupts other children while they are working.

Guadalupe feels alone because her husband has little patience with Jorge but refuses to admit that he is any different from most other boys his age. You are fairly certain that Guadalupe is describing behaviors consistent with attention deficit/hyperactivity disorder (ADHD).

Suggested answers can be found in Appendix D.

1 What other data would be helpful to you in making an accurate assessment of Jorge's problem?

2. If Jorge were experiencing conduct disorder (CD), what specific behaviors would you inquire about that separate it from ADHD?

3. What indications do you have that Jorge is not suffering from a pervasive development disorder, such as autistic disorder?

4. You can anticipate that Jorge's physician may place Jorge on a central nervous system stimulant for ADHD. Why is this the best choice of psychopharmacological interventions for Jorge's problem?

5. Select two interventions that you feel could be helpful for Jorge. Explain why you think those interventions will help Jorge.

Pervasive Developmental Disorders

Pervasive developmental disorders involve severe impairment of social interactions and imaginative activities. People with these disorders seldom develop the ability to communicate with others. At the same time, many basic areas of psychological development are affected.

Autistic Disorder (AD)

Autistic disorder is the model for the general category of pervasive developmental disorders, and it is the most severe example. AD usually becomes obvious between 18 and 36 months of age. Children with AD exhibit ritualistic behavior. Routines must be followed exactly; objects must be returned to their "rightful" place or the child will become agitated. They may spend hours in repetitive behavior such as stacking blocks or examining and fondling objects. Brightly colored moving objects are especially fascinating to these children.

Disturbances in motor behavior such as whirling, lunging, darting, rocking, and toe walking present a bizarre picture. Other stereotypical behaviors include hand flapping, twisting, and finger snapping. Some behavior may be self-mutilative, such as head banging or hand biting.

Communication with others is seriously impaired. Children with AD may be mute, may make unintelligible sounds, or may say words repeatedly. They may be unable to name objects and cannot use or understand abstract language. In addition, nonverbal communication is minimal or absent. Their moods are unpredictable, and they may cry or laugh uncontrollably and without apparent cause. These problems with communication and mood contribute to their failure to develop interpersonal relationships, leading to social isolation.

Autism is a lifelong disorder and most likely the result of multiple etiologies. Factors to be considered include genetics, infectious disease, metabolic disease, and structural abnormalities of the brain. Studies are focusing on excessive brain opiate activity, abnormal levels of oxytocin and vasopressin, structural abnormalities of the limbic system and cerebellum, delayed maturity of the frontal lobe between the ages of 2 and 4, and incomplete development of the frontal lobe (Ciaranello, 1996; Haznedar et al, 1997; Insel, 1997).

Tic Disorders

Included in this category are Tourette's disorder, chronic motor or vocal tic disorder, and transient tic disorder. These disorders involve sudden, rapid, recurrent, stereotyped movements or sounds. Stress exacerbates all forms of tics. More common in males, Tourette's occurs in approximately 4–5 people per 10,000 and may have an onset as early as 2 years. Associated features include obsessions and compulsions. Generally, the severity and frequency of symptoms decrease during adolescence and adulthood.

Concomitant Disorders

Children and adolescents with mental disorders often have two or three disorders at the same time. Depressed children and teens often experience oppositional defiant disorder and attention deficit disorders. In 40% of the cases of depression there is a concomitant anxiety disorder. In young people with ADHD, 44% have one other mental disorder, while 9% experience two other disorders. Conduct disorder and ADHD have a strong association with one another. Adolescents with conduct disorder frequently have a substance-use disorder. Concomitant disorders complicate both the treatment program and the prognosis of child and adolescent mental disorders (Hedaya, 1996; Wilens, 1997).

Psychopharmacological Interventions

In general, medications are used much less frequently with children than with adults. Because many of the psychotropic medications have side effects that slow cognitive functioning, they may interrupt the learning process—a major developmental task of childhood and adolescence. Most of the psychotropic medications have not had clinical trials with children and adolescents, and therefore the dosage has not been researched.

Antidepressants may be prescribed for children experiencing major depression. SSRIs and SNRIs such as Prozac (fluoxetine), Paxil (paroxetine), Zoloft (sertraline), and Effexor (venlafaxine) seem to be well tolerated in children and appear to have fewer side effects than other antidepressants. Other commonly prescribed drugs are Elavil (amitriptyline), Tofranil (imipramine), Aventyl (nortriptyline), and Wellbutrin (bupropion). Often lithium and Tegretol (carbamazepine) are combined in managing symptoms of bipolar disorder (Wilens, 1997).

In some cases, antidepressant medications are prescribed for children with ADHD, especially Effexor (venlafaxine) and Luvox (fluvoxamine). More commonly, central nervous system stimulants are prescribed. These medications increase the ability to focus attention by blocking out irrelevant thoughts and impulses. CNS stimulants lead to significant improvement in 70–75% of cases. The advantage of Ritalin (methylphenidate) and Dexedrine (dextroamphetamine) is that effectiveness is almost immediate, while the same effect with Cylert (pemoline) may take 6–8 weeks. Common side effects include pallor, a pinched facial expression, dark hollows under the eyes, anorexia, insomnia, headache, and dryness of the mouth. Toxic effects may include overstimulation or sedation (Wilens, 1997). See Table 20.2 for a description of these medications.

Multidisciplinary Interventions

Group therapy can be effective with both children and adolescents. In working with young children, the size of the group is usually limited to five. The length of the group session is determined by age and attention span. Group therapy with children is usually activity-oriented, for example, daily goal setting, art projects, music or movement therapy, and play therapy.

Because adolescents can reason and talk about their behavior, thoughts, and feelings, group therapy is a verbal process rather than the activity process used with children. Peers, as a source of support, feedback, and information, are very important in teenagers' lives. Group therapy with adolescents is often more productive than individual sessions.

The overall goals of group therapy are for the members to:

- learn to talk openly about themselves
- practice active listening
- give and receive feedback

Table 20.2 Medications to Treat ADHD

Generic Name	Trade Name	Recommended Dosage
dextroamphetamine	Dexedrine	Children 3 years and older: 2.5 mg in morning, at noon, and perhaps late afternoon. Increase dose by 5 mg weekly. Maximum total daily dose: 40 mg.
dextroamphetamine	Adderall	Children 3 years and older: 5–20 mg/day, od or bid.
methylphenidate	Ritalin	Children 6 years and older: 5 mg in morning, at noon, and perhaps late afternoon. Increase dose by 5–10 mg weekly. Maximum total daily dose: 60 mg.
pemoline	Cylert	Children 6 years and older: 18.75 mg in morning. Increase dose by 18.75 mg weekly. Maximum daily dose: 112.5 mg.

Sources: Goldstein and Goldstein, 1992; Sylvester and Nageotte, 1993.

- learn to help others
- learn new ways of relating through interacting in a safe environment

There is often a parallel group for the parents of children and adolescents so that the entire family can receive treatment simultaneously. Such a group enables the parents to support each other, learn growth and developmental stages, gain an awareness of their contribution to family dynamics, increase parenting skills, and explore their own needs and problems.

Behavior modification is quite effective with children and adolescents. On an individual basis, an undesirable behavior is identified. During an observational period, you record the number of times, and under which circumstances, the identified behavior occurs. Following this assessment, the data are analyzed, and a plan is developed to alter the behavior. The child/teen is told what is expected, what is not acceptable, and the consequences for undesirable behavior.

Community-based programs can help improve the mental health of children and adolescents. In adult mentor plans, such as Big Brothers and Big Sisters, the goal is to help children and teenagers succeed in school and the community. Youth organizations are largely recreational, but some are career-oriented or avocation-oriented, while others are politically or ethnically oriented. These youth organizations provide leadership experience, an opportunity to interact with and help others, and the chance to assume responsibility for oneself. Peer-helping programs have recently become popular. Older children and adolescents are trained in helping skills and assigned to work with peers or younger children. The helpers often gain as much from the experience as the recipients do.

Family therapy is often the preferred approach when there is a child or adolescent who is the identified client. Stressful events often disturb the equilibrium of the family system. Some families react by facing the challenge and adapting to it, which results in new ways of keeping the family system in balance. Other families find ways to avoid confronting the challenge in an effort to keep the status quo. These families often get "stuck" in familiar but dysfunctional ways of relating to one another and the external world.

Family therapists help family members look at a number of issues. They assess the family hierarchy, which defines power relationships among the members. They identify subsystems—groups of people within the family who join together to perform various functions—such as the parental or sibling subsystem. Therapists identify and discuss boundaries, which define the degree of emotional closeness among family members and subsystems (Wells, 1995).

The overall goals of family therapy are to:

- develop better parenting and nurturing skills
- reinstate generational boundaries in the family hierarchy
- assist adults to become more involved with each other
- decrease family reactions to symptoms to prevent inadvertent reinforcement of the problem

The Nursing Process

Assessment

The type of nursing assessment you conduct will depend on the child or adolescent's growth and developmental level. Observations of behavior and interactions with others may be the most important tool you will use. Play and art therapy techniques are often used in the assessment process. Family members must also be assessed if your data are to be accurate. Teachers often provide valuable data for a total assessment picture. Behavioral checklists from home and school are used in diagnosing ADHD. See the Focused Nursing Assessment table for general guidelines.

Diagnosis

Based on the assessment data, you will develop any number of nursing diagnoses for the individual child or adolescent as well as for the family. Some of the more common diagnoses are listed in the Nursing Diagnoses box.

Nursing Interventions

The accompanying box lists the nursing interventions classification (NIC) for children and adolescents.

Behavioral: Communication Enhancement

Active Listening

You may be wondering: How do I communicate therapeutically with a child or adolescent? What do I say? How can I get this person to talk to me? Start by asking yourself what you are feeling. In what context have you interacted with people in this age group before? What emotions does this child or teen stir up in you? What do you feel your role is when working with children or adolescents? Are you there to guide, direct, teach, advise, or protect? Answering these questions is the first step toward *communicating effectively* with children and adolescents.

Nursing Diagnoses

Children and Adolescents

Anxiety related to separation from parents; school phobia; unrealistic concerns over past behaviors and future events.

Fear of unfamiliar people and situations.

Impaired social interactions related to problems with peers; antisocial behavior.

Self-esteem disturbance related to low achievement in school; beliefs that others do not understand them; frequent criticism from others.

High risk for violence, directed at others, related to aggression; antisocial behavior.

High risk for violence, self-directed, related to poor impulse control leading to accidents; repetitive behavior such as head banging; suicide.

Impaired physical mobility related to unusual motor behaviors.

Altered thought processes related to loose association; poor concentration.

Impaired verbal communication related to an inability to formulate words; labile mood.

Altered family processes related to intensified parent-child conflict.

Rather than probing for details, listen for feelings. It is more important to help children learn how to interact effectively with you than to gather particulars. Children easily fall into superficially answering adults' questions and simply waiting for the next one. In this routine way, you set the pattern of a question-and-answer session. There are two problems with this pattern: The child will give you only short answers and not expand on the topic, and you will be frustrated when you run out of questions and haven't achieved any therapeutic purpose.

You will learn more by listening than by questioning. When you want information, use an open-ended format. For example, rather than asking, "Do you have friends?" say, "Tell me about the friends you like to do things with." Respect children's periods of silence. They may need this time to sort out thoughts and feelings and will be unable to do so if you bombard them with questions. Children soon dis-

Nursing Interventions Classification

CHILDREN AND ADOLESCENTS

DOMAIN: Behavioral

Class: *Communication Enhancement*

> **Interventions:** *Active Listening:* Attending closely to and attaching significance to a patient's verbal and nonverbal messages.
>
> *Socialization Enhancement:* Facilitation of another person's ability to interact with others.

Class: *Behavior Therapy*

> **Interventions:** *Play Therapy:* Purposeful use of toys or other equipment to assist a patient in communicating his/her perception of the world and to help in mastering the environment.
>
> *Art Therapy:* Facilitation of communication through drawings or other art forms.

Class: *Psychological Comfort Promotion*

> **Interventions:** *Simple Guided Imagery:* Purposeful use of imagination to achieve relaxation and/or direct attention away from undesirable sensations.

Class: *Coping Assistance*

> **Interventions:** *Self-Esteem Enhancement:* Assisting a patient to increase his/her personal judgment of self-worth.

Source: McCloskey and Bulechek, 1996.

---

cover whether or not you are a good listener. Some children do not respond to "talking" therapy because they have never experienced an adult really listening to them, they may not have been encouraged or allowed to express feelings, or they may not have the cognitive development to express their problems.

Children and adolescents recognize fake sentiments and insincere platitudes. They want to know that you are genuine, that you are trustworthy, and that your word is good. Explain what you expect of them and what they can expect from you. The clients you work with may have heard mixed messages throughout their lives and probably have learned to expect that adults make promises they do not keep. In working with young clients, you have an opportunity to model honest, adult behavior.

Socialization Enhancement

Social skills training (Bienert and Schneider, 1995) is beneficial for many children and adolescents with whom you will be working. The goal of social skills training is to increase the ability to negotiate stressful interpersonal situations with parents, peers, teachers, and others. Improving interpersonal skills helps alter negative self-perceptions. Skills include:

- self-expression skills
- using support systems
- seeing the perspective of others
- helping others
- assertiveness techniques such as peer-pressure resistance strategies
- social problem-solving techniques

Behavioral: Behavior Therapy

Play Therapy

Play therapy is especially helpful for children under 12 because their developmental level makes them less able to verbalize thoughts and feelings. You must establish

Text continues on page 496

Focused Nursing Assessment

CHILDREN AND ADOLESCENTS

Behavior Assessment	Affective Assessment	Cognitive Assessment
Do your friends comment that your behavior is in any way unusual?	Do your moods or feelings seem to change frequently?	How well do you think you are able to concentrate?
Do you see your behavior as being different from that of others your age?	Tell me what you worry about.	How difficult is it to get your attention?
Can you give me an example of ways you have gotten into trouble with your parents? Teachers? Other adults?	What kinds of fears do you experience?	Do others say they have trouble understanding you?
Have you been in trouble with the police?		

Social Assessment

Were there significant periods of time when you were separated from your parents?

Give me an example of the type of discipline used in the home.

Tell me how touch is used within the family.

Has there been increasing conflict with your parents or siblings?

Who do you get into physical fights with?

Are you having any problems with school? Attendance? Academic performance? Interactions with your friends?

Physiological Assessment

Do you have any problems moving around?

Have you had any changes in your eating patterns?

Have you had any changes in your sleeping patterns?

objectives for the use of play, as well as consider the age and needs of the child. Play therapy may be a one-to-one session, or it may be used with a group of children. The limits, discussed prior to the session, are that children are not allowed to hurt themselves or others, and they must not destroy any property. Within those limits, children are allowed to express any feelings and act out any of their experiences.

A typical play therapy room is equipped with a variety of toys and objects, including dolls of various sizes, shapes, and colors, a doll house, puppets, stuffed animals, clay, a sandbox, a sink for water play, toy cars and trucks, toy airplanes, blocks, soft balls, punching toys, soft foam bats, and magic markers or crayons. As you observe and interact with the children, you learn about family dynamics, conflicts, and traumas, as well as positive experiences and people in their life. Play therapy allows you to develop a sense of how each child perceives and experiences the world (Shirar, 1996).

The overall goals of play therapy are to:

- establish rapport with children
- reveal the feelings that children are unable to verbalize
- enable children to act out feelings of anxiety or tension in a constructive manner
- understand children's relationships and interactions with significant others in their lives
- teach adaptive socialization skills

Sand play is often used with children. It is a non-directive form of play therapy where the child is allowed to "play out" emotions and/or distressful situations in a sand box or sand tray. Being more directive, you can ask children to create a picture of anything they would like to and to put some toy animals or people in the scene. You then ask them to tell you about the picture, what is happening in the picture, how the people/animals feel, and what they would say if they could talk. You may wish to take a picture of the creation for future reference. Children need to be told that other children use the sand to express their feelings and so when they return, they will have a fresh box to express themselves. Otherwise, they will expect you to keep their "scene" exactly as they left it (Shirar, 1996).

Art Therapy

Art therapy is a way for children to express what is contained in the unconscious. You may ask them to draw or paint a picture themselves or tell you how to draw something. You may ask them to draw the family, draw themselves, draw feelings, draw what happened, draw a hero or an imaginary helper, or draw a nightmare. Art allows questions to be raised naturally. As children are engaged in creative art, you should observe them. Are they timid? worried about making mistakes? bold? haphazard? anxious or relaxed? Is the style small and neat or messy and careless? Art therapy provides information on how children perceive themselves and others and how they interact with significant people in their lives.

Behavioral: Psychological Comfort Promotion

Simple Guided Imagery

Guided imagery or *visualization* is an easily learned technique that can be used with children to facilitate coping and increase their sense of self-esteem. Children use their own imagination to create mental pictures using all the senses. It begins with a short relaxation exercise followed by general directions for the imagery. Children may imagine different ways of interacting with others, find heroes and heroines who will help them cope, or visualize themselves and their families as happy and joyful (Ott, 1996).

Behavioral: Coping Assistance

Self-Esteem Enhancement

Improving self-esteem is another goal of nursing interventions. You can provide opportunities for success. Praise and reinforce their behavior whenever possible. Focusing on positive characteristics and behaviors is often more helpful than focusing on limitations. Ask clients to draw up a list of all their strengths, for example: I am honest, I am a good friend, I can throw a ball, I can skip rope, I am a good big brother, and so on. You and your client can discuss this list and discover ways to use these characteristics in a positive manner. Another way to improve self-esteem is to allow children or teens to help someone else. The end result is usually that the helpers feel better about themselves.

Evaluation

In evaluating your nursing care, ask yourself if you have considered the child's or adolescent's cognitive level, emotional and social development, and physical abilities. Every client has unique characteristics and needs. Successfully meeting the outcome criteria depends on the individualization of standard intervention strategies.

Questions to guide the evaluation of the child or adolescent include the following:

1. Is the client exhibiting and verbalizing decreased anxiety?
2. Is the client interacting appropriately and safely with peers and adults?
3. Has the client's school performance improved?
4. Has the incidence of self-destructive behavior decreased?
5. Are the client's thoughts more coherent?
6. Is there less parent-child conflict?

Children and adolescents may have difficulty terminating the nurse-client relationship that lasts more than a short period of time. You may be one of the few adults in their lives who gives them undivided attention, honest communication, and respect. Plan the termination process in advance, and discuss it openly. Rehearse how they will react to problems in the future. Assure them that help is always available and that they are not being abandoned when the relationship ends.

Key Concepts

Introduction

- Although children and adolescents may experience some of the same mental disorders as adults, their symptoms are often determined by their developmental level. Other disorders may arise in childhood and continue on through adulthood.

Knowledge Base

- Like adults with OCD, the child with OCD tries to hide symptoms from others.

- Younger children with PTSD may repeatedly act out specific themes of the trauma.

- GAD is characterized by unrealistic concerns over past behavior, future events, and personal competency.

- Social phobia is a persistent fear of such things as formal speaking, eating in front of others, using public restrooms, or speaking to authorities.

- Separation anxiety is more common in children than in adolescents. The child may need to remain close to the parent, and their worries focus on separation themes.

- Selective mutism is the steady failure to speak in specific social situations where speaking is expected.

- Depression in infants may be exhibited with a frozen facial expression, weepy and withdrawn behavior, weight loss, and an increased incidence of infections.

- Depressed toddlers may appear sad or expressionless, experience delays or regression in developmental skills, become apathetic or more clingy, and have an increase in nightmares.

- Depressed preschoolers may have a loss of interest in newly acquired skills, make frequent negative self-statements and have thoughts of self-harm, or experience enuresis, encopresis, anorexia, or binge eating.

- School-age children who are depressed may have problems with depressed, irritable, or aggressive moods, academic difficulties, eating and sleeping disturbances, self-criticism, and suicidal ideation and plans.

- Adolescents who are depressed exhibit antisocial behavior, aggression, intense labile moods, difficulties at school, withdrawal, hypersomnia, and very low self-esteem.

- Seasonal affective disorder is more frequent after puberty, especially in girls.

- Bipolar disorder is frequently misdiagnosed as ADHD, conduct disorder, or schizophrenia when it occurs in adolescents.

- Children with ADHD have impulsive behavior and seek immediate gratification. Their emotions are labile, and they have difficulty maintaining interpersonal relationships. They have an extremely short attention span, which may be accompanied by learning disabilities.

- The exact cause of ADHD is unknown but it likely involves genetic factors, anatomical abnormalities, neurotransmission problems, and environmental factors.

- Children with ODD are disruptive, argumentative, hostile, and irritable. They have social problems with peers and adults and impaired academic functioning.

- Children with CD engage in antisocial behavior that violates the rights of others: physical aggression, cruelty, stealing, robbing, arson. Relationships with peers and adults are manipulative and used for personal advantage.

- Adolescent substance abuse may be related to genetic factors, parental modeling, teen rebellion, and self-medication to manage family dysfunction or symptoms of mental disorders.

- Children with AD spend hours in repetitive behavior, have bizarre motor and stereotypical behaviors, have severely impaired communication, and are often mentally retarded.

- Tic disorders involve sudden, rapid, recurrent, stereotyped movements or sounds.

- Child and adolescent onset disorders often have two or three other disorders going on at the same time.

Psychopharmacological Interventions

- Children suffering from major depression may be prescribed Elavil (amitriptyline), Tofranil (imipramine), Aventyl (nortriptyline), Effexor (venlafaxine), and Wellbutrin (bupropion). Lithium and Tegretol (carbamazepine) are combined in managing symptoms of bipolar disorder.

- Children experiencing ADHD may be prescribed Ritalin (methylphenidate), Dexedrine (dextroamphetamine), or Cylert (pemoline).

Multidisciplinary Interventions

- Play therapy is used to establish rapport with children, reveal feelings they are unable to verbalize, enable them to act out their feelings in a constructive manner, understand their relationships and interactions with others, and teach adaptive socialization skills.

- Group therapy gives children and adolescents the opportunity to learn to talk openly about themselves, practice active listening, give and receive feedback, learn to help others, and learn new ways of relating to others.

- Parents may be involved in a parallel group to learn growth and development stages, give and receive support, increase parenting skills, and explore their own needs and problems.

- Art therapy is a way for children to express what is contained in the unconscious.

- Guided imagery or visualization can facilitate coping and increase sense of self-esteem.

- Behavior modification identifies behaviors that are unacceptable, those that are acceptable, and consequences for undesirable behaviors.

- Community-based programs to improve the mental health of children and adolescents include adult mentor plans, youth organizations, and peer-helping programs.

- Family therapy can facilitate healthy functioning in the family.

Nursing Assessment

- Both the individual child or adolescent and the family members must be assessed according to growth and developmental levels.

Nursing Diagnosis

- Nursing diagnoses include *Anxiety, Fear, Impaired social interactions, Self-esteem disturbance, High risk for violence, Impaired physical mobility, Altered thought processes, Impaired verbal communication,* and *Altered family processes.*

Nursing Interventions

- Avoid asking multiple questions of children and adolescents. They respond better to active listening and undivided attention.

- Focusing on positive characteristics and behaviors will help clients improve their self-esteem.

- Social skills training includes self-expression skills, using support systems, seeing the perspective of others, helping others, assertiveness techniques, and social problem-solving techniques.

- Through the use of problem solving, older children and adolescents can locate information, design solutions, predict consequences, implement strategies, and confirm the outcomes.

- Homework assignments increase clients' active participation in the therapeutic process.

Evaluation

- Successfully meeting the outcome criteria depends on individualizing strategies according to cognitive level, emotional and social development, and physical abilities.

- Plan and discuss termination of the nurse-client relationship in advance.

Review Questions

1. Through your nursing assessment you have determined that Tanya has a social phobia. Which of the following behaviors supports your analysis? Tanya

   a. refuses to speak outside the home.

   b. is unable to eat in front of others.

   c. constantly is straightening and touching objects.

   d. acts out the theme of her fears.

2. Dick, age 14, has been diagnosed with bipolar disorder. You would expect to see which of the following problems?

   a. intense mood swings lasting only 1–2 hours

   b. inflated self-esteem

   c. spending sprees or sexual acting-out

   d. fire setting or gang behavior

3. Darryl is 3 years old and has been diagnosed with attention deficit/hyperactivity disorder. Which medication is most likely to be prescribed?

   a. Elavil (amitriptyline)

   b. Dexedrine (dextroamphetamine)

   c. Ritalin (methylphenidate)

   d. Cylert (pemoline)

4. One of the outcomes of play therapy is to enable children to

   a. act out feelings in a constructive manner.

   b. learn to talk openly about themselves.

   c. learn how to give and receive feedback.

   d. learn problem-solving skills.

5. Community-based, peer-helping programs provide adolescents with

   a. recreational activities.

   b. career-oriented activities.

   c. problem-solving practice skills.

   d. the opportunity to help others.

References

American Psychiatric Association. (1994). *Diagnostic and Statistical Manual of Mental Disorders,* 4th ed. Washington, D.C.: APA.

Bienert, H., & Schneider, B. (1995). Deficit-specific social skills training with peer-nominated aggressive-disruptive and sensitive-isolated preadolescents. *J Clin Child Psych, 24*(2), 287–299.

Black, B. (1995). Separation anxiety and panic disorder. In J. S. March (Ed.), *Anxiety Disorders in Children and Adolescents* (pp. 212–234). New York: Guilford Press.

Boris, M., & Mandel, F. S. (1994). Foods and additives are common causes of attention deficit hyperactive disorder in children. *Ann Allergy, 72*(5), 462–468.

Brage, D. G. (1995). Adolescent depression: A review of the literature. *Arch Psychiatr Nurs, 9*(1), 45–55.

Brown, A. (1996, Winter). Mood disorders in children and adolescents. *NARSD Research Newsletter,* pp. 11–14.

Ciaranello, R. D. (1996). Linkage and molecular genetics of infantile autism. In S. J. Watson (Ed.), *Biology of Schizophrenia and Affective Disease* (pp. 129–161). Washington, D.C.: American Psychiatric Press.

Costello, E. J., & Angold, A. (1995). Epidemiology. In J. S. March (Ed.), *Anxiety Disorders in Children and Adolescents* (pp.109–124). New York: Guilford Press.

Emslie, G. J. (1997). Children and depression. *Treatment Today, 9*(2), 10–11.

Goldstein, S., & Goldstein, M. (1992). *Hyperactivity.* New York: Wiley.

Goodyer, I. M. (1995). The epidemiology of depression in childhood and adolescence. In F. C. Verhulst & H. M. Koot (Eds.), *The Epidemiology of Child and Adolescent Psychopathology* (pp. 210–226). New York: Oxford Univ. Press.

Hartman, T. (1993). *Attention Deficit Disorder: A Different Perception.* Underwood Books.

Haznedar, M. M., et al. (1997). Anterior cingulate gyrus volume and glucose metabolism in autistic disorder. *Am J Psychiatry, 154*(8), 1047–1056.

Hedaya, R. J. (1996). *Understanding Biological Psychiatry.* New York: Norton.

Insel, T. R. (1997). A neurobiological basis of social attachment. *Am J Psychiatry, 154*(6), 726–735.

Johnston, H. F., & Fruehling, J. J. (1996). Bipolar disorders in children: A research update. *NAMI Advocate, 18*(1), 13–14.

Kazdin, A. E. (1995). Conduct disorder. In F. C. Verhulst & H. M. Koot (Eds.), *The Epidemiology of Child and Adolescent Psychopathology* (pp. 258–290). New York: Oxford Univ. Press.

Leonard, H., & Dow, D. (1995). Selective mutism. In J. S. March (Ed.), *Anxiety Disorders in Children and Adolescents* (pp. 235–250). New York: Guilford Press.

March, J. S. (Ed.). (1995). *Anxiety and Disorders in Children and Adolescents.* New York: Guilford Press.

Margolis, R. (1995). Adolescent chemical dependency. In A. M. Washton (Ed.), *Psychotherapy and Substance Abuse.* New York: Guilford Press.

McCloskey, J. C., & Bulechek, G. M. (Eds.). (1996). *Nursing Intervention Classification (NIC),* 2nd ed. St. Louis, MO: Mosby.

Milberger, S., et al. (1996). Is maternal smoking during pregnancy a risk factor for attention deficit hyperactivity disorder in children? *Am J Psychiatry, 153(9),* 1138–1142.

Ott, M. (1996). Imagine the possibilities: Guided imagery with toddlers and pre-schoolers. *Pediatr Nurs, 22(1),* 34–38.

Roberts, M. (1995). *Handbook of Pediatric Psychiatry* (2nd ed.). New York: Guilford Press.

Sherman, D. K., et al. (1997). Twin concordance for attention deficit hyperactivity disorder. *Am J Psychiatry, 154(4),* 532–535.

Shirar, L. (1996). *Dissociative Children.* New York: Norton.

Speier, P. L., et al. (1995). Depression in children and adolescents. In E. E. Beckham & W. R. Leber (Eds.), *Handbook of Depression* (2nd ed.) (pp. 467–493). New York: Guilford Press.

Swedo, S. E., et al. (1995). Rates of seasonal affective disorder in children and adolescent. *Am J Psychiatry, 152(7),* 1016–1019.

Sylvester, C., & Nageotte, C. (1993). Disorders in children. In D. Dunner (Ed.). *Current Psyciatric Therapy.* (pp. 421–426). Philadelphia: Saunders.

Wells, K. C. (1995). Family therapy. In J. S. March (Ed.), *Anxiety Disorders in Children and Adolescents.* (pp. 401–419). New York: Guilford Press.

Wilens, T. E. (1997). Brain disorders in children. *NAMI Advocate, 18(5),* 11–12.

Wilens, T. E., et al. (1996). Six-week, double-blind, placebo-controlled study of desipramine for adult attention deficit hyperactivity disorder. *Am J Psychiatry, 153(9),* 1147–1153.

Zealberg, J. J., & Santos, A. B. (1996). *Comprehensive Emergency Mental Health Care.* New York: Norton.

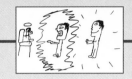

CHAPTER 21

Disorders of Older Adults

Karen Lee Fontaine

Objectives

After reading this chapter, you will be able to:

- Differentiate among the mental disorders that occur in older adults.
- Describe the use of medications in older adults.
- Design interventions specific to older adults.

Key Terms

ageism
pseudodementia

Over 13% of the American population is 65 years or older, and those over 85 make up the fastest-growing group. By the year 2030, older adults will comprise 22% of the U.S. population. In addition to medical care, older adults need mental health services. Studies indicate that 15–25% of older adults living in the community have symptoms of mental disorders. The prevalence rate escalates greatly among those who are in acute and long-term care settings. There has been an unfortunate lack of mental health care for this group of consumers related to hesitancy of the older population in seeking out psychiatric care, ageism, and lack of education for professionals in geriatric mental health (Bucholz et al, 1995; Rossen and Buschmann, 1995).

Although we actually begin to age from the moment of conception, we don't become aware of the effects of the aging process until mid-life and late adulthood. Older adults are confronted with many changes. In addition to physical illness, they experience sociocultural changes from alteration in self-concept, social roles, family support, occupational identity, and perhaps income. Loss is a predominant theme in many of their lives. In addition to this chapter, you will also find information on mental health issues and older adults in Chapters 15 (Cognitive Impairment Disorders), 16 (Grief and Loss), 17 (Suicide), and 18 (Domestic Violence).

Knowledge Base

Anxiety Disorders

Almost 20% of the population over 65 years experience significant anxiety. Panic attacks and phobic disorder often begin earlier in life and continue on in the older years, especially when those affected have received no treatment. Those who develop late-onset panic attacks, after age 55, have less avoidance behavior than person with early-onset panic attacks. Phobias remain quite common in later life. Sleep disturbances are common in persons with anxiety. Many have difficulty in getting to sleep and staying asleep, and have poor quality of sleep (Sheikh, 1994).

Anxiety is often associated with medical illness. The symptoms of cardiovascular disease, such as angina pectoris and myocardial infarction, may simulate panic attacks. Medications such as cold and allergy drugs, amphetamines, bronchodilators, and some calcium channel blockers may produce anxiety-like symptoms. Akathisia, a side effect of antipsychotic agents, is often indistinguishable from anxiety. Alcohol withdrawal and sedative/hypnotic withdrawal produce high levels of anxiety. There is a high prevalence of anxiety disorders in persons with Parkinson's disease. In addition, the medications used to treat Parkinson's may themselves cause anxiety. Often people suffering from dementing disorders experience concomitant anxiety (Sheikh, 1994).

Mood Disorders

Depression is the most common and troublesome mental disorder among older adults, who are at higher risk because of changes in self-concept and the multiple losses they have likely experienced. Many older people have an increase in stressful life events at the very time when they may have limited resources for managing such difficult circumstances. The more that stressful life events occur, the more their sense of helplessness becomes reinforced. If they reach the point of believing they have no control, they lose the will and the energy to cope with life, and depression frequently results.

Although depression is common, it may not be recognized and is frequently undertreated because health care professionals mistakenly view it as a "natural" part of aging. The consequences of this ageism include poor quality of life, cognitive impairment, nursing home placement, and increased risk of death by suicide. Of the older people living in the United States, about 4–15% are significantly depressed. For those living in residential care, the rate of depression is 15–20%. Some studies report that older adults experience symptoms of depression similar to those of younger adults. Other studies indicate that older people experience symptoms related to anxiety and somatic complaints rather than feelings of sadness. Older people with depression may exhibit signs of cognitive impairment leading to incorrect diagnoses of dementia. Symptoms include short-term memory problems, word-finding difficulty, confusion, and disorientation. Depression that simulates dementia is referred to as **pseudodementia.** This form of depression must be recognized and differentiated from irreversible dementia, and appropriate treatment measures must be implemented (Alexopoulos et al, 1996; Lebowitz, 1997; Reynolds et al, 1996).

People who have Parkinson's disease have a 35–50% chance of also having a major depression. Often the mood symptoms precede the motor changes, which suggests that the depression is not merely a reaction to the physiological changes of Parkinson's disease. Compared to other people with depression, these individuals are less guilty but more pessimistic, and have higher anxiety levels and more cognitive deficits (McGuire and Rabins, 1994).

Of people who have had a cerebral vascular accident, 20% experience depression with more symptoms of anxiety and cognitive impairment than is typical for people who become depressed after other medical diagnoses. Depression is more common with left hemisphere stroke, especially when located close to the frontal lobe. Other disorders contributing to depression include hypothyroidism, alcoholism, hypoglycemia, and multiple sclerosis (Alexopoulos, 1997; McGuire and Rabins, 1994).

While late-life depression can result from medical illness, it can also cause or magnify the effects of medical illnesses. For example, studies suggest that depression can accelerate osteoporosis in older women; it is also associated with increased incidence of heart attacks (Katz, 1997).

Bipolar disorder accounts for 5–10% of all mood disorders treated in the older population. Only a few of these individuals become ill for the first time after age 50. The cause of late-onset bipolar disorder is often a neurological disease. One common precipitant is a cerebral vascular accident in the right hemisphere affecting the limbic system. Other causes include hyperthyroidism; epilepsy; trauma; and degenerative, vascular, or neoplastic disease of the right hemisphere. Medications that produce manic symptoms include adrenal steroids, levodopa, antidepressants, bronchodilators, and decongestants (Devons, 1996; McGuire and Rabing, 1994).

Schizophrenia

Of older adults with schizophrenia, the majority have had the disorder since they were young. A number of these people show substantial improvement in symptoms, especially the positive characteristics, over the course of their lifetimes. Twenty-three percent of people with schizophrenia have a late-onset type, which occurs after age 45 and affects more women then men. The clinical picture is somewhat different than in early-onset schizophrenia. People with late-onset schizophrenia have more delusions, which are often persecutory and bizarre. They are more likely to exhibit vivid hallucinations but have fewer cognitive disruptions and negative characteristics compared to people with early-onset schizophrenia. Sensory impairment, such as hearing loss or cataracts, may increase the severity of the symptoms since environmental stimuli are often misinterpreted. In addition, people with hearing and vision loss tend to decrease social contacts and become socially isolated, which may increase suspicious thoughts. Medications are often effective, but lack of insight and suspiciousness can contribute to noncompliance (Finlayson, 1995; Pearlson and Petty, 1994).

Substance Use Disorders

Illicit drug use, such as cocaine or opiates, is unusual in older adults. However, alcohol abuse is a problem for 10–15% of older adults. Often they go undiagnosed because in old age the symptoms can be subtle or atypical, or mimic symptoms of other geriatric illnesses. Clients may present with erratic changes in mood or behavior; malnutrition; bladder and bowel incontinence; gait disorders; and recurring falls, burns, or head trauma. Older adults have less social, legal, occupational, and interpersonal consequences of their alcohol abuse because they are often not working and often live alone. Two-thirds of this group have had long-standing problems with alcohol and have multiple medical complications. One-third develop the drinking problem late in life, often in response to bereavement, retirement, loneliness, relationship stress, and physical illnesses. Denial of substance abuse is common at all ages but may be more intense in older adults because of memory problems and the shame-based belief of this generation that substance abuse is immoral (Atkinson and Ganzini, 1994; Zimberg, 1995).

Abuse of prescription drugs among the elderly is two to three times higher than the general population. Benzodiazepine dependence is most common and may have been prescribed for long periods of time. Of individuals who have a history of long-term use (more than one year), 70% are over the age of 50 and often have physical health problems. Among older people who are institutionalized, the abuse is even more widespread. Benzodiazepine abuse in the elderly results in excessive daytime sedation, ataxia which increases the risk of falls and accidents, and cognitive impairments such as attention and memory problems (Atkinson and Ganzini, 1994; Finlayson, 1995).

Culture-Specific Characteristics

By the year 2025 there will be 1 billion aged persons in the world, double the number in 1990. Of these, 72% will be living in "developing" countries. This population explosion means there will be an inevitable increase in age-related mental disorders such as dementias. Older persons with physical disorders often suffer mental distress when they lose self-esteem and independence. Social structures and values that once ensured care for the elderly are changing. Economic changes have made the inheritance of agricultural land or animals less valuable, resulting in loss of respect and care of older persons. The majority of migrants to the city are in their reproductive years, so the villages are populated predominantly by the elderly and very young, resulting in isolation and lack of adequate care. When the young are formally educated and their parents and grandparents are not, the young may not value the cultural traditions and customs. The potential mental health outcomes of these changes are increased depression, feelings of worthlessness, increased loneliness, and increased rates of substance abuse and suicide (Desjarlais et al, 1995).

Causative Theories

Neurobiological Theory

Genetic factors are significant for mood disorders among older persons. Twin and family studies indicate that the risk for first-degree relatives of people with bipolar disorder is four times higher than the general population. About 30% of the cases of depression are thought to have a genetic link. There are also age-related changes in neurochemisty. As we

age we have a decreased concentration of norepinephrine, dopamine, and serotonin. There is also a corresponding increase in monoamine oxidase, the enzyme involved in the breakdown of neurotransmitters. Structural changes contributing to depression include lowered frontal lobe volume and larger ventricular-brain ratios (Futterman et al, 1995; Katz, 1997; Rossen and Buschmann, 1995).

Psychosocial Factors

Self-concept is an organized set of thoughts about characteristics of the self: our beliefs about the type of person we are, how we relate to others, and our significance in our family and in the world at large. The many physical changes, social encounters, and psychological influences that occur with aging may be a threat to one's self-concept. The older person's self-definition also involves searching for the meaning of life and the meaning of death.

Self-concept is challenged when older people become victims of ageism. **Ageism** is a process of systematic stereotyping of and discriminating against older people simply on the basis of their age. Ageist attitudes categorize older adults as unnecessary and burdensome. Ageism is perpetuated whenever older people have diminished social status and reduced contact with younger people. It is maintained by people believing many myths about aging. Box 21.1 contrasts the fictions and the facts. (For a comparison of ageism with other forms of discrimination such as racism and sexism, see Chapter 3.)

Negative stereotypes hold that cognitive functioning in older adults is impaired. These stereotypes include the belief that, with age, thinking and problem-solving abilities become rigid, judgment is compromised, learning capacity is reduced, memory lapses are frequent, and severe mental confusion is inevitable. In fact, such stereotypical notions may be an accurate portrayal of the cognitive functioning of only 10–15% of the older adult population.

American culture is a youth-oriented culture. Old age is often portrayed solely as a time of dependency and disease. Movies, books, magazines, television, and jokes contribute to negative beliefs and attitudes about aging. Older people are viewed as asexual and physically unattractive. When they believe these stereotypes, they find themselves feeling helpless, hopeless, and depressed.

Box 21.1

Ageism: Fiction or Fact?

Fiction: Most older people are placed in institutions.

Fact: Only 5% are in institutions; 66% live in a family setting and 29% live alone.

Fiction: Old age brings senility and feeblemindedness.

Fact: Only 5% show serious mental impairment; only 10% suffer from mild to moderate memory loss.

Fiction: Older people cannot learn.

Fact: Learning is not impaired, though a longer period of time may be needed to respond to stimuli.

Fiction: All old people are similar.

Fact: There is a great deal of diversity in personalities, motivations, physical abilities, lifestyles, and economics among older adults.

Fiction: The next generation of older adults will be the same as the present generation.

Fact: The next generation will have more formal education and healthier lifestyle habits, be more youthful in appearance, have access to more technology, and be more assertive in its communication style.

Sources: Coffey and Cummings, 1994; Beresford and Gromberg, 1995.

Psychopharmacological Interventions

When administering any medication to older clients, you need to be aware of age-related physiological changes in absorption, distribution, and excretion of drugs. These changes can make older people especially prone to toxic effects, even at average dose ranges for the general population. Older people are also more sensitive to the side effects of psychotropic medications, especially sedation, psychomotor impairment, orthostatic hypotension, and anticholinergic side effects.

Short-acting benzodiazepines like Ativan (lorazepam) and Serax (oxazepam) are preferable in older clients. People with dementia, cerebellar disease, or psychomotor impairment may tolerate these drugs poorly. The preferred alternative is BuSpar (buspirone), which is nonaddictive, does not impair cognition or psychomotor function, and does not produce withdrawal symptoms.

Antidepressants are typically given in low doses and the dosage is increased very slowly. Tricyclic antidepressants are known to be effective in older clients, but they have side effects such as abnormalities of cardiac conduction and orthostatic hypotension that must be considered. Orthostatic hypotension is associated with increased falls, resulting in hip fractures and other injuries in older people. It is best to use tricyclics that are less sedating and less anticholinergic, such as Norpramin/Pertofrane (desipramine) or Aventyl/Pamelor (nortriptyline) with the older population.

The SSRIs have a much lower incidence of these troubling side effects. Drugs in this category include Prozac (fluoxetine), Paxil (paroxetine), Luvox (fluoxetine), Remeron (mirtzazpine), and Zoloft (sertraline). Their short half-lives make them especially useful for older people. The side effects most disturbing to older clients are nausea, insomnia, and restlessness. The newer SNRIs, Serzone (nefazodone), Effexor (venlafaxine), and Wellbutrin (bupropion), are also effective with older people; the main side effects are sedation and increased appetite (Harris, 1997).

Older persons are more vulnerable to the toxic effects of lithium. Renal function decreases as people age, and renal impairment leads to lithium accumulation. The cognitive changes of lithium toxicity may be mistaken for dementia in older people.

Some evidence suggests that psychostimulants may be helpful for older depressed clients who also have physical illnesses. Stimulants are especially helpful to those who are apathetic and unmotivated. Ritalin (methylphenidate) is the preferred stimulant for use in the older population and may be used alone or in combination with antidepressants.

Antipsychotic medications are effective for people with schizophrenia, bipolar disorder, and psychotic depression. They are frequently prescribed for older agitated clients or those experiencing behavioral problems associated with dementia. Side effects such as orthostatic hypotension, sedation, and memory impairment can be significant in this population.

Multidisciplinary Interventions

Physical restraints are applied in attempts to control behavior and maintain safety for older adults in residential or institutional settings. However, significant problems are associated with the use of restraints, such as increased agitation, confusion, incontinence, pressure sores, infections, feelings of anger and fear, and even death from accidental strangulation. In 1987 the Nursing Home Reform Law was enacted with the goal of reducing or eliminating physical restraint use in nursing homes and acute care hospitals. As facilities move toward restraint-free care, studies demonstrate increased staff interaction with residents, higher staff productivity, decreased resident agitation and drug administration, and fewer incident reports. Box 21.2 lists alternative measures to restraints (Mahoney, 1995; Sullivan-Marx, 1995).

Electroconvulsive therapy (ECT) is highly successful for the treatment of mood disorders, with a rapid therapeutic onset and a remarkable safety record. It is often the second treatment of choice when medications have not been effective or when the side effects are too severe. Antidepressants are 62% effective while ECT is 81% effective. ECT may be the first treatment choice in certain situations such as suicidality, severe malnutrition, medical contradictions to antidepressants, previous response to ECT, and client preference. ECT is also effective in depression associated with dementias, Parkinson's disease, and cerebral vascular accidents. Older people have more severe disorientation immediately after ECT; this usually clears in one to two hours (Butler and Lewis, 1995; Pritchett, Keller, and Coffey, 1994).

The Nursing Process

Assessment

Assessment of actual and potential problems with older clients requires an accurate perception of the situation from their viewpoint. Family or significant others should be asked for their perception and views. Because depression may exhibit as a pseudodementia, carefully assess mental status to differenti-

Box 21.2

Alternative Interventions to Restraints

Medications for pain relief

Recliners, chairs with deep seats, rockers

Sensory stimulation

Reality orientation

Structured daily routines

Physical exercise alternated with rest periods

Mattress on very low bed

Removal of unsafe obstacles to walking

Door alarms

Keypad locks for exit doors

Enclosed courtyards

Sources: Mahoney, 1995; Sullivan-Marx, 1995.

ate between dementia, delirium, and depression. Refer to Chapter 15 for assessment of cognitive disorders. Assess clients' ability to hear, since an undiagnosed hearing impairment could artificially increase your perception of psychopathology. The person who does not hear your questions may give incorrect or bizarre responses. Take an inventory of all current medications that clients are taking, since their difficulties may be related to polydrug intake.

Assessment includes determination of clients' functional abilities. Determine their ability to accomplish physical activities of daily living (ADLs) such as bathing, grooming, toileting, eating, and ambulating. Assess their abilities to do instrumental ADLs such as shopping, meal preparation, managing finances, housekeeping, using the telephone, and taking medications. The Focused Nursing Assessment table provides guidelines for the types of assessment questions to use with older adults.

Diagnosis

Nursing diagnoses are formulated on the basis of your assessment data. These diagnoses may be related to the behavioral, affective, cognitive, social, and physiological changes that have occurred with aging and life change events. The Nursing Diagnoses box lists some of the possible nursing diagnoses appropriate for older adults living in the community or in a residential setting.

Nursing Interventions

Ageism influences the attitudes of health care professionals and decision makers regarding the care of older adults. No matter what your clinical setting, you can combat subtle and overt ageism. Do not use chronological age to determine the type of care clients receive. Help both younger and older people modify their expectations, attitudes, beliefs, and feelings toward older adults in our culture. The box on page 510 lists the nursing interventions classification (NIC) for older clients experiencing mental disorders.

Physiological: Basic: Self-Care Facilitation

Self-Care Assistance
Some clients may need adaptive devices for personal hygiene, dressing, grooming, toileting, and eating. Help them establish a routine for self-care and provide only as much assistance as they need. Encourage clients to perform normal activities of daily living to the level of their ability. Families may need to be taught ways to provide appropriate assistance without forcing their loved ones into unnecessary dependence.

Behavioral: Behavior Therapy

Activity Therapy
Collaborate with occupational, physical, and/or recreational therapists, if appropriate, in planning and monitoring an activity program. Discover what are meaningful activities for each individual as well as their preferences for activities. Help them choose activities consistent with their physical, psychological, and social capabilities. Focus on skills they have rather than on deficits. Discuss with clients the scheduling of specific periods for diversional activity into their daily routine. Help them identify needed resources and to obtain transportation, as appropriate. Refer to community centers or activity programs. Instruct clients and families regarding the role of physical, social, spiritual, and cognitive activity in maintaining physical function and health and mental well-being.

Nursing Diagnoses

Older Adults

Altered role performance related to decreased strength and health changes.

Altered sexuality patterns related to nonacceptance of body image; loss of partner.

Body image disturbance related to multiple physiological losses.

Family coping, potential for growth, related to acceptance of wisdom and insight of older adults.

Family coping, potential for growth, related to finding satisfactory relationships with children, grandchildren, or other younger adults.

Fear related to the inevitability of mortality.

Hopelessness related to isolation from significant others.

Impaired adjustment related to retirement from active work responsibilities; nonsupportive relationships with significant others.

Ineffective individual coping related to unsuccessful attempts at forming a philosophy of life; multiple losses.

Powerlessness related to inadequate finances and economic burdens; inadequate societal provisions for older adults.

Self-esteem disturbance related to a lack of acceptance of the retirement role; continuous feelings of despair.

Spiritual distress related to the inability to find meaning in life; hopelessness and despair in the life review.

Substance Use Treatment
Chapter 13 covers interventions for clients with substance use disorders. Most older adults still resist referral to chemical dependency programs and are more comfortable in senior-oriented programs. In addition, a significant number of older people are unable or unwilling to leave their homes. Thus, programs must be specifically designed for older adults, including community outreach, home visitation, and social services. Alcohol problems should be presented to them in the context of problems of adjusting to aging.

Text continues on page 510

Focused Nursing Assessment

OLDER ADULTS

Behavior Assessment	Affective Assessment	Cognitive Assessment
What leisure and social activities do you participate in?	What do you worry about?	Describe how you feel about yourself in general.
What are your living arrangements? Independent? With family? Retirement center? Nursing home?	In what situations do you feel helpless? Hopeless? Anxious? Suspicious? Angry?	Are there any recent changes in your self-concept?
How well are you able to manage ADLs?	Do you have significant periods of loneliness?	How well are you able to make decisions? Solve problems?
In what way do you need assistance with ADLs?		Has there been any change in your attention span?
Have you experienced any recent changes in behavior?		How well are you able to communicate with others?
		Are you having any problems with memory?

Social Assessment

Describe your life in general, including both joyful and painful experiences.

What kinds of changes have you had to make in your lifestyle?

What social roles are you able to maintain?

Are you experiencing financial distress?

Describe the available support you have from family and friends.

Physiological Assessment

How physically active are you? Is this activity tiring?

Do you have any vision loss?

Do you have any hearing loss?

What chronic illnesses do you have?

Do you have any disabilities?

Are you experiencing pain?

Do you have any specific somatic complaints?

Have you had any changes in sleeping patterns?

Have you had any changes in eating patterns?

What medications, prescribed and OTC, are you taking?

Nursing Interventions Classification

OLDER CLIENTS WITH MENTAL DISORDERS

DOMAIN: Physiological: Basic
Class: *Self-Care Facilitation*
    Interventions: *Self-Care Assistance:* Assisting another person to perform activities of daily living.

DOMAIN: Behavioral
Class: *Behavior Therapy*
    Interventions: *Activity Therapy:* Prescription of and assistance with specific physical, cognitive, social, and spiritual activities to increase the range, frequency, or duration of an individual's (or group's) activity.
    Substance Use Treatment: Supportive care of patient/family members with physical and psychosocial problems associated with the use of alcohol or drugs.

Class: *Cognitive Therapy*
    Interventions: *Reminiscence Therapy:* Using the recall of past events, feelings, and thoughts to facilitate adaptation to present circumstances.

Class: *Communication Enhancement*
    Interventions: *Communication Enhancement: Hearing Deficit:* Assistance in accepting and learning alternative methods for living with diminished hearing.
    Socialization Enhancement: Facilitation of another person's ability to interact with others.

They may need special approaches such as slow-paced therapy and emotionally supportive therapy rather than the confrontive style used with younger adults. Social bonding with age peers often improves outcomes (Atkinson, 1995).

Behavioral: Cognitive Therapy

Reminiscence Therapy

Reminiscence is a guided recollection where clients are encouraged to remember the past and share their memories with either family, peers, or staff. Reminiscence focuses on strengths and does not encourage people to dwell on losses. It can raise self-esteem and increase social intimacy. When doing this, choose a comfortable setting and set aside adequate time. Encourage verbal expression of feelings of past events. Comment on the feelings that accompany the memories in an empathic manner. Use direct questions to refocus back to life events, if clients digress. Encourage clients to write about past events such as

traditional values, wisdom, and lessons learned (McCloskey and Bulechek, 1996).

By encouraging older adults to tell you about their lives, you can learn about where they have been and where they would like to go. In listening, you will learn about hope, grief, achievement, and loss. It is a way you can communicate caring while helping them maintain their sense of identity (Hirst and McKiel, 1997).

Behavioral: Communication Enhancement

Communication Enhancement: Hearing Deficit

It may be necessary to suggest a hearing examination if you suspect there is a hearing deficit. Discuss resources for hearing aids and telephones for the hearing impaired. Listen attentively, speak clearly, and refrain from shouting at people who have hearing deficits. Do not cover your mouth, talk with a full mouth, or chew gum when speaking. Use paper, pencil, or computer communication when necessary (McCloskey and Bulechek, 1996).

Socialization Enhancement

Maintaining social relationships is essential for the quality of life and mental health of older people. You can encourage clients to continue their involvement in already-established relationships as well as developing new relationships with people who have common interests and goals. Assist clients in finding meaningful social and community activities, remembering that the needs for support, belonging, self-expression and self-esteem can be met through social relationships (Cromwell and Phillips, 1995; McCloskey and Bulechek, 1996).

Evaluation

Evaluation of the outcome of specified interventions is the final stage of the nursing process. Successful outcomes of the nursing care of older adults include:

- satisfaction with home and leisure activities
- improved self-esteem
- improved communication with others
- improved social interactions
- finding meaning in life and death

Key Concepts

Introduction

- Studies indicate that 15–25% of older adults living in the community have symptoms of mental disorders.
- In addition to physical illness, older adults experience sociocultural changes from alterations in self-concept, social roles, family support, occupational identity, and perhaps income.

Knowledge Base

- Almost 20% of the population over 65 years experience significant anxiety which may be related to anxiety disorders or to medical illnesses.
- Although depression is common, it may not be recognized in older adults and may be confused with dementia.
- People with Parkinson's disease and cerebral vascular accidents are at risk for a concurrent depression.
- Most older adults who have schizophrenia developed the disorder when they were younger.
- Alcohol abuse is a problem for 10–15% of older adults and it is often undiagnosed.
- Benzodiazepine dependence results in excessive daytime sedation; ataxia, which increases the risk of falls and accidents; and cognitive impairments such as attention and memory problems.
- The population explosion of older adults means there is an inevitable increase in age-related mental disorders such as dementias.

- Aging causes a decrease in a number of neurotransmitters, which may be a factor in mood disorders among older adults.
- Ageism contributes to the incidence of depression among older people.

Psychopharmacological Interventions

- Older people are more prone to the side effects and toxic effects of many medications.

Multidisciplinary Interventions

- Physical restraints increase agitation, confusion, incontinence, pressure sores, feelings of anger and fear, and even death from accidental strangulation.
- ECT is highly successful for the treatment of mood disorders among older adults.

Nursing Assessment

- Carefully assess clients to differentiate between dementia, delirium, and depression.
- Clients who are hearing-impaired may give incorrect or bizarre responses when they do not hear questions.
- Assess for clients' ability to accomplish physical and instrumental activities of daily living.

Nursing Diagnosis

- Nursing diagnoses are related to the behavioral, affective, cognitive, sociocultural, and physiological changes that occur with aging and life events.

Nursing Interventions

- Help clients establish a routine for self-care and provide only as much assistance as they need.

- Help clients select and participate in meaningful activities to maintain physical function and health and mental well-being.

- Programs must be specifically designed for older persons with substance use disorders.

- Reminiscence therapy can raise self-esteem and increase social intimacy.

- If clients have hearing deficits, discuss available resources with them.

- Encourage clients to find meaningful social and community activities to meet their needs for support, belonging, self-expression, and self-esteem.

Review Questions

1. Which of the following demonstrates that your nursing care is based on stereotypes of older adults?

   a. In a community presentation, you say that most older adults live alone or in a family setting.

   b. You provide minimal client education because you believe that older people cannot learn.

   c. You expect that older adults will not be cognitively impaired.

   d. You expect that many nursing home residents have abundant interests in life, such as hobbies and other creative activities.

2. You decide that reminiscence therapy will be helpful for your client, Joe. You implement this by

   a. encouraging Joe to remember and discuss earlier life experiences.

   b. recommending Joe to a resocialization group.

   c. role-modeling adaptive ways to cope with aging.

   d. validating Joe's positive feelings about aging.

3. When Susan reviews her life, she despairs over the events and injustices that occurred, is unable to find any meaning in her life, and feels hopeless about the future. The most appropriate nursing diagnosis is

   a. *Potential for violence, self-directed.*

   b. *Altered role performance.*

   c. *Defensive coping.*

   d. *Spiritual distress.*

4. Mike has Parkinson's disease and a possible concurrent depression. During assessment, in what way would you expect Mike's symptoms of depression to differ from those of other people with depression? Mike is likely to have

   a. more pessimistic feelings.

   b. more guilt.

   c. lower anxiety levels.

   d. more cognitive deficits.

5. BuSpar (buspirone) is preferred over the benzodiazepines for older adults because BuSpar

   a. may lead to addiction.

   b. does not impair cognition.

   c. may interfere with psychomotor function.

   d. may produce withdrawal symptoms.

References

Alexopoulos, G. S., et al. (1996). Disability in geriatric depression. *Am J Psychiatry, 153*(7), 877–885.

Alexopoulos, G. S., et al. (1997). Clinically defined vascular depression. *Am J Psychiatry, 154*(4), 562–565.

Atkinson, R. M., & Ganzini, L. (1994). Substance abuse. In C. E. Coffey & J. L. Cummings (Eds.), *Textbook of Geriatric Neuropsychiatry* (pp. 298–321). Washington, D.C.: American Psychiatric Press.

Atkinson, R. M. (1995). Treatment programs for aging alcoholics. In T. Beresford & E. Gromberg (Eds.), *Alcohol and Aging* (pp. 186–210). New York: Oxford Univ. Press.

Beresford, T., & Gromberg, E. (Eds.). (1995). *Alcohol and Aging.* New York: Oxford Univ. Press.

Bucholz, K. K., et al. (1995). The epidemiology of alcohol use, problems, and dependence in elders. In T. Beresford & E. Gromberg (Eds.), *Alcohol and Aging* (pp. 19–41). New York: Oxford Univ. Press.

Butler, R. N. & Lewis, M. I. (1995). Late-life depression. *Geriatrics, 50*(8), 44–55.

Coffey, C. E., & Cummings, J. L. (Eds.). (1994). *Textbook of Geriatric Neuropsychiatry.* Washington, D.C.: American Psychiatric Press.

Cromwell, S. L. & Phillips, L. R. (1995). Forgetfulness in elders. *Geriatr Nurs, 16*(2), 55–59.

Devons, C. A. (1996). Suicide in the elderly. *Geriatrics, 51*(3), 67–72.

Desjarlais, R., et al. (1995). *World Mental Health*. New York: Oxford Univ. Press.

Finlayson, R. E. (1995). Comorbidity in elderly alcoholics. In T. Beresford & E. Gomberg (Eds.), *Alcohol and Aging* (pp. 56–69). New York: Oxford Univ. Press.

Futterman, A., et al. (1995). Depression in later life. In E. E. Beckham & W. R. Leber (Eds.), *Handbook of Depression (*2nd ed.) (pp. 494–525). New York: Guilford Press.

Harris, H. W. (1997). Pharmacological treatment of depression in late life. *Decade of the Brain, 8(*2), 6–8.

Hirst, S. P., & McKiel, E. (1997). The benefits of narrational relationships in the lives of older residents. *J Psychosoc Nurs, 35(*5), 40–43.

Katz, I. R. (1997). Biology of late-life depression. *Decade of the Brain, 8(*2), 4–6.

Lebowitz, B. D. (1997). Depression in late life: Progress and opportunity. *Decade of the Brain, 8(*2), 1–2.

Mahoney, D. F. (1995). Analysis of restraint-free nursing homes. *IMAGE, 27(*2), 155–160.

McCloskey, J. C., & Bulechek, G. M. (Eds.). (1996). *Nursing Interventions Classification* (2nd ed.). St. Louis, MO: Mosby.

McGuire, M. H., & Rabins, P. V. (1994). Mood disorders. In C. E. Coffey & J. L. Cummings (Eds.), *Textbook of Geriatric Neuropsychiatry* (pp. 244–260). Washington, D.C.: American Psychiatric Press.

Pearlson, G. D., & Petty, R. G. (1994). Late life onset psychoses. In C. E. Coffey & J. L. Cummings (Eds.), *Textbook of Geriatric Neuropsychiatry* (pp. 262–277). Washington, D.C.: American Psychiatric Press. 1994.

Pritchett, J. T., Keller, C. H., & Coffey, C. E. (1994). Electroconvulsive therapy in geriatric neuropsychiatry. In C. E. Coffey & J. L. Cummings (Eds.), *Textbook of Geriatric Neuropsychiatry* (pp. 634–659). Washington, D.C.: American Psychiatric Press.

Reynolds, C. F., et al. (1996). Treatment outcome in recurrent major depression. *Am J Psychiatry, 153(*10), 1288–1292.

Rossen, E. K., & Buschmann, M. T. (1995). Mental illness in late life. *Arch Psychiatr Nurs, 9(*3), 130–136.

Sheikh, J. I. (1994). Anxiety disorders. In C. E. Coffey & J. L. Cummings (Eds.), *Textbook of Geriatric Neuropsychiatry* (pp. 280–296). Washington, D.C.: American Psychiatric Press.

Sullivan-Marx, E. M. (1995). Psychological responses to physical restraint use in older adults. *J Psychosoc Nurs, 33(*6), 20–25.

Zimberg, S. (1995). The elderly. In A. M. Washton (Ed.), *Psychotherapy and Substance Abuse* (pp. 413–427). New York: Guilford Press.

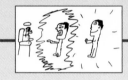

CHAPTER 22

Psycho-physiological Disorders

Leslie Rittenmeyer

Objectives

After reading this chapter, you will be able to:

- Explain the concept of psychophysiological disorders.
- Discuss the theory of stress.
- Describe psychoneuroimmunology.
- Implement the nursing process for clients with psychophysiological disorders.

Key Terms

complementary or alternative therapies
general adaptation syndrome (GAS)
psychoneuroimmunology

The correlation between the mind and the body fascinated the earliest scientists and continues to be an active area of scientific research today. The debate over whether or not a correlation exists is long past, but scientists still search for evidence to clarify the relationship between mind and body more precisely.

The mind-body correlation was initially recognized during the 1800s. Systems theory was developed as an attempt to give some organization to, and show connections between, concepts and scientific theories. It became a useful construct for understanding people, with all their complexities and intricacies. As a discipline, nursing has embraced the ideas of system theorists who believe that people are more than, and different from, the sum of their parts. This idea, an approach to viewing each person as a unique, complex individual, is known as *holism*. The relationship between psychological factors and medical conditions is complex and affected by many biological and psychosocial variables. Even the effects of stress have proven to be complex and difficult to measure. In fact, stress may have beneficial, negative, or mixed effects in a person. The concepts basic to this chapter include:

- A person is a totality of body, mind, and spirit.
- If there is an interruption in the homeostasis in one part of the person, all other parts will be affected.
- Illness and wellness result from the interaction of physiological, cognitive, and sociocultural phenomena.

Causative Factors

Many different factors are involved in the psychophysiological process of certain disorders. Those most relevant to nursing are biological, cognitive, and sociocultural. Figure 22.1 illustrates the interrelationship of these factors.

Biological Factors

Biological science attempts to explain how chronic physiological or psychological stress alters a person's internal environment, including cellular and hor-

monal changes. These changes determine where a person will be on the health-illness continuum.

Stress Theory

Contemporary stress theory as it relates to health is attributed to Hans Selye, who in 1950 published his now-famous work, *The Stress of Life*. Selye defined *stress* as the rate of wear and tear on the body (Selye, 1976). Examples are physical injury, disease, infection, and psychological and emotional tension. These demands are called *stressors,* and they have the potential to produce physical and chemical changes in the body to which the person must adjust. Selye named this stress response the **general adaptation syndrome (GAS)**.

The first stage in the GAS is the *alarm reaction*. The stressor is recognized, consciously or unconsciously, and the person is propelled into some type of action, the "fight-or-flight" response. Physiological changes are mediated through the autonomic nervous system. Hormone levels, blood supply, and oxygen are all increased. The person experiences an intensified level of alertness and anxiety.

In the *stage of resistance,* the second stage in the GAS, the body attempts to adapt to the stress. Hormone levels readjust, and the body achieves some level of homeostasis in the continued presence of the stress. The person relies on defense mechanisms and coping behaviors during this stage.

The third stage is the *stage of exhaustion*. Physiological resources are depleted, and the person is no longer able to resist the stress. The pituitary gland and adrenal cortex are unable to produce hormones, and the immune response becomes depressed. The person's thinking is disorganized, and there is a loss of contact with reality. If the stress continues, the person will eventually die (Wilson and Kneisl, 1996).

Psychoneuroimmunology

Psychoneuroimmunology is an area of scientific study that explores the damaging effects of chronic stress on the central nervous system, the body's defense against external infection, and aberrant cell division.

The immune system is a surveillance system that protects the body. The immune system responds to a person's internal and external environments. It must

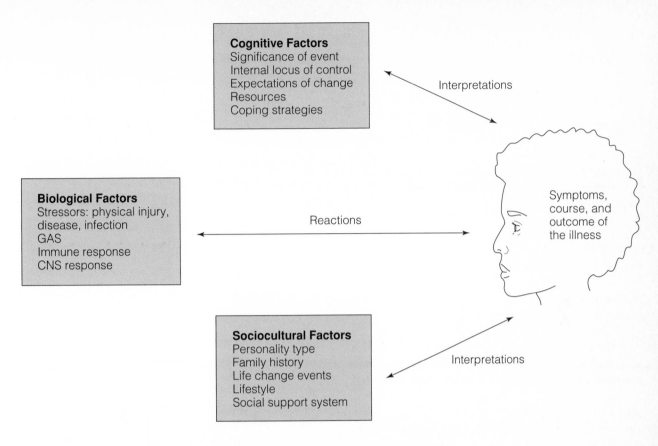

Figure 22.1 **The interrelationship of factors in psychophysiological disorders.**

Source: Wilson and Kneisl, 1992.

distinguish between normal cells and malignant cells, as well as identify and destroy foreign and disease-causing organisms. In autoimmune disorders, the immune system reacts inappropriately and attacks the body. Examples of autoimmune disorders are Graves' disease, rheumatoid arthritis, ulcerative colitis, ileitis, lupus, psoriasis, myasthenia gravis, and pernicious anemia. The immune system itself can be damaged, as in AIDS, or it can malfunction, as in allergies and cancer.

There are two types of immunity: innate and acquired. Innate immunity involves certain processes that do not depend on the person's having been previously exposed to a foreign agent. In innate immunity, foreign agents such as bacteria and viruses are attacked and destroyed by special cells of the body.

Innate immunity is supplemented by acquired immunity, which is a defense against specific pathogens. Every pathogen has a unique identifier called an antigen. When people are exposed to the antigen, by having the disease or by vaccination, they develop antibodies specific to the disease. Future exposure to the pathogen results in a fast and efficient defense by the body.

The tissues of the immune system include bone marrow, lymph nodes, spleen, thymus, and tonsils. The cells of the immune system communicate by neurotransmitters and an intricate network of immunohormones called interleukins. There are many ways the immune system can be disturbed. Immune cells, such as B cells and T cells, may be absent or defective, there may be an increased or decreased production of neurotransmitters and interleukins, or the body may attack its own normal cells (Hedaya, 1996; Soubervielle, 1994). The central nervous system and the immune system work as an integrated whole to maintain a state of healthy balance within the body. The pathways of communication are the autonomic nervous system and the neuroendocrine system. The autonomic nervous system innervates all the immune tissue and releases transmitters which activate the immune system. The other communication pathway involves hormone production by the hypothalamus and pituitary gland. These hormones are capable of altering the function of virtually every type of immune cell. The release of many of these hormones is significantly related to thoughts and feelings. Each thought and feeling has a chemical consequence within the brain relating to the production of neurotransmitters and neurohormones by the limbic system (Bennett, 1996; Hayes, 1995).

Cognitive and sociocultural stimuli are among the most potent factors in activating the biological responses to stress. An example is the effect of bereavement on a person's health. After the death of a spouse, the surviving spouse's risk of death is especially high during the first 6 months. This increased risk is thought to be related to a depressed immune system. Social isolation is another major risk factor for disease, expecially in the elderly and poor (Hayes, 1995).

Cognitive Factors

Lazarus (1968) has a different view of stress. According to his cognitive-phenomenological approach, neither the stimulus theories nor the response theories of stress sufficiently consider the individual differences of people. The emphasis of the cognitive approach is that people and groups differ in their vulnerability, interpretations, and reactions to certain types of events.

The perception of psychological stress is closely tied to the idea of control and of coping. The same stimulus presented to different individuals is perceived differently because of past experiences, as well as the ability to face or control the stressor. The focus is on the relationship between the cognitive process and the stressful event that causes certain reactions. Initially, the person must determine the personal significance of the event. The person must then identify options, constraints, and resources for coping with the stress. Some people are relatively resistant to the effects of

stress, while others are more susceptible (Akil and Morano, 1996). The cognitive factors that seem to buffer the effects of stress include:

- a belief in the ability to influence the course of events (internal locus of control)
- the expectation that change is normal
- the ability to mobilize resources
- the ability to use a wide range of coping strategies

Sociocultural Factors

People are influenced by their sociocultural environment. While some people have loving, nurturing surroundings, others live with abuse and hate. While some learn effective ways of coping, others struggle to merely survive.

Personality Type

Personality usually refers to a person's predictable response pattern to internal and external events. A person's usual behavior becomes more pronounced during periods of high stress. For example, when a highly independent person with a strong internal locus of control becomes ill, he or she may be incapable of participating in the collaborative relationships necessary to return to a healthy state. From this perspective, personality type can be an important determinant in coping ability.

Gender

Gender role socialization influences cognitive appraisal and coping, leading to gender differences in vulnerability to certain stressors. Coping strategies consistent with traditional female behaviors and values such as passivity, dependence, emotional reactivity, and self-deprecation may contribute to a decreased ability to effectively cope with stress. The majority of women who are employed outside the home continue to contribute tremendous hours to childcare and home maintenance. These excessive demands often exceed women's resources, limiting their ability to cope. In addition, women's work at home and on the job is often devalued. Stressors often identified by women are pay inequities, lack of affordable childcare, and fewer opportunities for advancement (Bennett, 1996).

Family History

Many of the coping skills brought to adult life are learned from the family. Issues such as dependency versus autonomy, communication patterns, attention-gaining behaviors, and secondary gains are a few of the factors that affect a person's ability to cope. Healthy families exhibit a productive interdependency, with shared responsibilities and roles that are adaptable and flexible to situational demands. Dysfunctional families are less adaptive and unable to teach effective coping behaviors.

The perception and appraisal of stressful situations may be correlated to a person's cultural background. Definitions of health and illness, health maintenance beliefs, and disease treatment are specific to cultural beliefs. What may be perceived as stressful in one culture may not be perceived that way in another.

Life Change Events

Although there is some debate about the most accurate way to measure life changes, it is agreed that when stressful life events occur, people are at increased risk for health problems. Most of us are aware that unpleasant events, such as hospitalization and family problems, are stressful. It is also true that pleasant events, such as vacations and holidays, are often stressful. If there are enough stressful events, the person's ability to continue to cope is compromised.

Socioeconomic Status

Socioeconomic status (SES) is inversely related to people's ability to manage stressful events. People suffering economic hardship experience more illness and have a shorter life expentancy. Because of its association with many chronic and devastating illnesses, stress is a major economic issue, costing the United States nearly $150 billion a year in illness, accidents, absenteeism, and substance abuse. Understanding stress and stress management has become a priority for many major corporations (Bennett, 1996).

Religious Involvement

For better or for worse, religion touches nearly every aspect of life: interpersonal interactions, family life, personality characteristics, socioeconomic status, and political activity. There are hundreds of published studies linking religious involvement and health and well-being, although this literature has been largely ignored. It is thought that the positive impact on physical and mental health involves the following (Levin et al, 1996):

- Avoidance of negative health behaviors such as substance abuse, smoking, and adolescent sexual activity.
- Practice of positive health behaviors such as proper diet and exercise as well as better self-care.
- Use of prayer to manage tension and anxiety.
- Help in searching for meaning in life events.

Medical Problems Masquerading as Mental Disorders

There are a number of medical disorders that may be mistaken for mental disorders. Without careful assessment, clients could be misdiagnosed and mistreated with potentially fatal results. Hedaya (1996) suggests using the acronym "THINC MED" during the assessment process. See Box 22.1 for a listing of these medical conditions.

Cardiovascular Disorders

There are psychological and behavioral factors that affect coronary artery disease, ventricular arrhythmias, and sudden death from cardiac problems. Physiological factors implicated in cardiovascular disorders include genetic predisposition; a high-calorie, high-fat diet; a sedentary lifestyle; cigarette smoking; and cardiovascular reactivity to environmental stimuli. Contributing affective states include anxiety, depression, and an acute situational disturbance. Type A behavior pattern, especially hostility, can increase the risk of cardiovascular disease. Sociocultural factors include high levels of life stress, work "overload," and lack of social support (Goldstein and Niaura, 1995).

A great deal of research has been done on the anxiety and stress levels of people who are predisposed to cardiovascular disorders. One thought is that people who are at risk are those who are never completely satisfied, even though they drive themselves hard, and those who experience hostility in response to stress. Chronic dissatisfaction with oneself and

Box 22.1

Medical Problems that Masquerade as Mental Disorders

Category	Medical Problem	Symptoms
T = Tumors	Frontal lobe	Abrupt personality change; flat affect
	Occipital lobe	Visual hallucination
	Parietal lobe	Sensory disturbances; agnosia; lack of awareness
	Temporal lobe	Mood and memory disturbances; hallucinations, paranoid delusions
H = Hormones	Hypothyroidism	Depression
	Hyperthyroidism	Anxiety disorder; manic episode
	Excessive cortisol	Anxiety disorder; manic episode; depression
	Decreased cortisol	Dysthymic disorder
I = Infections/ Immune Disease	AIDS, syphilis, herpes, TB, Lyme disease	Affect the CNS directly
	Epstein-Barr virus; hepatitis	Depression
	Lupus erythematosus	Cognitive defects; depression; severe anxiety; hypochondriasis
N = Nutrition	B_{12} deficiency	Mood disorders; paranoia; hallucinations; panic disorder
	B_1 deficiency	Dementia
M = Miscellaneous	Sleep disorders	Hallucinations; cognitive defects
E = Electrolytes	Altered levels	Confusion; irritability; delirium
D = Drugs	Medications, street drugs	Almost all drugs can cause psychiatric symptoms

Source: Hedaya, 1996.

hostility are often-linked maladaptive behaviors that predispose a person to disease. This combination of factors may contribute to the development of cardiovascular disorders.

Cancer

The role of psychosocial factors in the development of cancer is unclear at this time. Some studies are positive and some are negative for bereavement as a risk factor in cancer onset. Bereavement is associated with a significant increase in mortality in the first year of grieving in men younger than 75 years, but rather than cancer, the cause of death tends to be cardiovascular disease, accidents, and cirrhosis. Studies are also conflicting for an association between stressful life events and cancer onset. There is no association between the onset of cancer and depression. Whether or not depressive states influence cancer outcome is unknown at this time.

Recent studies indicate that cancer progression may be influenced by psychosocial factors. Certain characteristics help people who have cancer fight the effects of the disease process. For instance, the ability to be creative, to be receptive to new ideas, to grow intellectually, to have new experiences, and the motivation to seek the "best" medical care have all been identified as characteristics that increase remission rates. People who receive medical treatment and group psychotherapy have the longest survival rates. They also report improved mood, vigor, and quality of life (Levenson and Bemis, 1995).

The stress of cancer is quite different from everyday stress. There is the physical stress of the disease itself in the body. In addition there are the physical effects of treatment such as chemotherapy, radiation therapy, surgery, or hormonal treatment, all of which have serious side effects. The physical symptoms of cancer can trigger other psychological stresses. For example, stress is compounded when pain is interpreted as a possible indicator of recurrence or progression. People with cancer live with constant reminders that they have a serious and possibly terminal disease (Classen, Hermanson, and Spiegel, 1995).

Respiratory Disorders

Changes in the rate, regularity, and depth of respiration correlate with many emotional states. For example, a pain-stricken person gasps, a bored person yawns, a person in love or deeply sad sighs, and a highly anxious person hyperventilates. Changes in respiration are also symptoms of respiratory disorders. Of these disorders, asthma is the most widely studied from a psychophysiological perspective.

There are allergic, immunological, and psychological factors of asthmatic attacks. Psychological factors can directly alter the size of the bronchial tubes, leading to an acute asthmatic attack. Asthmatic attacks are extremely frightening, and this fear may contribute to feelings of helplessness and hopelessness. It is particularly terrifying to children and adolescents when friends or acquaintances who have asthma die from an acute attack. People with asthma often feel as if they are living with the daily threat of death.

Gastrointestinal Disorders

There are many behaviors connected to gastrointestinal functions. Changes in appetite, food intake, digestive functions, and elimination occur almost daily in relation to emotional stress. Disorders thought to have psychological factors include the following:

- esophagus: esophageal reflux, esophageal spasm
- stomach: hyperacidity
- intestines: constipation, chronic diarrhea, ulcerative colitis

Knowledge of the psychological and behavioral factors that may influence gastrointestinal disorders is far from conclusive. It appears that psychosocial stressors, the lack of social support, and a decreased sense of well-being may contribute to these disorders. High levels of anxiety or depression are frequently observed in this client population, as well as issues involving dependence and independence (Folks and Kinney, 1995).

The Nursing Process

Assessment

Important assessment areas are stress assessment, interpersonal assessment, assessment of anxiety, and assessment of secondary gains. The focus is on the sociocultural data, but remember to pay close attention to physiological problems as well. See the Focused Nursing Assessment table for guidelines.

Stress Assessment

Clients often need help in clearly identifying the source of their stress. Be careful not to make assumptions about the significance of the stress, because it is a very individual perception. It may help to begin with the precipitating event that brought the client into the health care system. As discussion continues, try to determine whether the present stress is an isolated episode or a culmination of many stressful events. Additional assessment data include the number of stressors and the duration of each one.

Explore with clients the available resources for dealing with stressful events in their lives. Assess their capacity for identifying problems and analyzing associated feelings. Determine whether the client is able to implement the problem-solving process or needs to be taught this approach. (Chapter 5 describes the problem-solving process in detail.)

Interpersonal Assessment

Nurses and clients work together to assess interpersonal and social skills. Ask direct questions about your clients' support systems of family and friends in the community. Do not assume that all social networks are supportive; some may be negative and draining.

Text continues on page 524

Focused Nursing Assessment

CLIENTS WITH PSYCHOPHYSIOLOGICAL DISORDERS

Behavior Assessment	Cognitive Assessment	Affective Assessment
What is your usual pattern for activities of daily living?	How frequently do you take the blame if something doesn't go right at home or at work?	What kind of situations cause you to feel anxious or angry?
How has your illness affected your usual level of functioning?	Do you tend to make decisions quickly or slowly?	What is your usual emotional reaction to stressful situations?
How much time do you spend at work versus leisure?	What decisions do you find easiest to make? Most difficult to make?	How do you express anxiety?
What are your leisure activities?	Would you describe yourself as a perfectionist at home and at work?	How do you express anger?
Would you describe yourself as an aggressive or a passive person?	How do you respond to criticism of your work?	What is your usual mood?
	How does disorderliness or messiness affect your stress level?	How has your diagnosis affected your usual mood?

Social Assessment

Who are the people you consider most significant in your life?

Do these people provide an effective support system?

Describe your relationships with other people.

What causes you to be upset with others?

Do you hold your feelings in when you are upset with others?

How do you resolve conflict with others?

Physiological Assessment

What physical symptoms worry you?

What medications are you taking?

What are your eating patterns?

What are your elimination patterns?

What are your sleeping patterns?

Is your lifestyle sedentary, moderately active, or active?

How do you feel after physical activity?

Does pain affect your daily activities?

Assessing the size of support systems tells you how many family members, close friends, and casual friends are available to the client. Assessing the frequency of contact tells you how often the client visits by phone or in person and thereby engages in social activities with family members and friends. Assessing reciprocity, the exchange of favors, tells you the ways in which the client is supportive to others and the ways in which others provide support to the client. Assessing forms of social support tells you the types of material support and kinds of advice the client receives. You can also determine who provides companionship and who provides love.

Assessment of Anxiety

Anxiety is an important area of assessment for clients with psychophysiological disorders. Some clients will show overt signs of anxiety, but many others manifest their anxiety in physical ways. Be alert for nonverbal cues. (To review basic guidelines for the assessment of anxiety, see Chapter 9.)

Many clients will have difficulty identifying with the word "anxiety." It may be more helpful for you to ask them about situations in which they feel uncomfortable or tense. Discuss how they typically manage these situations. Having clients identify how their family of origin dealt with anxiety may help determine learned patterns of behavior.

The discomfort of anxiety may be displaced onto others and expressed as anger or hostility, thereby making the client feel more in control of the situation. Be careful not to personalize this anger; learn to recognize it as a message from the client.

Assessment of Secondary Gains

When people are anxious or overwhelmed with stress, they will use both unconscious defense mechanisms and conscious coping behaviors to relieve their anxiety. These coping strategies may develop into secondary gains. For those who have a high level of dependency, the physical symptoms may get a great deal of attention and support from significant others. The sympathy and nurturing they receive may become a reason for continuing the disorder. The attention may be viewed as a reassurance of care and love. And, because ill people are often in a position of power, the disorder itself may be an unconscious attempt to gain control.

Diagnosis

In addition to nursing diagnoses related to the client's physiological responses to an illness, a number of nursing diagnoses are related to affective, cognitive, and sociocultural responses. These include:

- *Ineffective individual coping* related to unacknowledged secondary gains; inadequate support systems; unmet dependency needs; chronic dissatisfaction with oneself
- *Ineffective denial* related to avoidance of conflict
- *Self-esteem disturbance* related to external locus of control
- *Body image disturbance* related to disfiguring surgery
- *Anxiety* related to high stress levels; multiple life change events; unexpressed anger or hostility

Nursing Interventions

Interventions are designed to help clients meet the mutually agreed-upon goals and outcome criteria. Priorities of care are determined, with acute physiological needs taking precedence over sociocultural needs.

If you have identified deficits in the size, frequency, reciprocity, or forms of support systems, use the problem-solving process to help clients *improve their social competence*. Teach interactive skills such as effective communication and assertiveness techniques. Identify resources such as support groups, self-help groups, and special-interest clubs.

Progressive relaxation and *visual imagery techniques* help clients achieve or maintain more control over their body. Nursing research has shown that guided imagery influences the immune system in people with cancer. Clients also report improved quality of life and emotional state. Teach these techniques individually or in a group, reinforcing them with taped instructions. You may be more successful if you add music or soothing sounds. Help clients evaluate the differences they feel in their bodies, once they have mastered relaxation and visual imagery (Bennett, 1996).

Music therapy can influence our body, mind, and spirit. Studies indicate that music affects heart rate, blood pressure, respiratory rate, pain, anxiety, and mood states. It is also a way we can explore and express our feelings. Many clients find this an effective intervention in managing stress, anxiety, and pain (Covington and Crosby, 1997).

Dance and movement therapy may be very helpful for people experiencing medical problems. This therapy allows for the release of pent-up emotions, increases people's capacity to experience their bodies as the source of their creativity, and increases people's ability to play, to imagine, and to pretend. Dance and movement allow us to experience our inner feelings that cannot be rationally or verbally expressed. In a very real sense, dance and movement honors the connections between body, mind, and spirit.

The latest research suggests that prayer is not just salve for the soul—it may keep bodies healthy too. Prayer may reduce the adverse health effects of stress, improve recovery from surgery, decrease the death rate from coronary-artery disease, and lower suicide rate.

A powerful intervention for clients is *journal writing*. Encourage clients to write about their feelings, thoughts, and stressful events. Help them interpret their writing and evaluate their patterns of behavior. Even if clients choose not to share their journals with anyone else, catharsis and learning result from the writing itself.

Many people feel more in control of their lives when they exercise. *Exercise* has both physiological and psychological benefits. Depending on the client's physical condition and activity preference, suggest such exercises as yoga, walking, running, ballroom dancing, swimming, tennis, and so on. The best approach to planning an exercise program is multidisciplinary, designed for preferences, lifestyle, and the health needs of the individual client.

Humor has great healing power for the body, mind, and spirit. There is evidence that the therapeutic use of humor can affect the course of recovery from an illness. Recommend humorous books and movies. Most important, bring the humorous parts of yourself to the nurse-client relationship.

Complementary/Alternative Health Care Services

Western or allopathic medicine is the type of medicine with which we are most familiar. The focus is on specific parts of the body and has developed into the high technology of medical care in the United States. Allopathic medicine is extremely effective for trauma; infections; and acute, life-threatening, curable diseases. However, it has been less effective in chronic diseases. The model is one of external causes and the healer is in the position of power and control.

Homeopathic or traditional medicine, often referred to as complementary or alternative therapies, focuses on the entire person, is more gentle and natural, and is generally less invasive and less expensive. It relies on the self-healing capabilities of people and on the subjective aspects of the healer-client or nurse-client relationship. The model is one of internal causes and the healer is in the position of facilitator.

Integration of alternative medical practices is gaining greater acceptance from the public as well as the health care professions. As nurses, we need to know what our clients are doing in terms of their health care. We need to understand the principles of these therapies. In order to provide holistic nursing care we must understand and make use of our clients' belief system. Nursing schools are beginning to design courses in complementary/alternative medicine to meet this need. See Box 22.2 for a brief overview of some alternative medical practices.

Evaluation

Successful interventions result in the improved physical condition of clients with medical disorders. Improvement should also be noted in their affective, cognitive, and sociocultural responses to illness. Outcome criteria include:

- a decreased need for secondary gains
- adaptive means of meeting dependency needs
- the development of functional support systems
- the development of conflict-management skills
- evidence of an internal locus of control
- improved body image
- decreased anxiety
- implementation of stress-management techniques

Box 22.2

Complementary/Alternative Medicine

Acupuncture

The therapeutic goal of acupuncture is to regulate the qi (energy or life force). It is believed that when qi flows unimpeded the body is in a state of health. Often used for pain relief, improving well-being, and treating acute, chronic, and degenerative conditions.

Aromatherapy

Essential oils are extracted from plants and are massaged into the skin, inhaled, placed in baths, used as compresses, or mixed into ointments. The basis of action is thought to be the same as modern pharmacology, using smaller doses.

Ayurveda

The Indian system of medicine, Ayurveda, is at least 2500 years old. Illness is viewed as a state of imbalance among the body's systems. Nutritional counseling, massage, natural medicines, meditation, and other modalities are used to treat many disorders.

Chinese Medicine—Traditional

Chinese medicine has been developed over centuries. Practitioners are trained to use a variety of ancient and modern therapeutic methods, including acupuncture, herbal medicine, massage, heat therapy, and nutritional and lifestyle counseling. Chinese medicine seeks to balance the flow of qi, the energy or life force of a person. There are many different types of qi in the body; some nourish the body, some warm the body, some flow in channels, and some flow in the organs.

Chiropractic

Chiropractic is the third largest independent health profession in the Western world, after allopathic medicine and dentistry. It is based on the premise that the spine is literally the backbone of human health. Misalignments of the vertebrae caused by poor posture or trauma result in pressure on the spinal cord, which may lead to diminished function and illness.

Craniosacral Therapy

This is a manual procedure for correcting distortions in the structure and function of the brain and spinal cord, the bones of the skull, the sacrum, and interconnected membranes. It is used to treat chronic pain, migraine headaches, TMJ, and other conditions.

Herbal Medicine

This ancient form of healing is still widely practiced in much of the world. Plant material is used not only to treat disease but to enhance the quality of life both physically and spiritually.

Homeopathy

Practitioners use infinitesimal doses of natural substances, called remedies, to stimulate a person's immune and defense system.

Hypnotherapy

Therapists use a range of techniques to bypass the conscious mind and access the subconscious. Hypnosis may facilitate behavioral, emotional, or attitudinal change. It is often used in the treatment of phobias and stress, and to help people lose weight or quit smoking.

Jin Shin Jyutsu

This Oriental system is intended to harmonize the flow of energy to restore balance and reduce stress.

Kinesiology/Applied Kinesiology

In conjunction with standard methods of diagnosis, this system uses muscle testing to gain information about the general state of health. Treatments include nutritional supplements, muscle and joint manipulation, and lifestyle modification.

Massage Therapy

Massage has roots in both Eastern and Western cultures. It involves the process of kneading or otherwise manipulating a person's muscles and other soft tissues with the intent of improving well-being or health.

Meditation

Meditation includes a wide range of practices that involve training one's attention or awareness so that body and mind can be brought into greater harmony. Some seek to reduce stress or anxiety, while others seek a mystical sense of oneness with a higher power or the universe.

Naturopathy

Naturopathy is a primary health care system emphasizing the curative power of nature, working to restore and support the body's own healing ability using nutrition, herbs, homeopathic medicine, and Oriental medicine. It involves a 4-year course of study past the bachelor's degree, much like medical school.

QiGong

This involves manipulation of qi by means of physical exercises, mental exercises, and breathing.

Reflexology

Interventions are based on the idea that specific points on the feet and hands correspond with organs and tissues throughout the body. Pressure is applied to these points to treat a wide range of stress-related illnesses.

Rheiki

Rheiki is an ancient Tibetan healing system that uses light hand placements to channel healing energies to the client. It is commonly used to treat distress and acute and chronic problems, and to achieve spiritual focus.

Spiritual/Shamanic Healing

Practitioners regard themselves as conductors of healing energy or sources from the spiritual realm. They may call upon spiritual helpers such as power animals, angels, inner teachers, the clients' higher self, or other spiritual forces. Used for a wide range of emotional and physical illnesses.

Tai Chi/Martial Arts

The martial arts are perhaps best known as a means of self-defense, but they are also used to improve physical fitness and promote mental and spiritual development. The highly disciplined movements are thought to unite body and mind and bring balance to life.

Therapeutic Touch

Popularized by nursing professor Dolores Krieger, therapeutic touch is practiced by registered nurses and others to relieve pain and stress. The practitioner assesses where the person's energy field is weak or congested, and then uses her/his hands to direct energy into the field to balance it.

Yoga

Yoga is a range of body-mind exercise practices used to access consciousness and encourage physical and mental well-being.

Key Concepts

Introduction

- The relationship between psychological factors and medical conditions is complex and affected by many biological and psychosocial variables.

Causative Factors

- Stressors, such as physical injury, disease, infection, and psychological tension, have the potential to produce physical and chemical changes in the body.

- The stress response is referred to as the general adaptation syndrome (GAS), which consists of three stages: alarm, resistance, and exhaustion.

- In the alarm reaction stage, stress is recognized and the person is propelled into some type of action.

- The person then moves on to the stage of resistance, when the body attempts to adapt to the stress.

- If the stress continues, the person moves into the third stage, the stage of exhaustion. Thinking is disorganized, there is a loss of contact with reality, and the person ultimately risks death.

- Psychoneuroimmunology explores the damaging effects of chronic stress on the CNS, the body's defense against external infection, and aberrant cell division.

- The immune system is a surveillance system that distinguishes between normal and malignant cells and identifies and destroys foreign and disease-causing organisms.

- There are two types of immunity: innate and acquired. The cells of the immune system communicate by neurotransmitters and immunohormones called interleukins.

- The cognitive approach to stress emphasizes that people differ in their vulnerability to stress, in the significance of the event, and in reactions to the event.

- Cognitive factors that buffer the effects of stress are a belief in the ability to influence the course of events, the expectation that change is normal, the ability to mobilize resources, and the ability to use a wide range of coping strategies.

- Personality type may predict behavioral adaptations to stress. Characteristic behaviors are usually exaggerated under stress.

- The excessive demands on women often exceed their resources, limiting their ability to manage stress.

- Definitions of health and illness and the ways people are taught to deal with problems are specific to cultural beliefs.

- There are a number of medical disorders that may be mistaken for mental disorders.

Cardiovascular Disorders

- Risk factors for cardiovascular disorders include a genetic predisposition; type-A personality traits (especially hostility); high levels of stress; a high-calorie, high-fat diet; smoking; a sedentary lifestyle; anxiety and depression; and a lack of social support.

Cancer

- Recent studies indicate that cancer progression more than cancer onset may be influenced by psychosocial factors.

Respiratory Disorders

- Asthma attacks are extremely frightening, which may contribute to feelings of helplessness and hopelessness. People with asthma often feel as if they are living with the daily threat of death.

Gastrointestinal Disorders

- Traits such as perfectionism, an excessive need for affection, repression of negative emotions, and sensitivity to criticism are often correlated with gastrointestinal disorders.

Nursing Assessment

- Assessment includes identification of the sources of stress and the resources clients have to manage stress.

- Assess support systems for size, frequency of contact, reciprocity, and forms of support.

- Assess the client's level of anxiety. Some clients will show overt signs of anxiety, but many manifest their anxiety in physical ways.

- The presence of secondary gains must be determined during the assessment process.

Diagnosis

- Nursing diagnoses include *Ineffective individual coping, Ineffective denial, Self-esteem disturbance, Body image disturbance,* and *Anxiety.*

Nursing Interventions

- Use the problem-solving process to help clients improve their social competence.

- Clients can better manage their disorders by using progressive relaxation techniques and visual imagery techniques.

- Encourage clients to write in a journal about their feelings, thoughts, and stressful events.

- An exercise program should be designed around the preferences, lifestyle, and health needs of the individual client.

- The therapeutic use of humor can affect the course of recovery from an illness.

- Homeopathic or traditional medicine focuses on the entire person and relies on self-healing capabilities and on the subjective aspects of the nurse-client relationship.

Evaluation

- Outcome criteria include a decreased need for secondary gains, an adaptive means of meeting dependency needs, the development of functional support systems and conflict-management skills, evidence of an internal locus of control, improved body image, decreased anxiety, and the ability to implement stress-management techniques.

Review Questions

1. Which of the following is an example of a secondary gain?

   a. Marla initiates an exercise program to help her manage her hypertension.

   b. Jose uses denial to cope with the stress of being diagnosed with a substance use disorder.

   c. Sophie talks to her friends about the stress of being diagnosed with breast cancer.

   d. Michael enjoys the sympathy and nuturing he has received since his heart attack.

2. Gender role socialization is one factor contributing to the high level of stress in women. Which of the following statements supports this theory?

   a. Women's work at home and on the job is often devalued.

   b. Pay inequities for women are rapidly decreasing.

   c. Women have equal opportunities for professional advancement.

   d. Men assume responsibility for 50% of home maintaince chores.

3. Which of the following conditions may be mistaken for depression?

   a. occipital lobe tumor

   b. hypothyroidism

   c. hyperthyriodism

   d. altered electrolytes

4. In which of the following traditional therapies are interventions based on the idea that specific points on the feet and hands correspond with organs and tissues throughout the body?

   a. QiGong

   b. Naturopathy

   c. Reflexology

   d. Rheiki

5. Progressive relaxation techniques and visual imagery techniques help clients

   a. achieve or maintain more control over their bodies.

   b. relax, but they have not proven to be effective in any other way.

   c. evaluate their patterns of behavior.

   d. by ridding the body of all pathogens.

References

Akil, H., & Morano, M. I. (1996). The biology of stress. In S. J. Watson (Ed.), *Biology of Schizophrenia and Affective Diseases* (pp. 15–48). Washington, D.C.: American Psychiatric Press.

Bennett, C. (1996). Expanding the mind-body connection: Working women and stress. *Caps & Comments Psych Nurs, 2*(4), 249–254.

Classen, C., Hermanson, K. S., & Spiegel, D. (1995). Psychotherapy, stress, and survival in breast cancer. In A. Stoudemire (Ed.), *Psychological Factors Affecting Medical Conditions* (pp. 123–162). Washington, D.C.: American Psychiatric Press.

Covington, H., & Crosby, C. (1997). Music therapy as a nursing intervention. *J Psychosoc Nurs, 35*(3), 34–37.

Folks, D. G., & Kinney, F. C. (1995). Gastrointestinal conditions. In A. Stoudemire (Ed.), *Psychological Factors Affecting Medical Conditions* (pp. 99–122). Washington, D.C.: American Psychiatric Press.

Goldstein, M. G., & Niaura, R. (1995). Cardiovascular Disease. In A. Stoudemire (Ed.), *Psychological Factors Affecting Medical Conditions* (pp. 19–37). Washington, D.C.: American Psychiatric Press.

Hayes, A. (1995). Psychiatric nursing: What does biology have to do with it? *Archiv Psychiatr Nurs, 9*(4), 216–224.

Hedaya, R. J. (1996). *Understanding Biological Psychiatry.* New York: Norton.

Lazarus, R. S. (1968). Emotions and adaptation. In W. J. Arnold (Ed.), *Nebraska Symposium on Motivation.* Lincoln, NE: University of Nebraska Press.

Levenson, J. L., & Bemis, C. (1995). Cancer onset and progression. In A. Stoudemire (Ed.), *Psychological Factors Affecting Medical Conditions* (pp. 81–97). Washington, D.C.: American Psychiatric Press. 1995.

Levin, J. S. et al. (1996). Religious involvement, health outcomes, and public health practice. *Curr Issues Public Health, 2,* 220–225.

Selye, H. (1976). *The Stress of Life.* Highstown, NJ: McGraw-Hill.

Souberbielle, B. (1994). Anti-tumor immune mechanisms. In C. E. Lewis, C. O'Sullivan, & J. Barraclough (Eds.), *The Psychoimmunology of Cancer* (pp. 268–290). New York: Oxford Univ. Press.

Wilson, H. S., & Kneisl, C. R. (1996). *Psychiatric Nursing* (5th ed). Menlo Park, CA: Addison-Wesley.

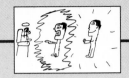

CHAPTER 23

Legal and Ethical Issues

Karen Lee Fontaine

Objectives

After reading this chapter, you will be able to:

- Distinguish between voluntary and involuntary admission.
- Integrate the concepts of competency and informed consent into nursing practice.
- Maintain confidentiality at all times.
- Institute precautions to prevent elopement.
- Discuss professional ethics in the mental health care setting.

Key Terms

commitment
competency
duty to disclose
elopement
informed consent
involuntary admission
voluntary admission

*M*any decisions nurses must make each day are affected by laws and ethical principles. It is important to be familiar with federal and state laws pertaining to nursing practice in general, and with those that have implications for the practice of psychiatric nursing in particular.

Mental disorders sometimes affect a person's ability to make decisions about his or her health and well-being. Whenever possible, client autonomy and liberty must be ensured by treatment in the least restrictive setting possible and by active client participation in treatment decisions. The challenge for nurses is maintaining the client's personal freedom in situations where public welfare and/or the client's best interests are threatened.

Types of Admission

Voluntary admission occurs when a client, for the purpose of assessment and treatment of a mental disorder, consents to confinement and signs a document indicating as much. If clients choose to leave the hospital, they must give written notice of their intention to leave the facility. The number of days between notice of intention and actual discharge is determined by individual states. This notification period provides the health care team with time to complete discharge arrangements or seek authorization for further hospitalization through the court system.

Commitment, or **involuntary admission**—detaining a client in a psychiatric facility against his or her will—may be requested in most states on the basis of dangerousness to self or others. A few states have altered their laws by including the criterion of prevention of significant physical or mental deterioration. Some groups are lobbying for additions such as "grave disability" (people are unable to provide for their basic needs such as food and shelter), "need for treatment," and "lack of capacity" (people are unable to fully understand and make an informed decision regarding the need for treatment).

In most states, adults can be held temporarily on an emergency basis until there is a court hearing. At the judicial hearing, the health care team must present clear and convincing evidence of dangerousness or need for treatment. Commitment is for a specific time period, which varies by state. Commitment may be for inpatient or outpatient treatment, the decision being made by the committing judge. At the end of the specified time, the health care team must discharge the client or petition the court for continued hospitalization (Jaffe, 1995; Kaplan, 1995).

Commitment is a controversial issue. In the United States, people have a fundamental right to make important decisions about their own treatment. At the same time, an individual may not be able to make treatment decisions when suffering from an acute episode of a mental disorder. There are legitimate concerns on both sides of the issue (Griffin-Francell, 1995; Jaffe, 1995).

Here are some of the reasons for commitment:

- Intervention will ease suffering and, in some cases, save lives.
- Commitment will alleviate embarrassment and rejection by the general public when grossly disturbed behaviors affect others.
- Commitment may reduce the length of a crisis, and that reduction seems to improve the prognosis for long-term recovery.
- In many instances, commitment is the only way to obtain treatment from the public mental health care system.
- In some cases, the family needs to protect itself against actual or threatened violence.
- The family may not be able to care for an acutely ill member and may see commitment as the only option.

Commitment is a very serious action because it restricts the freedom of someone who has not engaged in criminal activity. Here are some of the arguments against commitment:

- Commitment hearings are often perfunctory, and even though clients are entitled by law to an attorney, they often do not have one. Clients may not even be allowed to hear what is being said against them.
- The implicit promise of commitment is that the environment will be therapeutic, but many institutions dehumanize, degrade, and abuse clients.
- Because treatment is not consensual, it may not be effective.

- Commitment reinforces the stigma that mentally ill people are dangerous and unpredictable.
- It is a socioeconomic issue in that the majority of clients who are committed are poor and under-educated.
- If the family has requested commitment, the process damages trust among family members.

Commitment must never be viewed as a permanent or long-term solution. Alternatives must be explored. In some areas, mobile crisis teams or consumer-run services are offered as a substitute for hospital treatment. See Chapter 7 for further information on alternative treatments. Because severe mental illness is often cyclical, stabilized clients may sign advance directives indicating permission for treatment in the case of future incompetency. This plan is formulated between acute episodes and, while not legally binding in all states, advance directives assist family and caregivers who must make decisions for clients when they are unable to make them for themselves. Advance directives empower consumers who are psychiatrically disabled. Health care providers are given important information about the consumer's preferences for treatment. Family and friends experience less conflict and guilt during times of psychiatric crises.

The advance directive plan is initiated by the client and includes:

- symptoms which indicate that the person is not able to make decisions at this time
- the names and phone numbers of at least three people, including health care professionals and family members, who should make decisions in their behalf
- a listing of preferred, acceptable, and unacceptable medications, other treatments, and treatment facilities, including reasons

Competency

Competency is a legal determination that a client can make reasonable judgments and decisions about medical or nursing treatment and other significant areas of personal life. The principle is one of autonomy or self-determination. When a court rules an adult incompetent, it appoints a guardian or surrogate to make decisions on that person's behalf. Commitment is not a determination of incompetency. Clients who are committed for treatment are still capable of participating in health care decisions (Grisso and Applebaum, 1995).

Informed Consent

Informed consent is the client's right to receive enough information to make a decision about treatment and to communicate the decision to others. Clients may not be touched or treated without consent. If treatment is given without consent, the health care provider is held responsible for battery or offensive touching according to the law. In the event of an emergency situation with no time to obtain consent without endangering health or safety, a client may be treated without legal liability (Haas and Malouf, 1995).

Client Rights

Clients do not lose their constitutional or legal rights when they are admitted to a facility for treatment for a mental disorder. (For more information about mental health care consumers' rights, see Chapter 7.) Clients must be informed of the potential risks of psychotropic medications and the right to refuse such medications. If a client refuses medication and the physician believes it is essential for effective treatment, the physician may take the case to the courts for a decision. Figure 23.1 illustrates the outcomes of client decisions regarding their medications.

Confidentiality

The primary reason for confidentiality is to encourage clients to be honest and open, to facilitate accurate diagnosis and effective treatment. Confidentiality ensures that health care professionals, including nursing students, do not talk about clients with anyone who is not involved in their care. Going home and telling family members who is in the hospital and what happened on the unit is a serious breach of confidentiality. Discussing clients while in the hospital elevator or the cafeteria also breaches confidentiality. Nursing schools and hospitals have regulations

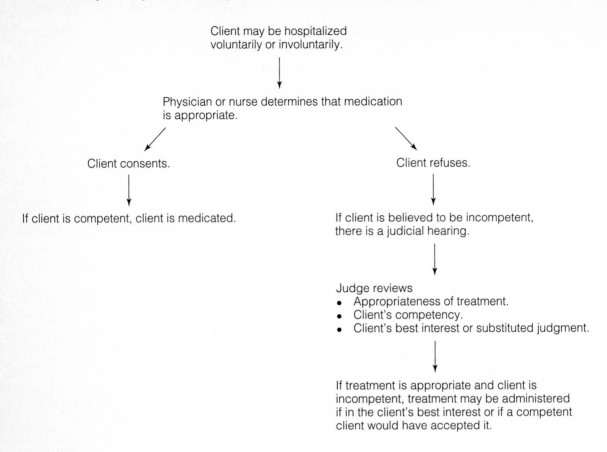

Figure 23.1 **Outcomes of client medication decisions.**

Source: Adapted from Applebaum, 1988.

regarding confidentiality. Breach of confidentiality is considered unprofessional conduct and is grounds for discipline by the state licensing board.

When you work with clients, you must discuss the subject of confidentiality. Explain to clients that what is discussed is shared only with the staff and the instructor. If you know the client from outside the hospital, reassure the client that his or her presence on the unit is absolutely confidential. In this situation, you should not provide care for this person nor read the chart.

There are federal regulations regarding chemical dependence (CD) programs. Everyone, including professionals and visitors, must sign a confidentiality statement before entering a CD unit. Staff members are not allowed to disclose any admission or discharge information. They may not even acknowledge whether the client is in the facility.

Legally, a child does not have the right to confidentiality. In most cases, the parents, as legal guardians responsible for the child, have the right to know what is going on in treatment. Parents usually desire information and some level of involvement in their child's treatment paln. They often seek advice on how to cope with the day-to-day challenges they face, what they might expect in the future, and sources of community support.

Many states have laws regarding when HIV test results and/or the diagnosis of AIDS may be disclosed. In many states, this information may not even be put in the medical record without the written consent of the client. In some states, clients must give written consent before HIV tests may be performed, while in other states, oral consent is sufficient. However, because oral consent is difficult to prove, most institutions require written consent.

Reporting Laws

All states make it mandatory for nurses to report suspected cases of child abuse or neglect. Failure to report these cases subjects the nurse to both criminal penalties and civil liability. Reporting protects the nurse from being sued by the parents or guardian. Many states have enacted adult abuse laws similar to the child abuse reporting laws. It is important that you know the laws for your state.

Duty to Disclose

The **duty to disclose** is the health care professional's obligation to warn identified individuals if a client has made a credible threat to kill them. The duty to disclose supersedes the client's right to confidentiality. In some states, the duty to disclose also includes threats against property. The general rule is to warn identified persons of believable threats when the client is not confined to the hospital.

Leaving Against Medical Advice (LAMA)

Some clients try leaving against medical advice, often called **elopement,** from the restrictive hospital setting. When a client successfully elopes, the staff notifies the physician, the hospital administration, and the family. If it is determined that the client is dangerous to self or others, local police are informed of the situation. A hospital can be sued when clients who elope commit suicide, are injured or killed in accidents, or injure or kill others while away from the hospital. The liability is determined on the basis of two elements. The first element is how much the staff knew or should have known about the level of danger to self or others. The second element is the appropriateness of precautions taken to prevent LAMA in light of that knowledge.

If you are assigned to a locked unit, you should take some basic precautions. Whenever entering or leaving the unit, look around and be aware of clients very near the door. These clients may slip out when the door is opened. If you leave the unit with other students, make sure that a client has not joined your group. When clients ask you to accompany them off the unit, check with the staff on each client's status for off-unit privileges.

Clients with Legal Charges

Some clients admitted to the psychiatric unit may have legal charges pending. You may have difficulty working with these clients when the behavior that resulted in the legal charges is in conflict with your personal values. Examples are a client admitted for severe depression with legal charges of sexually molesting his child, and a client admitted to a substance abuse program who hit a pedestrian while driving under the influence. When ethical dilemmas arise, you must identify your feelings and seek peer or supervisor advice in managing the situation and avoiding punitive reactions. Confidentiality is extremely important in such circumstances. Clients must also be informed that their medical records may be requested by the court and that staff members may be required to testify in court.

The Mentally Ill in Prisons and Jails

The number of mentally ill people in prisons and jails has increased over the past 30 years. Studies indicate that 10–15% of prison inmates suffer from a major mental disorder. With few long-term psychiatric facilities, many people who were previously cared for in state hospitals are now found in jails and prisons. The increase in numbers is also related to a lack of support in the community for the severely and persistently mentally ill population. About one-third of these individuals are homeless and victims of a cycle of mental hospitals, the street, and jail as a way of life over which they have no control. They may be jailed because no other agencies are available to respond to their psychiatric emergency. The jail has become the mental hospital that cannot say no. Often the crimes with which they are charged are misdemeanors resulting from their symptoms of mental illness, such as disorderly conduct, trespassing, and drunkenness. This "criminalization" of mental illness must be stopped. Under the 14th Amendment of the Constitution, mentally ill jail detainees have a right to mental health services. The reality is that psychiatric

Critical Thinking

Taneko is a 43-year-old lady who has been committed to a psychiatric facility by her husband. Taneko is very angry, sobbing hysterically, and screaming at Bill for bringing her to the hospital instead of her doctor's office. Bill maintains that Taneko is a danger to herself because she has been depressed for several months and this morning threatened suicide.

Taneko is seeing a psychotherapist on a regular basis and feels that her depression is related to her father's death, which occurred 9 months ago. Upon further assessment, the nurse learns that Taneko does not feel she is suicidal even though she made a statement to that effect earlier in the day. Taneko feels that she is being held against her will and wants to speak to an attorney. Bill is tired and frustrated. He does not want to take Taneko home because he does not feel that he can adequately take care of her.

1. Should Taneko be committed to the psychiatric facility or released? Defend your position.

2. One of Taneko's neighbors is a nurse working at the psychiatric facility where Bill took Taneko. What is the neighbor's responsibility, if any, toward Taneko now that she knows Taneko is a client there?

3. Even though Taneko is only being detained on a temporary basis, she has been placed on elopement precautions. Explain the rational for elopement precautions.

4. How will Taneko's rights be affected if she decides to stay hospitalized and undergo treatment for her depression?

5. As a mental health professional, how can Taneko's nurse show she cares? How can this best be achieved?

6. Elaborate on why Taneko and Bill's situation creates an ethical dilemma.

Suggested answers can be found in Appendix D.

status. Many mentally ill people suffer cruelty and abuse by other inmates, including torment, beatings, and rape. When an inmate needs someone to take the blame or punishment, the inmate who is mentally ill is easily manipulated into this position. Guards often place severely mentally ill prisoners in solitary confinement for misbehavior that is a product of their mental illness. Symptoms worsen with the prolonged social isolation, sensory deprivation, excessive use of force by guards, use of restraints as punishment, and inadequate medical care. Solitary confinement is no place for any prisoner, especially one who is seriously mentally ill (Peternelj-Taylor and Johnson, 1995; Teplin, Abram, McClelland, 1997). The suicide rate among jail inmates is eight times that of the U.S. population, with hanging being the most common method. The first 25 hours following the arrest is the period of highest risk. Adolescents may be especially vulnerable due to feelings of fear, humiliation, and isolation from their peer group. People charged with murder may be at highest risk due to a generalized impulsivity (Zealberg, Santos, 1996).

Caring: A Prerequisite to Ethical Behavior

People who are in a caring relationship are likely to behave in an ethical manner toward each other. Nurses have identified the following behaviors as being the most significant to a caring relationship (Wolf, 1986):

- attentive listening
- providing comfort
- honesty
- patience
- responsibility
- providing adequate information
- touch
- sensitivity
- respect
- calling the client by name

When clients are asked what they want from nurses, they respond with the following (Reilly, 1989; Sprengel and Kelley, 1992):

evaluation and intervention is haphazard at best (Rappaport, 1997). The prison subculture makes those who are seriously mentally ill more vulnerable to abuse and victimization by both inmates and guards, since those who are mentally ill hold low

- concern
- involvement
- sharing
- touching
- presence
- humor

Caring is being respectful of people's choices as to the best course of action to be taken. Caring is accepting people as they are and envisioning what they may become. Caring is honoring each person's wholeness of being—mind, body, emotions, and spirit.

Nursing Ethics

Nursing is a value-laden practice. We are required to make numerous ethical decisions every day. For example, we make ethical judgments when deciding to use prn medication, restraints, or seclusion for the client who is losing control.

The expectation that nurses will deliver competent care is fundamental to the notion of professional nursing practice. This is evidenced by the American Nurses Association Nursing Code of Ethics described in Box 23.1. Competence is both "knowing what" and "knowing how." It is not a permanent state achieved when you get your nursing license but rather a continuing process of improving and refining your skills and knowledge. Competence is both education and attitude. Education is the academic program you are enrolled in and continuing education throughout your years of practice. Attitude includes being open to criticism by colleagues, and a willingness to admit to lack of knowledge or error when appropriate. Competence is the recognition of one's limitations as well as one's strengths and skills. With the explosion of scientific information, competent nurses must stay current with developments in their areas of practice (Haas and Malouf, 1995).

Caring for clients whose values and lifestyles are similar to ours does not challenge us to make the choice to accept the client's inherent worth. As our society becomes more ethnically diverse and multicultural in character, the potential for rising ethical conflicts increases. When values and lifestyles are dissimilar, we are challenged to make caring, ethical decisions. Consider how each of the following clients might pose an ethical dilemma when admitted to a mental health care facility: a known drug pusher; a

Box 23.1

ANA Nursing Code of Ethics

1. The nurse provides services with respect for human dignity and the uniqueness of the client, unrestricted by considerations of social or economic status, personal attributes, or the nature of health problems.

2. The nurse safeguards the client's right to privacy by judiciously protecting information of a confidential nature.

3. The nurse acts to safeguard the client and the public when health care and safety are affected by the incompetent, unethical, or illegal practice of any person.

4. The nurse assumes responsibility and accountability for individual nursing judgments and actions.

5. The nurse maintains competence in nursing.

6. The nurse exercises informed judgment and uses individual competence and qualification as criteria in seeking consultation, accepting responsibilities, and delegating nursing activities to others.

7. The nurse participates in activities that contribute to the ongoing development of the profession's body of knowledge.

8. The nurse participates in the profession's efforts to implement and improve standards of nursing.

9. The nurse participates in the profession's efforts to establish and maintain conditions of employment conducive to high-quality nursing care.

10. The nurse participates in the profession's effort to protect the public from misinformation and misrepresentation to maintain the integrity of nursing.

11. The nurse collaborates with members of the health professions and other citizens in promoting community and national efforts to meet public health needs.

Source: American Nurses' Association, 1985.

mother who has killed her baby through physical abuse; a teenager who has sexually molested his sister; an adult daughter who has physically abused her elderly father; an accused rapist. As nurses, we must be able to respect the humanness of every client in spite of differences in values and lifestyles.

Traditionally, nurses have been taught ethics from the perspective of principalism. This is based on the belief that there are universal, objective principles that ought to govern the moral behavior of people. The principles are autonomy, beneficence, nonmaleficence, and justice. Autonomy is the right to make decisions for oneself. Beneficence is the performance of good acts that benefit others, in contrast to nonmaleficence, which is not acting in a way that would cause harm to self or others. The principle of justice states that people should be treated equally and people should be recognized for responsible behavior. The problem with the perspective of principalism is that socioeconomic and cultural contexts are completely ignored. They are also far too abstract to have any practical application in clinical practice (Artnak and Dimmitt, 1996; McGee, 1996).

Nursing is based on an ethics of care. We use many perspectives in the process of ethical decision making, which can be summarized in four categories: medical indications, client preferences, quality of life, and contextual factors. Medical indications include the diagnosis, prognosis, and treatment options with probable outcomes. Client preferences relate to the individuals' values and goals for life in general and their advance directives when they are acutely ill.

Quality of life involves clients' perceptions about what their life is like and what they would like it to be. Contextual factors include social and environmental details about the problem and how these affect treatment options (Artnak and Dimmitt, 1996).

The nursing profession places a high value on client autonomy and the client's right to participate in treatment planning and implementation, as reflected in the Nursing Code of Ethics. This code implies that one of the primary functions of the nurse is to be an advocate for the client's wishes. At times, you will function much in the same way as an advance directive. The Patient Self-Determination Act became federal law in 1990. This law states that clients have a right to participate in their own care. In addition, health care professionals are required to inform clients of the right to accept or refuse medical care, including medications.

Ethics is more a process than a set of answers. At the heart of every ethical dilemma is the potential for conflict—conflict within ourselves, conflict between nurse and client, or conflict among professionals. We must confront difficult ethical problems and arrive at options that best support the client's own values and wishes.

Key Concepts

Introduction

■ Whenever possible, client autonomy and liberty must be ensured by treatment in the least restrictive setting and by active client participation in treatment decisions.

Types of Admission

■ Voluntary admission occurs when a client consents to confinement in the hospital and signs a document indicating as much.

■ Commitment, or involuntary admission, may be implemented on the basis of dangerousness to self or others. Some states also have the criterion of prevention of significant physical or mental deterioration for involuntary admission.

■ Adult clients can be held temporarily on an emergency basis until there is a court hearing determining the need for commitment.

■ Commitment is for a specified period of time. At the end of this time, the client must be discharged or the court must be petitioned again for continued hospitalization.

■ Clients can initiate advance directives to guide families and caregivers in making decisions when they are unable to make them for themselves.

Competency

■ Competency is a legal determination that a client can make reasonable judgments and decisions about treatment and other significant areas of personal life.

- An adult is considered competent unless a court rules him or her incompetent. In such cases, a guardian is appointed to make decisions on that person's behalf.
- Clients who are committed are still capable of participating in health care decisions.

Informed Consent

- Informed consent is a client's right not to be touched or treated without consent. Clients must be given enough information to make a decision, must be able to understand the information, and must communicate their decision to others.
- In an emergency situation with no time to obtain consent without endangering health or safety, a client may be treated without legal liability.

Client Rights

- Clients do not lose their constitutional or legal rights when they are admitted to the hospital to treat a mental disorder.
- Clients have the right to refuse psychotropic medications.
- If the court finds the client to be incompetent and medications are in the client's best interest, the judge may order the client to take the medications.

Confidentiality

- Adherence to the principle of confidentiality is extremely important in the practice of psychiatric nursing.
- There are federal rules regarding chemical dependence confidentiality. Staff members are not allowed to disclose any admission or discharge information.
- Some states require written consent before HIV tests may be performed. States have laws regarding when HIV test results or the diagnosis of AIDS may be disclosed.

Reporting Laws

- All states make it mandatory for nurses to report suspected cases of child abuse or neglect. Some states have enacted similar adult abuse laws.

Duty to Disclose

- The duty to disclose is the health care professional's obligation to warn identified individuals if a client has made a credible threat to kill them.

Leaving Against Medical Advice (LAMA)

- Staff members must take precautions to prevent LAMA, or elopement, from the unit by those clients who are dangerous to self or others.

Clients with Legal Charges

- Clients who have legal charges pending against them must be informed that their medical records may be requested by the court.

The Mentally Ill in Prisons and Jails

- Clients with mental disorders may be jailed because their symptoms are mistaken for criminal behavior or there may be no other agencies available to respond to their psychiatric emergency.
- Clients with mental disorders who are imprisoned are vulnerable to abuse and victimization by other inmates.
- The suicide rate among jail inmates is eight times that of the U.S. population.

Caring: A Prerequisite to Ethical Behavior

- Caring behaviors include attentive listening; providing comfort, honesty, patience, and responsibility; providing adequate information, touch, sensitivity, and respect; and calling the client by name.

Nursing Ethics

- Nurses are required to make numerous ethical decisions every day. Client differences in values and lifestyles often present nurses with an ethical dilemma when clients are admitted to a mental health care facility.
- Competent care involves knowing what and how to do things, being open to criticism, and a willingness to admit to lack of knowledge or error when appropriate.
- The perspective of principalism in ethics ignores the socioeconomic and cultural contexts and is too abstract to have practical application in clinical practice.
- Nursing is based on an ethics of care, including medical indications, client preferences, quality of life, and contextual factors.

Review Questions

1. Commitment to a psychiatric unit

   a. involves the criminal justice system.

   b. is for an indefinite time period.

   c. is based on the principle of dangerousness.

   d. removes all client rights to autonomy.

2. Which of the following is an argument against commitment?

   a. The family may not be able to care for an acutely ill member.

   b. Interventions will ease suffering and in some cases, save lives.

   c. In many instances, it is the only way to obtain treatment from the public health care system.

   d. It reinforces the stigma that mentally ill people are dangerous and unpredictable.

3. Breach of confidentiality may mean

   a. no formal action will be taken.

   b. grounds for discipline by the state board of nursing.

   c. clients can sue nurses in the criminal justice system.

   d. failure of the nurse's duty to disclose.

4. The reason many mentally ill people end up in jail is that

   a. their symptoms are misjudged as criminal behavior.

   b. they are more likely to commit murder than other people.

   c. it is the only place their behavior can be controlled.

   d. their families request it to protect themselves.

5. Taking precautions against client elopement includes

   a. whenever entering or leaving a locked unit, looking around and being aware of clients who are very near the door.

   b. confining clients to their rooms or to the dayroom.

   c. allowing no clients to have off-unit privileges.

   d. placing clients in restraints if they are at risk for elopement.

References

American Nurses Association. (1985). *Code for Nurses with Interpretative Statements.*

Applebaum, P. S. (1988). The right to refuse treatment with antipsychotic medications. *Am J Psychiatry, 145*(1), 145–146.

Artnak, K. E., & Dimmitt, J. H. (1996). Choosing a framework for ethical analysis in advanced practice settings. *Arch Psychiatr Nurs, 10*(1), 16–23.

Griffin-Francell, C. (1995). Changing the involuntary commitment laws is not the answer. *NAMI Advocate, 16*(4), 18–21.

Grisso, T., & Appelbaum, P. S. (1995). Comparison of standards for assessing patients' capacities to make treatment decisions. *Am J Psychiatry, 152*(7), 1033–1037.

Haas, L .J., & Malouf, J. L. (1995). *Keeping up the Good Work: A Practitioner's Guide for Mental Health Ethics* (2nd ed.). Prof Resource Press.

Jaffe, D. J. (1995). Change involuntary treatment laws. *NAMI Advocate, 16*(4), 16–17.

Kaplan, R. J. (1995). New survey assesses outpatient commitment. *NAMI Advocate, 16*(4), 3–12.

McGee, G. (1996). Waiting for Godot: Where is the philosophy of nursing? *J Psychosoc Nurs, 34*(6), 43–44.

Peternelj-Taylor, C. A., & Johnson, R. L. (1995). Serving time: Psychiatric mental health nursing in corrections. *J Psychosoc Nurs, 33*(8), 12–19.

Rappaport, M. G. (1997). John Salvi III commits suicide. *NAMI Advocate, 18*(4), 3.

Reilly, D. E. (1989). Ethics and values in nursing. *Nurs & Health Care, 10*(2), 91–95.

Sprengel, A., & Kelley, J. (1992). The ethics of caring: A basis for holistic care. *J Holistic Nurs, 10*(3), 231–239.

Teplin, L. A., Abram, K. M., & McClelland, G. M. (1997). Psychiatric disorders among women in jail. *Decade of the Brain, 8*(2), 8–10.

Wolf, Z. (1986). The caring concept and nurse-identified caring behaviors. *Topics Clin Nurs, 8*(2), 231–239.

Zealberg, J. J., & Santos, A. B. (1996). *Comprehensive Emergency Mental Health Care.* New York: Norton.

Appendices

APPENDIX A

*DSM-IV Classification**

NOS = Not Otherwise Specified

Axis I

Disorders Usually First Diagnosed in Infancy, Childhood, or Adolescence

Mental Retardation[†]
Mild Mental Retardation
Moderate Mental Retardation
Severe Mental Retardation
Profound Mental Retardation
Mental Retardation, Severity Unspecified

Learning Disorders
Reading Disorder
Mathematics Disorder
Disorder of Written Expression
Learning Disorder NOS

Motor Skills Disorder
Developmental Coordination Disorder

Communication Disorders
Expressive Language Disorder
Mixed Receptive-Expressive Language Disorder
Phonological Disorder
Stuttering
Communication Disorder NOS

Pervasive Developmental Disorders
Autistic Disorder
Rett's Disorder

Childhood Disintegrative Disorder
Asperger's Disorder
Pervasive Developmental Disorder NOS

Attention-Deficit and Disruptive Behavior Disorders
Attention-Deficit/Hyperactivity Disorder
  Combined Type
  Predominantly Inattentive Type
  Predominantly Hyperactive-Impulsive Type
Attention-Deficit/Hyperactivity Disorder NOS
Conduct Disorder
Oppositional Defiant Disorder
Disruptive Behavior Disorder NOS

Feeding and Eating Disorders of Infancy or Early Childhood
Pica
Rumination Disorder
Feeding Disorder of Infancy or Early Childhood

Tic Disorders
Tourette's Disorder
Chronic Motor or Vocal Tic Disorder
Transient Tic Disorder
Tic Disorder NOS

Elimination Disorders
Encopresis
Enuresis (Not Due to a General Medical Condition)

Other Disorders of Infancy, Childhood, or Adolescence
Separation Anxiety Disorder
Selective Mutism

*Source: Adapted from American Psychiatric Association: *Diagnostic and Statistical Manual of Mental Disorders,* 4th ed. American Psychiatric Association, 1994.
†Note: These are coded on Axis II.

Reactive Attachment Disorder
of Infancy or Early Childhood
Stereotypic Movement Disorder
Disorder of Infancy, Childhood,
or Adolescence NOS

Delirium, Dementia, and Amnestic and Other Cognitive Disorders

Delirium

Delirium Due to . . . *[Indicate the
General Medical Condition]*
Substance Intoxication Delirium
Substance Withdrawal Delirium
Delirium Due to Multiple Etiologies
Delirium NOS

Dementia

Dementia of the Alzheimer's Type, With Early Onset
Uncomplicated
With Delirium
With Delusions
With Depressed Mood
Dementia of the Alzheimer's Type, With Late Onset
Uncomplicated
With Delirium
With Delusions
With Depressed Mood
Vascular Dementia
Uncomplicated
With Delirium
With Delusions
With Depressed Mood

Dementia Due to Other General Medical Conditions

Dementia Due to HIV Disease
Dementia Due to Head Trauma
Dementia Due to Parkinson's Disease
Dementia Due to Huntington's Disease
Dementia Due to Pick's Disease
Dementia Due to Creutzfeldt-Jakob Disease
Dementia Due to . . . *[Indicate the General
Medical Condition not listed above]*
Substance-Induced Persisting Dementia
Dementia Due to Multiple Etiologies
Dementia NOS

Amnestic Disorders

Amnestic Disorder Due to . . . *[Indicate
the General Medical Condition]*

Substance-Induced Persisting Amnestic Disorder
Amnestic Disorder NOS

Other Cognitive Disorders

Cognitive Disorder NOS

Mental Disorders Due to a General Medical Condition Not Elsewhere Classified

Catatonic Disorder Due to . . . *[Indicate the
General Medical Condition]*
Personality Change Due to . . . *[Indicate the
General Medical Condition]*
Mental Disorder NOS Due to . . . *[Indicate the
General Medical Condition]*

Substance-Related Disorders

Substance-induced disorders include withdrawal,
intoxication, delirium, dementia, psychotic disorder, mood disorder, anxiety disorder, sexual
disorder, and sleep disorder.

Alcohol-Related Disorders

Alcohol Use Disorders
Alcohol Dependence
Alcohol Abuse
Alcohol-Induced Disorders

Amphetamine (or Amphetamine-Like)– Related Disorders

Amphetamine Use Disorders
Amphetamine Dependence
Amphetamine Abuse
Amphetamine-Induced Disorders

Caffeine-Related Disorders

Caffeine-Induced Disorders
Caffeine Intoxication
Caffeine-Induced Anxiety Disorder
Caffeine-Induced Sleep Disorder
Caffeine-Related Disorder NOS

Cannabis-Related Disorders

Cannabis Use Disorders
Cannabis Dependence
Cannabis Abuse
Cannabis-Induced Disorders

Cocaine-Related Disorders
Cocaine Use Disorders
Cocaine Dependence
Cocaine Abuse
Cocaine-Induced Disorders

Hallucinogen-Related Disorders
Hallucinogen Use Disorders
Hallucinogen Dependence
Hallucinogen Abuse
Hallucinogen-Induced Disorders

Inhalant-Related Disorders
Inhalant Use Disorders
Inhalant Dependence
Inhalant Abuse
Inhalant-Induced Disorders

Nicotine-Related Disorders
Nicotine Use Disorder
Nicotine Dependence
Nicotine-Induced Disorder

Opioid-Related Disorders
Opioid Use Disorders
Opioid Dependence
Opioid Abuse
Opioid-Induced Disorders

**Phencyclidine (or Phencyclidine-Like)–
Related Disorders**
Phencyclidine Use Disorders
Phencyclidine Dependence
Phencyclidine Abuse
Phencyclidine-Induced Disorders

**Sedative-, Hypnotic-, or
Anxiolytic-Related Disorders**
Sedative, Hypnotic, or Anxiolytic Use Disorders
Sedative, Hypnotic, or Anxiolytic Dependence
Sedative, Hypnotic, or Anxiolytic Abuse
*Sedative-, Hypnotic-, or
Anxiolytic-Induced Disorders*

Polysubstance-Related Disorder
Polysubstance Dependence

Other (or Unknown) Substance–Related Disorders
Other (or Unknown) Substance Use Disorders
Other (or Unknown) Substance Dependence
Other (or Unknown) Substance Abuse
Other (or Unknown) Substance–Induced Disorders

Schizophrenia and Other Psychotic Disorders

Schizophrenia
  Paranoid Type
  Disorganized Type
  Catatonic Type
  Undifferentiated Type
  Residual Type
Schizophreniform Disorder
Schizoaffective Disorder
Delusional Disorder
Brief Psychotic Disorder
Shared Psychotic Disorder
Psychotic Disorder Due to . . . *[Indicate the
  General Medical Condition]*
  With Delusions
  With Hallucinations
  Substance-Induced Psychotic Disorder
Psychotic Disorder NOS

Mood Disorders

Depressive Disorders
Major Depressive Disorder
  Single Episode
  Recurrent
Dysthymic Disorder
Depressive Disorder NOS

Bipolar Disorders
Bipolar I Disorder
  Single Manic Episode
  Most Recent Episode Hypomanic
  Most Recent Episode Manic
  Most Recent Episode Mixed
  Most Recent Episode Depressed
  Most Recent Episode Unspecified
Bipolar II Disorder
Cyclothymic Disorder
Bipolar Disorder NOS
Mood Disorder Due to . . . *[Indicate the
  General Medical Condition]*
  Substance-Induced Mood Disorder
Mood Disorder NOS

Anxiety Disorders

Panic Disorder Without Agoraphobia
Panic Disorder With Agoraphobia
Agoraphobia Without History of Panic Disorder
Specific Phobia
Social Phobia
Obsessive-Compulsive Disorder
Posttraumatic Stress Disorder
Acute Stress Disorder
Generalized Anxiety Disorder
Anxiety Disorder Due to . . . *[Indicate the
    General Medical Condition]*
    Substance-Induced Anxiety Disorder
Anxiety Disorder NOS

Somatoform Disorders

Somatization Disorder
Undifferentiated Somatoform Disorder
Conversion Disorder
Pain Disorder
Hypochondriasis
Body Dysmorphic Disorder
Somatoform Disorder NOS

Factitious Disorders

Factitious Disorder
Factitious Disorder NOS

Dissociative Disorders

Dissociative Amnesia
Dissociative Fugue
Dissociative Identity Disorder
Depersonalization Disorder
Dissociative Disorder NOS

Sexual and Gender Identity Disorders

Sexual Dysfunctions
Sexual Desire Disorders
Hypoactive Sexual Desire Disorder
Sexual Aversion Disorder
Sexual Arousal Disorders
Female Sexual Arousal Disorder
Male Erectile Disorder

Orgasmic Disorders
Female Orgasmic Disorder
Male Orgasmic Disorder
Premature Ejaculation
Sexual Pain Disorders
Dyspareunia (Not Due to a
    General Medical Condition)
Vaginismus (Not Due to a
    General Medical Condition)
*Sexual Dysfunction Due to a
    General Medical Condition*

Paraphilias
Exhibitionism
Fetishism
Frotteurism
Pedophilia
Sexual Masochism
Sexual Sadism
Transvestic Fetishism
Voyeurism
Paraphilia NOS

Gender Identity Disorders
Gender Identity Disorder
    in Children
    in Adolescents or Adults
Gender Identity Disorder NOS
Sexual Disorder NOS

Eating Disorders

Anorexia Nervosa
Bulimia Nervosa
Eating Disorder NOS

Sleep Disorders

Primary Sleep Disorders
Dyssomnias
Primary Insomnia
Primary Hypersomnia
Narcolepsy
Breathing-Related Sleep Disorder
Circadian Rhythm Sleep Disorder
Dyssomnia NOS
Parasomnias
Nightmare Disorder

Sleep Terror Disorder
Sleepwalking Disorder
Parasomnia NOS

Sleep Disorders Related to Another Mental Disorder
Insomnia Related to . . .
Hypersomnia Related to . . .

Other Sleep Disorders
Sleep Disorder Due to . . . *[Indicate the General Medical Condition]*
    Substance-Induced Sleep Disorder

Impulse-Control Disorders Not Elsewhere Classified

Intermittent Explosive Disorder
Kleptomania
Pyromania
Pathological Gambling
Trichotillomania
Impulse-Control Disorder NOS

Adjustment Disorders

Adjustment Disorder
    With Depressed Mood
    With Anxiety
    With Mixed Anxiety and Depressed Mood
    With Disturbance of Conduct
    With Mixed Disturbance
    of Emotions and Conduct
    Unspecified

Other Conditions That May Be a Focus of Clinical Attention

Medication-Induced Movement Disorders
Neuroleptic-Induced Parkinsonism
Neuroleptic Malignant Syndrome
Neuroleptic-Induced Acute Dystonia
Neuroleptic-Induced Acute Akathisia
Neuroleptic-Induced Tardive Dyskinesia
Medication-Induced Postural Tremor
Medication-Induced Movement Disorder NOS

Relational Problems
Relational Problem Related to a Mental
    Disorder or General Medical Condition

Parent-Child Relational Problem
Partner Relational Problem
Sibling Relational Problem
Relational Problem NOS

Problems Related to Abuse or Neglect
Physical Abuse of Child
Sexual Abuse of Child
Neglect of Child
Physical Abuse of Adult
Sexual Abuse of Adult

**Additional Conditions That May
Be a Focus of Clinical Attention**
Noncompliance With Treatment
Malingering
Adult Antisocial Behavior
Child or Adolescent Antisocial Behavior
Borderline Intellectual Functioning
Age-Related Cognitive Decline
Bereavement
Academic Problem
Occupational Problem
Identity Problem
Religious or Spiritual Problem
Acculturation Problem
Phase of Life Problem

Axis II

Mental Retardation (see Axis I, Childhood)

Personality Disorders
Paranoid Personality Disorder
Schizoid Personality Disorder
Schizotypal Personality Disorder
Antisocial Personality Disorder
Borderline Personality Disorder
Histrionic Personality Disorder
Narcissistic Personality Disorder
Avoidant Personality Disorder
Dependent Personality Disorder
Obsessive-Compulsive Personality Disorder
Personality Disorder NOS

Axis III

Physical Disorders or Conditions

Axis III permits the clinician to indicate any current physical disorder or condition that is potentially relevant to the understanding or management of the case. These are the conditions listed outside the "mental disorders section" of ICD-9-CM. In some instances the condition may be etiologically significant (such as a neurological disorder associated with dementia); in other instances the physical disorder may not be etiologic, but it may be important in the overall management of the case (such as diabetes in a child with conduct disorder). In yet other instances, the clinician may wish to note significant associated physical findings, such as "soft neurological signs." Multiple diagnoses are permitted.

Axis IV

Psychosocial and Environmental Problems

Axis IV is for reporting psychosocial and environmental problems that may affect the diagnosis, treatment, and prognosis of mental disorders (Axes I and II). A psychosocial or environmental problem may be a negative life event, an environmental difficulty or deficiency, a familial or other interpersonal stress, an inadequacy of social support or personal resources, or other problem relating to the context in which a person's difficulties have developed. So-called positive stressors, such as job promotion, should be listed only if they constitute or lead to a problem, as when a person has difficulty adapting to the new situation. In addition to playing a role in the initiation or exacerbation of a mental disorder, psychosocial problems may also develop as a consequence of a person's psychopathology or may constitute problems that should be considered in the overall management plan.

When an individual has multiple psychosocial or environmental problems, the clinician may note as many as are judged to be relevant. In general, the clinician should note only those psychosocial and environmental problems that have been present during the year preceding the current evaluation. However, the clinician may choose to note psychosocial and environmental problems occurring prior to the previous year if these clearly contribute to the mental disorder or have become a focus of treatment—for example, previous combat experiences leading to Posttraumatic Stress Disorder.

For convenience, the problems are grouped together in the following categories:

- **Problems with primary support group**— e.g., death of a family member; health problems in family; disruption of family by separation, divorce, or estrangement; removal from the home; remarriage of parent; sexual or phsyical abuse; parental overprotection; neglect of child; inadequate discipline; discord with siblings; birth of a sibling

- **Problems related to the social environment**— e.g., death or loss of friend; inadequate social support; living alone; difficulty with acculturation; discrimination; adjustment to life-cycle transition (such as retirement)

- **Educational problems**—e.g., illiteracy; academic problems; discord with teachers or classmates; inadequate school environment

- **Occupational problems**—e.g., unemployment; threat of job loss; stressful work schedule; difficult work conditions; job dissatisfaction; job change; discord with boss or co-workers

- **Housing problems**—e.g., homelessness; inadequate housing; unsafe neighborhood; discord with neighbors or landlord

- **Economic problems**—e.g., extreme poverty; inadequate finances; insufficient welfare support

- **Problems with access to health care services**— e.g., inadequate health care services; transportation to health care facilities unavailable; inadequate health insurance

- **Problems related to interaction with the legal system/crime**—e.g., arrest; incarceration; litigation; victim of crime

- **Other psychosocial and environmental problems**—e.g., exposure to disasters, war, other hostilities; discord with nonfamily caregivers such as counselor, social worker, or physician; unavailability of social service agencies

Axis V

Global Assessment of Functioning (GAF) Scale*

Consider psychological, social, and occupational functioning on a hypothetical continuum of mental health–illness. Do not include impairment in functioning due to physical (or environmental) limitations.

Code   (Note: Use intermediate codes when appropriate, e.g., 45, 68, 72.)

100 | **Superior functioning in a wide range of activities, life's problems never seem to get out of hand, is sought out by
91 | others because of his or her many positive qualities. No symptoms.**

90 | **Absent or minimal symptoms** (e.g., mild anxiety before an exam), **good functioning in all areas, interested and
| involved in a wide range of activities, socially effective, generally satisfied with life, no more than everyday prob-
81 | lems or concerns** (e.g., an occasional argument with family members).

80 | **If symptoms are present, they are transient and expectable reactions to psychosocial stressors** (e.g., difficulty con-
| centrating after a family argument); **no more than slight impairment in social, occupational, or school function-
71 | ing** (e.g., temporarily falling behind in schoolwork).

70 | **Some mild symptoms** (e.g., depressed mood and mild insomnia) **OR some difficulty in social, occupational, or
| school functioning** (e.g., occasional truancy, or theft within the household), **but generally functioning pretty well,
61 | has some meaningful interpersonal relationships.**

60 | **Moderate symptoms** (e.g., flat affect and circumstantial speech, occasional panic attacks) **OR moderate difficulty
51 | in social, occupational, or school functioning** (e.g., few friends, conflicts with peers or coworkers).

50 | **Serious symptoms** (e.g., suicidal ideation, severe obsessional rituals, frequent shoplifting) **OR any serious impair-
41 | ment in social, occupational, or school functioning** (e.g., no friends, unable to keep a job).

40 | **Some impairment in reality testing or communication** (e.g., speech is at times illogical, obscure, or irrelevant) **OR
| major impairment in several areas, such as work or school, family relations, judgment, thinking, or mood** (e.g.,
| depressed man avoids friends, neglects family, and is unable to work; child frequently beats up younger children,
31 | is defiant at home, and is failing at school).

30 | **Behavior is considerably influenced by delusions or hallucinations OR serious impairment in communication or
| judgment** (e.g., sometimes incoherent, acts grossly inappropriately, suicidal preoccupation) **OR inability to func-
21 | tion in almost all areas** (e.g., stays in bed all day; no job, home, or friends).

20 | **Some danger of hurting self or others** (e.g., suicide attempts without clear expectation of death, frequently vio-
| lent, manic excitement) **OR occasionally fails to maintain minimal personal hygiene** (e.g., smears feces) **OR gross
11 | impairment in communication** (e.g., largely incoherent or mute).

10 | **Persistent danger of severely hurting self or others** (e.g., recurrent violence) **OR persistent inability to maintain
1 | minimal personal hygiene OR serious suicidal act with clear expectation of death.**

0 | Inadequate information.

---

*The rating of overall psychological functioning on a scale of 0–100 was operationalized by Luborsky in the Health-Sickness Rating Scale (Luborsky L: "Clinicians' Judgments of Mental Health." *Archives of General Psychiatry* 7:407–417, 1962). Spitzer and colleagues developed a revision of the Health-Sickness Rating Scale called the Global Assessment Scale (GAS) (Endicott J, Spitzer RL, Fleiss JL, Cohen J: "The Global Assessment Scale: A Procedure for Measuring Overall Severity of Psychiatric Disturbance." *Archives of General Psychiatry* 33:766–771, 1976). A modified version of the GAS was included in DSM-III-R as the Global Assessment of Functioning (GAF) Scale.

APPENDIX B

*NANDA-Approved Nursing Diagnostic Categories**

Activity Intolerance
Activity Intolerance, Risk for
Adaptive Capacity: Intracranial, Decreased
Adjustment, Impaired
Airway Clearance, Ineffective
Anticipatory Grieving
Anxiety
Aspiration, Risk for
Body Image Disturbance
Body Temperature, Risk for Altered
Bowel Incontinence
Breastfeeding, Effective
Breastfeeding, Ineffective
Breastfeeding, Interrupted
Breathing Pattern, Ineffective
Cardiac Output, Decreased
Caregiver Role Strain
Caregiver Role Strain, Risk for
Chronic Low Self Esteem
Chronic Pain
Colonic Constipation
Communication, Impaired Verbal
Community Coping, Ineffective
Community Coping, Potential for Enhanced
Confusion, Acute
Confusion, Chronic
Constipation
Constipation, Colonic
Constipation, Perceived
Decisional Conflict (Specify)
Decreased Cardiac Output
Defensive Coping
Denial, Ineffective

Diarrhea
Disorganized Infant Behavior
Disorganized Infant Behavior, Risk for
Disuse Syndrome, Risk for
Diversional Activity Deficit
Dysfunctional Grieving
Dysfunctional Ventilatory Weaning Response
  (DVWR)
Dysreflexia
Energy Field Disturbance
Environmental Interpretation Syndrome
Impaired
Family Coping: Compromised, Ineffective
Family Coping: Disabling, Ineffective
Family Coping: Potential for Growth
Family Process: Alcoholism, Altered
Family Processes, Altered
Fatigue
Fear
Fluid Volume Deficit
Fluid Volume Deficit, Risk for
Fluid Volume Excess
Functional Incontinence
Gas Exchange, Impaired
Grieving, Anticipatory
Grieving, Dysfunctional
Growth and Development, Altered
Health Maintenance, Altered
Health Seeking Behaviors (Specify)
Home Maintenance Management, Impaired
Hopelessness
Hyperthermia
Hypothermia

*Source: North American Nursing Diagnosis Association: *NANDA Nursing Diagnoses: Definitions and Classifications 1997–1998.*
North American Nursing Diagnosis Association, 1996.

Incontinence, Bowel

Incontinence, Functional

Incontinence, Reflex

Incontinence, Stress

Incontinence, Urge

Individual Coping, Ineffective

Infant Feeding Pattern, Ineffective

Infection, Risk for

Injury, Risk for

Knowledge Deficit (Specify)

Loneliness, Risk for

Management of Therapeutic Regimen: Community, Ineffective

Management of Therapeutic Regimen: Families; Ineffective

Management of Therapeutic Regimen: Individual, Effective

Management of Therapeutic Regimen (Individuals), Ineffective, Noncompliance (Specify)

Memory, Impaired

Nutrition: Less than Body Requirements, Altered

Nutrition: More than Body Requirements, Altered

Nutrition: Potential for More than Body Requirements, Altered

Oral Mucous Membrane, Altered

Organized Infant Behavior, Potential for Enhanced

Pain

Pain, Chronic

Parent/Infant/Child Attachment, Risk for Altered

Parental Role Conflict

Parenting, Altered

Parenting, Risk for Altered

Perceived Constipation

Perioperative Positioning Injury, Risk for

Peripheral Neurovascular Dysfunction, Risk for

Personal Identity Disturbance

Physical Mobility, Impaired

Poisoning, Risk for

Post-Trauma Response

Powerlessness

Protection, Altered

Rape-Trauma Syndrome

Rape-Trauma Syndrome: Compound Reaction

Rape-Trauma Syndrome: Silent Reaction

Reflex Incontinence

Relocation Stress Syndrome

Role Performance, Altered

Self-Care Deficit: Bathing/Hygiene

Self-Care Deficit: Feeding

Self-Care Deficit: Dressing/Grooming

Self-Care Deficit: Toileting

Self-Esteem, Chronic Low

Self-Esteem, Situational Low

Self-Esteem Disturbance

Self-Mutilation, Risk for

Sensory/Perceptual Alterations: visual, auditory, kinesthetic, gustatory, tactile, olfactory (Specify)

Sexual Dysfunction

Sexuality Patterns, Altered

Situational Low Self-Esteem

Skin Integrity, Impaired

Skin Integrity, Risk for Impaired

Sleep Pattern Disturbance

Social Interaction, Impaired

Social Isolation

Spiritual Distress

Spiritual Well-Being, Potential for Enhanced

Stress Incontinence

Suffocation, Risk for

Sustain Spontaneous Ventilation, Inability to

Swallowing, Impaired

Thermoregulation, Ineffective

Thought Processes, Altered

Tissue Integrity, Impaired

Tissue Perfusion, Altered: Renal, cerebral, cardiopulmonary, gastrointestinal, peripheral (Specify Type)

Total Incontinence

Trauma, Risk for

Unilateral Neglect

Urge Incontinence

Urinary Elimination, Altered

Urinary Retention

Violence, Risk for: Self-directed or directed at others

Addison-Wesley Nursing Drug Cards

Card Number	Generic Name	Trade Name(s)
1	alprazolam	Xanax
2	amitriptyline	Amitril, Elavil, Emitrip, Endep, Enovil
3	amoxapine	Asendin
4	benztropine	Cogentin
5	bupropion	Wellburtin
6	buspirone	BuSpar
7	carbamazepine	Tegretol
8	chlordiazepoxide	Librium
9	chlorpromazine	Thorazine
10	clonazepam	Klonopin
11	clorazepate	Tranxene
12	diazepam	Valium, Valrelease
13	diphenhydramine	Benadryl, Bendylate, Benylin, Compoz
14	disulfiram	Antabuse
15	fluoxetine	Prozac
16	fluvoxamine	Luvox
17	fluphenazine	Prolixin, Prolixin Decanoate, Permitil
18	haloperidol	Haldol, Haldol Decanoate

Generic name: alprazolam

Trade name: Xanax

Classification: Antianxiety, benzodiazepine

Common uses: Anxiety disorders, relief of anxiety associated with depression, panic disorder

Should not be used if: Client is pregnant or nursing, has glaucoma, has hepatic or renal disease.

Possible side effects: Drowsiness, fatigue, ataxia, dizziness, orthostatic hypotension, ECG changes, tachycardia, blurred vision, constipation, dry mouth, tolerance, physical and psychological dependency. May aggravate symptoms in some depressed clients.

Possible drug interactions: ↑ CNS depression from other drugs, including alcohol, antipsychotics, antihistamines, antidepressants, anticonvulsants, barbiturates, and narcotics. Nicotine, caffeine, valproic acid, and rifampin ↓ alprazolam's effectiveness.

Nursing considerations: Assess anxiety level, potential for addiction, history of allergies and/or medical problems. Watch for symptoms of overdose. Evaluate blood pressure lying and standing, blood studies, hepatic studies, I&O.

Usual dosage: 1.5–4 mg/day, should be gradually increased from 0.25–0.5 mg/day in 2–3 divided doses. Take with food to reduce GI symptoms.

Onset: 30–60 min; peaks in about 1 hr.

Generic name: amitriptyline

Trade names: Amitril, Elavil, Emitrip, Endep, Enovil

Classification: Antidepressant, tricyclic

Common uses: Major depression, depressive phase of bipolar disorder, chronic pain, and various types of headaches

Should not be used if: Client is taking MAO inhibitors, is pregnant or nursing or less than 12 yr old, has history of hypersensitivity to tricyclics, is in recovery phase of MI, has untreated glaucoma.

Possible side effects: Drowsiness, dizziness, orthostatic hypotension, tachycardia, hypertension, heart block, CHF, cardiovascular collapse, ECG changes, agranular cytosis, thrombocytopenia, leukopenia, dry mouth, constipation, increased appetite (weight gain), urinary retention.

Possible drug interactions: Potentiates CNS depressants, including alcohol, barbiturates, and benzodiazepines. Severe systemic reactions with MAO inhibitors: may cause hyperpretic crisis, severe convulsions, and death. Nicotine ↑ amitriptyline metabolism. Thyroid meds may interact to produce arrhythmias and tachycardia.

Nursing considerations: Assess initial VS and weight; monitor throughout therapy. Administer at bedtime or late in the day. Be aware of sudden mood changes. Evaluate for symptoms of blood dyscrasias, including sore throat, fever, malaise, unusual bleeding or bruising. Watch for symptoms of overdose.

Generic name: amoxapine

Trade name: Asendin

Classification: Antidepressant, tricyclic

Common uses: Major depression with psychotic symptoms, depression associated with organic causes, depressive phase of bipolar disorder, mixed symptoms of depression and anxiety

Should not be used if: Client is hypersensitive to tricyclics, is pregnant or nursing or less than 14 yr old, is currently taking a MAO inhibitor, is in an acute recovery period following an MI. Care should be taken with clients having history of seizures, prostatic hypertrophy, or cardiovascular, hepatic, renal, or respiratory difficulties; or with those who are elderly or debilitated.

Possible side effects: Drowsiness, dizziness, orthostatic hypotension, blurred vision, nasal congestion, tachycardia, MI, ECG changes, dry mouth, constipation, urinary retention.

Possible drug interactions: Potentiates CNS depressants, including alcohol, barbiturates, and benzodiazepines. Severe systemic reactions with MAO inhibitors. Nicotine ↑ amoxapine metabolism. Thyroid meds may interact to produce arrhythmias and tachycardia.

Nursing considerations: Assess initial VS and weight; monitor throughout therapy. Be aware of sudden mood changes. Evaluate for symptoms of blood dyscrasias, including sore throat, fever, malaise, unusual bleeding or bruising. Watch for symptoms of overdose.

Generic name: benztropine

Trade name: Cogentin

Classification: Antiparkinsonian, anticholinergic

Common uses: Parkinsonism, EPS associated with antipsychotic drugs (not including tardive dyskinesia), prevention of EPS

Should not be used if: Client is hypersensitive, is pregnant or nursing or less than 3 yr old, is routinely exposed to elevated external temps, has cardiac or GI problems, has glaucoma or urinary obstructions, has hypertension or hyperthyroidism.

Possible side effects: Drowsiness, dizziness, blurred vision, dry mouth, constipation, urinary retention, paralytic ileus.

Possible drug interactions: May ↑ CNS depression with alcohol, barbiturates, narcotics, and benzodiazepines. May ↓ antipsychotic effects of the phenothiazines or haloperidol. May ↑ anticholinergic effects of any other drug with anticholinergic properties.

Nursing considerations: Assess for symptoms of Parkinson's disease. EPS are similar with the addition of muscular weakness, restlessness, involuntary muscular movements, rolling back of the eyes, and bizarre facial and tongue and/or body movements. Evaluate for constipation, GI disturbance, or paralytic ileus, which may be life-threatening.

Generic name: bupropion

Trade name: Wellburtin

Classification: Smoking cessation

Common uses: To help individuals stop smoking

Should not be used if: Client is hypersensitive; is taking a MAO inhibitor; is pregnant or nursing or less than 18 yr old; has history of seizure disorder, cranial trauma, bulimia, or anorexia nervosa. Use caution if client has cardiovascular, hepatic, or renal problems; and if client is suicidal, psychotic, elderly, or debilitated.

Possible side effects: Agitation, insomnia, headache or migraine, tremors, seizures, blurred vision, hallucinations, impaired sleep quality, sedation, dizziness, tachycardia, dry mouth, constipation, nausea, vomiting, weight loss, anorexia, leukopenia, slight increase in BP, orthostatic hypotension.

Possible drug interactions: Drugs that alter hepatic enzyme activity may ↓ metabolism of bupropion. Levodopa may ↑ incidence of adverse effects. MAO inhibitors enhance toxicity of bupropion. Drugs that ↓ seizure threshold may ↑ risk of seizures.

Nursing considerations: Assess VS and weight, malaise. Evaluate history of seizures, allergies, glaucoma, alcohol/drug use.

Usual dosage: PO (adults), initially 200 mg/day given as 100 mg BID, increased to a maximum of 450 mg over several weeks of treatment with individual doses not to exceed 150 mg.

Generic name: buspirone

Trade name: BuSpar

Classification: Antianxiety, azaspirone

Common uses: Generalized anxiety states

Should not be used if: Client is hypersensitive, is using MAO inhibitors, is elderly or debilitated, is pregnant or nursing or less than 18 yr old. Use caution with clients who have hepatic or renal dysfunction. Clients should discontinue benzodiazepines or sedative/hypnotics before therapy with buspirone.

Possible side effects: Drowsiness, dizziness, insomnia, headache, nervousness, nausea.

Possible drug interactions: Use with MAO inhibitors may elevate blood pressure.

Nursing considerations: Assess extent of anxiety, lethality, presence of side effects. Evaluate history for allergies, contraceptive use, childbearing status, alcohol/drug use. Buspirone is less sedating than benzodiazepines.

Usual dosage: PO (adults), 5 mg TID, to be increased at intervals of 2–3 days, NTE 60 mg/day; usually effective dose: 20–30 mg/day.

Onset: Therapeutic levels may be reached in 7–10 days.

Generic name: carbamazepine

Trade name: Tegretol

Classification: Mood stabilizer, anticonvulsant

Common uses: Bipolar disorder, major depression, schizoaffective disorder, treatment-resistant schizophrenia, epilepsy, alcohol withdrawal

Should not be used if: Sensitivity to tricyclic antidepressants; baseline hematologic abnormalities or receiving other myelotoxic drugs; history of bone marrow depression. Use caution with history of cardiac damage, liver disease, ↑ intraocular pressure.

Possible side effects: Sedation, anticholinergic effects, dizziness, drowsiness, blurred vision, speech disturbances, abnormal antiarrhythmic action, antidiuretic effects, nystagmus, minor hematologic changes, hypotension, aggravation of hypertension, pruritus, photosensitivity, diaphoresis, chills.

Possible drug interactions: Serum concentrations of anticonvulsants may be ↓. Calcium-channel blocking agents (verapamil) may be ↑ to toxic level. Erythromycin ↓ clearance of carbamazepine. Doxycycline should not be given concomitantly. Serum concentration of warfarin ↓ MAO inhibitors, therefore, not recommended. Reliability of oral contraceptives may be adversely affected.

Nursing considerations: Tasks requiring mental alertness or physical coordination may become difficult. Assess for carbamazepine toxicity if erythromycin is also used. Discuss contraception. Assess elimination patterns. Assure proper hydration.

Generic name: diazepam

Trade names: Valium, Valrelease

Classification: Antianxiety, benzodiazepine

Common uses: Anxiety disorders, acute alcohol withdrawal, skeletal muscle spasms, convulsive disorders (adjunctive therapy), status epilepticus, preoperative sedation and relief of anxiety, anterograde amnesia

Should not be used if: Client is hypersensitive to benzodiazepines, is using other CNS depressants, is pregnant or nursing or an infant, is in shock or coma, or is elderly or debilitated. Use with caution if client has glaucoma, hepatic or renal dysfunction, history of drug abuse/dependence, or lethality.

Possible side effects: Drowsiness, fatigue, ataxia, dizziness, shock, cardiovascular collapse, agranulocytosis.

Possible drug interactions: Other CNS depressants have additive depressant effects. Cimetidine and valproic acid ↑ effects of diazepam. Oral contraceptives and antitubercular drugs have contradictory effects. Nicotine and caffeine ↓ effects of diazepam. Serum levels of phenytoin may be ↑. The effects of levodopa are ↓. Excretion of digoxin may ↑ potential for toxicity.

Nursing considerations: Assess VS lying and standing, lab values, level of anxiety, lethality, presence of side effects, childbearing status, contraceptive use. Evaluate for history of allergies, drug/alcohol use, glaucoma. May become habit-forming. Caution client that diazepam should not be used longer than 4 months unless directed

Generic name: diphenhydramine

Trade names: Benadryl, Bendylate, Benylin, Compoz

Classification: Antiparkinsonian, anticholinergic, antihistamine

Common uses: EPS, Parkinson's disease, motion sickness, nausea and vomiting, dizziness; for mild sedation

Should not be used if: MAO inhibitors have been used in previous 2 wk. Use caution with clients who are pregnant or nursing or less than 6 yr old, or who have asthma, heart or lung disease, glaucoma, ulcers, difficulty urinating, high BP, seizures, or hyperthyroidism.

Possible side effects: Sedation, dry mouth and mucous membranes, vision problems, difficulty urinating, muscle weakness, excitement (especially in children), nervousness.

Possible drug interactions: Potentiates alcohol and other CNS depressants. MAO inhibitors prolong and intensify anticholinergic effects.

Nursing considerations: If a dose is missed, do not double dose; caution advised in tasks requiring alertness, I&O.

Usual dosage: 50–300 mg/day; nighttime sleep aid dose: 25–50 mg.

Onset: Takes effect and peaks in 1 hr.

Generic name: disulfiram

Trade name: Antabuse

Classification: Alcohol deterrent, aldehyde dehydrogenase inhibitor

Common uses: Chronic alcoholism (aversion therapy)

Should not be used if: Client is hypersensitive to thiuram derivatives; has severe myocardial disease, coronary occlusion, psychosis; recently received or is receiving metronidazole, paraldehyde, alcohol, or alcohol-containing preparations. Use caution with clients who have hepatic or renal insufficiency, diabetes mellitus, seizure disorders, cerebral damage, history of rubber-contact dermatitis, chronic or acute nephritis, hepatic cirrhosis, abnormal EEG results, multiple drug dependence, hypothyroidism, or who are pregnant.

Possible side effects: Drowsiness; headache; metallic or garliclike aftertaste; hepatotoxicity; blood dyscrasias; disulfiram-alcohol reaction, which includes tachycardia, hypotension, flushing, dyspnea, headache, nausea and vomiting.

Possible drug interactions: Mild to severe life-threatening reactions with alcohol-containing preparations (including topical). ↑ effects of diazepam and chlordiazepoxide. Phenytoin intoxication, prolonged prothrombin time with oral anticoagulants. Unsteady gait or marked changes in behavior with isoniazid. Acute toxic psychosis with metronidazole. Additive CNS stimulation with marijuana. With barbiturates and paraldehyde, ↑ serum concentration and possible toxicity. Combination with tricyclic anti-

Generic name: fluoxetine

Trade name: Prozac

Classification: Antidepressant, SSRI

Common uses: Major depressive disorder, obsessive-compulsive disorder, bulimia

Should not be used if: Client is hypersensitive or is pregnant or nursing. Use caution if client has history of seizures, lethality, hepatic or renal insufficiency, drug abuse, a recent MI; or if client is underweight, elderly, or debilitated.

Possible side effects: Headache, nervousness, insomnia, drowsiness, anxiety, tremors, dizziness, fatigue, rash, nausea, diarrhea, dry mouth, sexual dysfunctions, anorexia, weight loss, anemia, thrombocytopenia, leukopenia, excessive sweating.

Possible drug interactions: Prolongs half-life of diazepam. Potential for hypertensive crisis with MAO inhibitors. There may be ↑ central and peripheral toxicity with tryptophan, agitation, restlessness, sudden elevation in mood, mental status, symptoms of blood dyscrasias.

Nursing considerations: Assess for lethality and sudden mood elevation that may precede suicide attempt, VS, weight. Evaluate history of glaucoma, alcohol/drug consumption.

Usual dosage: PO (adults), initial dose 20 mg/day given in the morning, may be ↑ after several weeks if no improvement is noted; doses above 20 mg/day should be

Generic name: fluvoxamine

Trade name: Luvox

Classification: Antidepressant, SSRI

Common Uses: Obsessive-compulsive disorder in adults and in children 8–17 yr old

Should not be used if: Client is pregnant or nursing; has known sensitivity to fluvoxamine

Possible side effects: Drowsiness, insomnia, nervousness, nausea, asthenia, low incidence of anticholinergic effects.

Possible drug interactions: Potential for hypertensive crisis with MAO inhibitors; ↓ theophylline clearance; not to be used with terfenadine, astemizole, and cisapride.

Nursing considerations: Drowsiness may impair driving or use of other machines; warn client to avoid alcohol which may ↑ drowsiness; teach diet considerations to minimize weight gain; assess for suicidal potential; evaluate effects of med on overall quality of life.

Usual dosage: 50–300 mg/day.

Onset: 1–4 wks.

Generic name: fluphenazine

Trade names: Prolixin, Prolixin Decanoate, Permitil

Classification: Antipsychotic, phenothiazine

Common uses: Acute and chronic psychotic disorders, schizophrenia

Should not be used if: Client is hypersensitive to phenothiazines, sulfites, or tartrazine; is comatose or CNS-depressed; is taking large amounts of CNS depressants; is hyper/hypotensive, pregnant or nursing, or less than 12 yr old; has bone marrow depression, subcortical brain damage, Parkinson's disease, or hepatic, renal, or cardiac insufficiency. Use caution with clients who have history of seizures, respiratory, renal, hepatic, thyroid, or cardiovascular disorders, prostatic hypertrophy, glaucoma, diabetes, hypocalcemia, history of severe reactions to insulin or ECT; those who are exposed to extreme temps or organophosphate insecticides; and those who are elderly or debilitated.

Possible side effects: Sedation, headache, EPS, tardive dyskinesia, blurred vision, NMS, orthostatic hypotension, skin rashes, photosensitivity, dry mouth, nausea, vomiting, ↑ or ↓ appetite, constipation, agranulocytosis, leukopenia, anemia, thrombocytopenia, pancytopenia, laryngeal edema, laryngospasm, bronchospasm, suppression of cough reflex.

Possible drug interactions: Cumulative effects with other CNS depressants. ↓ effects of levodopa. Additive anticholinergic effects, ↓ antipsychotic effects with anticholinergic agents. Barbiturates may ↓ effects of fluphenazine.

Generic name: haloperidol

Trade names: Haldol, Haldol Decanoate

Classification: Antipsychotic, butytrophenone

Common uses: Management of acute and chronic psychosis, control of Tourette syndrome, symptoms of dementia in older adults, short-term treatment of hyperactive children, prolonged treatment of chronic schizophrenia

Should not be used if: Client is hypersensitive to haloperidol or tartrazine; is comatose; is severely CNS-depressed; is taking other CNS depressants; is pregnant or nursing or less than 3 yr old; has bone marrow depression, blood dyscrasias, subcortical brain damage, Parkinson's disease, or hepatic, respiratory, renal, thyroid, or cardiovascular disorders; has severe hypo/hypertension. Use caution with clients who have history of seizure, prostatic hypertrophy, glaucoma, diabetes, hypocalcemia, acute illness or dehydration; those who are elderly, debilitated, or exposed to extreme environmental temps; and those who have severe reactions to insulin or ECT.

Possible side effects: Sedation, headache, EPS, tardive dyskinesia, blurred vision, NMS, orthostatic hypotension, photosensitivity, dry mouth, anorexia, constipation, paralytic ileus, impaired liver function, hypersalivation, agranulocytosis, leukopenia, anemia, cough reflex suppression, laryngeal edema, laryngospasm, bronchospasm, diaphoresis.

Possible drug interactions: CNS depressants have additive effect. Anticholinergic agents have additive anticholin-

Generic name: lithium carbonate

Trade names: Lithane, Eskalith, Lithonate, Lithotabs, Lithobid, Lithium Citrate, Lithonate-S

Classification: Mood stabilizer

Common uses: Bipolar disorder, maintenance therapy to prevent or diminish intensity of subsequent manic episodes, depression, schizoaffective disorder, treatment-resistant schizophrenia, alcohol withdrawal

Should not be used if: Client has severe renal or cardiovascular disease, dehydration, sodium depletion, brain damage, or is pregnant or nursing. Use caution with elderly clients; and with those with thyroid disorders, diabetes mellitus, urinary retention, or history of seizure disorder.

Possible side effects: Tremors, fatigue, dizziness, confusion, restlessness, headache, lethargy, drowsiness, ECG changes, acne, rash, hypothyroidism, excessive weight gain, anorexia, nausea, vomiting, diarrhea, dry mouth, thirst, polyuria, glycosuria, diabetes insipidus, reversible leukocytosis (WBC 10,000–15,000).

Possible drug interactions: Aminophylline, mannitol, acetazolamide, sodium bicarbonate, drugs high in sodium content may ↑ renal elimination and ↓ effectiveness of lithium. Haloperidol may cause encephalopathic syndrome and result in brain damage. Neuromuscular blocking agents prolong effects of skeletal muscle relaxation. Piroxicam, indomethacin, and nonsteroidal anti-inflammatory drugs produce significant ↑ in plasma lithium levels, thereby ↑ potential for toxicity. Thiazide diuretics ↓ renal clearance of lithium, thus ↑ risk of toxicity.

Generic name: oxazepam

Trade name: Serax

Classification: Antianxiety, benzodiazepine

Common uses: Anxiety, agitation during alcohol withdrawal

Should not be used if: Use caution if client is pregnant or nursing, has kidney or liver disease, or is allergic to aspirin.

Possible side effects: Drowsiness, muscle incoordination, fatigue, dizziness, confusion, restlessness, excitement, muscle spasms, nightmares, dose-dependent CNS adverse effects.

Possible drug interactions: Nicotine ↓ effectiveness. Alcohol potentiates sedation and dizziness. Levodopa-treated clients may experience ↓ control of parkinsonian symptoms. Closely observe clients on anticonvulsants.

Nursing considerations: Caution advised in tasks requiring alertness. May become habit-forming. If a dose is missed, do not double dose. Some evidence that ataxia and risk of falls is ↑ in older clients. The need for continued use should be reassessed regularly. This medication should not be abruptly discontinued.

Usual dosage: For severe anxiety, 30–60 mg/day. For agitation associated with alcohol withdrawal, 45–120 mg/day in divided doses.

Onset: 15–45 min.

Generic name: paroxetine

Trade name: Paxil

Classification: Antidepressant, SSRI

Common Uses: Obsessive-compulsive disorder; panic disorder

Should not be used if: Client is pregnant or nursing; known sensivity to mirtazapine.

Possible side effects: Drowsiness, low incidence of anticholinergic effects, sexual dysfunctions.

Possible drug interactions: Potential for hypertensive crisis with MAO inhibitors.

Nursing considerations: Drowsiness may impair driving or use of other machines; warn client to avoid alcohol, which may ↑ drowsiness; evaluate effects of med on overall quality of life.

Usual dosage: 50–200 mg/day.

Onset: 1–4 wk.

Generic name: phenelzine

Trade name: Nardil

Classification: Antidepressant, MAO inhibitor

Common uses: Atypical, nonendogenous, or neurotic depression; depression accompanied by anxiety; clients unresponsive to other antidepressants (usually not drug of choice)

Should not be used if: Client is hypersensitive to MAO inhibitors; has paranoid schizophrenia; is pregnant or nursing; has pheochromocytoma, CHF, disease of cardiovascular, renal, or hepatic system; has hypertension/history of severe headaches. Use caution with clients with history of seizures, lethality, schizophrenia, diabetes mellitus, angina pectoris, hyperthyroidism, and with those who are agitated/hypomanic, suicidal.

Possible side effects: Hypertensive crisis, dizziness, headache, drowsiness, blurred vision, orthostatic hypotension, hypertension, cardiac dysrhythmias, dry mouth, constipation, weight gain, photosensitivity, flushing, ↑ perspiration, urinary frequency, anorexia.

Possible drug interactions: Specific food (containing tyramine, tryptophan), drink, and other meds may cause severe reactions. Alcohol is to be avoided. OTC or prescription cold, hay fever, or weight-reducing med; other MAO inhibitor or tricyclic antidepressant; fluoxetine may result in severe adverse effects. May be additive with CNS depressants. ↑ BP with buspirone. Exaggerated effects of general anesthetics. Use caution with disulfiram.

Generic name: procyclidine

Trade name: Kemadrin

Classification: Antiparkinsonian, anticholinergic

Common uses: All forms of parkinsonism (adjunctive therapy), EPS (except tardive dyskinesia) associated with antipsychotic drugs

Should not be used if: Client is hypersensitive to anticholinergics; is less than 3 yr old; has angle-closure glaucoma, pyloric or duodenal obstruction, stenosing peptic ulcers, prostatic hypertrophy or bladder neck obstruction, achalasia, myasthenia gravis, ulcerative colitis, toxic megacolon, tachycardia secondary to cardiac insufficiency, or thyrotoxicosis. Use caution if client is elderly, debilitated, pregnant or nursing, or exposed to extreme environmental temps; has narrow-angle glaucoma; has hepatic, renal, or cardiac insufficiency; has hyperthyroidism, hypertension, autonomic neuropathy, or a tendency toward urinary retention.

Possible side effects: Drowsiness, dizziness, blurred vision, nervousness, dry mouth, nausea, constipation, paralytic ileus, urinary retention.

Possible drug interactions: Other drugs with anticholinergic properties ↑ anticholinergic effects, which may produce anticholinergic toxicity manifested by confusion, overt psychosis, visual hallucinations, hot dry skin, dilated pupils. ↓ absorption of levodopa and digoxin. ↑ CNS depressant effects. ↓ therapeutic effect of chlorpromazine, phenothiazines, and haloperidol. MAO inhibitors

Generic name:　propranolol

Trade name:　Inderal

Classification:　Antihypertensive, antianginal, anti-arrhythmic, beta-adrenergic blocker

Common uses:　Hypertension, angina pectoris, cardiac arrhythmias, migraine headaches, essential tremor, acute exacerbation of schizophrenic disorder and anxiety states, action tremors (drug-induced), tardive dyskinesia, acute panic symptoms, intermittent explosive disorder

Should not be used if:　Client is hypersensitive to beta-adrenergic blocking agents; is pregnant or nursing; has heart block greater than first degree, cardiogenic shock, CHF, overt cardiac failure, bronchial asthma, broncho-spasm, allergic rhinitis (pollen season), Raynaud's syndrome, malignant hypertension, or sinus bradycardia. Use caution if client has diabetes mellitus, myasthenia gravis, Wolff-Parkinson-White syndrome, thyrotoxicosis, impaired hepatic or renal function, inadequate cardiac function, sinus node dysfunction, or is undergoing surgery.

Possible side effects:　Dizziness, fatigue, insomnia, weakness, bradycardia, peripheral arterial insufficiency, hypotension, first- and third-degree heart block, nausea, diarrhea, depression, bronchial obstruction, broncho-spasm, laryngospasm, agranulocytosis.

Possible drug interactions:　Catecholamine-depleting drugs produce additive reduction in sympathetic tone, resulting in hypotension, bradycardia, vertigo, syncope. ↑ bradycardia. ↓ effects of sympathomimetics. Antimuscarinics and tricyclic antidepressants antagonize

Generic name:　risperidone

Trade name:　Risperdal

Classification:　Atypical antipsychotic

Common Uses:　Management of psychotic disorders; effective for both positive and negative symptoms

Should not be used if:　Client is pregnant or nursing.

Possible side effects:　Moderate sedative effects; few or no EPS; less tardive dyskinesia; postural hypotension early in treatment.

Possible drug interactions:　Alcohol may potentiate the CNS effects.

Nursing considerations:　Monitor BP; educate client about minimizing effects of postural hypotension; warn that alcohol and diazepam may potentiate hypotension.

Usual dosage:　4–16 mg/day given once a day.

Onset:　3–4 wk.

Generic name:　sertindole

Trade name:　Serlect

Classification:　Atypical antipsychotic

Common Uses:　Significant improvement in both positive and negative symptoms of schizophrenia

Possible side effects:　Nasal congenstion, dry mouth, postural hypotension especially early in treatment; ↓ ejaculatory volume; few or no EPS; ↓ tardive dyskinesia; minimal sedative or anticholinergic effects.

Possible drug interactions:　Alcohol may potentiate the CNS effects.

Nursing considerations:　Monitor BP; educate client about minimizing postural hypotension; warn that alcohol and diazepam may potentiate hypotension.

Usual dosage:　12–24 mg/day.

Onset:　4–8 wk.

Generic name:　sertraline

Trade name:　Zoloft

Classification:　Antidepressant, SSRI

Common uses:　Major depressive disorder

Should not be used if:　Client is hypersensitive or is pregnant or nursing. Use caution if client has history of seizures, lethality, hepatic or renal insufficiency, drug abuse, or a recent MI; or if client is underweight, elderly, or debilitated.

Possible side effects:　Headache, nervousness, insomnia, drowsiness, anxiety, tremors, dizziness, fatigue, rash, nausea, diarrhea, dry mouth, anorexia, weight loss, anemia, excessive sweating.

Possible drug interactions:　Prolongs half-life of diazepam. Potential for hypertensive crisis with MAO inhibitors. There may be ↑ central and peripheral toxicity with tryptophan, agitation, restlessness, sudden elevation in mood, mental status, symptoms of blood dyscrasias.

Nursing considerations:　Assess for lethality and sudden mood elevation that may precede suicide attempt, VS, weight. Evaluate history of glaucoma alcohol/drug consumption.

Usual dosage:　PO, 50–200 mg/day. Take in the morning.

Onset:　Takes effect in 3–5 wk.

APPENDIX C

Answers to Review Questions

Chapter 1

1. a
   Mental health is a growing toward potential with an inner feeling of aliveness.
   b. Absence of disease is not equivalent to health.
   c. Dissatisfaction is not an indication of health.
   d. Health has a general feeling of vitality.

2. a
   Rationalization is the justification of certain behaviors by faulty logic.
   b. Denial c. Repression d. Reaction formation.

3. c
   Feminist theory examines how gender roles limit the psychological development of all people.
   a. It is not an anti-male theory. b. It is done with individuals, couples and families. d. It may be used with battered women but is not exclusive to this group.

4. b
   Spirituality is the search for meaning and purpose in life.
   a. This illustrates an external locus of control.
   c, d. This is the psychosocial component of care.

5. c
   Circumstantiality is the overly detailed, tedious way of speaking that eventually reaches the goal.
   a. Confabulation is the unconscious filling in of memory gaps with imagined material. b. Blocking is a sudden stop in speech or train of thought. d. Loose association is a series of disconnected thoughts.

Chapter 2

1. b
   The enmeshed family is very close, very loyal, and highly dependent.
   a. The connected family has moderate to high closeness, high loyalty, and interdependence with more dependence than independence. c. The disengaged family has little closeness, little loyalty, and high independence. d. The separated family has low to moderate closeness, some loyalty, and interdependence with more independence than dependence.

2. d
   The rigid level of family functioning includes authoritarian leadership and strict discipline, and roles seldom change.
   a. Chaotic family b. Flexible family c. Structured family

3. a
   Sociocentric self is interdependent and interconnected and values cooperation, cohesiveness, group identity, and harmony with one's environment.
   b, c, d. These are characteristics of the egocentric self.

4. d
   Families that rate as high EE and AS are hostile, critical, emotionally over-involved, intrusive, and make guilt-inducing remarks during emotionally charged family discussions.
   a. Although the family may be dysfunctional, these characteristics have not been related to relapse. b, c. These are characteristics of functional families.

5. c
   These medications increase the risk of neural tube defects as well as neonatal hemorrhage due to low levels of vitamin K.
   a, b, d. These are risks associated with taking lithium during pregnancy.

Chapter 3

1. b
   Valuing diversity means helping people change only those patterns that are harmful.
   a. This is not related to diversity. c, d. This is forcing your values on those who are different.
2. d
   When prejudice is acted on, it becomes discrimination.
   a. Generalization b. Stereotypes c. Prejudice
3. a
   The emphasis is on power, status, and wealth.
   b. Individuals are more important than community. c. Solutions to problems are often based on short-term results. d. There is pressure to conform to the dominant group.
4. d
   Knowing ourselves is critical to becoming nonjudgmental of others.
   a. This is believing your personal values to be most important. b. This is believing your ethnic group values to be most important. c. Discrimination is a refusal to recognize that there are other points of view.
5. d
   This is seeing the world in absolutes of right or wrong.
   a, b, c. These do not relate to suicidal behavior.

Chapter 4

1. b
   Procedural memory involves the memory of motor skills and procedures.
   a, c, d. These are all declarative memory, which is memory for people and facts.
2. c
   The ability to be motivated and follow through on plans is centered in the frontal lobe.
   a. Parietal lobe dysfunction. b. Temporal lobe dysfunction. d. Occipital lobe dysfunction.
3. b
   The temporal lobe is the site of hearing.
   a. Visual hallucinations occur in the occipital lobe. c, d. The parietal and frontal lobes are not identified as sites of hallucinations.
4. a
   There is no apparent relationship between thoughts.

b. Tangential speech gets away from the main idea. c. Circumstantial speech adds unnecessary details. d. Concrete thinking is the inability to generalize.
5. d
   Serotonin influences the other neurotransmitters and is necessary for circadian rhythms.
   a. DA mediates abstract thinking, attention, and memory. b. NE regulates mood, memory, and cognition. c. ACH influences learning and memory.

Chapter 5

1. b
   These are common indicators of anger.
   a. Low self-esteem is expressed through minimal eye contact and a body posture of shrinking inward. c. Anxiety is expressed through restless movements and frequent eye blinking. d. Fear is expressed through rigid, tense body posture.
2. c
   You are asking the client to help you understand the progression of events.
   a. Exploring. b. Clarifying. d. Validating perception.
3. d
   Advising prevents clients from using the problem-solving process.
   a. "Why" questions force clients to explain and defend themselves. b. Disagreeing denies clients the right to think and feel as they do. c. Belittling is ignoring the importance of the client's problems.
4. b
   Being taken seriously validates our self-worth.
   a. The listener can hear the words but miss the message being communicated. c. The listener could ignore all other people but still be preoccupied with self, which interferes with listening. d. A good listener does not make assumptions.
5. b
   Brain-storming is the second step of problem solving.
   a. Identifying the problem precedes the implementation of the problem-solving process. c. First step. d. Third step.

Chapter 6

1. b
   A clue to auditory hallucinations is the client looking around to see who is speaking.
   a. Delusions are internal beliefs. c. Illusions are misperceptions of a real stimulus in the environment. d. There is no evidence of anxiety.
2. a.
   Listening to music may drown out the voices and distract from what the voices are saying.
   b. The voices may increase in volume in a quiet room. c. Focus on the hallucination may increase it. d. A person should not self-prescribe an increase in medication.
3. c
   Clients may act on beliefs that are harmful to the self or others.
   a. Delusions are fixed beliefs. b. Eliminating stressors is not related to the content of the delusion. d. The belief is real to the client.
4. b
   This is a symbolic act to prevent self-harm.
   a. The client is not hallucinating. c. This increases the client's shame. d. The client might be able to increase self-harm behavior in seclusion.
5. a
   Physical force is a type of violence that begets more violence.
   b. It may do this, but a is a better choice. c. All feelings are real and acceptable. d. Physical force takes control away from clients.

Chapter 7

1. b
   In milieu therapy the entire social structure of the residence or unit is designed to be part of the helping process.
   a, c, d. Therapeutic community is not a concept of these approaches.
2. a
   Decreasing sensory input may decrease anxiety or anger and help the client regain control.
   b. Seclusion should never be used for staffing ratios. c. Communication with others is part of milieu therapy. d. Seclusion takes away responsibility temporarily.

3. d
   Leaning how to interact with others is part of social skills training.
   a. Physical exercise is not related to social skills. b. This refers to self-help groups. c. This is part of family therapy.
4. b
   This interval is the standard to prevent physical injury from restraints.
   a. This interval will provide too much stimulus to the clients. c, d. These intervals are too long to prevent skin breakdown and circulation problems.
5. c
   ECT is contraindicated for a person with a recent MI.
   a, c, d. All of these people can receive ECT, which may be better for them than medications.

Chapter 8

1. a
   None of these foods contain tyramine and tryptophan.
   b, c, d. Food that must be absolutely restricted includes soy sauce, aged cheese, and cured meats.
2. d
   Benadryl is an anticholinergic agent for EPS.
   a. Paxil is an antidepressant. b. Ativan is an antianxiety agent. c. Clozaril is an antipsychotic.
3. b
   Serlect is a new atypical antipsychotic agent.
   a, c, d: These medications are all conventional antipsychotic agents which impact positive characteristics more than negative characteristics.
4. c
   Acute dystonic reaction has an abrupt onset with severe muscles spasms in the head and neck.
   a. Akathisia is the inability to sit or stand still. b. Tardive dyskinesia involves abnormal face, arm, and leg movements. d. Neuroleptic maligant syndrome includes hyperpyrexia, tachycardia, hypertension, confusion, and delirium.
5. c
   It usually takes 2–4 weeks for clinical improvement.
   a, b. These time periods are too short. d. This time period is too long.

Chapter 9

1. a
   Tofranil lowers the seizure threshold.
   b. Tofranil is not a CNS depressant. c. Tofranil does not alter blood glucose levels. d. Toranil takes 2-3 weeks before the client feels the effect.
2. b
   She needs much reassurance during this time.
   a. She fears being abandoned during a panic attack. c. Increased stimuli will increase her anxiety. d. Restraints will increase anxiety.
3. d.
   Secondary gains will maintain the disorder.
   a. She does not have difficulty making decisions. b. There is no evidence of obsessive compulsive behavior. c. Perfectionism is not a symptom of agoraphobia.
4. b.
   Repeated checking behavior is a form of OCD.
   a. Assessment of phobia. c. Assessment of PTSD. d. Assessment of somataform disorder.
5. c.
   Challenging thoughts is a part of cognitive restructuring.
   a. Mapping is an intervention for DID. b. This is client education. d. This is part of social skills training.

Chapter 10

1. d
   Dichotomous thinking is an all-or-none type of reasoning.
   a. Selective abstraction is focusing on certain information while ignoring contradictory information. b. Superstitious thinking involves believing in magic as an explanation for events. c. Overgeneralization occurs when a person takes information from one event and attaches it to a wide variety of situations.
2. a
   People with anorexia overexercise compulsively to increase weight loss.
   b, c, d. These patterns are more likely to occur in the general population or in those who have bulimia.
3. b
   This is a dangerously low level of potassium which could cause death.
   a, c, d. Are all within normal limits

4. d
   Antidepressants are the drugs of choice for treating bulimia.
   a, b, c. None of these medications is effective in treating bulimia.
5. b
   Help her identify that she is using the process of overgeneralization. She needs to recognize that weight loss will not solve all her problems.
   a. There is no evidence of secondary gains. c. There is no evidence of regression. d. Telling her what her problems are is nontherapeutic.

Chapter 11

1. c
   Postpartum depression begins within 2 weeks; lasts at least 2 weeks; person has feelings of despair.
   a. These feelings are not normal to the postpartum period. b. This begins on the first to fourth day; not as much despair. d. Psychosis includes hallucinations, and bizarre feelings and behavior.
2. a
   Anhedonia is the incapability of experiencing pleasure.
   b. Catastrophizing exaggerates failures in one's life. c. Somatization is the process by which psychological distress is experienced and communicated in the form of bodily symptoms. d. Secondary gains are the advantages from, or rewards for, being ill.
3. a
   Fluid loss (sweating) may lead to lithium toxicity.
   b, c, d. These activities are unlikely to increase fluid loss.
4. d
   These are all steps in the self-advocacy process.
   a, b, c. These are all interventions for someone who is depressed, but they are not part of self-advocacy.
5. c
   Exercise increases neurotransmitters which are at low levels during depression.
   a. Person may benefit from fresh air, but that, in itself, is not mood-altering. b. With enough diet and exercise, one's body shape might improve, which may indirectly improve one's mood. d. Diversional activity may be of benefit, but it will not directly lift depression.

Chapter 12

1. a
   Self-care is a behavior people usually engage in; negative characteristics are a loss of typical behavior.
   b. Delusions are positive characteristics. c. Hallucinations are positive characteristics. d. Hyperactive behavior is a positive characteristic.
2. c
   Somatic delusions are when someone believes something unusual is happening to one's body.
   a. This is an exaggerated sense of importance.
   b. The person believes that thoughts, feelings, and behavior are imposed by an external force.
   d. The person believes that remarks or actions are related to them when there is no connection.
3. b
   Command hallucinations can lead to suicide.
   a, c. Safety is a priority issue. d. There is no evidence of impaired social interaction.
4. a
   Symptoms of neuroleptic malignant syndrome include muscle rigidity, respiratory problems, hyperpyrexia, tachycardia, hypertension, confusion, and delirium.
   b. Dystonia is sudden muscle spasms, oculogyric crisis, and laryngospasms. c. Akathisia is feeling restless or jittery with a need to pace around.
   d. Tardive dyskinesia is involuntary movements of face and body, along with swallowing problems.
5. a
   Successful community living, the goal of rehabilitation, depends on the development of social and work skills.
   a. The administration of medications is not a major focus of rehabilitation. c. Clients should plan their own social activities in a rehabilitation program. d. Clients who are actively suicidal need more intensive care than rehabilitation.

Chapter 13

1. b
   European American women have an 8% rate of heavy drinking.
   a, c. African American and Hispanic American women have a 4% rate of heavy drinking.
   d. Asian American women have the lowest rate of alcohol consumption of all groups.

2. a
   A blackout is the inability to remember what occurred when under the influence of alcohol.
   b. Confabulation is making up information to fill gaps in memory. c. Wernicke's disease is ataxia and confusion. d. Korsakoff's syndrome is the loss of long-term and short-term memory.
3. d
   The hero acts like a surrogate parent
   a. The mascot uses comic relief. b. The lost child avoids the situation by withdrawal. c. The scapegoat acts out at home or in the community.
4. b
   It takes 14 days for Antabuse to be completely cleared out of the body.
   a. Antabuse does not cause photosensitivity.
   c. Antabuse does not cause sedation. d. Antabuse does not cause toxicity and is not measured by blood alcohol levels.
5. d
   Hyperthermia and seizures often accompany cocaine overdose.
   a. Esophageal varices occur from alcohol abuse.
   b. Cocaine is not taken orally. c. This intervention is appropriate for a person who has overdosed on hallucinogens.

Chapter 14

1. a
   These individuals crave solitude.
   b, c, d. Manipulation, sociability, and antisocial behavior are more common in Cluster B.
2. b
   Intense, labile affect is very common in Cluster B.
   a, c, d. These are characteristics of Cluster A.
3. a
   Fear of making the wrong decision leads to indecision.
   b, c, d. These are characteristics of Cluster A.
4. d
   Mood instability is a core feature of BPD.
   a, b, c. These diagnoses are more appropriate for Cluster A.
5. a
   Client's need for absolute guarantees interferes with the decision-making process.
   b. This is helpful for people who have a need for strict routines. c. This is helpful for people struggling with perfectionist behavior. d. This is helpful for people who have difficulty asking for help.

Chapter 15

1. b
   Apraxia is the inability to use objects properly.
   a. Agnosia is the inability to recognize familiar situations, people, or stimuli. c. Aphasia is the inability to communicate. d. Agoraphobia is a phobic disorder characterized by fear of being away from home.
2. d
   Confabulation is the filling in of memory gaps with imaginary information.
   a, b, c. While these are helpful interventions, they do not deal with the memory gaps.
3. a
   The alarm system will alert the family that she has successfully left the house.
   b. The use of restraints further confuses people. c. The neighbors will also be asleep at night. d. It is not realistic to expect the family to be awake all night.
4. a
   The family is feeling good about Moshe continuing to live in the home.
   b, c, d. In these statements the family is expressing frustration, helplessness, and hopelessness.
5. d
   Closed-ended questions are easier to respond to.
   a, b. The client may not understand what you are asking. c. Interpretations are not appropriate for someone who thinks concretely.

Chapter 16

1. c
   Each culture determines symbolic rituals of grief.
   a, b, c. Cultures define appropriate and inappropriate behavior.
2. a
   This is necessary to support ongoing family development to allow the other tasks to be accomplished.
   b, c, d. All of these tasks are accomplished after equilibrium is re-established.
3. d
   The relationship of a former spouse is not recognized.
   a, b, c. All of these relationships are recognized.

4. a
   Psychotic denial of death is not a part of uncomplicated grief.
   b, c, d. These are all symptoms of uncomplicated grief.
5. c
   These individuals experience discrimination in housing.
   a. They may have periods of hospitalization, but the goal is to live in the least restrictive setting. b, d. These rights are not automatically taken away when there is a mental illness.

Chapter 17

1. b
   European American men over the age of 65 have the highest rate of suicide.
   a. The only males with lower rates than African Americans are Chinese Americans. c. Women have lower rates than men; rates are highest in young adulthood. d. This group has the lowest rate of suicide.
2. d
   The client is experiencing auditory hallucinations that are giving him orders or commands.
   a. There is no evidence of hopelessness. b. There is no evidence of emotional pain. c. There is no evidence of delusions.
3. a
   This is a hint that things are going to change drastically or end fairly quickly.
   b. This is evidence of problem-solving behavior and the seeking of support. c. This is evidence of hopefulness and anticipation of pleasure in the future. d. Hallucinations are fading and having less influence in the person's life.
4. b
   The priority of care is protection to prevent further suicidal behavior.
   a, c, d. After her safety is assured, these goals would be appropriate.
5. d
   Reassuring her that you are not abandoning her and are interested in her welfare may ease her emotional pain.
   a. This is false reassurance. b. This invalidates and ignores her feelings. c. This may be seeking clarification but may also be heard as forcing her to defend her position.

Chapter 18

1. b

Ninety percent of teens killing their parents have been severely abused by the parents.
a, c, d. These factors are not related to teens killing their parents.

2. d

It is appropriate to use violence to make the child behave.
a. Effective communication decreases violence.
b. Hitting or spanking is not a democratic process.
c. Children are more likely to be hurt by family members than by strangers.

3. a

Spanking increases aggression in victims.
b. Spanking reduces the ability of parents to influence their children, especially when they are too big to control by physical force. c. It is no more unrealistic to expect parents not to hit a child than for a supervisor to never hit an employee. d. This teaches children that being extremely angry justifies hitting.

4. b.

Use of excuses accepts the blame but not the responsibility.
a. Justification accepts the responsibility but not the blame.
c. Minimization revolves around the extent, frequency, and effects.
d. Denial is stating that it never happened.

5. a

Clients must take charge of their own lives, something they have not been able to do in the abusive relationship.
b, c, d. All of these interventions are being in control of the client, which is similar to the abusive relationship.

Chapter 19

1. b

Masturbatory gestures would be considered an offensive working environment.
a, c, d. These are examples of quid pro quo type of harassment.

2. d

Inappropriate self-blame indicates a low self-esteem.

a, b, c. Although these are possible diagnoses for adult survivors, there is no evidence supporting these diagnoses.

3. b

If she can recognize that she is not responsible for the abuse, her self-esteem will improve.
a, c, d. Although you may do all these interventions, they do not apply to the diagnosis of low self-esteem.

4. a

Depersonalization is feeling as if one is detached or an outside observer.
b. Displacement is transferring emotional reactions from one object or person to another object or person. c. Identification is an attempt to handle anxiety by imitating the behavior of someone feared or respected. d. Projection is assigning blame to others for unacceptable desires, thought, or mistakes.

5. c

No other interventions can take place until she has been informed of her rights and has consented to all the other assessment procedures.
a, b, d. She must give informed consent for all these procedures. Telling clients their rights is the first step in obtaining consent.

Chapter 20

1. b

Fear of being judged while eating in front of others is a form of social phobia.
a. Refusing to speak in some situations and speaking in others is a form of selective mutism.
c. These are symptoms of obsessive compulsive disorder. d. These are symptoms of posttraumatic stress disorder.

2. a

Unlike adults with bipolar disorder whose moods last at least 5 days, adolescents have rapid mood swings.
b, c. These are characteristics of adults with bipolar disorder but not adolescents. d. This is characteristic of a person with conduct disorder.

3. b

Dexedrine is used for children 3 years and older.
a. This antidepressant is not typically prescribed for ADHD.
c, d. These drugs are used for children 6 years and older.

4. a
Play therapy helps children reveal feelings they are unable to verbalize.
b, c. These are skills learned in group therapy.
d. Problem solving is a cognitive activity, not a play activity.
5. d
Adolescents are trained in helping skills which provides opportunities to reach out to others.
a, b. These most likely occur in community youth organizations. c. It may utilize the problem-solving process, but it is not the main focus.

Chapter 21

1. b
One of the myths of aging is that older adults cannot learn.
a. Sixty-six percent of older adults live in a family setting and 29% live alone. c. Only 5% have serious cognitive impairment, and only 10% suffer mild to moderate impairment. d. Many people maintain old interests or find new activities as they age.
2. a
Reminiscence therapy is a review of past experiences of life.
b. This is group therapy. c, d. These typically occur with peers in a group.
3. d
Spirituality is related to a sense of fairness in life, as well as the ability to find meaning in life.
a. There is no evidence that she is suicidal.
b. There is no evidence she is having problems fulfilling her roles. c. She is not coping with her past life.
4. a
Pessimism is characteristic of people with both Parkinson's disease and depression.
b. They are usually less guilty. c. They have a higher level of anxiety. d. They have more cognitive deficits.
5. b.
BuSpar has little impairment of cognition.
a, c, d. All of these are side effects of the benzodiazepines.

Chapter 22

1. d
These are the rewards he gets for being ill.
a. Exercise is a form of coping behavior. b. Denial in an example of a defense mechanism. c. Talking to friends is a form of coping behavior.
2. a
Being devalued leads to decreased self-esteem and less of an ability to cope with stress.
b. Women continue to earn less than men for equal work. c. Men have more opportunity for professional advancement. d. Women continue to put in many more hours of work in the home than men do.
3. b
The lack of energy and mood changes associated with hypothroidism may be confused with depression.
a. An occipital lobe tumor may produce visual hallucinations. c. Hyperthroidism may be confused with anxiety or a manic episode. d. Altered levels of electrolytes can cause confusion, irritability, or delirium.
4. c
In reflexology, pressure is applied to points on the hands and feet to treat a wide range of stress-related illnesses.
a. QiGong involves manipulation of qu by means of physical and mental exercises and breathing.
b. Naturopathy is a primary health care system emphasizing the curative power of nature using nutrition, herbs, homeopathic medicine, and Oriental medicine. d. Rheiki uses light hand placements to channel healing energies to the client.
5. a
Research has demonstrated increased control over body processes.
b. These techniques alter body processes such as pulse, blood pressure, and immune response. c. These techniques are not related to insight into one's behavior. d. These techniques are not a cure for all infectious diseases.

Chapter 23

1. c

   Commitment is to protect the client and others.
   a. Being mentally ill is not a crime. Commitment takes place in the civil courts. b. Commitment is always for a specific time period. d. Clients do not lose their rights when they are committed.

2. d

   Involuntary admission increases the stigma against persons with mental illness.
   a, b, c. These are all arguments for commitment.

3. b

   Disciplinary action by the state board of nursing may occur.
   a. Formal action is often taken. c. Breach of confidentiality is a civil offense, not a criminal offense. d. Duty to disclose supersedes the client's right to confidentiality.

4. a

   Often the crimes for which they are charged are misdemeanors resulting from their symptoms of mental illness.
   b. They are most frequently charged with misdemeanors. c. A more appropriate placement would be a psychiatric facility. d. Families can request help from police, but families cannot make the decision for the person to be put in jail.

5. a

   Clients may quickly slip out the door as people enter and leave.
   b, c, d. All of these interventions are abusive to clients.

Suggested Answers to Critical Thinking in Action Questions

Note: These are just some of the possible responses. Other responses are possible and could also be correct.

Chapter 2

1. They have identified some problems and are working toward their goals.
2. Their relationship is similar to a social relationship in that both relationships take time, require commitment, and require caring. The differences are that the social relationship is reciprocal for both parties and involves meeting the individual needs of both. The nurse-client relationship is client-focused, therapeutic, directed toward client growth and adaptation, theory-based, and open to supervision.
3. Sara is demonstrating transference. She is unconsciously displacing her feelings about her father onto Bill.
4. Bill's response was therapeutic because it was nonjudgmental and demonstrated warmth and caring toward his client's feelings. Transference must be recognized and separated from the present situation.

Chapter 5

1. Mary used a non-judgmental approach by introducing herself, complimenting Ifle on her appearance, and explaining the length of her intended visit.

2. Mary told Ifle she would stay with her for an hour but left after 25 minutes. By Mary leaving early, Ifle may not believe Mary in the future when Mary specifies the length of the session. Mary made the assumption that Ifle was not in the mood to talk and did not validate her perception.
3. Ifle's rigid posture could indicate possible anger, fear, invasion of her personal space, or withdrawal. By avoiding eye contact with Mary, she possibly indicates shyness or low self-esteem. Her silence in the presence of Mary possibly indicates fatigue, not wanting to talk at the time, not knowing what to say, or not being comfortable talking.
4. Mary could have improved the interaction by staying for the entire hour, even though Ifle is silent, in order to demonstrate patience. She could have asked open-ended questions to encourage communication and to validate her perception of Ifle's silence.
5. Mary felt uncomfortable with Ifle's silence.

Chapter 8

1. Serotonin is an essential brain neurotransmitter. Prozac allows serotonin to remain in the area where it is most needed for a longer period of time, thus reducing the symptoms of depression.
2. Mrs. Salazar's symptoms will decrease and she will be better able to participate in other forms of treatment.

3. It was incorrect and inadequate. One aspect of the nurse's teaching was incorrect: Weight loss, not weight gain, is more common with Prozac, thus there is no need for Mrs. Salazar to be on a low-calorie, low-fat diet unless she is obese. Methods to counter or decrease side effects, the possible length of therapy, and the correct dosage and time schedule should have been included. Both Mrs. Salazar and her daughter should have been queried about their understanding and asked if they had questions.

5. Older adults are more sensitive than younger adults to antidepressant medications, and they may experience more side effects. The SSRI's may produce relief from depressive symptoms in a much shorter time period than other types of antidepressant drugs.

6. Because of her age and her depression, Mrs. Salazar may not be able to adequately understand or remember what she was taught about the drug.

Chapter 12

1. Ricardo possibly has the additional problem of depression coupled with his schizophrenia.

2. Positive characteristics are additional behaviors not generally seen in mentally healthy people. Negative characteristics are the absence of behaviors that are seen in mentally healthy adults.

3. Ricardo demonstrated the positive characteristics of schizophrenia, such as auditory hallucinations, inappropriate affect, and suspiciousness. Mohammed demonstrated the positive characteristics of delusions, visual hallucinations, and compulsive behavior.

4. Ricardo demonstrated the negative characteristics of schizophrenia, such as social withdrawal, minimal self-care, and hostility. Mohammed demonstrated the negative characteristics of social withdrawal and flat affect.

5. They will develop spastic facial distortions, frown, blink, grimace, lick, smack, have a protruding tongue, abnormal arm or leg movements, body rocking, or pelvic movements.

6. Stay with the client and ask him to describe what is happening. Also, explain to him what is actually happening and have him keep of diary of when his hallucinations occur and how long they last in order to identify a trigger.

Chapter 14

1. Marty most likely has an antisocial personality disorder, and he could benefit from treatment. There is hope that his behavior could be changed enough for him to lead a productive life.

2. Characteristics of Marty's disorder appeared prior to the age of 15, and he exhibited manifestations of lying, stealing, fighting, and aggression. He is unable to sustain employment or relationships, and he exhibits no guilt or concern for others.

3. Marty has developed a personality that puts himself and his needs before those of others or society. He needs immediate gratification and strives to meet his needs in spite of hurting others. According to social theory, this behavior may be in response to society's increasing complexity, which results in low self-esteem, and negative self-concept.

4. They may exhibit similar characteristics (aggression, manipulation, inability to accept responsibility, inability to care for or love another), therefore, interventions that worked for the previous client may be useful with Marty. These interventions include but are not limited to: a consistent, straight-forward, and business-like approach; group therapy; planning small steps together toward achieving therapeutic goals and setting limits on destructive behaviors.

5. Possible nursing interventions include: assertiveness training, encouraging independent functioning, and empathy.

Chapter 16

1. Mr. King may be experiencing complicated grief and may be developing depression. Data to support this includes: severe feelings of loss, seeing images and hearing voices of his dead wife, not participating in activities he previously enjoyed, and still crying for his wife 9 months after her death.

2. The risk factors include: the sudden unexpected death of his wife, long personal and business relationship with his spouse, having to cope with his own illness so soon after his wife's death, change in daily habits, and loss of home.

3. The signs Mr. King may be developing depression include his lack of interest in friends or family, not wanting to leave the house, and watching TV alone.

4. He has a very supportive family.
5. Mr. King lost his wife, therefore his loss is socially acceptable. People experiencing disenfranchised grief cannot be openly acknowledged and socially validated. In addition, they cannot mourn publicly because the relationship is not recognized, the loss is not recognized, or the griever is not recognized.
6. Unresolved complicated grief can lead to physical problems such as hypertension, cardiac problems, impaired immune function, or cancer. Mr. King's cancer may be the result of his grief due to impaired immunity.
7. There are many possible interventions. For example: encourage him to talk about his loss; help him identify his greatest fears about his loss; help him find new direction for his life; discuss potentially difficult times such as holidays and how to deal with such time; involve his family in his care, etc.

Chapter 18

1. Affective characteristics in Branko's behavior towards Drenko include: jealousy, possessiveness, forcing her to quit work, and forcing her to give up family and friends. Cognitive characteristics of his behavior include: unrealistically high standards, lack of flexibility, and blaming Drenko for his violence.
2. He most likely had a parent who was violent, and he is identifying with that parent.
3. Drenko submitted to the violence, feeling that she was at fault; therefore, the violence has become a way of relating for both her and Branko. His pattern of behavior will now be difficult to change.
4. Branko would likely speak for Drenko and criticize her answers or correct her. Drenko would seek direction from Branko prior to providing information about her injury. He may refuse to allow Drenko to be interviewed or cared for unless he was present.
5. The possible dangers to Drenko include severe emotional and physical injury, death, and abuse of their daughter.
6. Remain nonjudgmental when interacting with both Drenko and Branko. Assess the level of danger for Drenko and assess the level of danger to the child. Avoid offering quick or easy solu-

tions. Help Drenko develop an escape plan if her or her daughter's safety was threatened. Help Drenko identify interpersonal strengths to decrease her feelings of powerlessness. Report the violence if there is evidence that the child is being abused as well.

Chapter 20

1. Information on what behaviors Jorge displayed as an infant and as a small child would be helpful in making an accurate assessment. For instance, consider his ability to concentrate, ease of distractibility, overt acts of hostility, the manner in which he deals with frustration, and specific learning problems.
2. Severe and persistent antisocial behaviors would differentiate conduct disorder (CD) from ADHD. Behaviors include physical aggression and cruelty to people and animals, anger, and no indication of guilt or remorse for actions.
3. Jorge has the ability to communicate with others and is not severely socially impaired. He exhibits no ritualistic behaviors or unusual motor behaviors that are associated with autistic disorder.
4. Central nervous system stimulants increase the child's ability to focus attention by blocking out irrelevant thoughts and impulses. Some stimulants are effective immediately (Ritalin & Dexedrine), and they lead to significant improvement in 70 to 75% of ADHD cases.
5. There are several interventions that could be helpful for this client. Socialization enhancement will increase Jorge's ability to negotiate stressful interpersonal situations with his siblings, parents, and classmates. It will also help him develop a more positive self-perception. Self-esteem enhancement allows a shift in focus from negative behaviors to positive behaviors, making the client feel better about himself.

Chapter 23

1. There are many responses possible. Taneko is emotionally distraught and has threatened suicide–she may be dangerous to herself. Her husband is unable to care for her at this time, so Taneko should be held on a temporary basis until her need for treatment can be determined.

Taneko is capable of discussing her feelings even though she is emotionally distraught. She should not be detained just because her husband is tired of her depression. Further evaluation of the situation is, however, necessary.

2. The neighbor must maintain confidentiality; he must not disclose any information about Taneko's admission, treatment, or discharge from the facility.

3. The hospital can be sued when clients who elope from the facility commit suicide, are injured or killed in accidents, or injure or kill another person. Since the staff knows that Taneko has threatened suicide, they must assume that she is a danger to herself, especially during her highly emotional state. Therefore, they must take every precaution to prevent her from leaving the hospital and hurting herself.

4. All of her constitutional and legal rights will be maintained: the right to refuse medications, the right to be informed about treatments, etc.

5. Caring can be shown in many ways, including: listening, demonstrating concern, becoming involved with her care, staying with her, using touch, and using humor.

6. The situation creates an ethical dilemma because there is no law regulating the situation and because both parties have rights and needs; there is no one "right" answer.

APPENDIX E

Process Recordings

Table E.1 Process Recording of Client Interview with Student Nurse*

Student's name: Clare

Client's name/age: Val, 35 years

Client profile: Val presently lives in a supervised residential setting. Two weeks ago she began participating in the partial hospitalization program at the local mental health center. She has had many hospitalizations at the state hospital. The treatment plan goals include mood stabilization, medication compliance, learning independent ADLs, and learning appropriate coping skills. She has difficulty establishing relationships. She comes on strongly and then becomes so anxious that she withdraws. She has rapid mood swings from being very quiet to laughing inappropriately to putting her head down on the table. Although she smiles frequently, the behavior appears to be an anxious reaction more than an expression of happiness. She has been diagnosed with schizoaffective disorder.

Short-term goals for the one-to-one interaction: This is the first time I am meeting Val. My goal is to let her express her feelings and help her focus on one topic at a time.

Student's Communication	Analysis of Student's Response	Client's Communication	Analysis of Client's Response
"Could you tell me what your goals are for today?"	*Broad opening.*		
		"I don't know. I don't need to be here. I don't need mental help. People may think I'm crazy, but I'm not. I don't have any friends. Will you be my friend?" [The whole time she is rocking back and forth, changing positions. Her facial expression is changing from smiling to very serious and back to smiling. Her legs are crossed, and she is holding a soda can with both hands. She makes very little eye contact.]	*Appears to be very anxious and nervous. Her voice sounds like she is genuinely happy to have someone to talk to. The way she says she has no friends sounds like she is sad and has very low self-esteem. She is also using the defense mechanism of denial.*
"Yes, I'll be your friend." [Smiling.]	*Offering self. Even though I'm here in a professional role, I think she needs to hear the word "friend" at this moment.*		

*Contributed by Valerie Sheptock, Purdue University Calumet.

continued ➤

Table E.1 Process Recording of Client Interview with Student Nurse *continued*

Student's Communication	Analysis of Student's Response	Client's Communication	Analysis of Client's Response
		"Thank you. You're such a nice lady."	*Seems relieved that someone is being nice to her. Helps her feel better about herself.*
"You're welcome. What kind of groups are you in here?"	*Focusing. Then I try to get back to her goals.*		
		"I don't know. Here, you look." [Hands me her schedule.] "I don't need to be here. I'm going to Arizona to live."	*Unable to concentrate and remember, which makes her even more anxious. Flight of ideas.*
"You are? Are you going by yourself or with someone?"	*Changing the topic. I should have commented on how anxious she appears.*		
		"Yes, just as soon as my brother moves there. I'm going to live with him. I have no friends. I keep praying to God Jesus. I know he'll take care of me."	*Keeps repeating that she has no friends, which shows very low self-esteem and insecurity. She also has an external locus of control because she believes God will help her and she is helpless.*
"You think God is your only friend?"	*Reflection and clarifying.*		
		"Yep. Look at my legs. Do they look normal to you?" [She holds up one leg to show me.]	*Appears very concerned about her legs.*
"Yes, they look fine. Are they hurting?"	*Accepting and clarifying.*		
		"The inside of my legs were melting yesterday and I couldn't walk. I thought I was going to be a cripple, but I prayed to God Jesus and when I woke up today they were better. See, they filled back out." [Showing me her calves.] "I know you think I'm crazy, don't you? Well, oh, never mind. I can't wait to move to Arizona and see my dad."	*Has somatic delusions. She went with a group from the Center to the zoo the day before and never left the front gate because her "legs were melting." I believe she is so afraid of people and has such low self-esteem that the sight of all the people at the zoo triggered the delusion. She also seems to want to tell me more but changes her mind and starts talking about her dad.*
"Does your dad live there now?"	*Clarifying. Not very effective. It seems so important to her that she see her dad, I want to find out what that is about.*		

Table E.1 continued

Student's Communication	Analysis of Student's Response	Client's Communication	Analysis of Client's Response
		"No, he's going to move there with my brother. I don't need this mental health place. Nobody here likes me."	*Her anxiety level remains fairly high. The fact that she keeps telling me that no one likes her shows her vulnerability.*
"Why do you think no one likes you here?"	*Requesting an explanation. I should have asked, "What makes you think no one here likes you?"*		
		"They all make fun of me." [Looking at the floor with a sorrowful expression.]	*Appears sad and hurt.*
"What do they say to you?"	*Exploring.*		
		"Oh, I don't know. I guess stuff like I'm crazy. I'm going to go outside and have a cigarette." [Stands up and goes outside.]	*Her anxiety increases when I ask for an example. She finds an escape by going outside.*
"I'll come with you."	*Offering self. She may tell me she doesn't want me to come along.*		
		"Did you hear that bird? Do you know they can talk?"	*Very serious expression like she is trying to tell me something important.*
"They sound very pretty."	*Accepting.*		
		"No, I mean I can understand what they are saying. They really talk to me. People may think I'm crazy, but I'm not. I just keep praying to God Jesus. He's the only one who understands me. No one else will talk to me." [Sad expression.]	*She is experiencing auditory hallucinations. She sounds very sad and lonely. (Later in group, I learn she has auditory hallucinations that tell her no one likes her. She copes by praying.)*
"I'll talk to you."	*Offering self.*		
		"You're such a nice lady. What time is it?"	*Relieved that someone will talk to her. Aware that it is almost group time.*
"It's time to go to the first group. I'll go with you to your groups today and will be back next Tuesday to see you."	*Summarizing, closing.*		

Table E.2 Process Recording of Client Interview with Student Nurse*

Student's name: Jewell

Client's name/age: Connor, 17 years

Client profile: Connor has been admitted to the substance abuse program for poly-drug abuse. He lived with his parents until 3 weeks prior to admission, when he moved in with his sister because of conflicts with his parents relating to his substance abuse. He states, "They don't understand me or let me do what I want." He has a history of overdosing 2 years ago. He was hospitalized for depression when he was 10 years old. He describes his current drug use as marijuana daily, 6–7 beers a week, cocaine once a month, tranquilizers once a month, amphetamines 2–3 times a month, inhalants 2 times a month, and analgesics once a month. His goals are to live with his sister, go back to school for his GED, get a car, and get a job. He is still denying the significance of his substance dependence.

Short-term goals for the one-to-one interaction: My goal is to assist Connor in identifying ways drug-abusive behaviors control and interfere with his life and to identify behaviors needed to prevent relapse after discharge. The reason for my goal is to attempt to work toward the first step of accepting the fact that the problems are unmanageable.

Student's Communication	Analysis of Student's Response	Client's Communication	Analysis of Client's Response
[After he told me about past experiences with overdosing and rehab programs.] "So, why are you here this time?"	*I attempted a broad, open-ended question, but it really was requesting an explanation. Put Connor on the defensive.*		
		[Picking at his jeans, little eye contact.] "My parents brought me here."	*Used projection, probably because I put him on the defensive. Attempts to protect self-image; possibly embarrassed.*
"How did you feel about their decision?"	*Exploring feelings.*		
		[Looks up at me.] "Pissed off at first. But now I'm glad they did it. I have 10 more days to go, and if I could leave right now I wouldn't until my time was up."	*Identified positive and negative feelings but not specific. "Pissed" can be interpreted as resentment, disappointment, anger, etc. "Glad" can be interpreted as relieved, forgiving, etc.*
"What are your plans after you get out of here?"	*Exploring future expectations and goals.*		
		[Tossing head side to side on each statement, little eye contact.] "Live with my sister, go to school to get my GED, get a job, and get a car."	*Is able to identify goals established but appears bored as if telling me what he thinks I want to hear. Did not include treatment for abuse in plan.*
"Do you understand what your parents' reasons were for bringing you here?"	*Exploring. I changed the topic, but it was an attempt to assist Connor in identifying behaviors that lead to current rehab and unmanageable lifestyle.*		
		"They think I have a drug problem" [laughing]. "I guess they were right."	*Is trying to make himself believe; introjection of parents' values.*

*Contributed by Megan Parsanko, Purdue University Calumet.

Table E.2 continued

Student's Communication	Analysis of Student's Response	Client's Communication	Analysis of Client's Response
"Have you accepted that you have a drug problem?" [Pointing at his chest.]	*Clarifying. Helping Connor identify his beliefs.*		
		"Oh, I know I do." [Good eye contact.] "I tried to quit before for 6 months. The only reason I did was because they told me I was going to die."	*Honest. Admits but then changes the topic; avoidance by distraction.*
"Going through the first step is one of the hardest. It sounds like you're trying hard to do it. What made you come to that conclusion—that you have a problem?"	*Giving recognition. Exploring. Focusing.*		
		"A lot of things. I don't think I knew it before when I overdosed. I just thought I would die if I did it again. I found out I didn't die, so I kept using."	*Minimizing. He believes it is not that bad this time because he didn't overdose.*
"And now what do you realize?"	*Placing event in time and sequence. He went back to past experiences instead of focusing on the here and now.*		
		"Well, all my friends graduated yesterday except me. I have no education, no job, and no car. It sucks." [Jumps up to go inside, not waiting for me.]	*Avoiding by omission; talking about everything but using. Very low self-esteem. Attempting to withdraw and distance himself from me.*
[Followed him into lounge, sat on couch.] "Are you saying your life has become unmanageable, like the first step says?"	*Reflecting. Validating feelings.*		
		[Relaxed in his chair, sitting sideways facing me.] "Yeah, I guess."	*Showing interest and appears comfortable.*
"Can you tell me some things that brought about this unmanageable lifestyle?"	*Suggesting collaboration. Focusing.*		
		"Drinking and drugs." [Silence.] "I don't get along with my parents at all. They don't understand me."	*Denial by scapegoating and/or blaming. Projection.*

continued ➤

Table E.2 Process Recording of Client Interview with Student Nurse *continued*

Student's Communication	Analysis of Student's Response	Client's Communication	Analysis of Client's Response
"Connor, you told me what you're going to do after you get out of here. Do your plans include outpatient treatment?"	*Encouraging formulation of plan of action. May have been advising. I should have waited for Connor to mention outpatient treatment first.*	"Oh yeah, I'll be going to outpatient follow-up care. They want me to do 90 meetings in 90 days. But I think I'll just go when I need a meeting."	*Possibly accepted the need for treatment but minimizes the extent of the need for treatment. Still in denial.*
"When will you need a meeting?"	*Restating.*		
		"On my days off. I'll be working, and man, that's too much." [Shaking his head.]	*Overwhelmed.*
[Staff announced time for activities.] "Well, Connor, I hope you continue to recognize the reasons you are here now so you will be more successful in the program."	*Summarizing. Giving recognition. This was very difficult since he is obviously still in denial.*		

Table E.3 Process Recording of Client Interview with Student Nurse*

Student's name: Yolanda

Client's name/age: Luis, 23 years

Client profile: Luis has been admitted to the hospital for depression and to rule out schizophrenia. His mother died several years ago, and he lives with his grandmother, who is his only support system. His grandmother states he is a loner who has no friends. One month ago, Luis stopped taking his medication because he believes he does not need it. He stopped performing his ADLs, and his grandmother brought him to the hospital when he became almost immobilized.

Short-term goals for the one-to-one interaction: My long-term goal is to help Luis differentiate between reality and delusions. The purpose of this interaction is to help him accept that he has an illness and needs the help of doctors and medicine to function normally.

Student's Communication	Analysis of Student's Response	Client's Communication	Analysis of Client's Response
"What led up to your coming to the hospital?"	*Clarifying.*		
		"I quit taking my medication for about a month, and my grandmother made me come here. I didn't want to come here."	*Doesn't believe he needs to be in a hospital or needs medication. Denial. Feels forced into treatment.*
"What happened when you quit taking your meds?"	*Exploring. I hope to help him make a connection between stopping the meds and becoming ill.*		
		"I didn't want to do anything. Even watching TV got boring. I felt like nothing."	*Is unable to identify what feeling he had. He doesn't know whether he felt sad, hopeless, etc.*
"Did you feel sad or depressed?"	*Closed-ended questions. I might have asked, "Can you explain what you mean by 'nothing'?"*		
		"I just felt like nothing. I just sat there."	*Is unable to focus on feelings. I believe this is because it takes an effort to describe feelings, and Luis's depression depletes him of energy to accomplish this task.*
"Why did you stop taking your medicine?	*Requesting an explanation. I wanted to assess for the reasons he had. He did respond to my ineffective technique.*		

*Contributed by Harmony Gates, Purdue University Calumet.

continued ➤

Table E.3 Process Recording of Client Interview with Student Nurse *continued*

Student's Communication	Analysis of Student's Response	Client's Communication	Analysis of Client's Response
		"The Prozac makes me hyper or edgy, and sometimes I can't sleep. It also makes me dizzy at times. I used to self-medicate with alcohol and pot and that got my body off balance. I quit that and it took a while, but my body balanced itself out. So I figure that if I quit taking the Prozac for a while, the same thing will happen."	*Doesn't think he has an illness; it's just a temporary imbalance that can be cured with time. He may think he caused his illness by drinking and smoking pot. I believe Luis has delusional thinking in that he can fix himself if left alone. Possibly feels very powerful.*
"You think you don't need the Prozac and your body will eventually regulate itself?"	*Restatement.*		
		"Yes. The way I figure, you are not born with Prozac-producing cells, so you don't need it. I think that with these levels of it in my body, my cells quit producing things it could use instead."	*Has a logical and well-thought-through reason behind his delusions, but is unable to recognize that this is not the case. Feels like the doctor is worsening the problem by keeping him on the Prozac. Possible struggling for internal locus of control, which is difficult in the sick role.*
"Like negative feedback?"	*Clarifying. I thought he would understand this concept since he was a chemistry major in college.*		
		"Exactly." [Talks a little about his chemistry classes, etc.]	*Distracted by mention of something he remembers from school. Knows all about dopamine and other neurotransmitters. This encourages the use of rationalization.*
"How long do you think it would take for your body to balance itself?"	*Focusing.*		
		"Just a few weeks would probably be enough."	*Believes it would only be a few weeks to be normal, but he was in a catatonic state when not taking his medications for 1 month. Beliefs and reality are incongruent.*

Table E.3 continued

Student's Communication	Analysis of Student's Response	Client's Communication	Analysis of Client's Response
"You say it would only take a few weeks, but you were not taking your meds for a whole month before being admitted, and you were very sick. Could we talk about that?"	*Making an observation. I hope to help him make the connection between stopping the meds and becoming ill.*		
		"I was fine, I felt good. My grandmother made me come here. Two cops had to carry me in here. I didn't want to do anything, but I was fine. My grandmother noticed I wasn't eating enough, so she made me come here. She won't let me live with her anymore unless I take my medication."	*I think Luis is angry at his grandmother for making him come to the hospital and wanting him to take his medication.*
"If you leave here, will you stop taking your meds again?"	*Changing the topic. It would have been better if I had asked, "Are you angry with your grandmother?" or "How are you feeling about that decision?"*		
		"Yes, because my body will balance itself out."	*Delusional thinking that homeostasis can correct his illness. Perhaps a power struggle with his grandmother.*
"Last time you stopped taking your meds, you got very ill, but you believe that you will not get sick if you quit taking them again?"	*Clarifying, restatement.*		
		"If I gradually stop taking them, my body will be able to keep up."	*May be feeling very powerful or is struggling for control and thinks he can gain control if allowed to try.*
[Silence.]	*I think I have pushed him as far as I should for this session. He continues to deny the need for any medication. I'll try again tomorrow.*		

Table E.4 Process Recording of Client Interview with Student Nurse*

Student's name: Derek

Client's name/age: Marc, 30 years

Client profile: Marc has been admitted for major depression with suicidal tendencies. He is also slightly mentally retarded. He lives with his father, stepmother, and stepbrother. His parents divorced when he was 5 years old. His mother left at that time and has not stayed in touch. The last time Marc saw his mother was 10 years ago at his brother's funeral. He thinks his stepmother is to blame for all his problems. Prior to admission, he had a fight with his stepmother and tried to commit suicide by stabbing himself with a screwdriver. He has a history of suicide attempts when confronted with situations involving conflict. He just found out yesterday that his family is moving and he is not going with them.

Short-term goals for the one-to-one interaction: To let Marc vent his feelings in order to reduce his high level of tension and anxiety.

Student's Communication	Analysis of Student's Response	Client's Communication	Analysis of Client's Response
		[Right arm and leg are continuously moving; appears very anxious.] "I'm really agitated today. I'm sorry, but I'm a little crabby today."	*Expresses feeling of agitation. Nonverbal and verbal are congruent.*
"It's okay to be agitated. Do you want to talk about it?"	*Accepting, broad opening.*		
		"Well, it's my stepmother. I'm not going back there. She turned my father against me. He never said I was retarded or anything like that. Then he called me an a--hole. She put it into his head. I love my father. You know, he's my blood. I love my father. I don't know what I'll do if something happens to him."	*Projection. Blaming stepmother for everything father does. Doesn't want to think father would ever do anything to hurt him. Thinks blood relatives are all good and other relatives are all bad.*
"Do you think something is going to happen to him?"	*Exploring his fears.*		
		"Yes, I know something is going to happen to him. God tells me when something is going to happen to him. God told me he was going to be in an accident. I knew it before it happened. My cigarette went down— that's how I knew something happened. My neighbor told me and I knew it already happened. It was a bad wreck. He's okay now, but I know something is going to happen to him."	*Delusions of grandeur— God speaks to him. Marc sees the cigarette as a communication from God. Reaction-formation. Rather than feeling anger toward his father about the move, he expresses exaggerated worry and concern for his father.*

---

*Contributed by Beverly Gill, Purdue University Calumet.

Table E.4 continued

Student's Communication	Analysis of Student's Response	Client's Communication	Analysis of Client's Response
"What do you think will happen to him?"	*Exploring.*		
		"I don't know. He's sick. He's a diabetic. He has bad nerves, too. I just don't know what I'll do without him. But I won't go back there. She just puts bad things in his head. She is bad to me. She pinches me and hits me. I won't go back there. No one will make me. Mary is making plans for Social Security."	*Rationalization. His father told him they were moving and he wasn't coming along. Instead Marc makes it his choice not to go back so he will not feel abandoned by his father.*
"Who is Mary?"	*Clarifying.*		
		"Mary is my caseworker. She's making plans for Social Security. She's getting me into a residential home. It's an emergency, so I will get in. Mary will take care of my money. She'll take care of everything. Nobody can make me go back. I can't sleep at night. I see my loved ones. Last night [pauses, looks around], don't say anything, but I saw my brother last night. I saw him in the window. It was beautiful. I miss him so much. He's my blood. I love him so much."	*Dependent on Mary. Mary will take over and protect him when everyone else has abandoned him. High anxiety and lack of sleep may contribute to visual hallucinations. Doesn't want anyone to know about the hallucinations.*
"Where is your brother?"	*Clarifying. I don't know if he is talking about the brother who died or if this is a different brother.*		

continued ➤

■ *Table E.4* Process Recording of Client Interview with Student Nurse *continued*

Student's Communication	Analysis of Student's Response	Client's Communication	Analysis of Client's Response
		"He died about 10 years ago. I miss him so much. He's my blood. Tommy, he's my stepbrother. He called me stupid. I'm not stupid. They're not my blood. My father would never hurt me. He loves me. She pinches me and tries to control me. I won't go back there. Nobody can make me go back. I'll kill myself if I have to go back there. Nobody can make me go back."	*Expresses sorrow over loss of brother. Again, blood relatives are all good, others are all bad. Can't believe father would hurt him so stepmother must not want him—rationalization. Expresses a desire to commit suicide if he has to go back; maladaptive coping. Even though he is not going back, he still is trying to convince himself this is his decision.*
"No, nobody can make you go back there."	*Reassuring. I hope this is true and not false reassurance. I want to support his defenses.*		
		"They can't? They can't make me go back?"	*Seems to feel relieved.*
"No, that is your choice. You seem to have already established a plan so you won't have to go back."	*Reassuring. Supporting his plan of action.*		
		"Yes, Mary is taking care of it. She's going to get me an apartment and take care of my money. I won't go back there. I get so angry there."	*Mary seems to be his new focus for support. Needs new external locus of control, someone he can trust.*
"What do you do to help relieve your anger?"	*Focusing.*		
		"I pace a lot. I used to smoke five packs of cigarettes a day. Now I smoke one pack a day."	*Is able to identify ways he relieves his anger.*
"Do you have any activities that calm you?"	*Focusing.*		
		[Seems to be calming down, sitting back on sofa, leg not bouncing.] "I like to swim. I was in the Special Olympics for swimming. I like to swim. I like to play basketball. I won medals for swimming."	*Is very proud of his accomplishments. This increases his self-esteem, which is very threatened right now by abandonment issues.*
"You seem very proud of that."	*Recognition.*		
		"Yes, I was a hero, standing up there with all those medals." [Marc received a phone call, and we ended our conversation.]	*Marc is very proud. Associates medals with being a hero. Attempts to re-establish self-esteem.*

Table E.5 Process Recording of Client Interview with Student Nurse*

Student's name: LaChanda

Client's name/age: Sue, 24 years

Client profile: Sue presently lives with her roommate, Shirley, in an apartment. She has been working in a small grocery store which recently closed and is concerned that she will not be able to find another job. Shirley states that Sue has become more depressed and often is unable to leave the apartment to look for work. When Shirley returned home from work three days ago, she found Sue stuporous and incoherent from taking "too many" Valium in an attempt to kill herself.

Short-term goals for the one-to-one interaction: This is the first time I am meeting Sue. My goal is to help her discuss her feelings about what led up to her suicide attempt.

Student's Communication	Analysis of Student's Response	Client's Communication	Analysis of Client's Response
"Sue, can you tell me what brought you here?"	*Focusing.*	(arms folded across chest; looks down at legs, one of which is shaking)."I guess I can. It is a real long story. Are you sure you want to hear it?"	*She appears distant and cool; unsure if she can trust me. Low self-esteem makes her doubt I would be interested in her.*
(leaning forward, attempting to make eye contact; lightly touch her hand to draw attention toward me). "Absolutely, Sue. I have the morning to sit and talk if you wish."	*Offering self.*		
		(position remains the same; voice emotionless) "That might be nice. I might feel better if I talk about how I feel, but I doubt it."	*She has not felt better for a long time and doubts that anything could help. Still mistrustful and unsure of me.*
Sometimes, Sue, talking about how we feel inside and getting it outside helps us see our feelings in a different way and we can understand them better.	*Encouraging action.*		
		(makes eye contact) "I hope so, I really do. I have been so miserable. I'm so depressed that I tried to kill myself.	*She feels her life is valueless; she is weary from carrying her burdens around inside of herself.*
"Sue, could you tell me what was happening when you tried to kill yourself?"	*Exploring.*		
		(rocking in chair) "I hate myself, I really do. Bad things happen to me because of the things I do."	*Anxiety increasing as she begins to speak of things she has avoided for a long time.*

*Contributed by Cathy Sartain, Purdue University Calumet.

continued ➤

■ *Table E.5* Process Recording of Client Interview with Student Nurse *continued*

Student's Communication	Analysis of Student's Response	Client's Communication	Analysis of Client's Response
(maintaining eye contact and leaning forward) "Sue, it must be very difficult for you to tell me that you hate yourself. Can you tell me more about the way you feel and the bad things that have happened to you?"	*Accepting, exploring.*		
		(hands gripping the arms of chair; knuckles are white) "My brother molested me from the time I was 4 until I was 13. My Mom caught us once and whipped me. She took me to church and told everyone. They pointed their fingers at me and said 'Shame on you'."	*Watching me to see my reaction. She is embarrassed and worried that I will feel differently about her now. Reliving the horror of that time is very anxiety-producing.*
"What an awful experience."	*Accepting; acknowledging feelings.*		
		(breaks eye contact and hangs head) "Yes, I don't know why my Mom did me that way. I guess it was my fault."	*Believes she deserved the things that happened because she is unworthy of anything better.*
"I'm not sure why she did that, either. Do you think you did something to have this happen to you?"	*Exploring.*		
		"Yes, but I don't know what it was. I did everything I could to stay out of his way. He always came looking for me. I never, never wanted to be touched by my brother."	*Confused because for so long she has felt responsible and how she can't think of a single things she did to deserve the abuse. Increased turmoil as old thoughts conflict with new ideas.*
"I hear you saying that you didn't do anything to cause the abuse. Is this correct?"	*Clarifying.*		
		"I didn't do anything. Maybe it's not my fault after all."	*Searching for confirmation of her thoughts.*
"No, Sue, it wasn't. Your brother is responsible for his behavior, not you."	*Validating perception.*		
(Sue has a long way to go before she will be able to let go of feeling responsible for her abuse. Perhaps this is the first little step.)		(face devoid of emotion; rocking in chair) "It's not my fault. I'm glad. I can like myself better knowing its not."	*The beginning of an improved self-esteem.*

APPENDIX F

*Nursing Interventions Classification (NIC)**

DOMAIN: Physiological: Basic

Class: *Activity and Exercise Management*

> **Interventions:** *Exercise Promotion:* Facilitation of regular physical exercise to maintain or advance to a higher level of fitness and health

Class: *Elimination Management*

> **Interventions:** *Constipation Management:* Prevention and alleviation of constipation

Class: *Immobility Management*

> **Interventions:** *Physical Restraint:* Application, monitoring, and removal of mechanical restraining devices or manual restraints which are used to limit physical mobility of patient

Class: *Nutritional Support*

> **Interventions:** *Eating Disorders Management:* Prevention and treatment of severe diet restriction and overexercising, or binging and purging of food and fluids
>
> *Nutritional Management:* Assisting with or providing a balanced dietary intake of food and fluids

Class: *Physical Comfort Promotion*

> **Interventions:** *Progressive Muscle Relaxation:* Facilitating the tensing and releasing of successive muscle groups while attending to the resulting differences in sensation
>
> *Simple Massage:* Stimulation of the skin and underlying tissues with varying degrees of hand pressure to decrease pain, produce relaxation, and improve circulation.

Class: *Self-Care Facilitation*

> **Interventions:** *Self-Care Assistance:* Assisting another to perform activities of daily living
>
> *Sleep Enhancement:* Facilitation of regular sleep/wake cycles

*Source: McCloskey, J. C., & Bulechek, G. M. (1996). *Nursing Interventions Classifications (NIC)*, 2nd ed. St. Louis: Mosby.

DOMAIN: Behavioral

Class: *Behavioral Therapy*

Interventions: *Activity Therapy:* Prescription of and assistance with specific physical, cognitive, social, and spiritual activities to increase the range, frequency, or duration of an individual's (or group's) activity

Animal Assisted Therapy: Purposeful use of animals to provide affection, attention, diversion, and relaxation

Art Therapy: Facilitation of communication through drawings or other art forms

Assertiveness Training: Assistance with the effective expression of feelings, needs, and ideas while respecting the rights of others

Behavior Management/Overactivity: Provision of a therapeutic milieu which safely accommodates the patient's overactivity while promoting optimal function

Behavior Management: Self-Harm: Assisting the patient to decrease or eliminate self-mutilating or self-abusive behaviors

Behavior Management: Sexual: Delineation and prevention of socially unacceptable sexual behaviors

Behavior Modification: Promotion of a behavior change

Behavior Modification: Social Skills: Assisting the patient to develop or improve interpersonal social skills

Limit Setting: Establishing the parameters of desirable and acceptable patient behavior

Milieu Therapy: Use of people, resources, and events in the patient's immediate environment to promote optimal psychosocial functioning

Music Therapy: Using music to help achieve a specific change in behavior or feeling

Mutual Goal Setting: Collaborating with patient to identify and prioritize care goals, then developing a plan for achieving those goals through the construction and use of goal attainment scaling

Patient Contracting: Negotiating an agreement with a patient which reinforces a specific behavior change

Play Therapy: Purposeful use of toys or other equipment to assist a patient in communicating his/her perception of the world and to help in mastering the environment

Self-Responsibility Facilitation: Encouraging a patient to assume more responsibility for own behavior

Substance Use Prevention: Prevention of an alcoholic or drug use lifestyle

Substance Use Treatment: Supportive care of patient/family members with physical and psychosocial problems associated with the use of alcohol or drugs

Substance Use Treatment: Alcohol Withdrawal: Care of the patient experiencing sudden cessation of alcohol consumption

Substance Use Treatment: Drug Withdrawal: Care of a patient experiencing drug detoxification

Substance Use Treatment: Overdose: Monitoring, treatment, and emotional support of a patient who has ingested prescription or over-the-counter drugs beyond the therapeutic range

Class: *Cognitive Therapy*

    Interventions: *Anger Control Assistance:* Facilitation of the expression of anger in an adaptive nonviolent manner

    Cognitive Restructuring: Challenging a patient to alter distorted thought patterns and view self and the world more realistically

    Reality Orientation: Promotion of patient's awareness of personal identity, time, and environment

    Reminiscence Therapy: Using the recall of past events, feelings, and thoughts to facilitate adaptation to present circumstances

Class: *Communication Enhancement*

    Interventions: *Active listening:* Attending closely to and attaching significance to a patient's verbal and nonverbal messages

    Socialization Enhancement: Facilitation of another person's ability to interact with others

Class: *Coping Assistance*

    Interventions: *Anticipatory Guidance:* Preparation of patient for an anticipated developmental or situational crisis

    Coping Enhancement: Assisting a patient to adapt to perceived stressors, changes, or threats which interfere with meeting life demands and roles

    Counseling: Use of an interactive helping process focusing on the needs, problems, or feelings of the patient and significant others to enhance or support coping, problem solving, and interpersonal relationships

    Crisis Intervention: Use of short-term counseling to help the patient cope with a crisis and resume a state of functioning comparable to or better than the pre-crisis state

    Grief Work Facilitation: Assistance with the resolution of a significant loss

Guilt Work Facilitation: Helping another to cope with painful feelings of responsibility, actual or perceived

Mood Management: Providing for safety and stabilization of a patient who is experiencing dysfunctional mood

Recreation Therapy: Purposeful use of recreation to promote relaxation and enhancement of social skills

Self-Esteem Enhancement: Assisting a patient to increase his or her personal judgment of self-worth

Spiritual Support: Assisting the patient to feel balance and connection with a greater power

Therapy Group: Application of psychotherapeutic techniques to a group, including the utilization of interactions between members of the group

Class: *Patient Education*

    Interventions: *Teaching: Disease Process:* Assisting the patient to understand information related to a specific disease process

Class: *Psychological Comfort Promotion*

    Interventions: *Anxiety Reduction:* Minimizing apprehension, dread, foreboding, or uneasiness related to an unidentified source of anticipated danger

Calming Technique: Reducing anxiety in patient experiencing acute distress

Distraction: Purposeful focusing of attention away from undesirable sensations

Simple Guided Imagery: Purposeful use of imagination to achieve relaxation and direct attention away from undesirable sensations

Simple Relaxation Therapy: Use of techniques to encourage and elicit relaxation for the purpose of decreasing undesirable signs and symptoms such as pain, muscle tension, or anxiety

DOMAIN: Safety

Class: *Crisis Management*

Interventions: *Rape-Trauma Treatment:* Provision of emotional and physical support immediately following an alleged rape

Suicide Prevention: Reducing risk of self-inflicted harm for a patient in crisis or severe depression

Class: *Risk Management*

Interventions: *Abuse Protection:* Identification of high-risk, dependent relationships and actions to prevent further infliction of physical or emotional harm

Abuse Protection: Child: Identification of high-risk, dependent child relationships and actions to prevent possible or further infliction of physical, sexual, or emotional harm or neglect of basic necessities of life

Abuse Protection: Elder: Identification of high-risk, dependent elder relationships and actions to prevent possible or further infliction of physical, sexual, or emotional harm, neglect of basic necessities of life, or exploitation

Area Restriction: Limitation of patient mobility to a specified area for purposes of safety or behavior management

Delirium Management: Provision of a safe and therapeutic environment for the patient who is experiencing an acute confusional state

Delusion Management: Promoting the comfort, safety, and reality orientation of a patient experiencing false, fixed beliefs that have little or no basis in reality

Dementia Management: Provision of a modified environment for the patient who is experiencing a chronic confusional state

Elopement Precautions: Minimizing the risk of a patient leaving a treatment setting without authorization when departure presents a threat to the safety of patient or others

Hallucination Management: Promoting the safety, comfort, and reality orientation of a patient experiencing hallucinations

Seclusion: Solitary containment in a fully protective environment with close surveillance by nursing staff for purposes of safety or behavior management

DOMAIN: Family

Class: *Life Span Care*

Interventions: *Caregiver Support:* Provision of the necessary information, advocacy, and support to facilitate primary patient care by someone other than a health care professional

Family Involvement: Facilitating family participation in the emotional and physical care of the patient

Family Mobilization: Utilization of family strengths to influence patient's health in a positive direction

Family Therapy: Assisting family members to move their family toward a more productive way of living

Glossary

abstract thinking The ability to generalize information, make predictions, build on prior memory, and evaluate the effects of decisions.

acquaintance rape   *See* date rape.

affect Immediate emotional expression; what others observe.

ageism The process of systematic stereotyping of and discriminating against older people simply on the basis of their age.

agnosia An inability to recognize familiar situations, people, or stimuli; not related to impairment in sensory organs.

agoraphobia A phobic disorder characterized by fear of being away from home and of being alone in public places when assistance might be needed.

agraphia An inability to read or write.

alexia An inability to identify objects or their use by sight; also called visual agnosia.

alexithymia An inability to analyze, interpret, and name physical feelings and emotions.

anger rape Rape characterized by physical violence and cruelty to the victim; the ability to injure, traumatize, and shame the victim provides the rapist with an outlet for his rage and temporary relief from his turmoil.

anhedonia The state in which a person is unable to experience pleasure.

anorexia nervosa An eating disorder in which a person attempts to lose weight by dramatically decreasing food intake and increasing physical exercise.

antisocial personality disorder (ASPD) A disorder beginning in childhood and continuing into adulthood characterized by a pattern of irresponsible and antisocial behavior.

anxiety (1) A feeling of tension, distress, and discomfort produced by a perceived or threatened loss of inner control rather than from external danger. (2) Emotion in response to the fear of being hurt or losing something valued.

aphasia Loss of the ability to understand or use language.

apraxia An inability to carry out skilled and purposeful movement; the inability to use objects properly.

astereognosia An inability to identify familiar objects placed in one's hand; also called tactile agnosia.

autistic Relating to a preoccupation with one's own thoughts and feelings that interferes with effective communication with others.

avoidant personality disorder (APD) A disorder characterized by timidity, fear of negative evaluation, and social discomfort.

biogenic theory A theory that focuses on how genetic factors, neurotransmission, and biological rhythms relate to the cause, course, and prognosis of mental disorders.

bipolar disorder A mood disorder characterized by alternating depression and elation, with periods of normal mood in between; also called manic-depressive disorder.

blocking A disruption in the thinking process; thoughts suddenly stop and do not continue for a period of time.

borderline personality disorder (BPD) A disorder characterized by a pattern of instability in self-image, interpersonal relationships, and mood.

bulimia nervosa An eating disorder in which a person attempts to manage weight through dieting, binge eating, and purging.

catastrophizing A distorted thinking process that exaggerates failures in one's life.

circadian rhythms Regular fluctuations of a variety of physiological factors over a period of 24 hours.

circumstantial speech Speech that includes many unnecessary and insignificant details before arriving at the main idea.

Cluster A A category of personality disorders characterized by eccentric behavior and social withdrawal; disorders are paranoid, schizoid, and schizotypal.

Cluster B A category of personality disorders characterized by dramatic, emotional, or erratic behavior; disorders are antisocial, borderline, histrionic, and narcissistic.

Cluster C A category of personality disorders characterized by anxious and fearful behavior; disorders are avoidant, dependent, and obsessive-compulsive.

codependency Non–substance-abusing partners who enable their partners to continue to abuse alcohol or drugs.

cognitive processes In Sullivan's social-interpersonal theory, the development of thinking progresses from unconnected to causal to symbolic.

commitment Detaining a client in a psychiatric facility against his or her will, requested on the basis of dangerousness to self or others; also called involuntary admission.

compensation Covering up weaknesses by emphasizing a more desirable trait or by overachievement in a more comfortable area.

competency A legal determination affirming that a client can make reasonable judgments and decisions about treatment and other significant personal issues.

compulsion A repetitive behavior or thought used to decrease the fear or guilt associated with an obsession.

concrete thinking Focused thinking on facts and details, a literal interpretation of messages, and an inability to generalize or think abstractly.

confabulation Filling in memory gaps with imaginary information.

conscious The aspect of consciousness that encompasses all things that are easily remembered.

conversion disorder A somatoform disorder characterized by sensorimotor symptoms.

coping mechanism A conscious attempt to manage stress and anxiety; may be physical, cognitive, or affective.

countertransference A nurse's emotional reaction to a client based on significant relationships in the nurse's past; the process may be conscious or unconscious, and the feelings may be positive or negative.

crisis A turning point in a person's life at which usual resources and coping skills are no longer effective and the person enters a state of disequilibrium.

cyclothymic disorder A mood disorder characterized by a mood range from moderate depression to hypomania, which may or may not include periods of normal mood.

date rape Rape characterized by a perpetrator who is known to the victim; also called acquaintance rape.

declarative memory Memory relating to people, places, and objects; the verbal expression of memory.

defense mechanism An unconscious attempt to deny, misinterpret, or distort reality to alleviate anxiety.

delirium An acute, usually reversible brain disorder characterized by clouding of the consciousness (decreased awareness of the environment) and a reduced ability to focus and maintain attention.

delusion A false belief that cannot be changed by logical reasoning or evidence.

delusions of grandeur *See* grandiosity.

dementia A chronic, irreversible brain disorder characterized by impairments in memory, abstract thinking, and judgment, as well as changes in personality.

denial An attempt to screen or ignore unacceptable realities by refusing to acknowledge them.

dependent personality disorder (DPD) A disorder characterized by an inability to make everyday decisions without an excessive amount of advice and reassurance from others.

dichotomous thinking Distorted, all-or-none reasoning involving opposite and mutually exclusive categories.

displacement The transferring or discharging of emotional reactions from one object or person to another object or person.

dissociative amnesia Loss of memory in response to trauma; may be localized, selective, generalized, or continuous.

dissociative disorders A category of anxiety disorders characterized by an alteration in conscious awareness of behavior, affect, thoughts, and memories, and an alteration in identity, particularly in the consistency of personality.

dissociative fugue A rare dissociative disorder in which people, while either maintaining their identity or adopting a new identity, wander or take unexpected trips.

dissociative identity disorder (DID) A dissociative disorder characterized by the existence of two or more personalities in the same individual.

dual diagnosis The concurrent presence of a major psychiatric disorder and chemical dependence.

duty to disclose A physician's obligation to warn identified individuals if a client has made a credible threat to kill them.

dynamism In Sullivan's social-interpersonal theory, a long-standing pattern of behavior.

dysthymic disorder A mood disorder similar to major depression but remaining mild or moderate.

ego In intrapersonal theory, the component of the personality that mediates the drives of the id with objective reality in a way that promotes well-being and survival.

ego-dystonic behavior Behavior that is inconsistent with one's thoughts, wishes, and values.

ego-syntonic behavior Behavior that conforms to one's thoughts, wishes, and values.

electroconvulsive therapy (ECT) The introduction of an electric current through one or two electrodes attached to the temple or temples, as treatment for depression.

elopement Leaving a psychiatric facility against medical advice.

enabling behavior Any action by a person, called a codependent, that consciously or unconsciously facilitates substance dependence.

extrapyramidal side effects (EPS) Side effects caused by antipsychotic medications, which include dystonia, pseudoparkinsonism, neuroleptic malignant syndrome (NMS), and tardive dyskinesia.

gang rape Rape characterized by a number of perpetrators; may be part of a group ritual that confirms masculinity, power, and authority.

general adaptation syndrome (GAS) The structural and chemical changes produced by stress to which a person must adjust; the GAS occurs in three stages: alarm, resistance, and exhaustion.

generalized anxiety disorder (GAD) A chronic disorder characterized by persistent anxiety without phobias or panic attacks.

grandiosity An exaggerated sense of importance or self-worth usually accompanied by the belief of having magical powers; also called delusions of grandeur.

hallucination The occurrence of a sight, sound, touch, smell, or taste without any external stimulus to the corresponding sensory organ; the experience is real to the person.

histrionic personality disorder (HPD) A disorder characterized by showing excessive emotion for the purpose of gaining attention.

hyperetamorphosis The need to compulsively touch and examine every object in the environment.

hyperorality The need to taste, chew, and examine any object small enough to be placed in the mouth.

hypochondriasis A somatoform disorder characterized by the belief of having a serious disease despite all medical evidence to the contrary.

id In intrapersonal theory, the biological and psychological drives with which a person is born; its major concern is the instant gratification of needs.

idea of reference A cognitive distortion in which a person believes that what is in the environment is related to him or her, even when no obvious relationship exists; also called personalization.

identification An attempt to manage anxiety by imitating the behavior of someone feared or respected.

illogical thinking Thinking in which ideas are inconsistent, irrational, or self-contradictory.

illusion A sensory misperception of environmental stimuli.

informed consent A client's right to receive enough information to make a decision about treatment and to communicate the decision to others.

intellectualization A mechanism by which an emotional response that normally would accompany an uncomfortable or painful incident is evaded by the use of rational explanations that remove from the incident any personal significance and feelings.

introjection A form of identification that allows for the acceptance of others' norms and values into oneself.

involuntary admission *See* commitment.

loose association Thinking in which there is no apparent relationship between thoughts.

magnification A cognitive distortion in which much importance is attributed to unpleasant occurrences.

major depression A mood disorder characterized by loss of interest in life and unresponsiveness, moving from mild to severe, severe lasting at least 2 weeks; also called unipolar disorder.

manic-depressive disorder *See* bipolar disorder.

mental status examination An assessment procedure that provides information about a client's appearance, speech, emotional state, and cognitive functioning.

minimization Not acknowledging the significance of one's behavior.

mood A sustained emotional state; what the person describes.

narcissistic personality disorder (NPD) A disorder characterized by a pattern of grandiosity, hypersensitivity to evaluation by others, and lack of empathy.

negative characteristics The absence of behaviors normally seen in mentally healthy adults, such as minimal self-care, social withdrawal, blunted or flat affect, anhedonia, concrete thinking, symbolism, and blocking; typically occur during the prodromal and residual phases of schizophrenia.

neologism A meaningless word created specifically to express a certain idea.

nerve tracts Groups of nerve fibers carrying signals to and from the same area.

nuclei Dense collection of nerve cells with common specific functions.

obsession An unwanted, repetitive thought.

obsessive-compulsive disorder (OCD) An anxiety disorder characterized by unwanted, repetitious thoughts and behaviors.

obsessive-compulsive personality disorder (OCPD) A disorder characterized by perfectionism and inflexibility.

overgeneralization A cognitive distortion in which information is taken from one situation and applied to a wide variety of situations.

panic attack The highest level of anxiety, characterized by disorganized thinking, feelings of terror and helplessness, and nonpurposeful behavior.

panic disorder A progressive anxiety disorder characterized by sudden and unexpected panic attacks; may or may not be accompanied by agoraphobia.

paranoid personality disorder A disorder characterized by a tendency to interpret the actions of others as deliberately demeaning or threatening.

perseveration phenomena Continuous, repetitive behaviors that have no meaning or direction.

personalization *See* idea of reference.

personification In Sullivan's social-interpersonal theory, an image people have of themselves and others.

phobic disorder An anxiety disorder characterized by a persistent disabling fear of an object or situation; when the object or situation cannot be avoided, the person responds with panic.

phototherapy Exposure to full-spectrum fluorescent lamps for the treatment of seasonal affective disorder.

pleasure principle In intrapersonal theory, the tendency for the id to seek pleasure and avoid pain.

positive characteristics Behaviors not normally seen in mentally healthy adults, such as delusions, hallucinations, loose association, inappropriate affect, and overreactive affect; typically occur during the active phase of schizophrenia.

posttraumatic stress disorder (PTSD) An anxiety disorder characterized by a constant anticipation of danger and a phobic avoidance of triggers that remind the person of the original trauma; other characteristics include irritability, aggression, and flashbacks.

potency The power to produce the desired effects per milligram of medication.

power rape Rape characterized by the rapist's intent to command and master another person sexually, not to injure the victim.

preconscious The aspect of consciousness that encompasses thoughts, feelings, and experiences that have been forgotten but that can easily be recalled to consciousness; sometimes called subconscious.

pressured speech Tense, strained speech that is difficult to interrupt.

procedural memory Memory of motor skills; the behavioral expression of memory.

projection A process in which blame for unacceptable desires, thoughts, shortcomings, and mistakes is attached to others or the environment.

proprioception The ability to know where one's body is in time and space, and the ability to recognize objects and their functions.

pseudodelirium Symptoms of delirium without any identifiable organic cause.

pseudodementia A disorder, frequently depression, that simulates dementia.

psychosexual development In intrapersonal theory, the process by which personality develops from birth to adolescence.

psychosis A state in which a person is unable to comprehend reality and has difficulty communicating and relating to others; often accompanied by hallucinations and delusions.

psychotropic medications Medications that affect cognitive functions, emotions, and behaviors.

rape Any forced sexual activity.

rape-trauma syndrome Symptoms of, or specific responses to, the experience of being raped; also, a nursing diagnosis.

rationalization Justification of certain behaviors by faulty logic and ascription of motives that are socially acceptable but that did not, in fact, inspire the behavior.

reaction formation A mechanism that causes people to act exactly opposite to the way they feel.

reality principle In intrapersonal theory, the ability of the ego to delay the immediate achievement of pleasure.

receptor agonist Substance other than the specific neurotransmitter that is capable of stimulating the receptor.

receptor antagonist Substance that blocks a receptor site, inhibiting or eliminating neurotransmission.

regression Resorting to an earlier, more comfortable level of functioning that is characteristically less demanding and responsible.

repression An unconscious mechanism by which threatening thoughts, feelings, and desires are kept from becoming conscious; the repressed material is denied entry into consciousness.

ritual abuse Emotional, physical, and sexual abuse that occurs in a ceremonial or systematic form by a specific group.

Russell's sign A callus on the back of the hand, caused by forcing vomiting.

sadistic rape Rape distinguished by brutality as a necessary ingredient for the rapist to become sexually excited.

schizoaffective disorder A disorder characterized by symptoms that appear to be a mixture of schizophrenia and mood disorders.

schizoid personality disorder A disorder characterized by a pattern of indifference to social relationships and a restricted range of emotional experience and expression.

schizophrenia A disabling major mental disorder characterized by distortions in thinking, perceiving, and expressing feelings.

schizotypal personality disorder A disorder characterized by peculiarities of ideation, appearance, and behavior that are not severe enough to meet the criteria for schizophrenia.

seasonal affective disorder (SAD) A mood disorder characterized by depression during fall and winter and normal mood or hypomania during spring and summer.

secondary gain An advantage from, or reward for, being ill.

selective abstraction A cognitive distortion that focuses on certain information while ignoring contradictory information.

self-mutilation The deliberate destruction of body tissue without conscious intent of suicide.

somatization Process by which psychological distress is experienced and communicated in the form of somatic (bodily) symptoms.

somatization disorder A somatoform disorder characterized by multiple physical complaints involving several body systems.

somatoform disorder An anxiety disorder characterized by physical symptoms that have no underlying organic basis.

somatoform pain disorder A somatoform disorder characterized by pain that cannot be explained organically.

sublimation Displacement of energy associated with more primitive sexual or aggressive drives into socially acceptable activities.

substance abuse The purposeful use, for at least 1 month, of a drug that results in adverse effects to oneself or others; does not meet the criteria for substance dependence.

substance dependence The habitual use of a drug that continues despite adverse effects.

substitution The replacement of a highly valued, unacceptable, or unavailable object by a less valuable, acceptable, or available object.

sundown syndrome The intensification of behavioral symptoms during the late afternoon or early evening hours; seen in dementia and delirium.

superego In intrapersonal theory, the component of personality that is concerned with moral behavior.

superstitious thinking A cognitive distortion in which a person believes that some unrelated action will magically influence the course of events.

symbolism A type of thinking in which an object or idea comes to represent a different object or idea.

tangential speech Thoughts veer from main idea and never get back to it.

therapeutic alliance The conscious process of nurse and client working together toward mutually established goals.

therapeutic milieu An active part of the treatment plan, which includes the physical environment as well as all interactions with staff members and other clients.

transference A client's unconscious displacement of feelings for a significant person in the past onto the nurse in the current relationship; the feelings may be positive or negative.

unconscious The aspect of consciousness that encompasses thoughts, feelings, experiences, and dreams that cannot be brought to conscious thought or remembered.

undoing An action or words designed to cancel some disapproved thoughts, impulses, or acts in which the person relieves guilt by making reparation.

unipolar disorder *See* major depression.

voluntary admission The process through which a person consents to confinement for the purpose of assessment and treatment of a mental disorder.

withdrawal A syndrome that occurs after reducing or terminating the intake of alcohol or a psychoactive substance.

Index